C000185493

Child Health
A Textbook for the DCH

For Churchill Livingstone

Publisher: Georgina Bentliff
Project Editor: Elif Fincanci-Smith
Editorial Co-ordination: Editorial Resources Unit
   Copy Editor: Pat Croucher
Production Controller: Nancy Henry
Design: Design Resources Unit
Sales Promotion Executive: Hilary Brown

Child Health
A Textbook for the DCH

Edited by

David R. Harvey MB FRCP DCH
Senior Lecturer in Paediatrics, Institute of Obstetrics and
Gynaecology; Consultant Paediatrician, Queen Charlotte's
and Chelsea Hospital, London and St Mary's Hospital,
London

and

Ilya Z. Kovar MB FRCP FRCPC FAAP
Senior Lecturer in Child Health, Charing Cross and
Westminster Medical School; Consultant Paediatrician,
Charing Cross Hospital, London

SECOND EDITION

CHURCHILL LIVINGSTONE
EDINBURGH LONDON MELBOURNE NEW YORK AND TOKYO 1991

CHURCHILL LIVINGSTONE
Medical Division of Longman Group UK Limited

Distributed in the United States of America by Churchill
Livingstone Inc., 1560 Broadway, New York, N.Y. 10036,
and by associated companies, branches and representatives
throughout the world.

© Longman Group Limited 1985
© Longman Group UK Limited 1991

All rights reserved. No part of this publication may be
reproduced, stored in a retrieval system, or transmitted in
any form or by any means, electronic, mechanical,
photocopying, recording or otherwise, without either the
prior permission of the publishers (Churchill Livingstone,
Robert Stevenson House, 1–3 Baxter's Place, Leith Walk,
Edinburgh EH1 3AF), or a licence permitting restricted
copying in the United Kingdom issued by the Copyright
Licensing Agency Ltd, 90 Tottenham Court Road, London,
W1P 9HE.

First edition 1985
Second edition 1991

ISBN 0-443-04026-5

British Library Cataloguing in Publication Data
Child health. — 2nd ed.
 1. Paediatrics — manual
 I. Harvey, David, 1936 — II. Kovar, Ilya
 618.92

Library of Congress Cataloging in Publication Data
Child health: a textbook for the DCH/edited by David
 Harvey and Ilya Kovar. — 2nd ed.
  p. cm.
 Includes bibliographical references and index.
 ISBN 0-443-04026-5
 1. Pediatrics. I. Harvey, David (David Robert)
 II. Kovar, Ilya.
 [DNLM: 1. Pediatrics. WS 100 C5363]
 RJ45.C533 1991
 618.92—dc20
 DNLM/DLC
 for Library of Congress   90-15109
                                  CIP

Produced by Longman Singapore Publishers (Pte) Ltd.
Printed in Singapore

Preface to the Second Edition

We were very pleased by the reception given to this book. There have been important and exciting changes since the first edition was published. The position of community paediatrics has been greatly strengthened in recent years. In the United Kingdom, consultant paediatricians with a special interest in community child health have been appointed in a large proportion of health districts; we hope that this will ensure there will be further improvement in prevention of accidents and other serious problems of childhood, and also in the care of handicapped children.

It is very encouraging that so many general practitioners are now taking on child health surveillance. This means that the DCH is even more important as an examination for those entering general practice.

Since the last edition we are sad that Christine Cooper has died. Jane Wynne has joined our team to enlarge the section on child abuse as this subject has become of such great importance in clinical paediatrics. Sheila Tyrrell was a pioneer in community child health and we are sad that she also has died since the first edition. Marion Miles and Stuart Logan have taken on the clinical and epidemiological sections of the chapters she wrote. Neil Frazer, Cathy Haworth and Christopher Kelnar have joined us to write on general practice, haematology and endocrinology.

We are very grateful to our contributors for the revisions they have made to their chapters and to the new contributors who have worked so hard in writing their sections. We were very interested to receive a number of letters giving us useful tips for the book, and should be happy to hear from any readers who have comments about it.

London
1991

D.R.H.
I.Z.K.

Preface to the First Edition

This book is intended primarily for doctors interested in preparing for the Diploma in Child Health examinations. We hope that family doctors, even if not taking the examination, will also find it useful in their everyday practice. We have asked contributors to include sufficient information on hospital practice so that general practitioners will know the sort of management their patients may receive if referred to a paediatric department.

Since this book began its gestation there have been several changes in the regulations, and aims, of the various diplomas of child health; the London examination is now supervised by the Royal College of Physicians, while there is a totally new examination of community child health in Edinburgh. The new regulations stress the importance of community child health and the role of both preventative and therapeutic aspects of primary care. The DCH has assumed a useful and important place in the training and accreditation of general practitioners and community paediatricians and is no longer to be regarded as a mini MRCP.

We thank our contributors and the staff at Churchill Livingstone for their patience; we hope that the reader will find the information from the various contributions on general practice, development and the subspecialities useful.

London   D.H.
1985   I.K.

Contributors

M. J. Brueton MSc MD MRCP DCH
Reader in Child Health, Charing Cross and
Westminster Medical School, London, UK

Sarah Bundey MB FRCP DCH
Senior Lecturer in Clinical Genetics,
Birmingham Maternity Hospital, Birmingham, UK

Andrew M. Butterfill MB MRCP DCH
Consultant Paediatrician, County Hospital,
Hereford, UK

Michael C. K. Chan MD FRACP
Senior Lecturer, School of Tropical Medicine,
University of Liverpool, UK

Mary Cummins MB MRCP DCH
Consultant Paediatrician, Ealing Hospital,
London, UK

Professor Sir John Dewhurst MD FRCS FRCOG
Emeritus Professor of Obstetrics and
Gynaecology, Institute of Obstetrics and
Gynaecology, Queen Charlotte's and Chelsea
Hospital, London, UK

James A. S. Dickson FRCS
Consultant Paediatric Surgeon, Children's
Hospital, Sheffield, UK

Robert Dinwiddie MB FRCP DCH
Consultant Paediatrician, The Hospital for Sick
Children, Great Ormond Street, London, UK

Elspeth Earle MB MRCPsych DPM
Formerly Consultant Psychiatrist, Queen
Charlotte's and Chelsea Hospital, London, UK

Neil Frazer BA BM BCH MRCGP
General Practitioner, Grove Health Centre,
London, UK

Janet Goodall MB FRCP DCH
Formerly Consultant Paediatrician, City
Hospital, Stoke-on-Trent, UK

Anthony W. Goodwin MB MRCP DCH
Senior Registrar in Paediatric Cardiology
Newcastle General Hospital, UK

David R. Harvey MB FRCP DCH
Consultant Paediatrician, Queen Charlotte's and
Chelsea Hospital; Consultant Paediatrician, St
Mary's Hospital; Senior Lecturer in Paediatrics,
Institute of Obstetrics and Gynaecology,
London, UK

Cathy Haworth MRCP MRCPath
Senior Lecturer in Haematology, Charing Cross
and Westminster Medical School, London,
UK

Archibald S. Hunter MB MRCP DCH
Paediatric Cardiologist, Freeman Hospital,
Newcastle-upon-Tyne, UK

Christopher J.H. Kelnar MA MD MB FRCP DCH
Consultant Paediatrician, Royal Hospital for
Sick Children, Edinburgh, UK

Ilya Z. Kovar MB FRCP FRCPC FAAP
Senior Lecturer in Child Health, Charing Cross
and Westminster Medical School; Consultant
Paediatrician, Charing Cross Hospital, London,
UK

Thomas J. Lissauer MB FRCP
Consultant Paediatrician, St Mary's Hospital,
London, UK

S. Lingam MD (Hons) MRCP DCH
Consultant Paediatrician in Community Child
Health; Honorary Senior Lecturer, Haringey

District Health Authority, Community Child Health Unit, St Ann's General Hospital, London, UK

Stuart Logan MB BCh MRCP
Senior Lecturer in Paediatric Epidemiology, Institute of Child Health, London, UK

J. Mackinnon BSc MB MRCP
Formerly Consultant Paediatrician, Sydenham Children's Hospital, London, UK

Marion Miles MB FRCP DCH
Consultant Community Paediatrician, St Mary's Hospital, London, UK

Patricia Morris-Jones MB FRCP DCH
Reader in Paediatric Oncology, University of Manchester, UK

George W. Rylance MB MRCP
Consultant Paediatrician, Children's Hospital, Birmingham, UK

Richard S. Trompeter MB BS FRCP
Consultant Paediatrician, The Hospital for Sick Children, Great Ormond Street, London, UK

Sheila Wallis MB MRCP DCH
Consultant Paediatrician, Royal Berkshire and Battle Hospitals, Reading, UK

J. O. Warner MD FRCP
Professor of Child Health, University of Southampton, UK

A. Whitelaw MD FRCP
Consultant Neonatologist, Hammersmith Consultant Paediatrician, Oslo, Norway

Jane Wynne MB ChB MRCP
Consultant Paediatrician, Leeds General Infirmary, Leeds, UK

Contents

1. Epidemiology and demography

S. G. Logan

There have been major social and demographic changes in Britain over the past forty years. Overall living standards have risen dramatically, although in recent years unemployment has widened the large discrepancies between the richest and poorest. The proportion of the population under 15 has dropped from over 35% in 1941 to less than 20% in 1986, while the proportion belonging to ethnic minority groups has risen from 0.4% to 4.3%.

Patterns of illness have changed too, largely as a consequence of social change. Advances in medical technology, particularly the development of immunisation and antibiotics, have also had their effects. Diseases such as tuberculosis, once the scourge of Europe, have dwindled to insignificance. As recently as 1955, tuberculosis killed 148 children and acute poliomyelitis 72 children compared with three and none respectively in 1985. Accidents, perinatal disease, congenital abnormalities and sudden infant death syndrome now dominate the childhood mortality statistics. Health services with their strong hospital base have not always developed in a way appropriate to the changing situation.

EPIDEMIOLOGY

Epidemiology is the study of the patterns and determinants of disease in populations. The science of epidemiology has two functions, first to provide the ground rules for the conduct of research, and secondly to locate our knowledge of disease within its social and environmental context. Important terms used in epidemiology include:

Incidence rate. This is the number of new cases of a condition occurring in a defined population during a specified period. For example, the incidence of tuberculosis amongst children aged 10–14 in the UK was 5.9 cases per 100 000 per year in 1984.

Prevalence. This is the number of cases of a condition in a defined population at one moment in time. This reflects the pool of cases in the population and is a useful measure when considering chronic conditions. For example, the prevalence of diabetes mellitus amongst children from a birth cohort at 10 years of age was 1.3 cases per 1000 children.

Mortality rates. These are a special kind of incidence rate. There are a number of specific mortality rates that are important in paediatrics (Fig. 1.1).

Types of study

Most studies carried out by epidemiologists fall into one of three categories:

Cross-sectional studies. A population, or a sample of the population, is examined in order to determine the prevalence of a particular condition. Associations between the disease and other factors may be sought, giving clues about causation.

Cohort studies. Here a group of individuals is studied over time, having been assigned at the beginning of the time period to the case or control group depending on known exposure to the factor or disease of interest. Differences in outcome between cases and controls allow inferences to be drawn about the effects of the exposure. Such studies provide the strongest evidence of a possible causal association as well as data about the natural history of the disease. Unfortunately such studies are expensive and are unsuitable for the study of

1

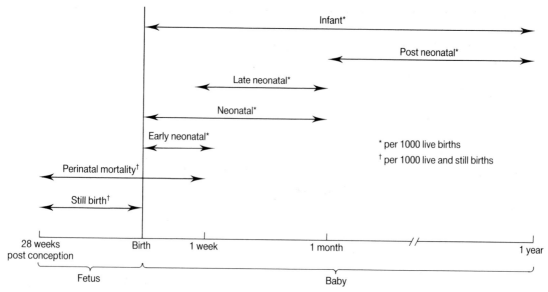

Fig. 1.1   Definitions of important mortality rates.

rare outcomes or of diseases with a long latency period.

Case control studies. A group of cases with a particular condition and a group of controls without the condition in question are studied to determine the relative frequency of the particular exposures of interest in the two groups. A greater frequency amongst the case group may suggest an association between the factor and the disease. This technique is relatively quick and cheap, and is useful for studying rare diseases, but may be subject to bias and does not give information about the natural history of a disease.

DEMOGRAPHIC CONSIDERATIONS

The average female life expectancy at birth in 1901 was 48 years; by 1982 it was 77 years. For males both figures are a little lower. Mortality rates have fallen at all ages but especially in younger age groups (Fig. 1.2). It is clear from the graph that the major fall in mortality rates for all ages preceded the appearance of most modern medical technology. The much decreased chance of death in childhood has itself helped to bring down the fertility rates as parents now expect their children to survive into adulthood. Smaller families and longer life expectancy have resulted in a rising

proportion of the population in the older age groups and relatively less children.

The proportion of children born outside of marriage has been rising steadily in recent years (19.2% in 1985), as has the number of divorces and remarriages. Many children live in single-parent households which has important health implications as they tend to be poorer, and there-

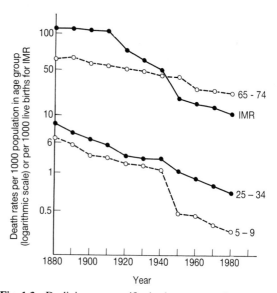

Fig. 1.2   Declining age-specific death rates over time.

fore more vulnerable to illness. The average age of first pregnancy has risen steadily, although the number of very young women having children remains worryingly high.

Inevitably these changes are reflected in changes in the pattern of the health of children.

PATTERNS OF MORTALITY

Patterns and rates of mortality give important information about the overall health of the population. Mortality statistics for England and Wales are published annually by the Office of Population Census Surveys (OPCS) and for Scotland and Northern Ireland by their respective Registrars General. Included in these reports are breakdowns of the death rates by cause and by factors such as social class, maternal age and place of residence.

In England and Wales 40% of all childhood deaths occur in the first month and 70% during the first year of life. Although only 7% of children weigh less than 2.5 kg at birth, 48% of all infant deaths occur in this group (Fig. 1.3). A large proportion of deaths in the first year are due to *perinatal problems* (37%), including those associated with prematurity, *congenital abnormalities* (26%) and *sudden infant death syndrome* (18%) (Fig. 1.4).

Between the ages of 1 and 14 'injury and poisoning' is by far the most important single cause of death, causing over one-third of all deaths in this age group in 1985. Although accidents were already the leading cause of death during the 1950s, infectious diseases were much more important than they are now: pneumonia alone was responsible for 8.2% of all deaths in this age group (Table 1.1). Numerically accidents are equally important in children under 1 year but proportionately they are overshadowed by other conditions (Fig. 1.4).

PATTERNS OF MORBIDITY

Morbidity data is more difficult to obtain and to interpret than mortality data which is easily available and reasonably reliable. However, if one wishes to build up a picture of the health of a community such information is obviously vital. Disease in a population may be regarded as a pyra-

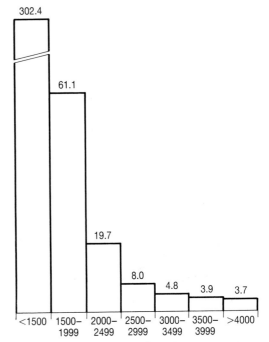

Fig. 1.3 Birth weight-specific infant mortality rates (England and Wales 1985).

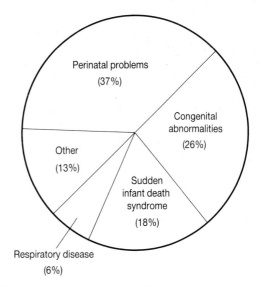

Fig. 1.4 Causes of infant mortality.

mid with mortality at the apex (Fig. 1.5); moving down the pyramid the layers consist of increasing numbers of less serious conditions. In the UK we are fortunate in having some information on childrens' health in each layer of the pyramid.

Table 1.1 Deaths in children aged 1–14 in 1955 and 1985 for some important categories in order of frequency

1955		1985	
Category	Deaths (%)	Category	Deaths (%)
Injury and poisoning	25	Injury and poisoning	33.6
Respiratory disease	13*	Congenital abnormalities	15.3
Malignant disease	11.7	Malignant disease	14
Infectious disease	9.4	Diseases of the CNS	9.4
Congenital abnormalities	8.7	Respiratory disease	6.2*
Diseases of the GIT	4.1	Infectious disease	4

* Includes deaths from pneumonia
Note: Changes in the International Classification of Disease mean that categories are not strictly comparable over time.

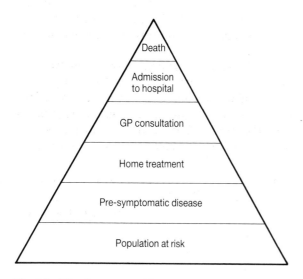

Fig. 1.5 The disease pyramid.

SOURCES OF INFORMATION

In addition to mortality data derived from death certificates, OPCS collects and publishes other information. This includes basic information about the size and composition of the population, socio-economic data broken down by area and some morbidity data.

Details on all deaths and discharges from hospital are coded on a regional basis by specialty to form the Hospital Activity Analysis (HAA) which is held by the Regional Health Authorities. The OPCS Hospital Inpatient Enquiry (HIPE) codes 10% of these discharge diagnoses across the country which provides a useful picture, especially of changes over time. Unfortunately the data is not linked to individuals so that it is not possible to distinguish between one person being admitted on a number of occasions and a number of people being admitted once.

Information about GP consultations is available from two surveys conducted in sentinel general practices by the Royal College of General Practitioners in 1970–72 and in 1980–82. About 50 general practices were involved in each study. Unfortunately it is likely that those practices were not representative of the country as a whole but rather of those run by enthusiastic GPs.

Perhaps the best overall picture of the health of children in the community was provided by three birth cohort studies. All (or a weighted sample in the first study) children born in one particular week in England and Wales in 1946, 1958 and 1970 have been followed up since birth. They have been sent questionnaires or examined at regular intervals with data being collected on social factors, educational achievements and health status. Unfortunately because each of the cohorts has been followed separately the results are not always comparable. None the less they do provide a unique picture of the prevalence and natural history of a vast number of diseases in childhood and their relation to social and environmental factors.

Certain infectious diseases are notifiable and this information is collected by OPCS. Inevitably these notifications are far from complete, particularly for less serious diseases. In addition the Centre for Disease Surveillance and Control (CDSC) registers laboratory reports of the isolation of specific organisms.

For some conditions registers are maintained by OPCS or other bodies. For instance OPCS has registers of cases of malignant disease and of congenital abnormalities (compiled from voluntary notifications by midwives), the UK Childhood Cancer Research Group registers childhood malignancies, collecting data from a number of sources to supplement that from OPCS, while the National Congenital Rubella Surveillance Programme monitors cases of congenital rubella. Since 1986 the British Paediatric Surveillance Unit, sponsored by the British Paediatric Association, has been using a system of monthly notifications by paediatricians to allow researchers to monitor the incidence of rare conditions in childhood.

DETERMINANTS OF HEALTH IN A POPULATION

- Age and sex structure
- Genetic factors
- Physical environment
- Social factors
- Availability and use of medical services

Gender

Sex differences in mortality and morbidity rates are apparent at all ages (Fig. 1.6). For children in the UK a considerable part of this difference is explained by differences in the rate of injury.

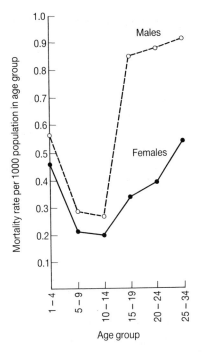

Fig. 1.6 Age-specific mortality rates for males and females (England and Wales 1985).

Injuries and poisoning are overall about twice as common in boys as in girls. For most other categories of disease, although there are some differences, they are of much smaller magnitude.

Genetic factors

Apart from the effects of certain specific conditions (e.g. sickle cell anaemia), there is little evidence that genetic factors have a major impact on the health experience of different populations. Table 1.2 lists some of the common genetically determined abnormalities. Numerous studies of immigrant groups have suggested that the longer they spend in a new country the more nearly their pattern of disease resembles that of the host population, suggesting that the environment has more impact than genetic factors. An interesting, and as yet unexplained, exception is the behaviour of hepatitis B virus. The risk of transmission from mother to child appears to vary with ethnic group, being highest in ethnic Chinese and lowest in white mothers, irrespective of the country of residence.

In 1985 4.3% of the population of England and Wales described themselves as belonging to an ethnic minority group. Of these 52% described themselves as belonging to a group originating from the Asian subcontinent, of whom 35% were born in the UK. A further 22% were West Indian,

Table 1.2 Birth prevalence per 1000 live births of some serious Mendelian disorders (UK)

Disorder	Birth prevalence/1000
Familial hypercholesterolaemia	2.0
Polycystic disease of the kidney	0.8
Cystic fibrosis	0.5
Non-specific mental retardation	0.5
Huntington's chorea	0.5
Neurofibromatosis	0.3
Congenital deafness (recessive form)	0.2
Dominant childhood deafness	0.1
Phenylketonuria	0.1
Sickle cell anaemia*	0.1
β-thalassaemia*	0.05

* An approximate estimate based on gene frequencies in immigrant populations.

of whom 50% were born in the UK. There is relatively little information about health patterns in these groups, although some figures suggest quite significant differences between the UK-born population and those born outside the country (Table 1.3). It seems likely however that these differences are largely the result of differences in material well-being and culturally determined behaviour rather than of genetic differences.

Physical environment

While some specific environmental hazards have been identified, a link between others, such as damp and overcrowded housing and poor health, has been difficult to determine. Many of the possibly disadvantageous circumstances tend to occur in combination, making the effect of any one difficult to elucidate. Other suggested hazards such as environmental pollutants may be so widespread that investigation is difficult. It can be argued that in these circumstances it may be appropriate to accept a much lower order of evidence before proceeding to action than one would require before accepting the validity of a scientific theory.

Social factors

Certain behaviours such as smoking and excessive alcohol intake (both by parents and children) are unequivocally associated with adverse health outcome. Harmful effects of behaviours such as lack of exercise and poorly balanced diets have also been suggested but remain unproven.

Table 1.3 Perinatal infant mortality rates by mother's country of birth: 1986

Mother's country of birth	Perinatal mortality rate* (per 1000 live and still births)	Infant mortality rate (per 1000 live births)
All	9.5	9.4
UK	9.4	9.4
West Indies	12.5	10.3
Pakistan	16.9	14.8
India	10.5	9.0
East Africa	11.9	10.2
West Africa	11.4	10.5

The most powerful social predictor of health outcome is social class. In the UK social class is usually classified by means of the Registrar General's classification of occupations. This scheme, devised in 1912 and repeatedly revised since, assigns all occupations to one of six social classes (Table 1.4). Children and married women are classified according to the social class of their father or husband; there are unresolved problems with the classification of single women and illegitimate children in this system, although most researchers use the woman's most recent occupation.

The differences between the health of children from different social classes are striking. Perinatal and infant mortality rates are almost 60% higher in the children of mothers in social class V than in those of social class I (Figs 1.7 and 1.8). Although mortality rates have been falling in all social classes in recent years the differentials remain. To some extent this is due to the higher proportion of low birthweight babies born to mothers in the less advantaged social groups. However, even amongst babies weighing less than 1500 g, there is a far higher death rate in those from poorer social classes.

As always morbidity data is more difficult to obtain but a number of studies have shown that children from the less advantaged social groups are on average smaller and are more likely to be admitted to hospital than those from more privileged groups. At age 20 there is a 6-cm difference in mean height between men in social classes I and V.

Because of the problems with the use of occupation as a means of classifying social class, various other measures have been used including the level

Table 1.4 The Registrar-General's classification of social class

I	Professional occupations
II	Intermediate occupations (including most managerial occupations)
IIINM	Non-manual skilled occupations
IIIM	Manual skilled occupations
IV	Partly skilled occupations
V	Unskilled occupations

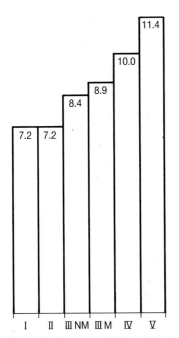

Fig. 1.7 Perinatal death rate per 1000 total births by social class (England and Wales 1986).

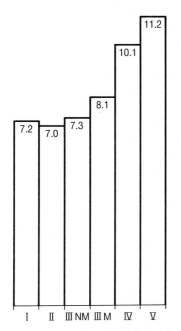

Fig. 1.8 Infant mortality rate per 1000 live births by social class (England and Wales 1986).

of parental education, access to amenities and absolute income. Whichever scheme is used, children from the more advantaged groups do far better on all measures of health status.

Social class is not an attribute, merely a convenient abstraction, so it cannot be said to cause anything. The differences in health experience must partly reflect the effects of material deprivation, but this is not the whole explanation. There is a gradation in mortality and morbidity rates across the social classes, not a sudden increase in the lowest one or two groups (Figs 1.7 and 1.8). Presumably social class acts as a marker for a constellation of adverse factors reflecting both deprivation and culturally determined behaviour patterns.

Medical services

There is surprisingly little evidence that the availability of medical services is an important determinant of the health of populations. Indeed in 14 of the world's richest countries the number of doctors per head of population correlated negatively with outcome measures such as infant mortality rate. This result may well be an artefact due to the difficulty of comparing such disparate countries, but it is clear that the major determinants of health lie outside the realm of medicine. It should also serve to remind us of the importance of the continual evaluation of medical practice. All too often ambitious schemes are started on slender evidence and without the mechanisms for audit.

THE FUTURE

Evaluation is gradually coming to be seen as an integral part of good practice. The development of the national child health computer system in the UK will help paediatricians to achieve this goal. Eventually information should be available nationally in a form which will allow the comparison of immunisation rates and the proportion of children covered by preschool and school surveillance programmes in different districts and even by individual child health clinics and GPs. However, if we want to evaluate the effectiveness of the system, and not simply measure what is being done, then clinicians will have to be prepared to define their goals much more clearly in terms of the health needs of the population they serve. At the same time the needs of research will need to be weighed against the need to preserve confidentiality. New measures of efficiency which are consumer oriented and health rather than disease based will have to be developed. Most importantly, doctors, particularly those working outside hospitals, will have to learn to think about populations and their needs as well as individual patients.

2. History-taking: clinical examination and basic investigations

M. Cummins

INTRODUCTION

The aim of history taking and clinical examination in paediatrics is the total assessment of the child and his physical complaint in the context of his family and social circumstances. Any medical problem is greatly affected by previous illness, family relationships, housing conditions and schooling difficulties.

HISTORY TAKING

The correct diagnosis and comprehensive management of illness is impossible without an accurate history. In children, this is usually obtained from the mother or father. As soon as they are old enough, children should be encouraged to give their own account of the problem; even a young child can, for example, identify the site of pain. During the interview the child should gain confidence from watching friendly communication between the doctor and his parents. Appropriate toys and a small table should be available in the consulting room. All but the illest child will enjoy some distraction. The doctor may gain valuable information about the child's abilities and general state by simple observation during this period.

It is important to learn and listen carefully. One should remember that the parents are usually right, they have had much more time to watch the child than the doctor.

Outline of history

1. Name and personal details of child including school and local child health centre where appropriate.
2. Name and relationship of informant.
3. Referring doctor or agency.
4. Presenting complaint.
5. Details of present complaint.
6. Direct systematic questioning.
7. Recent contact with infectious disease.
8. Past history:
   a. Birth history
   b. Feeding history
   c. Medical history
   d. Hospital admissions
   e. Development
   f. Immunisations
9. Family history: names, ages, occupations of immediate family.
Illness in family. Is there any consanguinity?
10. Social history: details of housing and particularly bathroom and cooking facilities. Facilities for play. Number of bedrooms. Financial situation. Behaviour and relationships.
11. Schooling: performance, attendance, difficulties, special teaching required.

Model history

Rosemary X (known as Rosie)
58 Hamilton Road,
London W6
Date of birth 6.2.80
Age 10 months
Referred by Dr Y
Informant — mother. Rosie's sister also present.

Presenting complaint

Cough for 5 days.

History of present complaint

Well until 5 days ago when she developed a cough. Appetite decreased for 3 days when wheezing began. Listless and febrile for 24 hours. Rubbing right ear. Sister aged 3 also has a cold. No diarrhoea or vomiting. Drinking fairly well but not eating. Micturition normal.

Past history

Birth. Born at Fishpool Hospital after a normal pregnancy, normal delivery at 41 weeks' gestation, induced because of poor weight gain. Birthweight 2.8 kg. No neonatal problems. Forty-eight hour discharge.

Illnesses. Recurrent chestiness since the age of 3 months. Occurs about every month with colds. Treated with antibiotics and cough linctus on several occasions. Well in between attacks. Mild eczema since 2 months old. No other illnesses. No operations. No hospital admissions.

Immunisations. BCG given at birth because of family history of tuberculosis. Triple and polio aged 3 months and 5 months. Third injection recently delayed by a cold.

Development. Smiled at 5 weeks. Sat at 7 months. Pulls to standing. Cruises around furniture. Babbles. Waves bye-bye. Plays pat-a-cake. Has passed 8 month developmental test at local clinic and hearing test from health visitor.

Feeding. Breast fed for 3 months. Mixed feeding at 4 months. Now eats family food, and drinks 'red top' cow's milk not boiled.

Family and social history

Family. Mother aged 22, single, English, healthy. Father aged 24, single. Works on a building site, healthy. Sister: Jane, aged 3 years (same father).

Family illnesses. Maternal grandfather had tuberculosis 2 years ago treated at the local chest clinic. Her mother had bronchitis and eczema as a child. There is no diabetes, epilepsy, or other disease in the family.

Social. Rosie and her sister live with their mother in a two-bedroomed council flat on the fifth floor of a block which has its own kitchen and bathroom. Rosie sleeps in bed with her mother; she wakes frequently at night. Their father visits erratically and provides no financial support. Both children go to day nursery. The health visitor sees children regularly. The family had social work help in the past but not at present. Grandparents live locally but both work and do not have much time for the children.

At the end of a well-taken history the doctor should be able to form a list of problems and differential diagnostic possibilities. The clinical examination should then confirm or support one of the possibilities and leave the doctor with a working diagnosis which is then confirmed by further investigation or by response to a clinical trial of therapy.

PHYSICAL EXAMINATION

The methods of examination vary considerably with the age of the child and the clinical situation. Knowledge of what is normal for children of different ages is essential in order to distinguish that which is abnormal (Table 2.1). It is not appropriate to assess the development of an acutely ill child other than by means of the history, whereas a well 4 year old can co-operate with a detailed neurological examination. Unpleasant procedures are sensibly left to the end of the examination, e.g. examination of ears, throat, rectum. Weighing and measuring of toddlers and infants many be classified as 'unpleasant', but are usually carried out before seeing the doctor. The undressing and dressing involved is not appreciated by children.

Most toddlers are happiest sitting on their

Table 2.1 Normal values for physiological measurement is at different ages

	Birth	6 weeks	1 year	5 year	10 years
Respiratory rate (per minute) (mean)	30	30	25	22	20
Heart rate (per minute) (mean)	140	135	115	100	90
Systolic blood pressure (mmHg) (mean)		95	95	100	105

mother's knees but may lie on the examination couch once they have gained confidence. Infants should be examined naked; an irreducible inguinal hernia may be missed as the cause of persistent crying, or an undescended testicle may remain undiagnosed if the napkin is not removed. Older children may be embarrassed if completely naked.

General condition

The general condition of the child should first be considered in the light of the particular clinical situation. The alertness, responsiveness, hydration, state of nutrition, colour and temperature must be noted. It is useful to make the general comment whether or not the child 'looks ill'. The skin should be examined closely for rashes and other lesions; for example, it is vital not to miss the petechial rash of meningococcal infection.

Weighing and measuring

These can be distressing for young or ill children. The measurements are, however, essential. Infants must be weighed naked, while older children may keep on underclothing. Length is measured using an infant measuring table up to 2 years of age and height with a standiometer in older children. The measurements should be plotted on a percentile chart.

The head

The size of the head is measured around its maximum circumference using a paper or metal tape measure; plastic tape measures stretch and should not be used. The size of the head must be related to the child's height and weight and plotted on the appropriate percentile chart (Figs 2.1, 2.2).

Size and shape

A big head may be found in a big child, as a familial trait, in hydrocephalus, megalencephaly, subdural effusion or space-occupying lesion. A small head is found in a small child, mental retardation, as a familial tendency and in craniostenosis. Unusual head shape may be related to preterm birth, baby's posture or Down's syn-

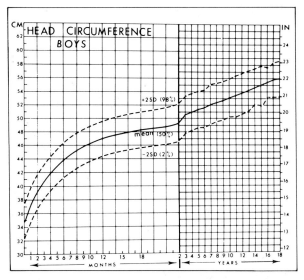

Fig. 2.1 Head circumference for boys from birth to 18 years (from Nelhaus (1968) with permission).

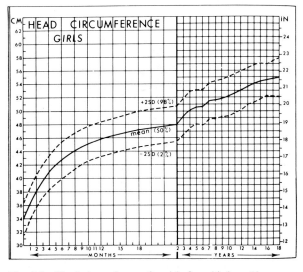

Fig. 2.2 Head circumference for girls from birth to 18 years (from Nelhaus (1968) with permission).

drome. Preterm infants have increased anteroposterior diameter (dolichocephaly); cranial asymmetry is commonly seen in normal infants (plagiocephaly); reduced anteroposterior diameter (brachycephaly) is associated with Down's syndrome.

The fontanelles

The fontanelles should be palpated. The anterior fontanelle is normally flat and pulsation can be felt. Bulging and loss of pulsation in the resting state suggest raised intracranial pressure. Other signs of raised intracranial pressure are separation of the skull suture lines and the sun-setting sign. The anterior fontanelle usually closes between 10 and 18 months of age, but there is a very wide normal variation. Premature closure, however, occurs in craniostenosis and microcephaly; delayed closure is associated with hydrocephalus, hypothyroidism, rickets and cleidocranial dysostosis. The posterior fontanelle is usually palpable for the first 1 or 2 months of life. The third fontanelle is a normal variant and lies between the anterior and posterior fontanelles; it occurs more commonly in Down's syndrome than among the general population. Craniotabes or softening of areas of the skull is also common in normal infants but is found frequently in rickets.

The eyes

Convergent squint is abnormal after 6 months of age, (See Ch. 26) and ophthalmological referral is indicated. Severe squint may require expert opinion in infants less than 1 month old. Wide epicanthic folds may cause an apparent convergent squint, but asymmetrical reflection of a light shone into the pupils is seen in true squint. Sticky eyes are common in the first year of life. Gentle bathing with moist cotton wool is usually sufficient treatment. Examination with the ophthalmoscope will exclude lens and vitreous opacities and refractive errors. Examination of the fundi may be difficult and dilatation of the pupils needed. In young infants, it is best to do the examination during sleep. Older children can have their gaze attracted by a toy. Where there is suspicion of a non-accidental injury, retinal haemorrhages may be seen without skull fractures. Congenital ptosis is seen frequently but acquired ptosis suggests third nerve palsy and possibly raised intracranial pressure. Nystagmus is frequently associated with severe visual defect, but may also have a neurological cause. Screening for refractive errors should be a routine part of the developmental examination using Stycar equipment in infants and young children.

The face

The features may be very helpful in diagnosing generalised conditions such as Down's syndrome, hypothyroidism or Hurler's syndrome. Abnormal shapes and relationships of the facial features are described in many congenital syndromes.

The ears

The ears must be inspected for external abnormalities. They are low set if the upper border of the lobe is below a line drawn from the lateral angle of the eye to the external occipital protruberance. Low-set ears are found in Down's and other congenital syndromes. It is essential to examine the ears of all sick children with an auriscope. The mother should hold the child firmly (Fig. 2.3), otherwise pain may be caused. The largest speculum possible is used to avoid both discomfort and pushing wax inwards. The ear lobe should be pulled gently outwards. Otitis media causes an inflamed, thickened, immobile, bulging or perforated drum. The symptoms are varied, inconsolable crying, fever, head banging, feeding

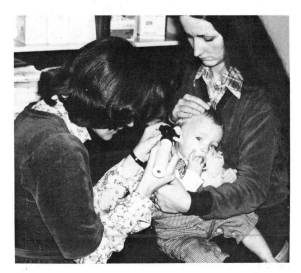

Fig. 2.3   The auriscope examination of a young child.

difficulties or rubbing ears. Hearing tests appropriate for age should be carried out after recovery.

The mouth and throat

This is best left to the end of the examination if tongue depression is needed (Fig. 2.4). Many children will provide a good view of their throats by tilting their heads back, protruding the tongue and saying 'aah'. When the tongue depressor is correctly used gagging is not inevitable. The palate, mucosae and teeth should also be inspected. Tonsillitis may cause abdominal pain, difficulty in swallowing and even respiratory obstruction if there is gross tonsillar enlargement. It is impossible to differentiate bacterial from viral tonsillitis on clinical grounds — viruses are the cause in around 90% of cases. The throat should not be examined in the presence of stridor as respiratory obstruction may be precipitated. Dental infections may cause facial pain or swelling, ear ache and submandibular swelling.

The neck

In Turner's syndrome the neck is short and webbed. Swellings may be due to lymph node enlargement, salivary gland enlargement, goitre, branchial cyst or cystic hygroma. The latter transilluminates. Torticollis in an infant may be due to sternomastoid tumour which is usually palpable around the midpoint of the muscle. Neck retraction may be present in severe respiratory distress in an infant or at any age due to meningism.

The lymph nodes

Lymph nodes are frequently enlarged in response to local or generalised infection. Occasionally, more sinister conditions are responsible. Resolution to normal size may take several months. The groin glands may be palpable without evidence of recent infection.

The chest

The shape and symmetry of the chest should be noted. Pigeon chest or barrel-shaped chest are associated with chronic undertreated asthma. Sternal depression (pectus excavatum) may be familial. Gynaecomastia is not uncommon in boys at puberty, and the two breasts may be asymmetrical in girls. Wide-spaced nipples are seen in Turner's syndrome.

Respiratory distress

Signs of this are tachypnoea (Table 2.1), cyanosis, flaring of the alae nasi, use of accessory muscles, intercostal and subcostal recession and pulsus paradoxus. Impaired percussion note may be due to a collection of fluid or gross pulmonary consolidation. Auscultation is often unhelpful, and cold stethoscope can cause crying. The most ill asthmatics have silent chests but all other signs of severe respiratory distress. Classical signs of consolidation are unusual in childhood, and a chest X-ray must be carried out if pneumonia is suspected. Added sounds heard on auscultation frequently transmitted from the throat, musical added sounds and coarse crepitations are common in toddlers with upper respiratory tract infection, and do not usually indicate pneumonia or the need for antibiotic treatment.

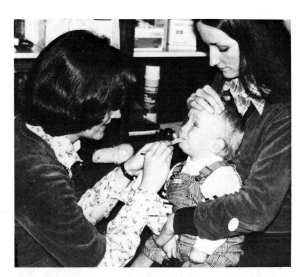

Fig. 2.4 The examination of the mouth and throat of a young child.

The heart

Palpation of the pulse for rate and rhythm should routine. Sinus arrhythmia may be marked and extra-systoles are not unusual. Oedema, clubbing and cyanosis should be sought and the femoral pulses palpated. Blood pressure is measured at rest with the appropriately sized cuff (Table 2.2). The precordium may bulge with cardiac enlargement and palpation may reveal abnormal ventricular impulses and thrills. Heart sounds and murmurs should be listened for carefully. Murmurs are graded from one to six and are timed. Innocent murmurs are common and are accentuated by fever.

The abdomen

Inspection may reveal distension, visible peristalsis, outline of organs, umbilical or inguinal herniae, distended veins and scars. Abdominal breathing is normal in infants, loss of this may indicate peritonitis. The child should be examined lying on a bed or in the mother's arms; flexion of the hips and knees is helpful. The ability of the child to blow out and suck in the abdominal wall freely helps to exclude peritoneal irritation. The child's face should always be watched so that tenderness may be detected. Abdominal organs should be palpated, warm hands are essential. In infants, the normal liver is palpable up to 2 cm below the costal margin and the spleen tip may be felt when the abdominal wall is lax. Rectal examination should be carried out in cases of rectal bleeding, constipation, suspected intussusception and in children with acute abdominal pain.

The genitalia

Male

Both testes are usually descended at birth and are of equal size. Scrotal swelling may be due to hernia, hydrocele, cyst of the cord, etc. Hydroceles are common, non-tender, transilluminate and often resolve spontaneously. Inguinal herniae will be tender if irreducible or strangulated. Torsion of the testis or epididymites produces a swollen tender scrotum. The foreskin cannot normally be retracted in babies, it can usually be retracted after

Table 2.2 Practical aspects of blood pressure measurement

1. Child at rest

2. Cuff: depth at two-thirds length of the upper arm, and bladder length should be the circumference of the arm

3. Technique:

ultrasonic	— correlates best with intra-arterial pressures
auscultation	— for older children
palpation	— inaccurate
flush method	— inaccurate

the age of 6 years. Testes are frequently retractile in older children. If examination is carried out with the boy's hips and knees flexed as in a squatting position, the testes will lie in the scrotum.

Female

The examination of girls' genitalia has assumed great importance with the emergence of child sexual abuse as a common problem during the 1980s. There are few descriptions of normal variants. The subject is dealt with in Chapters 8 and 22.

The skeleton

Knock knees, bow legs, intoeing gait and flat feet are common in infancy, and rarely require treatment. Pain in the knee may be referred from the hip. Limp may originate from the hips, the knees, the spine and intra-abdominal conditions. The spine should be examined. Scoliosis developing during adolescence may require urgent treatment. Minor anomalies of the hands and feet, e.g. extra digits, simian crease, curvature of fifth finger and syndactyly, particularly of the second and third toes are common.

The nervous system

The techniques of examination vary enormously with the age of the child, his developmental progress and his state of general health. In addition to standard equipment for neurological examination, it may be useful to have some coloured 1-inch (2.5 cm) cubes, a bell and a Manchester rattle (for hearing tests). In very young children, seedless raisins may be used to test fine motor skills and very small cake decorations (hundreds and thousands) to test near vision. Small toys and picture books may also be helpful. Observation alone will give a great deal of information, particularly in young or mentally retarded children. Behaviour, apparent intelligence, gait, co-ordination, power and speech may be assessed by observation.

Full neurological examination includes the state of consciousness and orientation, emotional state and intelligence. Speech, comprehension, reading and writing should also be assessed when appropriate. The cranial nerves, gait, posture, power, tone, co-ordination, sensation and reflexes are also examined. It may require more than one consultation to complete the examination in detail. Examination methods have been standardised for different age groups and for detecting minor neurological abnormalities (Paine & Oppe 1975).

BASIC INVESTIGATIONS

It is important to remember that even minor procedures may be alarming for young children and their parents. No investigation should be carried out without good reason. When taking blood, all the necessary tests should be made with one venepuncture wherever possible. It is best if a parent holds the child during painful procedures when this is technically possible. Doctors must become accustomed to the presence of parents at such times.

Urine samples for culture are collected as midstream or clean catch specimens. Urine collected into bags stuck on to the perineum is suitable for biochemical testing but not for culture because of contamination with skin organisms. Suprapubic aspiration of the bladder may be necessary in the young infant with suspected urinary tract infection.

It is very important to know or to have access to normal values for investigations which may vary with age (see Appendix).

Laboratory investigation for some common conditions

1. Enuresis:
   urine culture
   urine glucose

2. Recurrent abdominal pain:
   urine culture
   sickle test (in children from ethnic groups in which sickle cell disease is common)
3. Diarrhoea:
   stool culture for bacteria, microscopy for parasites and electron microscopy for rotavirus. Blood urea and electrolytes (if evidence of dehydration). Test stool for reducing substances if symptoms persistent
4. Failure to thrive:
   urine sugar and protein, urine culture and microscopy, haemoglobin, blood urea and electrolytes, stool microscopy and culture
5. Before general anaesthesia:
   haemoglobin and sickle test (when ethnic origin indicates)
6. Febrile convulsion:
   lumbar puncture essential if child less than 18 months old, or if any clinical suspicion of meningitis
7. Convulsion without fever:
   blood glucose and haemoglobin, plasma calcium, urea, amino acids, skull X-ray and EEG
8. Recurrent wheezing:
   plasma IgE, blood eosinophil count, chest X-ray, Mantoux test, skin tests.

REFERENCE

Paine R S, Oppe T E 1975 Neurological examination of children, 5th edn. (Clinics in Developmental Medicine No 20/21). Spastics International Medical Publications with Heinemann Medical, London.

FURTHER READING

Apley J, MacKeith R 1978 The child and his symptoms, 3rd edn. Blackwell Scientific, Oxford
Illingworth R S 1987 The normal child, 9th edn. Blackwell Scientific Publications, Oxford
Illingworth R S 1988 Common symptoms of disease in childhood. Churchill Livingstone, Edinburgh
Nellhaus G 1968 Head circumference from birth to eighteen years; practical composite international and interracial graphs. Pediatrics 41: 106–114
Pain R S, Oppe T E 1975 Neurological examination of children, 5th edn. Clinics in Developmental Medicine 20/21. Spastics International Medical Publications with Heinemann Medical Books, London

3. Growth and development

S. Wallis

Growing up is one of the essential features of childhood. Growth and development usually occur in harmony, each influencing the other. The effects of a loss of this harmony can be clearly seen with the premature onset of puberty in a 6-year-old girl, or the mentally retarded 15-year-old boy, taller than his mother, but with the abilities and understanding of a naughty 3 year old.

GROWTH

Cell and tissue growth

Three phases of tissue growth have been postulated. In the first phase all cells multiply; during the second phase some cells multiply, but they also increase in size due to the addition of cytoplasm, while in the final phase cell multiplication halts and only cell enlargement occurs. Some cells, such as those of skin and blood, continue to multiply and replace themselves throughout life. Other tissues such as brain, muscle, and lung have only a limited phase when cell multiplication can occur and, therefore, are more vulnerable to insults at this time. Animal research has shown that if the supply of nutrients is limited during the whole of this sensitive growth phase then the relevant organ (e.g. the brain) remains small and does not catch up in growth later; if it is only affected for part of the time, catch-up can occur.

Attempts have been made to apply these principles to human growth. It is known that some babies who grow slowly before birth catch up, while others remain small. The evidence suggests these babies are more likely to remain small if slow growth has been severe (affecting head as well as body growth) and prolonged (starting before 34 weeks' gestation).

Patterns of human growth

The curve of growth is a continuous process, extending from fetal life through birth and childhood into adult life.

Prenatal growth

Data about prenatal growth have been obtained by carefully examining fetuses aborted because either the fetus or the uterus was defective. Recently, ultrasound has enabled us to measure the fetus in utero. During the first trimester of pregnancy crown–rump measurements are very accurate, from about 13 weeks' gestation biparietal diameter measurements of the head can be made, and from midterm head and abdominal circumference measurements. Growth curves have been compiled using this data, and it is clear that growth in utero is extremely rapid with little variation between infants until the last trimester of pregnancy. The first indication of slow growth is a reduction in abdominal circumference, and if very severe, head growth slows. It is suggested that an early ultrasound measurement before 20 weeks to confirm dates, and measurement of head diameter and abdominal circumference at 32 weeks, would detect 90% of all small-for-dates infants.

Variations in fetal growth depend not only on the fetus, but also the mother and the environmental and nutritional circumstances in which she lives. Probably, maternal size has the greatest constraining influence on fetal growth, for the obvious reason that a small mother would have difficulty delivering a large baby. Studies where Shire horses were crossed with Shetland ponies clearly demonstrated this; the foals whose mothers were Shire horses were much larger than those whose mothers were Shetland ponies.

Maternal size is affected by race, health, nutrition and socio-economic factors which date back to the mother's own childhood. There are growth charts which allow for the mother's height and weight when assessing the baby's weight. Small-for-dates babies are born more frequently into those families where smoking, pre-eclampsia and short stature are more common.

Maternal health in pregnancy is important. Most problems such as hypertension and pre-eclampsia result in slow growth because they impair the supply of nutrients to the fetus; poorly controlled maternal diabetes, however, results in overweight babies because the baby responds to the high maternal blood sugar levels transmitted across the placenta by secreting extra insulin which, in turn, promotes the deposition of fat.

Of fetal factors which affect growth the baby's sex is the most important, male babies are heavier than female babies. Intrauterine infection, chromosomal, genetic and congenital malformations usually slow fetal growth. Transposition of the great arteries is a notable exception, these babies are often heavier than expected at birth. Multiple pregnancy also affects fetal growth because the nutrients must be shared, in twin pregnancy, slowing of growth starts around 33 weeks' gestation.

Postnatal growth

After birth the growth velocity of the majority of body tissues tends to follow a general curve similar to that of height and weight (Fig. 3.1). Growth of the brain and head, however, continues as rapidly as before birth, only slowing at about 4 years, and then halting long before other tissues stop growing. Reproductive tissue starts its growth spurt much later, coinciding with the pubertal increase in height.

Increase in size is rapid in the first 2 years of life, and during this period the child moves onto his genetically inherited growth curve, catching up

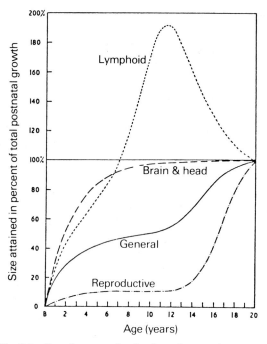

Fig. 3.1 Growth curves showing how the growth patterns of the brain and head, reproductive and lymphatic tissues vary from the general growth curve of the rest of the body (from Tanner (1962) with permission).

from any constraints during fetal life such as small maternal size. From 2 years, growth continues steadily until puberty. Most children have growth curves which follow the centile curves on the growth chart. During this period it is important to allow for parental height when considering whether a child is growing normally.

At puberty there is a sudden increase in growth velocity, the boys start their growth spurt about 18 months later than girls and ultimately achieve a greater height. There is a very wide variation in the time of onset of puberty, and to a lesser extent in the sequence of events. In girls, the first event is usually breast enlargement (range 9–13 years), followed closely by growth of pubic hair; in one-third of girls pubic hair appears before the breast bud. Menarche occurs relatively late in puberty (range 11–15 years) and growth continues after menarche; on average girls gain a further 6 cm in height. The time taken to complete pubertal changes may be as short as 18 months or extend for 5 years or more. In girls, puberty is defined as precocious if the onset is before 8 years and is regarded as delayed if there are no signs of puberty by 13 years, or menarche has not occurred by 16.5 years. In boys, the first sign of puberty is enlargement of the testes accompanied by changes in the skin of the scrotum which reddens and alters in texture (range 10–13.5 years). The growth spurt and changes in body dimensions, including growth of the penis and development of pubic hair, start about 1 year later and reach a peak over a 12-month period coinciding with the first seminal emissions. Growth of facial and axillary hair and breaking of the voice occur relatively late in puberty, the latter is due to lengthening of the vocal cords with the sudden growth spurt of the larynx. The breast also undergoes changes with increase in size of the areola. Up to one-third of boys develop a distinct enlargement of the breast in mid-puberty, this usually disappears spontaneously over the following year. Puberty in boys is said to be precocious if it occurs before 10 years, and delayed if there are no signs by 15 years.

Measurement and use of growth charts

Growth is always assessed by measuring height (length in children under 2 years), (Figs 3.2, 3.3), weight and head circumference, and also on the stage of pubertal development where appropriate (Table 3.1). Sometimes where body proportions are disturbed, measurements of sitting height and limb length are made, e.g. in achondroplasia where the limbs are short. Special equipment is needed to measure height, but if it is not available a rough measurement obtained from a growth screening wall chart is useful for detecting those children who need more detailed measurement.

The best standards for assessing growth of British children are those designed by Tanner (1987) from measurements of many hundreds of British children at different ages. Charts are available for plotting height, weight, head circumference and growth velocity. The height charts for boys and girls are illustrated in Figures 3.4(a) and (b). Each chart shows a series of centile curves. The 50th centile gives the median value for height of children at each age, that is half the children in the sample measured were taller than the 50th centile at each age, and half the children shorter. Similarly for the third centile, 97% of children were

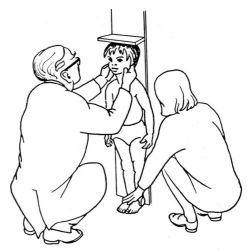

Fig. 3.2 Measuring the child's height. Make sure the child stands with the feet together, heels touching the ground and the heel plate. Young children tend to stand with their feet apart and to go up on tiptoe, they may need to have their feet held. The head should be in the Frankfort plane (so that a line drawn from the lower border of the eye to the upper margin of the external auditory meatus is horizontal), this avoids flexion of the neck. Encourage the child to stretch up to maximum height by gentle upward pressure on the bony mastoid processes, just behind the ears.

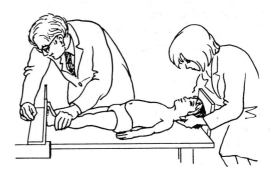

Fig. 3.3 Measuring a baby's length (length should be measured in children under 2 years). The baby lies on his back. One person holds his head in the Frankfort plane, and gently pulls to extend the baby to his full length. A second person straightens the baby's legs, so they lie flat on the table, and then brings a moveable footboard up against the heels. Length is often difficult to measure because babies prefer to lie curled up.

taller at each age and 3% were shorter. The third and 97th centile curves, or the two standard deviation lines, are regarded as the limits of normal, and children whose measurements fall outside this range may need to be studied. It is important to remember, however, that three normal children

Table 3.1 Stages of pubertal development

Boys: genital development
Stage 1 Preadolescent; the testes, scrotum and penis are the same size and proportions as in early childhood
Stage 2 The scrotum and testes grow, and the skin of the scrotum reddens and changes in texture
Stage 3 The penis begins to grow longer
Stage 4 Growth continues; the penis broadens and the glans develops, the testes and scrotum enlarge and the scrotal skin darkens
Stage 5 The genitalia are adult in size and shape

Girls: breast development
Stage 1 Preadolescent; only the papillae are raised
Stage 2 Formation of the breast bud; the breast and papilla become elevated into a small mound, and the areola enlarges
Stage 3 Further enlargement and elevation of breast and areola
Stage 4 The areola and papilla project to form a secondary mound above the level of the breast
Stage 5 Mature stage, only the papilla projects, the areola recedes to the general contour of the breast

Both sexes: pubic hair
Stage 1 Preadolescent; no pubic hair
Stage 2 Sparse growth of long pigmented downy hair, sometimes curly, at the base of the penis or along the labia
Stage 3 Hair spreads sparsely over the junction of the pubes and is coarser, darker and more curled
Stage 4 Hair is now adult in type, but has not spread to the medial surface of the thighs
Stage 5 Hair is adult in type and in distribution, having spread to the medial surface of the thighs. Spread up the linea alba occurs much later

out of every 100 will have measurements below the third centile, and a further three normal children will be above the 97th centile.

When assessing height it is important to allow for parental height, tall parents tend to have tall children, and short parents have short children. There are special charts which allow for midparental height, or as a quick check the child's height centile can be compared with those of his parents. The heights can be plotted on the child's growth chart as if they were aged 19 years. When plotting maternal height on a boy's chart, add 13 cm (the average difference between men and women's height) or subtract 13 cm from the father's height for the girl's chart. The midpoint between the parental height is then found on the chart, this is the midparental height centile, and a line extending 8.5 cm up and down from it will indicate the range of heights within which 95% of their children

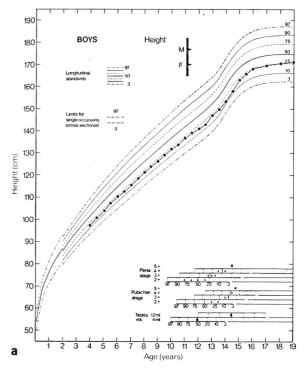

a

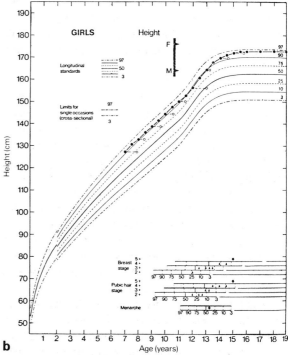

b

Fig. 3.4 Growth charts showing centiles for height and pubertal development. There are separate charts for boys (**a**) and girls (**b**) (from Tanner & Whitehouse (1978) with permission).

should come. If parental height is allowed for in this way, a short child with short parents may move from below the third to the 50th centile, whereas a child of average height with tall parents may move from the 50th to below the third centile.

Single measurements of height, weight and head circumference give limited and often misleading information; it is much more useful to plot a series of measurements on the growth chart to ascertain the pattern of growth. Most children's growth curves tend to follow centile curves without crossing them, except in the first year of life, and at puberty. Children who are exceptionally large or small, taking into account parental size, or who have one growth parameter which differs greatly from the others, such as a large head circumference or short stature, or whose growth curves cross centile lines, may need investigation.

DEVELOPMENT

The study of child development is rather like looking down a series of increasingly powerful microscopes, the closer one looks the more detail emerges. Knowledge of detail is essential in order to help the handicapped child achieve various skills despite his handicap; for instance, helping the blind child learn to reach towards the sound made by a toy which he cannot see. The sooner difficulties are recognised, the sooner appropriate help can be given. Traditionally doctors and health visitors have attempted to detect handicap by carrying out developmental assessments of all children at specified ages, but it is usually parents who are the first to suspect abnormality in their child's development. It is now thought that after the 6-week check it is more sensible for doctors and health visitors not to attempt to screen all children but rather to give their time to those children where there are special concerns.

It is important to take a full developmental history and to observe closely the child's spontaneous play so as to be able to recognise delay or atypical developmental patterns. Developmental charts and scales are helpful for learning the extent of normal ranges and patterns of development. The following charts and notes outline development at key ages

when children have commonly been seen, and give age ranges for the acquisition of many skills.

The developmental assessment should be brief as young children can and will only concentrate for short periods, 15 minutes or less is usually recommended. Severe delay in motor development should become obvious in the first year, while most cases of cerebral palsy are detected by 18 months. It is hoped to identify the deaf child early, but many are only recognised because of poor speech development, by which time they are usually 2 or 3 years old. Parents are often aware that something is wrong and their anxieties should be taken seriously. The milder forms of mental handicap also become apparent around 2–3 years, with immature patterns of play and poor language skills being present. Special help at home, or in a nursery group should be made available, starting soon after the handicap is recognised.

Selected school entry medical examinations are carried out where there are no preschool records or inadequate documentation or a special request has been made by parents or school staff. It is hoped this will allow more time for those children with less obvious neurodevelopmental disorders who will need special help at school. About 5% of children in normal schools have significant learning difficulties and up to 20% are said to need extra help at some stage of their schooling.

Notes on development (Fig. 3.5):

6 weeks

Many treatable disorders can be detected at this age. Always enquire whether there are any parental concerns, particularly regarding hearing and vision. Physical examination should include measurement of weight and head circumference, and a careful check for abnormalities of the eyes, heart, hips and testes.

Motor

At this stage one is looking for abnormalities of posture, muscle tone, and strength but it is very difficult to ascertain their significance. The following are always abnormal: persistent and marked asymmetry, e.g. torticollis or spinal curvature, ex-

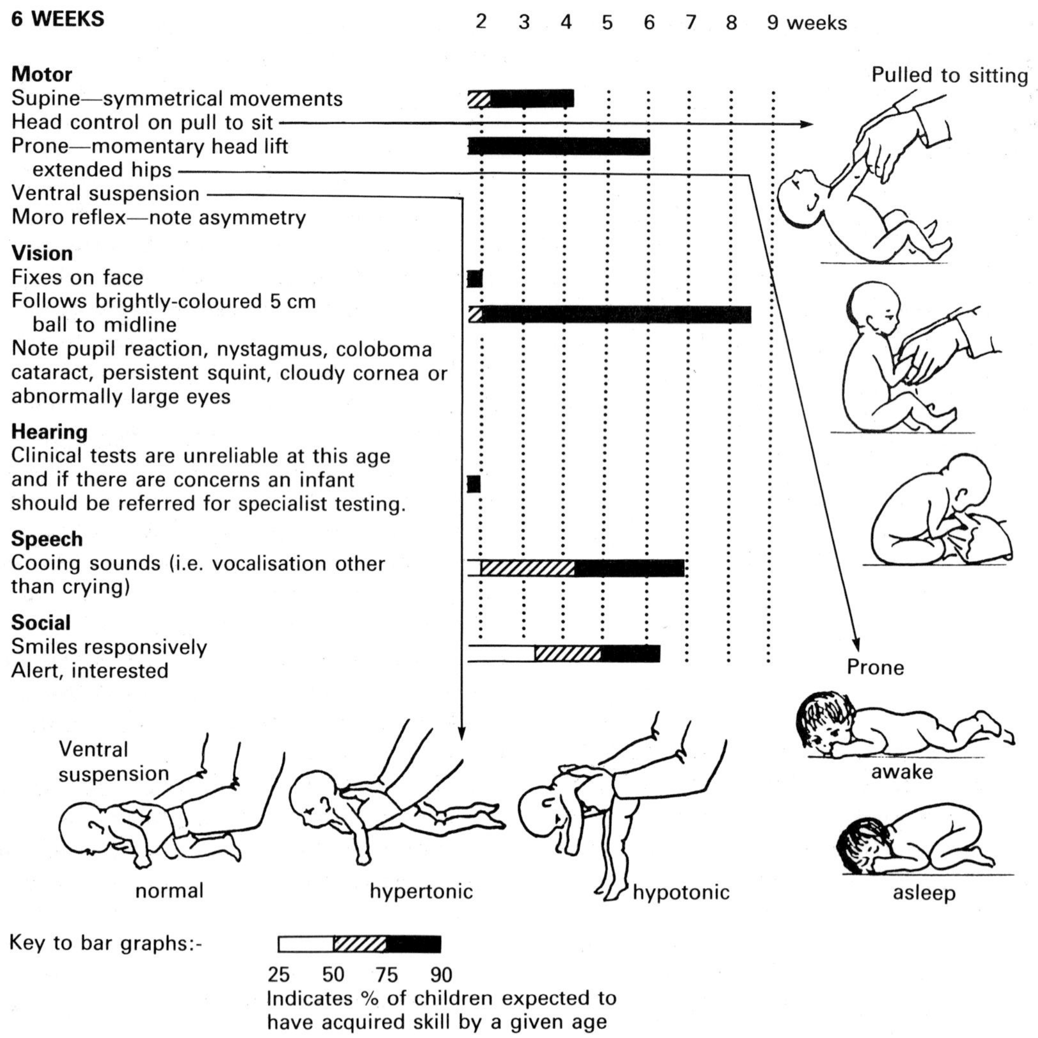

6 WEEKS　　　　　　　　2　3　4　5　6　7　8　9 weeks

Motor
Supine—symmetrical movements
Head control on pull to sit ————————→ Pulled to sitting
Prone—momentary head lift
　extended hips ————
Ventral suspension —
Moro reflex—note asymmetry

Vision
Fixes on face
Follows brightly-coloured 5 cm
　ball to midline
Note pupil reaction, nystagmus, coloboma
cataract, persistent squint, cloudy cornea or
abnormally large eyes

Hearing
Clinical tests are unreliable at this age
and if there are concerns an infant
should be referred for specialist testing.

Speech
Cooing sounds (i.e. vocalisation other
than crying)

Social
Smiles responsively
Alert, interested　　　　　　　　　　　　　　Prone

Ventral
suspension

normal　　　　hypertonic　　　hypotonic　　　awake / asleep

Key to bar graphs:-

　25　50　75　90
Indicates % of children expected to
have acquired skill by a given age

Fig. 3.5 Development at 6 weeks.

treme hypotonia, extensor spasm and inability to lift the limbs against gravity.

Supine. Lies with head to one side and arm and leg on that side more extended (asymmetric tonic neck reflex or ATNR).

Prone. Less flexed than at birth, when awake hips are extended and pelvis is low on the couch, the sleeping baby often reverts to newborn flexed posture.

Head control is beginning to develop. When prone, the baby briefly lifts his head and turns his face to the side. On pull to sit the head lags until the body is nearly vertical when it is held momen-

tarily erect before flopping forwards. Marked hip flexion when prone, and excessive head lag are abnormal.

Ventral suspension. If the infant is suspended with a hand under his abdomen, he momentarily holds his head level with his body, and his hips, knees and elbows are partially flexed. In hypertonia, the head is held above the line of the trunk and cannot be flexed, and the hips and knees are fully extended in line with the trunk. The hypotonic infant limply hangs over the hand and is unable to lift head or limbs.

Neonatal reflexes should be present and symmetrical, but obligatory responses which do not fade on repetition are abnormal.

Vision

Mothers usually know whether their babies look at them intently during feeds. Nevertheless, always inspect eyes and test vision; it is important to recognise severe visual defects quickly as some benefit from early surgery, e.g. removal of cataracts, congenital glaucoma. Babies who fail to visually fix or follow a bright-coloured object, or who have nystagmus, persistent squint, absent red reflex or other ocular abnormality should be urgently referred to an ophthalmologist. Visual information is important for early learning and early developmental guidance is thought to help if there is poor vision.

Hearing

Hearing is difficult to test in the young infant. Loud sounds, at least 60 dB, are often needed to elicit a response at this age. Several special techniques have been developed and evidence so far suggests they allow recognition of severe hearing loss in the first weeks of life. The auditory response cradle measures behavioural response to sound whereas measurement of cochlear emissions and brain stem evoked response audiometry give an objective measure. Children known to have an increased risk of sensorineural hearing loss should be referred for testing: this includes those with a positive family history, evidence of a dysmorphic syndrome or congenital infection, and those who have received exchange transfusions or neonatal intensive care.

Social

A baby's alertness and interest is shown by his ability to imitate and his responses to social stimuli. No smile by 8 weeks is cause for serious concern, unless the baby was preterm. Sometimes babies of this age are hungry or uncomfortable at the time of testing, and are not very responsive. If you have to rely on the history, ensure that the mother understands you are referring to a smile in response to a social overture, rather than a smiling expression during sleep.

7–9 months (Fig. 3.6)

Motor

Head control is achieved by 4 months. In prone, head and chest should be lifted off the bed. In supine, the baby is starting to lift the head off the pillow and by 7–8 months there should be no head lag, shoulders should be braced and elbows flexed on pull to sit. Hypotonia is obvious, but if there is increased extensor tone, the child may rise to his feet when pulled to sit.

Sits alone for a few seconds with a straight back. Control of trunk muscles develops from above downwards, initially the back is C-shaped when sitting, then the thoracic spine straightens and finally the lumbar curve is lost.

Sitting balance. Two responses are required to balance the trunk upright against gravity; the truncal righting response, involving tilting of the trunk and head to correct the loss of upright position, and protective responses where the hands are put out to prevent falling over. Forward balance develops first, then sideways and finally backwards balance which is usually achieved by 12 months. A child cannot sit or walk alone until he has both balancing and protective reactions, they are often slow to develop in cerebral palsy.

Mobility. The infant is starting to move around usually by rolling, some are already pivoting or creeping on their stomachs, the average age for crawling on hands and knees is 10 months. No mobility by 10 months should cause concern.

Neonatal reflexes should have disappeared, persistence is a serious sign of delay.

Manipulative and adaptive skills

Reaching develops in several stages. Initially there is a phase of hand regard, when the infant waves his hands in front of his eyes, pronating and supinating them at the wrists; this should have stopped by 5 months. During the next stage the infant looks excitedly at an object, moulding his hand as if to grasp it. Initially, reaching and touching the object occurs by accident, and is

7–9 MONTHS

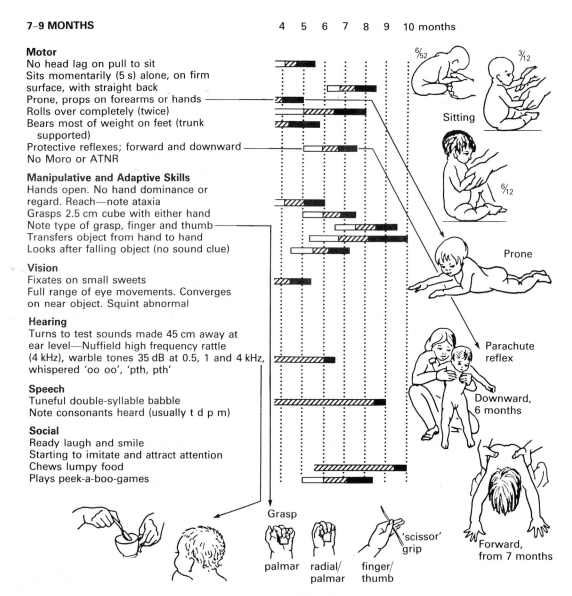

| | 4 | 5 | 6 | 7 | 8 | 9 | 10 months |

Motor
No head lag on pull to sit
Sits momentarily (5 s) alone, on firm surface, with straight back
Prone, props on forearms or hands
Rolls over completely (twice)
Bears most of weight on feet (trunk supported)
Protective reflexes; forward and downward
No Moro or ATNR

Manipulative and Adaptive Skills
Hands open. No hand dominance or regard. Reach—note ataxia
Grasps 2.5 cm cube with either hand
Note type of grasp, finger and thumb
Transfers object from hand to hand
Looks after falling object (no sound clue)

Vision
Fixates on small sweets
Full range of eye movements. Converges on near object. Squint abnormal

Hearing
Turns to test sounds made 45 cm away at ear level—Nuffield high frequency rattle (4 kHz), warble tones 35 dB at 0.5, 1 and 4 kHz, whispered 'oo oo', 'pth, pth'

Speech
Tuneful double-syllable babble
Note consonants heard (usually t d p m)

Social
Ready laugh and smile
Starting to imitate and attract attention
Chews lumpy food
Plays peek-a-boo-games

Sitting

Prone

Parachute reflex

Downward, 6 months

Forward, from 7 months

Grasp

palmar   radial/palmar   finger/thumb   'scissor' grip

Fig. 3.6 Development at 7–9 months (For key to bar graph, see Fig. 3.5, p. 22).

probably helped by the ATNR where the arm is extended in the direction the child is looking. Gradually, voluntary reaching occurs but is very ataxic to begin with. By 8 months the infant should have a steady accurate reach with either hand, good head and shoulder control is essential. Use of only one hand may indicate hemiplegia.

Grasp. The grasp reflex should be fading by 4 months, so that the hands lie open and can be used to grasp objects. Initially objects are grasped in the palm for a few moments, but by 8 months there is a secure radial palmar grasp. There is also an awareness of holding an object, so it is briefly looked at, transferred from hand to hand, then explored in the mouth and if dropped watched as it falls to the ground (average age 6 months). Later, the interest in objects extends to looking for them when they disappear from view — the concept of permanence of objects expected by 9 months. One inch (2.5 cm) cubes are the correct size of toy for the infant to grasp in his palm, smaller toys will be lost, and the hand is not big enough for larger toys.

Vision

Note visual interest for near and distant objects. Good head control leads to macular fixation and binocular vision, that is both eyes move together in all directions — test by moving a light from side to side and watching reflections of light in the eyes. Demonstrate convergence by persuading the child to look at a small sweet. Squint is abnormal. Obvious squints are detected by asymmetrical reflection of the light in the pupils. Less obvious squints are detected with the cover test, the infant is persuaded to look at a small toy (not a light), and then one eye is covered by moving a hand in front of the eye. A squint is present if the *uncovered* eye then moves to take up fixation on the toy. Squints are often only present intermittently, so parental concern, particularly if there is a family history of squint, should lead to referral.

Hearing

Parental anxiety should always be taken seriously. Ask parents for examples of sounds their child responds to, such as smiling in response to a quiet voice, looking towards the door when he hears it opened quietly, or excitement when he hears food being prepared or a bath run. In some districts all parents are given a printed hearing check list after their baby's birth. Hearing tests are difficult to carry out accurately in a clinic. Distraction-type tests are used, where the child is only scored as passing if he turns and localises the sound. Localisation skills develop from reflex eye movements, where the eyes move towards the ear in which the sound is heard loudest. Sounds are first localised at ear level, then below and finally above ear level (localisation behind or above the head is very difficult and not achieved until much later). By 8 months the majority of children can localise quiet sounds or voice at ear level, whereas a number of these may have failed at 6 months. After 10 months they are less easily distracted by a new stimulus and may fail to turn to the test sounds in spite of normal hearing. Success is more likely if interesting test sounds are used, particularly those familiar to the child, they should not be louder than 35 dB. Warble tones are more successful than pure tones at this age.

Distraction tests are often carried out by specially trained health visitors — two work together, one produces the test sounds and the other distracts the child. It is often difficult to produce standardised test sounds at the correct frequencies and sufficiently quiet, and so many health visitors use special machines calibrated to produce warble tones at 35 dB at 0.5, 1 and 4 kHz frequencies.

Speech

The sounds a baby makes are an indication of the sounds he hears and is trying to imitate. By 9 months he should enjoy making tuneful babble including consonants, for example 'adadadada' and 'umumum'. Parents of deaf children often comment on the striking lack of baby sounds made by their deaf child, compared with his normally hearing siblings.

Social

Lack of interest in surroundings, infrequent smiles and failure to imitate are cause for concern, and may indicate intellectual delay or sometimes social deprivation.

18 months (Fig. 3.7)

Motor

During the second year children become increasingly adept at motor skills. The majority can walk alone, balance momentarily on one leg to kick a ball, or walk upstairs, but they crawl downstairs backwards. Children who cannot walk alone, must be examined carefully for signs of cerebral palsy, muscle disorder or intellectual delay. One-third of these children are found to have some abnormality, most of them have been recognised earlier. Some, who are not walking, may be moving around in other ways, such as rolling, creeping, or bottom shuffling. There is often a family history of moving in the same way. These children are slow to sit alone, although most do so by 15

18 MONTHS

15 16 17 18 19 20 21 months

Motor
Stands alone well
Walks alone at least 10 steps
Stoops and recovers
Kicks ball forward

Manipulative and Adaptive Skills
Note reach, grasp and release use of both hands
No mouthing, casting or drooling
Fine pincer grasp
Stacks two 2.5 cm bricks (imitates)
Dumps raisin from bottle (imitates)
Books—turns two or more pages at once
Looks at pictures

Vision
Near vision—'hundreds and thousands' (1 mm sweets)
Distant vision—mounted or rolling ball test; should see 3 mm ball at 3 m. Cover test for squint

Hearing and Language
Real objects (sock, shoe, brush, cup, spoon); child should point to each on naming
Note appropriate manipulation of objects and whether named spontaneously
Points to one named body part—hair, eyes, feet, nose, teeth
Says 3 words with meaning (other than 'Mama' and 'Dada')
Combines two different words
Obeys simple commands—'Give me'; 'Sit down'; 'Come here'

Social
Drinks from cup (open top)
Uses spoon, spilling little
Imitates housework
Enjoys nursery rhymes
Removes garment

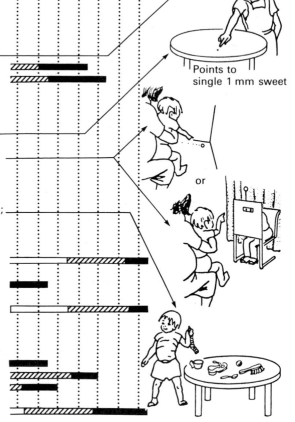

Points to single 1 mm sweet

or

Fig. 3.7 Development at 18 months (For key to bar graph, see Fig. 3.5, p. 22).

months, and are slow to walk alone, this is usually achieved by 26–28 months.

Manipulative and adaptive skills

Manipulative skills. By 18 months a child should have developed accurate reach and a mature voluntary grasp and release. Stacking bricks tests the accuracy of reach, grasp and release; the use of a raisin or tiny sweet demonstrates index pointing and fine pincer grasp between the tip of the thumb and first finger.

Play. During the second year children can concentrate on tasks of their own choice, but cannot use, or tolerate any intervention, or attempts to modify the task. Their understanding is shown by attempts to stack bricks, dump the raisin from a narrow-necked bottle after being shown, and interest in books and pictures. By 18 months children should indicate their understanding of familiar lifesize objects by using them appropriately in play, e.g. brushing hair with the brush or putting a spoon in the cup and feeding themselves.

At this age children are not easily distracted from their play, they tend to rigidly fix their attention on the activity of their own choice and often cannot tolerate intervention or assistance from an adult without a tantrum. For this reason formal tests are difficult and more is seen by watching the child playing spontaneously.

Ataxia or tremor when reaching, immature grasp, and obvious hand preference are abnormal, and suggestive of cerebral palsy. The mouthing of toys and drooling seen in the first year should have disappeared; so should casting, which is the deliberate throwing of toys onto the floor in a repetitive manner normally seen between 12 and 15 months — persistence of any of these suggests intellectual delay, as does failure to define objects by use or fleeting attention control.

Vision

Visual acuity is difficult to test accurately at this age.

Near vision is crudely assessed using hundreds and thousands, small round coloured cake decorations, which are about 1 mm in diameter. One or two sweets are discretely dropped onto a felt-covered table top of contrasting colour, taking care not to indicate the position of the sweets with the hand or eye. To pass, the child should point to a sweet or try to pick it up.

Distance vision is not routinely tested at this age. The Stycar tests designed by Mary Sheridan can be used to give a rough measure of acuity in handicapped children where other methods are precluded. The tests use white balls of graded sizes from 6 cm down to 3 mm in diameter. These balls are either rolled along the ground, or mounted on sticks and shown from behind a screen 3 (or preferably 6) m from the child. The balls should always be shown against a plain, black background. By watching the child's eyes, one can detect whether he has seen the balls. He should see the smallest 3 mm ball at a distance of at least 3 m.

Cover test should always be done, as squints can appear at any time during the preschool years. They are sometimes more obvious on distance vision tests, particularly when there is a defect of distance vision in one eye.

Hearing and language

Hearing tests are difficult to carry out accurately at this age. Parental concern about hearing, failure to respond to spoken commands or poor vocalisation, are indications for a formal hearing test.

Comprehension of spoken language can be tested by asking the child to select the appropriate lifesize object on naming, e.g. 'where's the shoe'?, 'where's Teddy?' or asking him to point to different parts of the body. Differentiation of the sounds in the words 'sock' and 'shoe', or 'feet' and 'teeth', demonstrate not only the ability to hear high frequency sounds, but also to subtly discriminate between them.

Expressive language is less easy to elicit in a strange place. Toddlers often chatter when they are happily playing and this should be listened for. There is usually a lot of tuneful jargon, with some words said clearly with meaning. Familiar lifesize objects such as a cup, brush and spoon, and Ladybird pictures are useful aids for eliciting language. By 2 years children are using plurals, e.g. biscuits, and are putting two words together, e.g. 'Daddy car' or 'Sara bikit' (= biscuit). Phrases such as 'all gone' do not count as they are learnt as a single word.

Social

Social skills such as drinking from a cup, or using a spoon depend on whether the child has been allowed to try and feed himself. Most toddlers want to imitate adults and are keen to test their independence. They sometimes refuse to feed if parents insist on helping them to ensure a good food intake or to avoid mess. As a result temper tantrums, and feeding, sleeping, or bowel problems are particularly common amongst toddlers.

2.5–3 years (Fig. 3.8)

Motor

The 2.5-year-old child walks well with a steady even stride, feet fairly close together; he goes up and down stairs, two feet per step holding the bannister, and by 3 years many go upstairs alternate feet to each step. Balance and running skills have improved. Initially the child runs well indoors in a straight line, and later develops the ability to negotiate objects whilst running. Jumping and climbing are practised in play, and peddling a tri-

2.5–3 YEARS

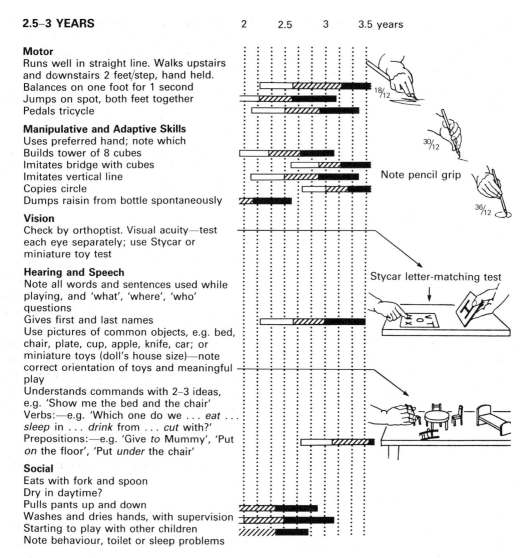

Motor
Runs well in straight line. Walks upstairs and downstairs 2 feet/step, hand held.
Balances on one foot for 1 second
Jumps on spot, both feet together
Pedals tricycle

Manipulative and Adaptive Skills
Uses preferred hand; note which
Builds tower of 8 cubes
Imitates bridge with cubes
Imitates vertical line
Copies circle
Dumps raisin from bottle spontaneously

Vision
Check by orthoptist. Visual acuity—test each eye separately; use Stycar or miniature toy test

Hearing and Speech
Note all words and sentences used while playing, and 'what', 'where', 'who' questions
Gives first and last names
Use pictures of common objects, e.g. bed, chair, plate, cup, apple, knife, car; or miniature toys (doll's house size)—note correct orientation of toys and meaningful play
Understands commands with 2–3 ideas, e.g. 'Show me the bed and the chair'
Verbs:—e.g. 'Which one do we ... *eat* ... *sleep* in ... *drink* from ... *cut* with?'
Prepositions:—e.g. 'Give *to* Mummy', 'Put *on* the floor', 'Put *under* the chair'

Social
Eats with fork and spoon
Dry in daytime?
Pulls pants up and down
Washes and dries hands, with supervision
Starting to play with other children
Note behaviour, toilet or sleep problems

Note pencil grip

Stycar letter-matching test

Fig. 3.8 Development at 2.5–3 years (For key to bar graph, see Fig. 3.5, p. 22).

cycle shows the ability to coordinate alternate leg movements.

Manipulative and adaptive skills

From 18 months children start to demonstrate hand preference. The other hand is still used co-operatively for bimanual tasks such as threading beads, or building a three-brick bridge. Exclusive use of one hand is suggestive of hemiplegia. The pencil grip matures from the initial palmar grasp in the midshaft of the pencil, with a movement of the whole arm at 18 months, to an early tripod grip by 2.5–3 years. The pencil is held near the point between the thumb and first two fingers permitting finer movements of the hand and forearm.

Play. In the third year a child's attention control is still single-channelled and given to one task at a time, but much more flexible; so that once his full attention has been obtained he can be given directions to carry out a task, and then must be encouraged to transfer his interest back to the task. The child's ability to carry out some of the manipulative and linguistic test items, will give a measure of his attention level. When he is asked to imitate a bridge made of cubes, the bridge is built in front of him, and then he is asked to make another. Copying is more difficult, for example the circle is dawn out of his sight, he is then shown the circle and asked to copy it.

Vision

In some parts of the UK, orthoptists routinely see children to check for less obvious squints and refractive errors. By 3–3½ years the majority of children are able to co-operate with their tests, and this is thought to be a good age for screening.

In the Stycar letter matching tests the children are shown single letters at a distance of 3 m, and asked to point to the matching letter on the card in front of them. It is important to check that they are able to match the letters correctly close up, before testing at a distance — 80% of 3 year olds can do this. Children who fail to match the letter size 4 (equivalent to Snellen 6/9) with each eye separately, should be referred to an ophthalmologist. If the child cannot match letters, he can be asked to match specially standardised pictures of familiar toys or objects (Kays pictures) from a distance of 3 m or 6 m.

Hearing and language

It is important to check language skills carefully as delay may be the first indication of poor hearing, intellectual retardation, or less commonly a specific language disorder. Inability to communicate in the presence of normal intelligence leads to great frustration, and the children often resort to gesture and mime. If any abnormalities are found formal hearing tests should be carried out.

The child of 2.5–3 years should understand pictures and that doll's-house-size miniature toys represent real objects and play meaningfully with them; failure to do so suggests intellectual delay. Verbal comprehension can be tested with pictures or miniature toys; at 2 years most children can relate two ideas together or carry out a command containing two information-carrying (or operative) words, e.g. 'put the spoon in the box', and by 3 years, four ideas together, for example 'put the cup on the table and put the baby in the bath'.

Most children chatter continuously whilst playing and have a vocabulary of at least 200 words. By 2 years they are using plurals and putting two words together in phrases, e.g. 'baby bath', 'Daddy go'; and by 3 years are putting three words together in short sentences consisting of subject — verb — object, for instance, 'Sara eat cake'. The pronouns 'I', 'me' and 'you' are used correctly by 3 years, as are most prepositions. Persistent and frequent 'what', 'where', 'who' questions are a feature of this age.

Social

Some children are starting to attend nursery at the age of 3 years, they need to be able to separate from their parents and to have achieved some independance in daily living skills. Feeding, washing and dressing are carried out increasingly skilfully, and most children like to do everything without help. The majority of children are dry in the daytime, and some are also dry at night. It is again important to enquire about behaviour problems, one study found they occurred in 18% of children over 2 years old and were frequently associated with maternal depression.

4.5–5 years (school entrance examination)
(Fig. 3.9)

Motor

There is a wide variation of normal motor skills, but a number of children, particularly boys, are significantly slow in motor development and appear clumsy compared with their more agile peers. If clumsiness is severe, or is associated with poor skills in other areas, educational difficulties are likely; otherwise the majority of clumsy children seem to cope. A number of physiotherapists have developed therapy programmes to help these children become more aware of their body images, and the position of their joints and limbs. At present it only seems practicable to refer the most severely affected children for this type of help.

Manipulative and adaptive skills

In order to cope at school a child must be able to

4.5–5 YEARS

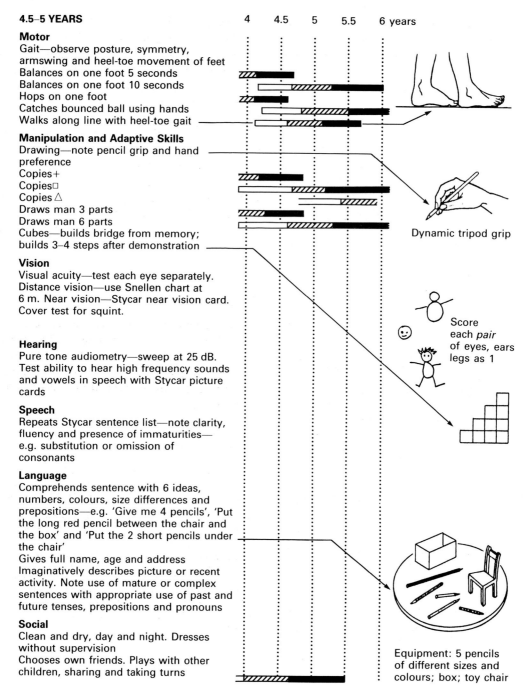

Motor
Gait—observe posture, symmetry, armswing and heel-toe movement of feet
Balances on one foot 5 seconds
Balances on one foot 10 seconds
Hops on one foot
Catches bounced ball using hands
Walks along line with heel-toe gait

Manipulation and Adaptive Skills
Drawing—note pencil grip and hand preference
Copies+
Copies□
Copies △
Draws man 3 parts
Draws man 6 parts
Cubes—builds bridge from memory; builds 3–4 steps after demonstration

Dynamic tripod grip

Vision
Visual acuity—test each eye separately. Distance vision—use Snellen chart at 6 m. Near vision—Stycar near vision card. Cover test for squint.

Score each *pair* of eyes, ears legs as 1

Hearing
Pure tone audiometry—sweep at 25 dB. Test ability to hear high frequency sounds and vowels in speech with Stycar picture cards

Speech
Repeats Stycar sentence list—note clarity, fluency and presence of immaturities—e.g. substitution or omission of consonants

Language
Comprehends sentence with 6 ideas, numbers, colours, size differences and prepositions—e.g. 'Give me 4 pencils', 'Put the long red pencil between the chair and the box' and 'Put the 2 short pencils under the chair'
Gives full name, age and address
Imaginatively describes picture or recent activity. Note use of mature or complex sentences with appropriate use of past and future tenses, prepositions and pronouns

Social
Clean and dry, day and night. Dresses without supervision
Chooses own friends. Plays with other children, sharing and taking turns

Equipment: 5 pencils of different sizes and colours; box; toy chair

Fig. 3.9   Development at 4.5–5 years (For key to bar graph, see Fig. 3.5, p. 22).

control his focus of attention and integrate information from several sources at once. For instance, the teacher may be speaking about an object and the child needs to be able to look at it and listen to the teacher at the same time. This is called multi-channelled attention control. He should be able to hold a pencil in a mature tripod grip, thus enabling him to make small controlled movements of his hand, and to put even pressure on the pencil. He should also be able to copy shapes as a preliminary to writing, and demonstrate his visual perception of people in a drawing. Construction of three-dimensional shapes from a model is tested.

Vision

Visual defects can appear at any stage of childhood due to growth of the eyeball, this usually causes shortsightedness (myopia) and therefore visual acuity should be checked every couple of years at school. About 7% of 5-year-olds are found to have a squint, some previously unrecognised; a tendency to tilt the head to one side should raise suspicions.

Hearing

Hearing is tested in two ways. First, the ability to hear quiet sounds at different frequencies is tested with an audiogram. Second the ability to listen to sounds and discriminate between them is tested with the Stycar picture cards for high and low frequency sounds. The latter test is more likely to be failed by children with poor ability to listen, in spite of normal hearing. Some of these children have a history of fluctuating hearing loss due to glue ear.

Speech and language

Speech should be clear, fluent and easily understood by persons other than members of the family. Some minor immaturities such as substitution of the consonants R, L, W or Y and S, F or Th are still common and usually disappear by 7 years. Encourage the child to talk by asking him about a recent outing, or to describe a picture.

Write down some examples of what he says. He should speak imaginatively using mature sentences, containing two clauses joined by 'and', for example, 'I went shopping and Mummy stayed at home'; or complex sentences containing a subordinate clause such as 'I didn't go shopping because I was ill'. Past, present and future tenses of verbs, prepositions and pronouns should be used appropriately. Children who have poor linguistic skills at school entry, frequently have difficulty with learning, in particular with learning to read. They urgently need assessment of hearing and speech therapy advice. Ideally these problems should be recognised at the 2.5–3-year examination, so the children can be helped before starting at school.

Social

A child needs to be independent in daily living skills, feeding, dressing, washing and toileting, to manage at school. In addition, he should separate easily from his family, and make friends with other children, understanding the need to share and take turns in games.

FURTHER READING

Bryant G J, Davies K J, Newcombe R G 1979 Standardisation of the Denver developmental screening test for Cardiff children. Developmental Medicine and Child Neurology 21: 353–364
DHSS 1976 Fit for the future. DHSS, London
Hall D M B 1984 The child with a handicap. Blackwell Scientific, Oxford
Holt K S 1977 Developmental paediatrics. (Postgraduate Paediatric Series) Butterworths, London
Sheridan M D 1975 Children's developmental progress from birth to five years: the Stycar sequences. NFER Publishing Company Ltd, Windsor
Tanner J M 1978 Foetus into man. Open Books Publishing, London

4. Prevention of illness and care of the normal child

N. Frazer

INTRODUCTION

A general practitioner (GP) looks after a defined list of patients and functions as a generalist working with all ages and seeing conditions which are frequently ill defined and undifferentiated. He is responsible chiefly to his patients: the public may choose their own doctor rather than have him allocated to them according to the street in which they live. The advantage of this system is that both parties can work together in a mutually acceptable personal relationship; the disadvantage is that the state cannot organise preventive measures as easily as in some other systems. This aspect of care is the one that is most often neglected in British general practice, where care has mostly been offered on a haphazard, reactive basis.

The leaders of the profession have recognised for some time that to improve the health of the nation as a whole, and children in particular, requires a more proactive approach to health. This sort of approach should be relatively easy for the GP as the defined list enables one to identify a targetable population (Table 4.1).

Opportunistic screening of adults has proved reasonably successful when dealing with conditions such as hypertension. The time-course of childhood and the understanding that those families in greatest need are frequently those who require most help in the way services are provided suggest that a planned approach to screening is more appropriate.

Any worthwhile programme needs to be organised correctly: this requires a suitable information handling system. In the past very good results have been obtained in many practices using manual records such as age–sex registers and

Table 4.1 Model for preventive care and its integration into the GP's range of services

REACTIVE Tertiary prevention	ACUTE CONSULTATION (at home or in the surgery) Acute otitis media
OPPORTUNISTIC Secondary prevention	FOLLOW UP Hearing test 6 weeks after
PROACTIVE Primary prevention	COLD CONSULTATION Routine hearing test for babies at 7 months

disease indexes. In the future the advantages of computerised systems mean that much more information can be stored and recalled. A practice can discover the effectiveness of their cervical smear system and highlight any shortcomings and target their energies more appropriately. Abnormalities can be followed up using the information stored. This situation also operates for more complex topics such as the setting up of a paediatric surveillance clinic or an immunisation programme.

The concept that a practice can act as a unit to generate and maintain certain levels of preventive care is relatively new. Increasing numbers of practices have taken this role seriously and publish, primarily for their own internal audit, their practice reports.

It is difficult to be certain how much the immunisation programmes have contributed to the considerable improvements in infant mortality and postneonatal death in the past 60 years. There have been tremendous improvements in the living conditions of a large part of the population, and these have probably been of overriding importance. This country's figures are no longer thought of as being particularly good, and the possibility remains that if our immunisation rates do fall then the herd immunity to life-threatening diseases such as poliomyelitis or whooping cough will fall to the extent that epidemics may occur. The incidence of whooping cough notifications went up considerably after the public debate regarding the potential side-effects in the early 1980s, when the frequency of whooping cough vaccination fell.

Before considering the ways in which GPs can set about providing preventive services, it is helpful to consider the ways in which prevention can be defined.

CLASSIFICATION OF PREVENTIVE MEASURES

Primary prevention aims to prevent the occurrence of a disease.

Secondary prevention aims to detect a disease early or at a presymptomatic stage when its effects can sometimes be reversed and its progress halted.

Tertiary prevention aims to halt the development of complications in a previously recognised disease.

The types of prevention are shown in Table 4.2.

Secondary prevention of a disease can be undertaken by screening a population. For this to be effective the disease must satisfy the following criteria:

1. Untreated, it must have potential serious consequences.

2. It must be easily and reliably recognisable at an early or presymptomatic stage.

3. Effective treatment must be easily and economically available.

The prevention of illness in general practice can be considered under the headings detailed below.

Prevention of genetic and congenital disease

Most congenital disease occurs sporadically. In some situations, for example where there is a family history or even where the parents are affected or have had an affected child, parents can be given genetic counselling. A couple may decide not to have children (primary prevention), or accept that the risk of having an affected child is low enough to be worth accepting, especially if the condition

Table 4.2 Developmental surveillance regime (as in Hall 1989)

Neonatal	Full family history, obstetric and birth history. Full examination including weight and measurement. Hips, eyes and testes. Phenylketonuria (PKU) and thyroid stimulating hormone (TSH) tests
On return home	Re-check hips
6 weeks	History, parental concerns. Examine and measure. Hips. Ask about sight and hearing. Inspect eyes
7–9 months	Parental concerns. Ask about sight and hearing. Observe for squint. Distraction hearing test. Check for congenital dislocation of the hip and testes
18–24 months	Parental concerns especially behaviour, vision and hearing. Observe child walking with normal gait. Saying a few words and understanding more. No suitable sight or hearing screen, so if in doubt refer. Iron deficiency anaemia in risk groups or faddy eaters
36–42 months	Vision, squint, hearing, behaviour and development. Indications of special educational problems. Height on chart. Re-check testes hearing test if indicated
School entry — 5 years	Parents' or teachers' concerns. Physical including heart sounds. Plot height. Snellen test for vision. Sweep hearing test
School	Visual acuity — 8, 11, 14 years. Colour vision testing with Ishihara charts at 11 years. Repeat height if there are concerns

like Down's syndrome can be detected early enough in pregnancy to allow a termination (secondary prevention). Congenital toxoplasmosis if detected early enough can be modified if the mother is given treatment whilst she is pregnant. This may reduce the degree of handicap from which the baby suffers as the harmful effect of toxoplasmosis may be limited by the appropriate drug regimen (tertiary prevention).

The prevention of illness in the newborn is one of the main aims of antenatal care. Prompt detection of disorders such as pre-eclampsia, placental insufficiency or maternal diabetes mellitus can significantly reduce morbidity in the baby. Premature labour can sometimes be averted, and neonatal asphyxia prevented by careful antenatal care. A mother who is Rhesus-negative can be given anti-

D gamma globulin within 24 hours of the birth of a baby or after a miscarriage. This should help prevent the development of Rhesus disease in subsequent pregnancies.

Prevention of metabolic and nutritional disorders

One of the best established biochemical screening tools is the Guthrie test, which detects high levels of phenylalanine in blood taken by a heel prick between the sixth and fourteenth days of life. Once diagnosed, profound mental handicap can be avoided if the child is kept on a diet low in phenylalanine. Testing for hypothyroidism on the same blood sample has been introduced more recently; the detection of high levels of TSH is now well established (pp. 264).

Pure nutritional diseases are not common in children in the UK. Babies of Asian origin are now recognised as at greater risk of iron deficiency in the first 3 years of life. Prolonged milk feeding, late weaning and the possibility that there is a greater loss of blood through the intestine in these children are all possible aetiological factors. Asian children are also at greater risk of developing rickets: the peak incidence is in the second and third years of life when they have been changed from artificial formula milk which is enriched with vitamin D to a mixed solid diet and unmodified cows' milk. Older Asian children also show an increased incidence of rickets. There is a complex interaction between the poor ability to synthesise active metabolites of vitamin D when there is limited exposure to the sun, reduced amount of vitamin D in the diet and a further reduction in the amount absorbed associated with the presence of phytate in chapati flour. In Glasgow the 'Stop Rickets' campaign has shown how effective a biochemical screening programme can be.

Iron and vitamin D deficiency also occur in preterm babies.

Prevention of handicap

Antenatal and intrapartum care contribute considerably to the primary prevention of mental or physical handicap in childhood. Secondary prevention of recognisable conditions such as squint, congenital dislocation of the hip, and undescended testes in their early stages can prevent lifelong morbidity.

Developmental surveillance of children at regular intervals may demonstrate that particular children are not developing as quickly as their contemporaries. Potentially reversible conditions may be discovered such as conductive deafness. Even if irreversible conditions such as sensorineural deafness or blindness are revealed, a child can be helped by being directed, early, towards the appropriate form of therapy so that his future development can be facilitated.

Prevention of accidents

The most important cause of death in England and Wales in children between the ages of 1 and 14 years is accidents: roughly half occur as a result of road traffic accidents, and another quarter as a result of accidents in the home. There is increasing publicity about the dangers for children of their riding in the front seats of the car, and there is an increasing campaign to make it compulsory for children to wear seat belts in the back of cars. Many domestic accidents occur because there is inadequate supervision. Children may be left in rooms where there are unguarded fires, or where there are potentially scalding hot fluids within reach of an inquisitive toddler. Drugs, and chemicals such as bleach or weed-killer, are all potentially lethal to children. Some parents need help in appreciating that very young children are not capable of understanding potential danger, and that natural curiosity tends to be a particularly strong impulse. Unfortunately, an accident can occur in a fraction of a second. At the same time parents must not be overprotective and stop their children taking part in appropriate play.

Prevention of psychiatric and emotional disorders

Serious psychiatric diseases in childhood are uncommon. Behavioural and emotional disorders including overactivity, poor impulse control and conflicts over sleep and appetite are much more common; 7% of 3 year olds show some sort of moderate or severe adjustment problem. Behavioural disturbances persist in up to two-thirds of these children at the age of 8 years. The family doctor may be able to spot these sorts of behaviour pattern early and bring them to the attention of other members of the caring professions, who have the relevant skills and the time to deal with them. Social services, health visitors, housing departments and advice bureaux may all need to be involved, in addition to child psychiatrists and psychologists. The material and emotional environment within a family can be improved considerably to the benefit of young children.

Prevention of infectious disease

Classically the control of infectious disease has been based on four principles:

1. Isolation of infected patients from those at risk of the disease.
2. Eradication of factors that transmit the infection.
3. Elimination of infecting organisms.
4. Increasing the resistance of the host.

The isolation of infected patients (quarantine) is a time-honoured way in which disease spread can be limited. Patients in hospital suffering from life-threatening infections are barrier nursed; children suffering from infections such as measles in the community are kept away from school, and anyone who is thought to be suffering from rubella is kept away from pregnant women. The regulations relating to notification are an integral part of the way in which we manage illnesses. A family who suffers from an attack of salmonella food poisoning is kept in effective quarantine until cleared. In addition the notification procedures provide a basis for the compilation of statistics relating to infection. (Table 4.3).

Transmission agents can be identified and controlled. Clean water helped to eliminate the occurrence of typhoid and cholera in this country, and the testing and slaughter of affected cows reduced the incidence of bovine tuberculosis. The correct design and maintenance of water cooling plants will limit the spread of legionella. Scrupu-

Table 4.3 Notifiable diseases (as at 1 October 1988) as defined in the Public Health (Infectious Disease) Regulations 1988

Cholera, plague, relapsing fever, smallpox, typhus

Acute encephalitis

Acute poliomyelitis

Anthrax

Diphtheria

Dysentery (amoebic or bacillary)

Leprosy

Leptospirosis

Malaria

Measles

Meningitis

Meningococcal septicaemia (without meningitis)

Mumps

Ophthalmia neonatorum

Paratyphoid fever

Rabies

Rubella

Scarlet fever

Tetanus

Tuberculosis

Typhoid fever

Viral haemorrhagic fever

Viral hepatitis

Whooping cough

Yellow fever

lous attention to handling body fluids is now thought to be essential in dealing with patients with hepatitis B or with AIDS.

The most dramatic success with any infectious illness has been seen with smallpox: it has been completely eradicated. Similarly there is the potential to raise the herd immunity to measles to such an extent that its prevalence in the community drops to a level that it should never cause outbreaks.

As the fall in the incidence of many infections began before immunisation programmes were instituted, it is clear that this was not solely responsible for the improvement. Proper nutrition, good general hygiene and suitable housing conditions are all important in improving the ability of the host to fight off infection. That we do not have all these factors under our complete control is seen from the fact that there are variations in the occurrence of infections such as scarlet fever. In Utah in the USA there has been a sudden resurgence of rheumatic fever. We do not know if this will cross over to the UK.

IMMUNISATION AGAINST INFECTIOUS DISEASE

Immunisation against particular infectious diseases is only appropriate when lasting immunity is obtained from a single episode of the specific illness. Attempts to manufacture effective influenza vaccine or a vaccine against malaria have been hampered by the regular alteration in the antigenic make-up of the infecting organism. There has been some limited success in producing vaccines against particular strains of *Neisseria meningitidis* and *Streptococcus pneumoniae* but their clinical use is limited. In the UK therefore, there has been remarkably little change to the diseases which are targeted in the childhood immunisation programme. The way in which the injections are spaced has been altered however. There is no universal agreement as to the single best regimen — in the USA four rather than three injections are given in the first year of life, with the first injection being given rather earlier than here. The differences in the final immunity achieved are probably imperceptible and probably much more important to the relative success of any immunisation programme is the take-up rate. In most states in France and the USA, it is more or less compulsory for parents to have their children immunised if they are to be eligible for child benefit or allowed to enter into state school at 5 years. As a result they attain high take-up rates. This is in obvious contrast to this country where there have been instances of the rates falling. This is partly explained on the basis that parents have become increasingly anxious about the possibility of serious side-effects and that there has been a degree of complacency among parents and professionals as the memory of outbreaks of illnesses such as diphtheria and polio become fainter.

There is probably very little prospect of immunisation being made compulsory in this country. Such a law would be distasteful and punish children rather than parents. The main way of improving the uptake rates must be through better education and motivation of parents and professionals.

For a practice to provide a good immunisation service surprisingly little in the way of organisational back-up is required. It is necessary to have an up-to-date register of children under the age of 5 years. This can be maintained manually or on computer. If the practice's paediatric population is served by attached health visitors it is likely that they will be maintaining a good current register of their client group. They may also have the advantage that the health visitor records frequently arrive some months before the general practice records when a child changes registration. A practice may take on itself the load of summoning children to the immunisation clinic or it may rely on the district, and, in the future, the national computer to call for children to attend. Unfortunately all such systems, manual or computer based, are fallible — they depend chiefly on the quality of the information fed in. Children who do not attend must be followed and issued with further invitations. The child's health visitor may wish to follow it up herself. If all else fails the child's notes can be flagged so that the appropriate doctor sees it when the child next attends for whatever reason. The GP's task is further complicated by the fact that there are possibly three or four, or even five, records of the child's immunisation status:

1. The GP record.
2. The Health visitor record.
3. The mother's record.
4. The Family Health Service Authority (FHSA) record.
5. The District or National Computer record.

Some considerable amount of time may be wasted trying to tie all these together but the GP should aim for 95% acceptance rates on his records. This allows for those whose parents are adamantly against immunisation and for a very few who have absolute contraindications.

Table 4.4 shows a typical immunisation schedule.

Contraindications are now much more narrowly defined. There is unfortunately considerable dis-

Table 4.4 Routine immunisation schedule

Vaccine	
1st DTP and oral polio	2 months
2nd DTP and oral polio	3 months
3rd DTP and oral polio	4 months
MMR vaccine	12–18 months
Booster DTP and oral polio (if a child has not had pertussis or MMR vaccine it can be offered now and given at the same time)	4–5 years
Rubella vaccine for girls (the need for this will cease when those children now being given MMR at 1+ reach the age of 10)	10 years onwards
BCG if tuberculin negative	10–14 years
Tetanus toxoid + oral polio	School leaving (15–18 years)

information as to what are and what are not contraindications.

General contraindications

1. Do not immunise during an acute illness (i.e. a fever >38.5°C). Snuffly noses are not a contra-indication, otherwise some children will never be immunised. Taking an antibiotic is not a contra-indication provided the child is afebrile

2. Request specialist advice from your local expert whenever you are concerned or unsure, especially if the child suffers from conditions such as malignancy, haemophilia, is on steroids, or is immunosuppressed (including HIV+). These conditions are rare in most practices, so it is not an admission of defeat to ask!

3. If an earlier injection has produced a severe local or general reaction within 7 days it is safest to ask for specialist advice.

Pertussis

Considerable work has gone into attempts to try and elucidate what are the real contraindications to pertussis vaccination. Suggestions that asthma or a family history of allergy are reasons for not giving pertussis have, like many others, been totally discredited. Contraindications are:

1. A child with a personal history of idiopathic epilepsy, or similar in a very close family member — a parent or sibling.

2. The child has had neurological problems neonatally.

3. The child has an active neurological disorder.

Measles, mumps and rubella

This vaccination was launched in October 1988 in this country, having been used in other countries for some years. When introduced into Australia there was a 10% increase in the uptake rate for all immunisations. It will gradually replace the rubella programme given to girls around their tenth birthday, as it has already replaced the measles injection given between 1 year and 14 months. Contraindications are:

1. It should not be given to immunosuppressed children.

2. It should not be given to a child who has had a serious anaphylactic reaction to egg, kanamycin or neomycin.

A personal or family history of convulsions is not a contraindication. Such children should be encouraged to come as they may be at increased risk of febrile convulsions when they develop the illness.

Some children get a mild measles-like illness about 5–7 days after the injection. Much less commonly there is a salivary gland swelling at the same time. Rubella vaccination is sometimes followed by the development of a mild transient arthralgia and faint rash.

Poliomyelitis

The live, oral drops should not be given to any child who has impaired immunity, or in a household where someone suffers from any form of immunosuppression. The alternative, inactivated Salk injection should be used. Any parent or sibling who has not been immunised should be given vaccine at the same time as any child who is being given the Sabin vaccine.

Additional vaccines

Increasing travel means that there is a frequent need to consider the use of additional vaccines, such as typhoid and cholera. The combination of additional vaccines depends on the exact destination, and up-to-date information should be sought. Illnesses such as typhoid and malaria are quite commonly seen in people returning to the Indian subcontinent — they are unaware that the immunity which they took for granted when they were living in that environment eventually fades. Some parents do not appreciate that their children who have been brought up in the UK have no immunity at all, and are at serious risk.

Whilst these services involve some organisational back-up within a practice, there is a continuing need to provide a service which is personal and user friendly. It takes time to develop good relationships with families, but once these become established the newer proactive services should be seen even amongst the most suspicious of parents as being helpful rather than intrusive.

REFERENCES

General Medical Services of the British Medical Association and the Royal College of General Practitioners 1988 Handbook of preventive care for preschool children, 2nd edn. RCGP Publications, London
Hall D (ed) 1989 Health for all children. Oxford Medical Publications, Oxford
Immunisation against infections diseases 1990 HMSO, London

5. Caring for children in general practice

N. Frazer

The Working Party of the Royal College of General Practitioners (RCGP) in their report 'Healthier children: thinking prevention' quote the earlier recommendations of the controversial Court Report that in the UK a general practioner (GP) is ideally placed to deliver most community-based paediatric services. The document produced by the RCGP goes to some length to demonstrate why a GP should be seen as the overwhelmingly important provider of child health services. The argument is made persuasively, acknowledging the often real criticisms of the opponents of such a view. The evidence of the Royal Commission into the NHS given by the RCGP includes this statement: 'Our main liability is poor care. Our picture of the assets of good general practice must be balanced by the frank recognition that care by some doctors is mediocre and by a minority is of an unacceptably low standard.'

The services provided at present to children would seem to provide an adequate basis for the provision of child health care. Unfortunately it seems that they often fail to deliver what they claim. Reading the reports after events such as the death of an abused child, or the Cleveland Inquiry into Child Sexual Abuse gives an understanding of the way in which the different parts of the services become fragmented and the way in which our failings can irreparably affect the lives of children. Seeing an account of 'the pathology' probably gives a better idea than any description of the theoretical beauty of the body of the services that are provided.

That there is room for improvement in the health of British children cannot be denied. Comparing data demonstrates this: the proportion of British children dying in the first year of life is much greater than in Japan or in Scandinavian countries. The figures from Japan show that they have achieved a remarkable turn around, to the extent that they have overtaken us. In different parts of the UK there are persistent differences. The South of England has a much lower mortality ratio than the North, or Scotland. Similarly in different social classes there have been longstanding differences in mortality: in 1931 twice as many babies died in social class V homes as compared with social class I. The Black Committee report in 1980 stated that a child born to professional parents provided he or she was not socially mobile could expect to spend about five or more years as a living person than a child born in an unsheltered manual household. Even more disturbingly, the same report drew attention to the fact that the infant mortality rate in social class V as compared to social class I had widened to 2.5:1. More recent figures suggest an improvement.

GENERAL PRACTICE STATISTICS

In the UK there are around 32 000 GPs, with an average list size of just over 2000. Each GP is responsible either personally or in conjunction with his partners for the care of the patients on his defined list size 24 hours a day and for 365 days a year. He is the doctor of first contact, and his patients can see him at their own instigation, without referral.

The way a GP organises himself to provide cover is largely, for the time being, up to the individual. He can provide care through rotas within his partnership or with the co-operation of other local doctors. In some parts of the country, commercial deputising services may also be available for a fee for which the doctor is responsible.

It is likely that a GP will be looking after more than one member of a family, and often three and sometimes four generations of the same family. Some doctors feel that this function is so important that they have a policy of only registering whole households rather than individuals. A GP should, through repeated, short contacts over a number of years, develop an understanding of a family, its environment and the variety of personalities within it.

Organisation of the GP's work

A family doctor needs to ensure that he is available continuously, or that he can make arrangements to provide cover when he is not available personally. His services will be required in an emergency, to treat episodic illness and to follow the course of chronic problems. In order to provide services that are convenient for himself and for his patients most doctors now work appointment systems. Whatever system he does operate, he must make certain that it allows sick children to be seen as promptly as possible. To run such a system means that receptionists must be trained not to see themselves as barriers between the patient and the doctor.

Parents do not seek help for all a child's illnesses: 40% of problems are managed within the family or by seeking the advice of a local chemist. Nevertheless in one year, three out of four children below the age of 15 will see their GP, and on average, each will have about four consultations every year with their doctor. In the first year of life a child will be seen about eight times by the doctor, but this includes visits for preventive measures such as immunisation, and developmental surveillance. In one year, 90% of all children under the age of 5 years see their doctor — the figure for the whole population is 67%. Socially deprived families make more use of their GP for the treatment of episodic illness, but, unfortunately, make less use of the preventive services.

The British GP will, on average, have around 2000 consultations with children in any year, amounting to about 40 in a week. This will occupy almost one-third of his time. The commonest reasons for children seeing the doctor are shown in Table 5.1. Referral to a hospital occurs after only a small percentage of consultations: the large majority of episodic illness is managed by GPs. His management depends on the nature of the problem, but after carefully taking a history from the parents, and if possible the child, and after a clinical examination, he is less likely to reach a firm diagnostic label, less likely to prescribe medication and more likely than his hospital colleagues to use simple discussion and reassurance. This is partly a function of the different spectrum of disease that he is seeing but also a function of the fact that he can review a sick child many times over a number of days, or can advise the parents on signs which might suggest that he should be contacted again. In this way he can avoid unnecessary treatment, and help parents to cope with the anxieties of dealing with a sick child. Against this he must feel sure that he is in a position to make a diagnosis early in those less common situations where a child needs urgent attention. Most junior doctors coming into general practice for the first time tend to deal with a problem from a hospital view-point; some continue to investigate unnecessarily, whilst a few begin to feel that what they are seeing is not really illness at all, but 'just a lot of snotty-nosed children'. Unfortunately into this are interspersed the cases of early meningitis, the children with occult urinary tract infections, or the very rare child whose recurrent 'chesty cough' turns out to be cystic fibrosis. In acutely ill young children he must be prepared, therefore, to wait and not give an antibiotic without good clinical grounds, to consider the possibility of the less obvious, and to concern himself with providing evidence that may

Table 5.1 Commonest reasons for children consulting their GP (Court report)

Reason	%
Respiratory disease including asthma	28
Ill-defined symptoms	13
Infectious diseases	11
Skin disease	10
Preventive procedures	10
Accidents	10

prove or disprove any hypothetical diagnosis. There are no safe short-cuts. In more chronic problems he must weigh the evidence for any diagnosis in the light of background features, such as a child's development and growth. Some conditions do not fit simply into the categories of acute or chronic; asthma has both acute and chronic phases. Short-term life-saving decisions need to be made and longer-term problems need to be addressed. Levy's study of children in his practice suggested that in many children the diagnosis of asthma was applied later than it should, as a high proportion of such children had been seen frequently for problems such as recurrent nocturnal cough.

A GP will also need to advise on problems relating to a child's emotional and behavioural life. Just as he needs to acquaint himself with key physical signs that are markers for serious physical illness, he will need to recognise behavioural clues to suggest which child with, for instance, school refusal needs referral for the opinion of a child psychiatrist rather than simple reassurance. A thorough knowledge of developmental norms is vital when making any assessment of the age appropriateness of a child's behaviour.

There are groups of children in most practices who, because of the presence of chronic illness or handicap or other special need, tend to become detached from the normal running of the practice. They may often be referred amongst various departments within the hospital and may be encouraged, particularly in the inner cities, to seek their primary care at the local casualty department where the 'paediatrician' (this is the usual way of referring to the senior house officer on call) will be called down to advise. Whilst this is obviously unsatisfactory for the GP, it should also be seen that this is not in the best interests of the hospital nor most importantly the patients. Once this sort of situation has become established it is difficult for the GP to break it, chiefly because of the difficulty in explaining this to our hospital colleagues.

Quantifying referral rates as a way of measuring the quality of a practice is fraught with difficulty; overall, practices may vary by as much as a factor of 20 times. Referral to a paediatric outpatient clinic occurs in less than 5% of consultations with children. In group practices where one or more partners have a special interest in paediatrics, referral rates are much lower: less than 1% end in referral. However, a practice which has recently set up its own developmental clinic may reasonably expect to use hospital paediatric services more for the first few years while their confidence grows.

THE PRIMARY HEALTH CARE TEAM:

One of the main developments within the NHS since its inception in 1948 has been the integration of and increased co-operation of the various professionals involved in the primary health care team. Curtis Jenkins (1987) has reviewed the way in which the general practice child health services and health visitor services arose historically, separately and randomly in the first half of the century. Repeatedly, it seems that reports have recommended that community child health services be focused in general practice. It is a condemnation of our predecessors that this has still not been achieved. The future depends on the enthusiasm of the present generation of GPs in accepting this responsibility. The introduction of the new 1990 contract gives some limited financial encouragement to GPs to be more active in child health.

Child health services will always need to take into account the autonomy of the different professionals. Each has a separate training and role that should be respected. Health visitors are Registered General Nurses who have undergone further professional training. A health visitor is not actively involved in performing technical procedures, but her role is to prevent ill health in the community. She has been trained to identify most health and social problems, to recognise needs and to mobilise appropriate resources. Although largely identified with their work with the under-fives, health visitors also work with the elderly. She has a statutory requirement to visit every newborn baby at the age of around 10 days. It is to be hoped that she will have met the mother during the antenatal period, and may have already played a part in health education. During the first few weeks and months of a baby's life she will be an invaluable source of advice for the mother on parentcraft, infant feeding, immunisation, and all aspects of a baby's growth and development.

Where GPs have worked with health visitors who are attached to their practice's patients as opposed to patients living within a tightly defined area, they are convinced of the way in which their work is mutually complementary. Face-to-face informal communication, as can only occur where people are working from a shared base, leads to the development of trust and mutual respect. Each member may feel a sense of support from discussion with other team members, and may be alerted to and deal with a family's problems with a more complete understanding of what is the matter. Patients also benefit from consistent handling and advice where members agree on a policy and maintain loyalty to each other.

Unfortunately the traditional authoritarianism of the medical profession has led to a situation where many health visitors are nervous that an attached role is by necessity a subservient one. This ought not to be the case but some doctors do stick to old ways. Sadly the question of attachment is still a real issue: not only with health visitors but also with midwives and district nurses. The decision that community nursing should be based on neighbourhood patches as opposed to the practice-based team seems to be a retrogressive step as far as child health services are concerned.

Home visits

A long-standing feature of British general practice is the home visit. Home visits are now rare in North America, but up to the 1960s about 40–60% of a British GP's time was spent making visits. Nowadays, home visiting rates vary between 10% and 20% and seem to be rather higher in rural areas, and in the North of England. The population is now more mobile; there are more private cars, and many GPs insist on a geographically more defined practice area. One of the contributing factors has been the growing confidence that feverish children do not come to harm, if taken to the doctor's surgery, any more than they might if taken to the local hospital. It might also be explained by the notion that the premises occupied by most GPs are better equipped than they once were. A doctor can make a more efficient use of his time — roughly five people can be seen in

the surgery in the time taken for one home visit, depending on the distance travelled.

Set against this, one of the proudest claims of the traditional family doctor is that of knowing his patients and knowing their homes. A home environment may have a considerable effect on a person's health. Observation of a household may give invaluable information about a family's way of life and their relationships. A home may be untidy, overcrowded and without basic amenities. There may be inappropriate heating; there may be no toys or books. The television set may be left on at all times, even while the doctor attempts to conduct an examination. There may be illness in other family members or in other dependants. A doctor may notice unexpected dangers, and offer appropriate advice. A profusion of books on baby-care may alert the visitor to the probable expectations of the parents and their high level of anxiety. Although a doctor can, if sensitive to this sort of factor, pick up useful information in the surgery from a patient's speech and clothing, and their use of verbal and non-verbal language, a much more impressive amount of information can be gathered in the home.

The consultation and what can be achieved

Dealing with each problem in either the context of the home or the surgery, in normal working hours or out of hours is the normal role of the GP. This traditional, reactive approach is regarded nowadays as being too limited a view of the part a GP

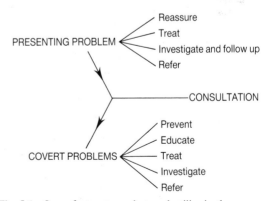

Fig. 5.1 Some factors to explore and utilise in the 6-minute general practice consultation

can play. Increasingly higher expectations within the profession, and by our patients, require that additional functions be fulfilled: these are embodied in the concepts of prevention or the *proactive* approach.

Any improvement in the health of our children necessitates our actively seeking out children to screen for diseases before they cause irreparable morbidity lasting into adult life (e.g. undescended testes, or squint). Equally important but rather less glamorous is the process of maintaining and possibly improving upon the percentage of children we immunise. That the GP, if adequately trained, is the most suitable person to deliver these services is acknowledged in the Court Report, and by the British Paediatric Association and RCGP. There is not yet universal agreement within the profession as to what sort of training doctors should receive, nor is there universal agreement as to what sorts of screening examinations should be performed on children. Since the new contract, each FHSA has been required to maintain a list of doctors approved for payment for carrying out paediatric surveillance.

Within the context of general practice there is even some discussion about the need for setting aside separate sessions dedicated to surveillance. Some doctors feel that they can perform all the necessary tasks in normal, acute surgery time. This means that a GP relies on his ability to pick up abnormalities of development during consultations for intercurrent illness. The statistics relating to the frequency with which children attend may lend some support for this. This form of opportunistic screening for conditions such as high blood pressure in adults seems to work in some well-organised practices. Probably most successful practices make use of a mixed policy; in addition to dedicated sessions, the doctor selects children, such as those suffering from otitis media, to return at a later stage for hearing tests. However most GPs who take the responsibility to offer screening services believe that setting aside separate sessions is in the interests of children and their parents, and benefits the rest of the primary care team. A good clinic that is functioning well is likely to benefit from the presence of a health visitor: high-quality record keeping demands the attention of a good clerical back-up, undistracted by the demands of a busy surgery.

However these services are delivered, they will involve extra work for the practice. Doctors who are not interested in providing these services sometimes point out that there is little financial incentive to take on the extra work: there are studies which suggest that those practices who have a good child-care programme have reduced consultation rates for acute illnesses and have fewer out-of-hours calls. In any event a doctor has the opportunity to perform a number of different tasks when a child is brought to the surgery. One disappointing aspect of the revised GP contract is that a GP may find it more difficult to maintain his income doing child surveillance than if he spends his time on other less important practice activities.

PREVENTING ILLNESS

To argue that illness is preventable does not mean that it can easily be prevented. This is particularly true in primary care paediatrics; many of the factors that are responsible are social and environmental. Parental smoking can have a significant effect on the chances of a child developing frequent respiratory problems. Housing and the family's income have an effect on a child's health in a number of ways. It is more or less impossible for a doctor to affect either of these two factors directly. He can have a significant effect on some factors however.

Accidents

The commonest cause of death in children between the ages of 6 months and 15 is accidents. A third of all deaths in this age group are as a result of accidents. Similarly lifelong disability can ensue after injury in road accidents or after burns. Accidents in the home are disproportionately represented in children under the age of five. Sadly there is an alarming difference between the mortality rate in the lower social classes: five times as many poor children die. This suggests that many deaths might be prevented by providing better accomodation. There is evidence to suggest that health-care workers can help. Studies suggest that parents can be educated to make their children wear seat-belts in cars. The number of accidents can also be reduced by frequent visiting of families in their homes, by giving advice opportunistically and by following up to ensure that potential dangers have been eliminated from the home. Normally this role is performed chiefly by the health visitor, but a GP can offer useful support.

Other environmental factors

Many environmental factors affect the health of children. It is still worrying that so many dwellings do not have sole access to a bath or shower or have no bathing facility at all. About 10% of social class V families do not have sole use of an inside WC. There are more health problems in families living in the upper floors of high-rise buildings. It has now been shown that damp increases the chances of a vulnerable child developing exacerbations of recurrent respiratory illness. Many parents in these circumstances feel undeniably concerned about it as a factor in a child's ill-health. The local environmental health office may also bear witness to the presence of damp and co-existing moulds. Communication with the local housing department is under present circumstances, with their own very limited resources, largely ineffective. Smoking remains one of the few factors that a family doctor can affect. The importance of doing this can be seen from studies suggesting that children brought up in a household where there are smokers are on average shorter. This is in addition to the well-known effect on the number of respiratory infections.

PRACTICE RECORDS

A prerequisite of good general practice is good record keeping. This is particularly true of paediatric practice: not even the most gifted doctor is likely to have total recall for important details like a child's height and weight at different ages. Many GP's notes are still badly disorganised. Most regions now have as one of the basic criteria for aspiring trainers that notes be filed in order with letters tagged separately, and that each patient's notes contain an up-to-date summary. It is unfortunately the case that candidates still fail this rather basic standard.

At their best, notes are clear, legibly written (typed if possible), possibly problem orientated, with separate summary cards The RCGP has produced paediatric cards which can be folded into the existing out-dated Lloyd-George envelope. Some practices use A4 records: these require more storage space and are more expensive for a practice to install and to run. It is to be expected that more records will be kept on computer in the future.

Any practice interested in providing good care for children should be able to measure the height and weight of children. Once measured any figures need to be stored in an appropriate way. Centile charts can be obtained commercially, or the small charts on the RCGP preschool record cards can be used.

Many different ways of attempting to acknowledge the importance of health problems in other members of the family have been used over the years. Keeping these up to date and arranging for any record other than the patient's personal card at the time of a consultation is sometimes a problem. Some GPs file a family's records together and arrange for them all to be pulled together when any member sees the doctor. A family record card is a useful refinement.

A working age–sex register allows a doctor to take the initiative and provide preventive care for

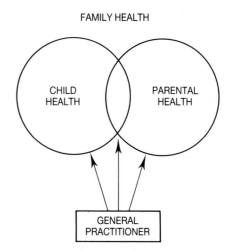

Fig. 5.2 Parents or children may present to doctors, who may influence parental, child or family health.

selected age groups of patients. Disease indexes are particularly useful to arrange for the monitoring of chronic diseases such as asthma, diabetes and thyroid disease. Computers are increasingly replacing manual registers; although few practices have exploited these to their full potential, a willingness to invest time and energy, in addition to the necessary money, should lead to their soon being regarded as an indispensable tool for a modern practice.

PRACTICE REPORTS

Many practices produce a practice report. It is now mandatory to do so. The production of practice reports started long before such an idea was raised. McGuinness in Cheshire was the earliest pioneer. He showed that producing such a report served as a means of identifying the way in which a practice had functioned in the preceding year and the way in which it might be improved in subsequent years. Practice reports so far have been of individual design and content, reflecting the special interests and skills of the GPs who compile them. Most reports — a selection of which can be seen through the Regional Adviser in General Practice's office or at the Royal College of General Practitioners library — collate statistics such as a practice's immunisation rates. Some also produce statistics relating to the outcome of their practice-based developmental clinic, or analyse the outcome of the mothers for whom they provided

antenatal care. Since their production is now a statutory requirement, most FHSAs are committed to offering useful advice. It seems likely that those practices who have the organisational skills and the enthusiasm to produce such statistics are in the best possible position to maintain high levels of care and, if possible, to improve them. The widest discrepancies relate to the uptake rate for measles immunisation. In 1986 the uptake for measles vaccine was 71%, with 22 districts achieving rates of over 85%. It is not known what percentage of GPs attain these figures, but certainly some practices can and some better them. The introduction of MMR from late 1988 may be associated with an increase in the rates by as much as 10%, as was the experience in Sweden and Australia.

For those practices who are keen to explore the possibility of auditing their immunisation rates, or other practice activity, the Practice Activity Analysis sheets devised by the Birmingham Research Unit of the RCGP are a useful starting point. Those practices who are associated to their local, district computerised call and re-call system may be able to obtain their figures direct.

Practices which are interested in proactive or preventive medicine are more likely to be held in respect by their patients. As attitudes and social conditions improve, the expectations of the quality of care may reasonably continue to rise. Those practices which manifest high-quality preventive services whether it relate to immunisation rates, paediatric surveillance or the prompt provision of

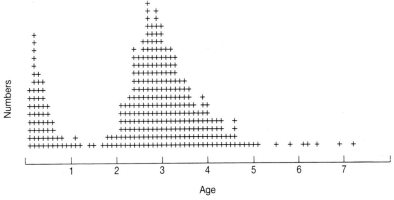

Fig. 5.3 One doctor's personal list profile. As a doctor ages, so the patients on his list tend to be older. Within this practice, the doctor is seeing a relatively high proportion of children and very few elderly people.

appointments and out-of-hours care provide a bulwark of reassurance to their patients. The practice report may reasonably be thought of as a tool for self-audit. That GPs are concerned for the quality of care they offer rather than the financial exploitation of their list size may be a useful indicator to parents about to choose a doctor.

Another way in which a GP may improve the way in which his practice looks after children's health is in the provision of advice leaflets for parents. Morrell developed simple leaflets which, when given to parents, seemed to help their understanding of their child's illness to the extent that they managed the initial stage of minor illness with greater confidence.

ANTENATAL CARE

The unique advantage that the family doctor has over his colleagues is that he will have looked after the mother during the course of her pregnancy. In 1970 over 90% of GPs were involved in antenatal care. During this time, in addition to satisfying the requirements of good technical care, a GP will ensure that he develops a sound understanding of the patient's personality and her needs, and that she becomes well acquainted with the members of the practice team and the way in which the practice works. There should be close liaison in the practice team — most obviously the health visitor and midwife, but also the more sensitive receptionist may be able to play an important role.

In the antenatal period it may be possible for a team to identify those mothers who are at high risk of developing problems after delivery, including postnatal depression. Formal questionnaires are available to screen women antenatally and postnatally, but many GPs prefer to rely on their own informal assessment, having a general discussion with a mother with a few favourite questions that he feels appropriate yet not too intrusive. It appears that once again there are significant social class differences: working class mothers with preschool children are much more likely to become depressed than their middle class counterparts — up to 42% as opposed to 5%. Depression is also much less common in mothers with older children.

Many GPs aim to visit a mother as soon as possible after delivery. This may have little direct clinical benefit, provided that the baby has already been examined by a doctor and the midwife is happy with the mother's condition, but it may still be highly effective. It shows that the doctor is prepared to take time when there is no apparent medical need. This sort of attitude can benefit a mother and help her to gain confidence in her carers.

The technical aspect of antenatal care should not be forgotten. The large majority of women attending a GP for shared care will, by definition, have uncomplicated pregnancies. The GP must be alert to the development of complications such as preeclampsia which are hazardous to the fetus. Congenital rubella still occurs. More attention to educating mothers as to the hazards of alcohol and tobacco use may have lifelong benefits to the health of a child.

General practitioner intrapartum care is now less common. A GP taking on the responsibility of delivering a baby at home or in a GP–obstetric unit may, according to his technical skill, put the baby at risk. The standard of most GP–obstetrics is high, but even the most accomplished GP must be aware of his own technical limitations.

SPECIAL CARE BABIES

An increasing number of babies born either prematurely or at low birthweight for other reasons now survive. Once released from hospital this group have very special needs from their GP. It is likely that the families of these children have witnessed sudden dramatic changes in their baby's condition which have required urgent, 'high-tec' intervention from the neonatal paediatricians. The more intelligent may be liable to overinterpret minor changes in a baby's behaviour, and to misinterpret the 'masterly inactivity' of their GP as a reflection of incompetence. To stop this sort of situation happening a GP should try and become involved early, show that he understands their concerns and be prepared to discuss a child and to refer to the paediatricians at a lower threshold than usual. Progressive attempts can be made to wean parents off their reliance on hospital services. If a GP has some experience of neonatology he may feel confident in doing this: his confidence may also come over to the parents. Where the GP is unhappy about his clinical acumen, early referral will be needed. In the future he should encourage the parents to communicate direct with him rather than the hospital, and attempt to discuss a child with the hospital as often as possible to acquaint himself with any potential management problems.

The bonding that occurs in a neonatal unit may be a two-way process. Just as parents become reliant on the care of the neonatal unit, the staff may find it difficult to let go the families with whom they have shared stressful times. Reactions may be, at times, extremely rewarding. The offer of a first-name relationship with the junior paediatric staff and the very occasional extension of the relationship so that the hospital staff have been known to visit at home 'to see how you're getting on' may be in marked contrast to the role played by many GPs.

Parents will more or less carry on attending hospital outpatients for neonatal follow-up; the frequency depending on the presence of any at-risk factors. Playing an active part may mean that a GP can reduce the need for non-planned attendances at hospital. Discussion with senior paediatric colleagues to obtain adequate advice about the timing and indications for immunisation should mean that the GP feels confident to discuss these issues with the parents and be prepared to immunise these children in the surgery. Immunisation is currently recommended to be carried out at the appropriate and usual postnatal age.

CHILD ABUSE (see Ch. 8)

The GP's role in the management of potential child abuse is complex. Estimates vary, but if 5000 children a year are victims of non-accidental injury a GP will only see a case every 5 years. About 10% of battered children die and another 10% are left with residual brain damage. These statistics hide the many probable children who are subject to less obvious physical, or sexual or emotional abuse.

Abuse tends to occur at times of stress, especially if the parents are unhappy, young or socially isolated. The abusers may be incapable of expressing frustration other than physically. Frequently such parents may have been the subject of abuse in their own childhood. Even prior to their identification as a problem family they frequently fail to keep appointments at the antenatal clinic, with the health visitor, or to attend regularly for immunisation sessions. On the other hand, they may make frequent demands for help on an apparently impulsive basis. They may well be unreasonable and rude. These patients, who are probably making a cry for help, need to be treated with extreme patience.

The GP in conjunction with the other members of the primary health care team, but most particularly the health visitor, is in an ideal position to spot a family at risk or in trouble and to attempt to provide support before abuse happens. A mother or father may feel able to admit to negative feelings towards their child in the course of a consultation with their own doctor in the confidence that he is acting as their agent. At this stage, just unloading their feelings may prevent abuse from occurring. If appropriate, together with the health visitor and social services, he may provide more formal counselling, help with re-housing, and obtaining access to day nursery places.

Once abuse is suspected, the GP should arrange for the child to be taken to a place of safety as soon as possible. Most frequently this is done by arranging admission to hospital through the paediatrician, but in some circumstances he may need to inform the social services direct.

A GP needs to remember that the needs of the child are overriding, and that this duty is more important than all other considerations. Any concern regarding the confidentiality of a consultation with a parent who may or may not be abusing their child should take second place. (If anxious about this the doctor should discuss it with his defence society.) At the same time he should attempt to adopt a non-judgemental attitude to the parents. He may need to deal with his own feelings of distaste and anger as calmly as he possibly can. The family may still need his services to discuss their guilt and recriminations.

Because of the recurrent publicity about these matters there are overriding pressures on those with statutory responsibilities to appear to behave quite rigidly. It may seem to parents and to the GP that social services are over-reacting. Under such circumstances he may be able to counsel parents and console them when they become angry and verbally aggressive.

Most local authorities have developed procedures so that the role of any professional is outlined. Although this sort of procedure is most relevant to those members who have statutory obligations, GPs should acquaint themselves with local advice. In an emergency, when in difficulty he should contact a senior colleague, or a member of his local medical committee for advice.

The recent spate of deaths and the ensuing inquiry reports make harrowing reading. Although not openly criticised as frequently as some of the other professions concerned, it is disturbing to see how commonly the absence of an adequate GP seems to be a factor. The Jasmine Beckford Inquiry report suggests that GPs seeing newly registered patients or registering them as temporary patients, may be at particular risk of missing background clues. Any small child attending as a temporary or as a new patient needs to be assessed, even if in only the broadest terms, for growth and developmental status. GPs should also consider contacting the 'previous' GP when he has any concern about a child he is seeing for the first time.

CHILD SEXUAL ABUSE (see Ch. 8)

Publicity has also drawn attention to the frequency of the sexual abuse of children. The family doctor needs to bear the diagnosis in mind when dealing with children complaining of non-specific abdominal pains, with behaviour disorders or where a child has apparently started to do less well at school without reason. The child may make a disclosure giving cause for concern to the mother, to the teacher, health visitor, or to the doctor. Under these circumstances the GP's role is to take a careful history, and to conduct a brief general examination. A visual inspection only of the genital area may be appropriate, but this should be avoided if there seems the slightest distress on the child's part. The GP should make arrangements normally through the social services so that the child can be examined jointly by the appropriately experienced paediatrician and forensic medical examiner (formerly known as a police surgeon). Forensic exhibits may be important: a child who has been abused in the preceding 72 hours should be asked not to wash or to change clothes until formally examined. It is possible that a GP unused to examining the genitalia of a child may misinterpret his findings, and may destroy invaluable forensic evidence, so the specialist team should be contacted if there is any doubt.

The GP who becomes involved in cases where abuse is an issue needs to be confident that he has made adequate, contemporaneous notes. He should retain a due sense of modesty in interpreting his findings, in that at a later date he may have to justify his remarks in court. It is likely that any child will be examined by more experienced paediatricians, who may be in a better position to discuss the different causes of any injury.

IMMIGRANT FAMILIES

It has been said that between 3% and 4% of the UK population are of New Commonwealth origin. An increasing number of people of Afro-Caribbean or Indian subcontinent origin are black British — about half or more having been born in this country. It is increasingly difficult to talk of these people as a homogeneous group: they represent a wide variety of different countries of origin, of religion, of diet, and social attitude.

Social factors

Most immigrant groups were attracted from developing to developed countries as a cheap labour force. In addition to intrinsic health problems of their own, such as tuberculosis in Asian communities or sickle cell disease in Afro-Caribbean peoples, they frequently acquire some of the less favourable social and environmental conditions found in deprived socioeconomic groups. Poor overcrowded housing and lower paid jobs seem to be common problems. Frequently both parents are working to support the family and, in some families, money is still being sent 'home' to provide for relatives who are living in even worse conditions. The work of Pollak, based on her experience in a South London general practice, shows how the absence of books and toys may result in the understimulation of children and possibly lead to the perpetuation of social class and racial distinctions. The quality of child-care facilities is vitally important to families of low income where both parents are working: no one can be very happy with the present provision. In addition to the problems of deprivation, there is conflicting pressure on adolescents of Asian origin — particularly girls — where there may be a stark contrast between the lifestyles and moral values of their peer group and their parents. Behavioural and emotional problems may occur and their GP needs to be aware of this. Afro-Caribbean adolescents frequently encounter far-reaching educational and employment disadvantages. A GP needs to be aware of the social milieu in which he works and the realities of the lives his patients lead when confronted with someone expessing symptoms.

Figures published by the OPCS relating to 1985 suggest that cultural habits may still be relevant. There are still differences in the proportion of babies born illegitimate in different racial groups. It is not a doctor's concern to decide whether illegitimacy remains a valid concept. However, where there are statistical grounds for relating illegitimacy to lack of financial support to a mother and baby, it would seem that those groups might have greater need of health provision than others.

Intrinsic problems

In addition to the problems of deprivation there are particular medical problems within many immigrant populations. A GP needs to be aware of the possibility of sickle cell disease and its often subtle manifestations. It presents most frequently in children between the ages of 6 months and 2 years — a GP may have the advantage of knowing the mother's sickle status. Similarly in the Cypriot and eastern Mediterranean population there is an increased risk of thalassaemia. Other associations such as that between coeliac disease and people originating in the West of Ireland are much less tight.

The increased prevalence of rickets in Asian children has arisen because of the way their lifestyle has interacted with the environment. Vitamin D metabolism is affected by diet, by sunlight and by skin pigmentation. As a result of the understanding of these complex processes it should now be preventible.

The unique position of the family doctor makes him aware of health problems in the various generations of a family. When he sees their parents or grandparents he may be able to predict the pattern of illness that children are likely to develop in their own adult life. This is true of all sectors of the community: dietary habits in childhood affect the chances of developing ischaemic heart disease, acquiring a smoking habit in adolescence may affect cardiovascular and respiratory disease in later life. The increased incidence of and death rate from diabetes in Asians living in this country should increase the amount of time spent by members of the primary health care team discussing dietary issues with Asian mothers.

SUDDEN INFANT DEATH SYNDROME (SIDS)

Sudden unexpected death in infancy, or cot death is defined 'as the sudden death of any infant or young child, which is unexpected by history and in which a thorough autopsy fails to demonstrate an adequate cause for death'. The incidence in the UK is about 1 in 500 live births. SIDS affect all social classes, but like all postneonatal deaths are more common in the lower social classes. Because of changes in the pattern of other components of postneonatal mortality SIDS are a rising percentage of the total. The number of children dying as a result of congenital abnormalities has remained constant but the number who die as a result of well-defined infectious illnesses has fallen. As there has been a fall in postneonatal mortality, there is an apparent increase in the proportion, if not the real numbers, of children dying as a result of SIDS. The average family doctor is likely, during the course of his professional life-time, to deal with this problem only once in every 5–10 years.

The definition of the disorder underlines the difficulty in deciding upon its aetiology. Some of the many and varied suggestions as to its cause (not listed in any order of probability) are:

1. Congenital cardiovascular abnormality.
2. Disorders of breathing.
3. Overwhelming viral infection.
4. Congenital enzyme deficiency.
5. Disorders of temperature control.
6. Gastro-oesophageal reflux.
7. Sleeping position.
8. Suffocation (including that done deliberately by parents).

It is more or less certain that there is not one underlying cause that can account for all events, and it is probable that in many instances a number of factors may play a part.

Statistically a number of studies have suggested some risk factors that may underlie cot deaths (Table 5.2), although these give little help in understanding the aetiology of the condition. There is an increased risk associated with prematurity, and a slightly increased risk in a family which has already lost a child with SIDS (this rises in subsequent children by only about 1%). Epidemiological factors can indicate about half of all babies who will die as a result of cot death. About 15% of all births in these studies fell into their high-risk groups. So as a test for a doctor dealing with any particular child they are of low sensitivity and low specificity.

Among the very many babies and young children who present to a GP with mild, non-specific illnesses, there may be one or two who are in the early stages of a serious illness. The GP is obviously concerned to be sure that he does not miss a potentially extremely ill child. As he assesses the child he will take into account the generalised background problems that he is aware of in the family. He will also need to look at a child to make some assessment of whether there are any obvious indicators of serious illness. Unless he can satisfy himself that there are convincing signs or symptoms of a localised, defined illness he may wish to consider referral. A baby whose behaviour displays sinister features such as apathy, listlessness, pallor, floppiness or poor feeding should be assessed very carefully. The combination of dopiness and irritability is an especially strong indicator for referral to a paediatrician. The difficulty faced by GPs is illustrated by the assertion made by one of the

Table 5.2 Epidemiological factors associated with SIDS

Maternal factors	Young mothers, low social class
	Close spacing between pregnancies
	Smoking
	Artifical feeding
Factors in the baby	Low birthweight
	Male
	Winter months
	Age 2–4 months

most distinguished professors of paediatrics since the war, that GPs should arrange for all first-born baby boys brought to the doctor between the ages of 3 and 6 months to be admitted when presenting with symptoms in the winter months. This certainly overstates the case, would add a significant workload to the hospital and probably overestimates the capabilities of our paediatric colleagues.

Prevention of cot death

Without a clear idea as to what causes cot deaths, it is impossible to take steps which can be relied upon to prevent them. However, there are two ways in which investigators have tried to reduce their frequency. The study performed in Sheffield involved targeting those groups which had already been identified as being at greater risk of SIDS. This higher risk category of baby was provided with more intensive health visitor support than a control group, and it appeared that this reduced their chances of dying as a result of cot death. This particular study, however, was not large enough to show a statistically significant difference.

The other main attempt to reduce the frequency of SIDS has been to pay particular attention to groups of babies who might, as individuals, be thought of as being at special risk. One of the most attractive theories to explain SIDS has been the idea that children suffering from cot death might be at risk because of prolonged episodes of apnoea. It has been recorded that normal babies may stop breathing for periods of about 15 seconds. It was felt that babies who stopped breathing spontaneously for 30 seconds or more might be about to die ('near-miss' SIDS). Viral infections may lengthen the duration of apnoeic episodes. Some babies have recurrent apnoeic or cyanotic episodes, and some of them appear to be at higher risk of death. Unfortunately, this has not turned out to be useful. In the USA, out of 400 consecutive cot death victims, only 1.5% had a medically recorded apnoeic episode, and in only another 7.5% had their parents had a recollection of some sort of appropriate event.

On the basis of the hypothesis that disordered respiration was responsible for some deaths, it was decided to try providing apnoea alarms to babies who were thought to be at special risk. Some parents have felt strongly reassured by using this sort of device, especially when they have found that their baby has stopped breathing and recovered when stimulated. There is, however, the considerable drawback that the alarms are not mechanically perfect, and that there are frequent false-positive and false-negative signals — any movement a baby makes may be misinterpreted as a breathing movement. Obstructive apnoea, where a baby continues to make respiratory movements in the presence of upper airways obstruction, is also not detected.

Apnoea monitors seem to make many parents more anxious. In some situations babies have died despite having had their apnoeic episode detected and attempts made to resuscitate them.

Optimism that apnoeic monitors might be a significant advance has been replaced with a rather more cautious view of their role, so that they are rarely used now. Sometimes a family who have already lost a child as a result of SIDS may request a monitor. Oximetry, which measures continuously the oxygen saturation of the blood, may prove to be a better method of monitoring, but is at present very expensive.

Dealing with SIDS

The family doctor's role in the events that ensue after a cot death is as important and possibly easier to prepare for. It is likely that parents in their desperate attempts to resuscitate their baby will take him to hospital rather than wait for the doctor to call. The GP will probably hear the news from the hospital, and should be prepared to visit the family in their home as soon as possible. The bereavement process is likely to be intense and protracted. In some areas there are teams set up who, in addition to providing counselling skills, will provide practical help regarding funeral arrangements and coroners courts. The fact that the police need to be involved at some stage in any unexpected death will come as a shock to grief-stricken parents. Unfortunately as part of the natural process of mourning parents will often experience a very strong feeling of guilt: one mother wrote of her repeated recall of the incident, with the true

sequence only altered by her taking note of the baby's cry in the night so that she was able, in her dreams, to pick him up and save him. The police and the local newspaper may comment in such a way that they actively increase the parents' sense of guilt.

We are all now rather more aware of the stages of mourning: that anger is an integral part of mourning is now widely understood. In the 1980s however we have little experience of death in childhood; this accentuates the difficulties for parents and for their doctors. The parents may feel they have failed their child and the doctor may feel that he has failed the parents. Families may direct anger towards the doctor if they think that he has let them down. The incidence of symptoms in the week before has been compared in babies who died and in controls: symptoms such as cough, diarrhoea and vomiting were all slightly more common, but these symptoms are so non-specific as to be useless to the doctor. Unfortunately they may have led to the parents having requested advice from the doctor whose reassurances seem inappropriate in the light of subsequent events. Paediatric staff may have wittingly or not added to their sense of grievance. Under these sort of circumstances it is likely that the parents will wish to see another doctor in the future. Meanwhile the doctor needs to control his own feelings, and provide support to the family as long as they require it.

Parents will need to ask questions repeatedly. They may want to know whether anything was found at the autopsy, whether the baby felt pain, whether he choked or overheated. They may ask whether factors such as laying him on a particular surface may have caused it, whether breastfeeding may have helped and what can be done in the future to prevent a recurrence in other children.

Self-help groups may be invaluable. The Foundation for the Study of Infant Deaths produces leaflets for parents and professionals that are excellent. Again, the special advantage of the family doctor is that of continuity. Of all the professionals involved in a mother's life during the course of her pregnancy and then the birth and tragic death of her child, the GP is the person who is most likely to be involved in the next pregnancy, birth and childhood. If he has supported the parents through the events of a cot death, he can be of tremendous help to them in subsequent times.

REFERENCES

Curtis Jenkins G 1987 Child health in general practice. In: Macfarlane J A (ed) Progress in child health, vol 3. Churchill Livingstone, Edinburgh
Working Party of the Royal College of General Practitioners 1982

Healthier children — thinking prevention. Royal College of General Practitioners, London

FURTHER READING

Investing in the future: child health ten years after the Court report 1987 National Children's Bureau, London
Hall D (ed) 1989 Health for all children. Oxford Medical Publications, Oxford
Milner A D 1987 Apnoea monitors and SIDS. In: RCGP year book 1987. RCGP Publications, London

6. Child health care in the community

M. Miles

Parents, or others acting as parents, provide the greater part of health care for children. Statutory and voluntary services offer resources which are designated to support parents in this role. The relationship between professionals and parents should be one of partnership rather than supervision, if the parents are to be able to make the best use of the services available.

DEVELOPMENT OF THE CHILD HEALTH SERVICE

The general practitioner service evolved in the second half of the nineteenth century following increased specialisation of the hospital service. Both these services responded to patient demand and were mainly concerned with the treatment of illness. Preventive services began when at the end of the nineteenth century the first training course for health visitors was established. School attendance became compulsory in 1870 and this exposed the extent of physical ill health among children. School doctors were rapidly appointed during the next few years and, subsequently, dentists as well.

A major step forward was taken in 1918 with the Maternity and Child Welfare Act which encouraged the development of health services based at welfare centres. Child guidance clinics were established with the aim of preventing emotional and behavioural difficulties; these services blossomed in the 1920s and 1930s, and the 1940s saw the emergence of the newly named school health service.

The National Health Service Act 1946 led to the establishment of the NHS in 1948 with the inten-tion to provide free, comprehensive health services for everyone. Unfortunately, it consolidated a tripartite structure of GP, hospital specialist and local health authority services. Within the latter, health services for children under five were administered separately from the education authority's school health service. In 1974, with the first NHS reorganisation, the services were brought together, incorporated into the NHS, and all became the responsibility of the health authority. However, the opportunity to establish a single comprehensive child health service was not taken and preventive child health care remained separate from therapeutic care. The Brotherston Report (1973) relating to Scotland and the Court Report (1976) relating to England and Wales considered child health services and both recommended the provision of a single child health service within which the delivery of preventive and curative health care would be integrated at primary and secondary care level. The Court Report stressed the need for greater emphasis on prevention and deplored the distinction made between treatment and prevention which was potentially confusing for parents seeking a combination of both. Regrettably, to date, the recommendations have not been implemented and the service remains fragmented. GPs undertake the larger part of treatment for children and a varying amount of preventive care. The hospital service provides specialist secondary care which may be delivered both within and outside of hospital. The community child health service contributes to both primary and secondary health care and is responsible for most preventive care, including the school health service.

WHAT IS PREVENTION?

Prevention occurs at primary, secondary or tertiary level. For discussion see Chapter 4.

The artificiality of separating prevention from treatment is obvious. However, since the community child health service is predominately concerned with prevention, its definition serves to demonstrate both the extent and importance of that service.

CHILD HEALTH SURVEILLANCE

The health authority is responsible for ensuring that an appropriate surveillance programme is offered to all children and that it is monitored effectively. The Court Report identified five activities to be undertaken by health professionals engaged in the delivery of a surveillance programme. They are as follows:

1. Oversight of health and physical growth of *all* children.
2. Monitoring the developmental progress of *all* children.
3. Providing advice and support to parents and, when necessary, arranging treatment or referral of the child.
4. Providing a programme of effective infectious disease prophylaxis.
5. Participation in health education and training in parenthood.

They are as relevant today as when described over a decade ago and define the aims of the community child health service in relation to surveillance precisely. From these aims specific objectives for the service can be designed whereby it can be seen whether the desired outcome has been achieved or not. The objectives would need to be reviewed and revised at regular intervals to ensure that they reflect the changing needs of the children concerned. The emphasis on the content of the health surveillance changes as the child gets older and can be conveniently considered for the preschool child and school child separately.

PRESCHOOL SERVICE

For most children, preschool surveillance is undertaken in child health clinics organised by the child health services.

During this period of a child's life specific physical and sensory abnormalities such as congenital dislocation of the hip, undescended testes, congenital heart lesions, growth disorders, visual and hearing defects should be identified.

In order to meet the needs of children under the age of 5 years, the 1981 Education Act places a duty on the health authority to bring to the attention of the local education authority any child who has, or is likely to have, special educational needs. It must first inform the parents of the concern. A surveillance programme should therefore include oversight of developmental progress including the development of language and play. Whether this is best achieved by application of routine developmental screening tests is debatable since many of the screening procedures in current use have not been adequately researched and would not meet the criteria usually applied to screening programmes. Their predictive value is unsatisfactory since many children who fail them eventually make normal progress and some who pass are found to have problems at a later date. Most serious impairments are usually identified by anticipation, the child being closely reviewed following neurological insult, or by parents or other caregivers. A view is emerging that developmental progress is usually best monitored by ensuring that all health professionals involved in the process have good understanding of child development and are thus able to respond appropriately to parents or caregivers expressing concern about a child's development. A more selective approach could be reserved for families where the parents are unable or unwilling to identify developmental problems. If consideration of developmental progress is included in all contacts with children rather than limiting it to routine checks, the danger of it becoming a 'box ticking' exercise is avoided. A pass-or-fail approach should be discontinued and more time devoted to listening to parents and discussing with them their child's performance and encouraging the development of observation skills.

The content and timing of surveillance programmes vary considerably from district to district. Recommendations for future practice have been made following a review of the subject by a working party comprised of representatives from the British Medical Association, the Royal College of General Practitioners, the Health Visitors Association, the Royal College of Nursing, and the British Paediatric Association.

Surveillance encompasses much more than just screening and a high standard should be maintained to ensure the appropriate delivery of advice and intervention at an early age. Each district should take account of local factors and tailor its surveillance programme, so that the needs of children to whom it is being delivered are met (Hall 1989).

Delivery of preschool surveillance

Health visitors and doctors work together to ensure that effective surveillance takes place. In many districts a major part of the programme is undertaken by health visitors; the community child health doctor being responsible for examination of babies around 6 weeks of age and selectively thereafter. Increasingly, general practitioners are undertaking surveillance of health and development and are ideally placed to do so, since they can integrate prevention and treatment. The introduction of the 1990 contract for general practitioners, whereby suitably trained GPs can offer a child health surveillence programme in accordance with that offered by the health authority or board, should result in an acceleration of this process.

At the same time, the parental contribution to surveillance should be acknowledged, as they are often the first to recognise a problem or disability. Their observations are invaluable and can be encouraged by the use of checklists; a highly successful hearing checklist has been devised by McCormick* and has proved to be reliable.

THE SCHOOL HEALTH SERVICE

Health surveillance for schoolchildren is undertaken by the school health service. In many

* Hints for Parents by Barry McCormick. Children's Hearing Centre, General Hospital, Nottingham

districts this service relates specifically to children of primary school age and older, the children under five receiving the preschool service even if attending a nursery school.

Background and objectives

The school health service was founded in 1907 and at that time was chiefly concerned with the identification and correction of physical ill health. The years since then have seen the development of educational medicine which is defined as 'the study and practice of child health and paediatrics in relation to the processes of learning'. The Court Report goes on to say that 'it requires an understanding of child development, the educational environment, the child's response to schooling, the disorders which interfere with a child's capacity to learn, and the special needs of the handicapped. Its practitioners need to work cooperatively with teachers, psychologists and others who may be involved with the child and to understand the influences of family and social environment.' Five objectives were listed which remain totally relevant to current needs.

1. To promote the understanding and practice of child health and paediatrics in relation to the process of learning.

2. To provide a continuing service of health surveillance and medical protection throughout the years of childhood and adolescence.

3. To recognise and ensure the proper management of what may broadly be described as medical, surgical and neurodevelopmental disorders insofar as they may influence, directly or indirectly, the child's learning and social development, particularly in school but also at home.

4. To ensure that parents and teachers are aware of the presence of such disorders and of their significance for the child's education and care.

5. To give advice and services to the local education authority as required in the Education Act and NHS Reorganisation Act.

The school health service is available to all children attending state schools, in some districts independent schools are similarly served. Although all children have access to primary health care from their GPs, it is not possible for all family doctors to carry this service into the school setting. Each school needs to relate to a single doctor who has adequate time and the necessary skills to be able to consider the health and development of children in the context of education. The emphasis is on prevention and the service must meet the needs of the children, their parents and the school staff. The school doctor is well placed to collaborate with GPs to provide an integrated service.

Service patterns

The pattern of health surveillance delivered in schools is variable. In most primary schools all children are offered a school entry medical examination around the age of 5 years. This examination is not compulsory. In some districts, where an efficient preschool surveillance programme has been established, there is a move towards selective medical examinations at this age; selection depending upon the needs of the individual children. In any case, subsequent examinations are best performed on a selective basis including a request from the school nurse, parents, the child or other agencies including the school.

Regular health interviews are undertaken by the school nurse and questionnaires may provide a useful way of monitoring health progress and generating specific health input.

The school health surveillance programme should ensure that the hearing of all children is screened on entry to primary school. Further testing should be related to the needs of individual children with special reference to those with learning or behavioural difficulties or those for whom there is no record of previous testing.

Vision screening also takes place at school entry and thereafter at regular intervals. Since defects of colour vision may affect career planning, screening is best performed on entry to secondary school to take account of this. There is debate about the value of routine screening of near vision, but it should be included in the assessment of any child if a visual difficulty is suspected.

School health surveillance also includes the monitoring of growth and ensuring the completion of immunisation programmes.

Health education

The school health team is available to make a contribution to health education either by direct contact with individual children or by participation in health education programmes included in the school curriculum. The need to develop effective programmes involving both the health and educational authorities is self-evident when consideration is given to the problems of tobacco, alcohol, solvent and other drug abuse which affect children. Prevention is an objective which has not yet been achieved. One hopes that some of the initiatives being introduced will have good results.

Children with special needs

When the special educational needs of a child aged 5 years or more are assessed under the 1981 Education Act, the local education authority must seek medical advice about that child. The advice is sought via the doctor designated by the health authority who is responsible for coordinating all relevant medical information including that provided by the school doctor. The school nurse also contributes information and advice relevant to the assessment.

As the integration of handicapped children into ordinary schools progresses, the school health team has an important contribution to make. Members of the school staff need adequate information, advice and support about health problems if the educational needs of the children are to be met.

Service delivery

The delivery of a health service in schools is most efficiently and effectively achieved when all schools, whether primary, secondary or special, have a named school doctor and nurse who work closely together as a school health team. The doctor should be appropriately trained in educational medicine and in an ordinary school is usually a community child health doctor, but may be a GP working in the community child health service.

Much of the routine surveillance is undertaken by the school nurse who is the key member of the team.

Children with more severe handicaps usually attend special schools where the school doctor may be a senior clinical medical officer or a consultant paediatrician with a special interest in community child health.

All school health teams should be able to respond promptly to health matters affecting education whether the concern is expressed by children, their parents or their teachers.

OTHER ASPECTS OF SPECIALIST CARE

In addition to the school health service, a wide range of other specialist and secondary health care is provided by senior clinical medical officers and consultant paediatricians working in the community child health service. The doctors concerned may operate from a community or hospital setting since old physical boundaries are fast disappearing. Sometimes they work as members of a child development team or district handicap team contributing, with other professionals, to the assessment and management of children with overt or suspected handicaps. Unfortunately, so far only two-thirds of districts have such a team. Many teams contain doctors with a special interest in audiology or social paediatrics or other aspects of child health.

Audiology

In most districts the community child health service provides an audiology service whereby senior child health doctors undertake further assessment of children identified by hearing screening programmes.

Up to 25% of preschool children have episodes of conductive hearing loss, usually due to secretory otitis media. The progress of these children can be monitored by this service and the need for further intervention evaluated. Although the effect of this condition on the development of speech, learning and behaviour is still unclear, it can adversely affect them all, particularly in the presence of other disabilities. There are some children who are at risk of developing severe conductive problems; they include children with cleft palate, Down's syndrome, Turner's syndrome and facial malformation syndrome. By working in association with

district otolaryngological colleagues, an effective service can be delivered whereby appropriate treatment for these children is ensured. The oversight of children with sensorineural hearing loss is usually maintained by an audiological physician.

Social paediatrics

The Adoption Agencies Regulations 1983 require the appointment of a medical adviser to the agency's adoption panel. The 1988 DHSS document, *Working Together* — a guide to arrangements for interagency co-operation for the protection of children from abuse — recommends that each health authority should identify a doctor to coordinate the provision of advice to social services departments.

INFORMATION COLLECTION AND RECORDS

Since the intention of the community child health service is to reach all children for whom the health authority is responsible, there has to be a system whereby the service is monitored to ensure that the aim is achieved. Information is collected centrally in order to assess the outcome of service programmes and to assist in the future planning of the service.

Supporters of a computerised information system, such as the Child Health System which was produced within the NHS and designed by the Child Health Computing Committee, would claim that its use should enhance the performance of the service. Certainly, the use of a nationally agreed system should ensure the transmission of information from one district to another. However, there is concern that such a system lacks flexibility and it does not allow interrogation at the point when a child is seen.

Since 1 April 1988, information relating to immunisation and child health surveillance programmes has been collected under the terms of the Körner Committee's Fifth Report (Körner 1985). This should greatly assist the evaluation of services.

Child health care is shared between parents and many different professionals, consequently information is not always readily available when required, and is frequently difficult to locate for children from socially mobile groups. There is, therefore, a strong case to be made for the identification of a record card, for national use, which can be held by parents or caregivers. The record would hold information relating to surveillance, illnesses and accidents and could be added to by parents and professionals. There is considerable debate about this proposal and lack of agreement about how much additional health information should be recorded elsewhere and by whom. However, there is widely held support for the principle, and the use of such a record was recommended in the National Children's Bureau report *Investing in the Future* (1987). Hopefully progress will soon be made on this subject.

SERVICE MANAGEMENT

The Griffiths NHS Management Inquiry Report was published in 1983. It proposed a radical programme intended to promote a stronger management process which was seen by the professionals concerned as a threat to clinical freedom. The stated aim was to move from consensus as a management style to the establishment of general management which would bring together the organisation, planning responsibility, implementation and control of performance. Thus responsibility would be pushed to the point where action could be taken. The general manager is accountable to the health authority at district and regional levels and the various unit managers to the district general manager.

The restructuring of management provided an opportunity to integrate the child health services delivered by the hospital and the community within one district unit of children's services. However, this opportunity has rarely been taken and in many districts children's health services are fragmented into at least two units. It follows therefore that the provision of services becomes the responsibility of more than one unit manager. In most districts the community child health service is managed within the same unit as the health visiting service, along with other community services directed at other age groups.

The community unit manager is responsible for the delivery of the community child health service and advises the district management group and health authority who, together with the regional health authority, has ultimate responsibility for the planning of child health services. Each district in England and Wales has a Joint Care Planning Team (JCPT) which identifies gaps in provision relating to community care including children and families with special needs. The JCPT can recommend projects which, if locally approved by the health and social services authorities, can be funded from a special fund allocated by the Department of Health to regional authorities. Subsequent long-term funding may be accepted by the health or social services authority.

Specialists in community medicine contribute to the planning and monitoring of child health services, taking account of epidemiological, social and other factors.

The clinical management of the community child health service varies from district to district. Each year sees the appointment of more consultant paediatricians with a special interest in community child health, ensuring that the service is consultant led. In other districts senior clinical medical officers co-ordinate the service. The budget for the service may be held by a clinician but more usually by a service manager.

PEOPLE IN THE COMMUNITY CHILD HEALTH SERVICE

There is now general agreement that every district should have a consultant-led community child health service. Many consultant community paediatricians have a special interest in learning, language or motor disorders or the problems presented by children who have been abused or seek permanent substitute families. Their work lies mainly outside hospital but many contribute to hospital-based services, thus promoting the integration of child health services.

Senior clinical medical officers provide secondary care in many different ways.

Clinical medical officers usually provide primary care delivered through child health clinics and in schools.

Until recently there was no nationally recognised training programme for doctors working in community child health. Currently posts are being identified and approved to provide appropriate higher specialist training.

The *health visitor* is a nurse who usually has obstetric training and has completed one of several courses which lead to registration as a health visitor by the UK Central Council for Nursing, Midwifery and Health Visiting. Health visitors are highly trained and have the advantage of working both in a clinic or practice setting and the child's home. Their skills are extensive and positively directed to the promotion of health and the prevention of mental, physical and social ill health. They do not undertake technical nursing procedures.

The *school nurse* is the key health professional in the school setting and is able to maintain contact with children, their parents and their teachers. The integration of handicapped children into ordinary schools has widened the role of the school nurse, especially when the children have specific health problems.

The *community dental service* provides for the routine examination of children's teeth and subsequent treatment at community clinics if required. During the decade 1973–83 the proportion of 5 year olds with no dental decay rose from less than 30% to 52% and for 12 year olds from 8% to 21%. Reasons for these improvements include a greater public awareness of the need to care for teeth, generated by health education campaigns, and the use of fluoride in water and toothpaste. Changes in dietary habits have also made an important contribution.

An *education social worker*, previously known as an education welfare officer, is a trained social worker employed by the local education authority. The education social work service is particularly concerned with the promotion of school attendance. Since school absence has many causes the education social worker is likely to be involved in a wide range of welfare issues and to be called upon to exercise broadly based, social work skills. It is only in a minority of cases that work with children and their parents results in court proceedings; the emphasis is rightly on early preventive work.

SPECIAL ISSUES

Many districts have a client group faced with particular difficulties which present a challenge to the community child health service.

Clinic non-attenders

These are not confined to any one social class although the reason for associated poor uptake of services may vary from one client group to another. Non-attendance is a problem of rural areas as well as inner city ones.

Homelessness

This is a social problem but it exposes the children involved to increased health risks and makes the co-ordination and delivery of a preventive service more difficult. There is no generally accepted policy as to how services should be made available to them. Some districts offer the same facilities to non-residents as residents. In other districts the view is taken that the responsibility for surveillance cover rests with the authority whose care they have temporarily left. Consequently, the children, often severely disadvantaged, receive only a minimal input.

Accidents

Accidents are still the most common cause of death among children over the age of 1 year. Much progress has been made through legislation to improve the situation, although direct approaches to improve home safety have been disappointing. Most injured children present at accident and emergency departments or their GP's surgeries, but the community child health service has an important role to play both in the prevention of accidents and the co-ordination of the follow-up of these children.

CHILD HEALTH IN ETHNIC MINORITIES

Over the past four decades Britain has become a multiracial society. Since surveillance involves whole populations, the health needs of children from ethnic minority groups must be met without discrimination. Professionals working with immigrant families must familiarise themselves with the different pattern of lifestyle presented. They may find that Asian women communicate through their husbands; the women may become isolated and sometimes depressed. Community services need to make special provision in order to surmount language barriers. Advice and treatment must be offered in such a way as to take account of the context in which they will be acted upon.

Frequently there is confusion relating to the records of Asian and Muslim children. The absence of a surname and lack of understanding about titles accorded to women generate unnecessary problems, since, with consideration, the father's family name can be used to identify members of the same family.

There are some specific health and developmental items that warrent identification and can be addressed by the community health staff.

Growth

Many Asian and Chinese babies are smaller at birth than white and Afro-Caribbean babies. Similarly, older children are often lighter and shorter than their peers. To avoid generating unnecessary monitoring of growth, and thereby anxiety, these facts need to be borne in mind.

Diet

Dietary habits have resulted in deficiencies of iron and vitamin D intake and the development of anaemia and rickets. The health visitor is well placed to help in the reduction of these particular problems and to promote more satisfactory practice generally, including breast feeding, either by direct contact or through the mother and baby or toddler groups which she organises.

Infection

Asians are susceptible to tuberculosis and there is a higher incidence of infection in immigrants from that continent. Newly arrived Asian children should be identified and vaccinated if they have a negative skin test. Older members of such families may have undetected tuberculosis. Thus, when non-immune children from the UK make a visit to relatives in Asia they may be at particular risk and should be protected before travelling.

Infestation

Intestinal infestation occurs in children coming from Asia and the West Indies either for the first time or on return from holiday. Health visitors and school nurses can promote better understanding of the health risks involved and assist in the early identification of infestation when it is likely to occur.

Development

Many children from ethnic minorities live in poor households which have inadequate play space and play material. Some West Indian children have been reported to receive care from many different people, including relatives and minders, and may lack a clear mother or father figure. They may be encouraged to grow up quickly and there is sometimes no tradition of play between mother and child during early years. These practices may predispose to the development of language and behavioural problems; professionals delivering surveillance programmes must offer appropriate advice and support. These cultural patterns are modifying; play material can be provided by toy libraries while mother and toddler groups encourage play activities. Day nursery or play group attendance may be indicated and can be particularly beneficial to the child if the mother's involvement is also encouraged.

By contrast, Asian mothers are very close to their children, often to the point of limiting play because they are overprotective. However, there may still be a lack of toys in the home and the health visitor and doctor are faced with the problem already described.

Health education and advice

Cultural attitudes within Asian and Muslim families do not encourage the discussion of sexual matters. School programmes relating to sex education and sexual health, complemented by advice from the school health service, are particularly important for these teenagers who take part with parental consent.

Haemoglobinopathies occur more commonly in the children of immigrants from the West Indies,

Cyprus and Asia. Since these conditions are genetically determined, the school health service could encourage the identification of carriers so that genetic counselling can be offered. In the past, screening procedures have proved unpopular but could be considered and operated in a caring sensitive manner set in the context of health education.

REFERENCES

Brotherston Report 1973 Towards an integrated child health service. Chairman JHF Brotherston. HMSO, Edinburgh
Court Report 1967 Fit for the future: the report of the Committee on Child Health Services. Chairman SDM Court. HMSO, London
Hall D 1989 A programme for child health surveillance. Oxford University Press, Oxford.
Körner E 1985 Fifth report of the Steering Group for Health Services Information. HMSO, London
National Children's Bureau 1987 Investing in the future: child health ten years after the court report. Chairman P Graham. National Children's Bureau, London

FURTHER READING

Black J 1987 The new paediatrics: child health in ethnic minorities. British Medical Journal, London
British Paediatric Association 1987 Report on the school health services. BPA, London
de Lobo E H 1978 Children of immigrants to Britain. Hodder and Stoughton, London

7. Adoption and children in care

M. Miles

All children benefit from living in a family which is able to provide care and security. Unfortunately, for a variety of reasons, some natural parents are either unable to provide appropriate care for their children or do not wish to do so. Under these circumstances, while the child's future is being decided, there is a danger that the child will be exposed to repeated changes of caregiver. Care fragmented in this way can adversely affect all aspects of the child's development and should be avoided by provision of a permanent family placement at the earliest opportunity. Adoption is likely to be the best way of ensuring both security and commitment, especially for young children and babies.

ADOPTION

From early times people have cared for children who were not born to them. Legal adoption as it is known today only began in this century, even though it was known in Roman times, and reflects western traditions.

Definition

Adoption transfers the legal rights and duties of the natural parent to the adopters. It is legally permanent and irrevocable. The child takes the adopters' surname and inherits in the same way as a natural child.

Until relatively recently, adoption was seen as a solution to the problems of illegitimacy on the one hand and infertility on the other. When many healthy babies were available for adoption, adopters could select the child they wanted for reasons that would not always be acceptable today. Now the needs of the child are carefully assessed and a family has to be able to meet them before placement can take place.

Adoption practice

A child is always placed for adoption by an agency, unless a close relative wishes to adopt or the child comes from abroad. There are many adoption agencies: most are based in local authority social services departments; others are voluntary agencies such as Barnardo's and National Children's Home.

In order to adopt, applicants have to be at least 21 years old. There is no legal upper limit but most agencies set their own limits depending on the age and needs of the child concerned. A single person can adopt, married couples adopt jointly and a natural parent can adopt his or her own child.

An application for an adoption order is made to a court. Before the order can be made, the court has to be satisfied that the parent or parents understand and agree to adoption. When agreement is not forthcoming, the court can dispense with that agreement; usually, this is in cases of child abuse. A mother cannot agree to adoption before her baby is 6 weeks old.

Once an adoption order is granted, a copy of the entry in the Adoption Register is issued to replace the original birth certificate, access to which can be obtained by an adopted child once he reaches the age of 18 years.

Adoption trends

In England and Wales, adoptions were at their

maximum of approximately 25 000 annually in the late 1960s. Babies less than 1 year of age, who were placed with non-relatives, accounted for 75% of these. Since then the number of adoptions has declined. In particular, the number of healthy babies available for adoption has fallen. This drop is due to several factors — more efficient contraception, access to abortion, and better support for single parents.

In the early 1970s, step-parent adoption was popular and by 1974 accounted for over 60% of all adoptions. This practice is less favoured now, but still represents about 50% of adoptions.

By 1984, the total number of adoptions for that year had fallen to 8648. Roughly half were non-relative adoptions and of these 1814 (43%) involved babies under 1 year of age while 1396 (30%) concerned children aged 5 years or more. In 1984, 127 000 children, roughly 1% of all children aged 17 and under, had been adopted. Over the next decade the expectation is that the number of adopted children will continue to fall and that fewer children will have been adopted as babies. The implications for the children concerned, adopters and professionals involved are considerable.

Placement needs

Currently, while there are very few healthy babies available for adoption, there are many thousands of older children who could be placed. Most of these children have special requirements. They may be emotionally disturbed or have physical or mental handicaps. Additional factors which have to be considered include the existance of siblings. Until recently it was considered acceptable to place children, who were black, Asian or of mixed parentage, in white families in order to ensure experience of secure family life. Now more concerted efforts are made to place children in a family with a cultural and ethnic background similar to their own. Unfortunately, the recruitment of families able to meet the special needs of many of these children is slow and the waiting which ensues denies the children the security they need. However, facilities for finding families for children with special needs are improving and some agencies, such as Parents for Children, specialise in this work.

Since there are very few healthy babies available, some adopters look abroad, often to poorer countries, for a child. However, there is no organisation which brings babies into the UK from abroad, and such adoption can present formidable problems.

Adoption panel

The adoption panel considers both the children needing placement and prospective adopters. In the UK, the Adoption Agencies Regulations 1983 required adoption agencies to set up adoption panels and specify their membership. The maximum number of panel members is 10, the minimum seven, and there must be at least one man and one woman member. Two panel members have to be social workers employed by the agency and there has to be a management representative. A medical adviser has to be appointed as a panel member and at least two members have to be independent of the agency. The agency also has to identify a chairman. Most panels seek to appoint a representative from an ethnic minority group and an adoptive parent. A legal adviser is not required as a panel member, but is usually present since so many cases present legal complexities.

Medical adviser's role

The British Agencies for Adoption and Fostering (BAAF) has long recognised the significance of the health and developmental issues presented by children in care. Through its medical group, BAAF has recommended and promoted standards of good practice and has encouraged the involvement of doctors with a wide knowledge of child health care in this work. The 1983 regulations in turn recognise this contribution and hence the inclusion of a doctor in the panel. The medical adviser's role is comprehensive; it involves an evaluation of the health information about the children, their natural parents, and the prospective adoptive parents and advice to the panel about the implications. The medical adviser arranges the medical examination and many advisers undertake the clinical work themselves. Before undertaking the examination, information is obtained about the child's birth, subsequent care, health, development, behaviour and school progress. Thus a comprehensive assessment of the child's health and developmental status, prognosis and needs can be compiled to assist in the identification of a family able to meet the child's long-term needs. Additional contributions from a psychologist, psychiatrist and other consultants may be required to complete a profile on a child who requires specific treatment or who has special educational needs. Health and developmental information thus collated is given to the adopters and their GP. If the child has special needs the medical adviser liases with other health and educational professionals as required.

BAAF has produced report forms which cover all the health matters required and their use is recommended by the 1983 Adoption Agencies Regulations.

As more children with special needs are being placed for adoption the demand for skilled paediatric advice at primary and secondary care level grows. Frequently, the children concerned have been exposed to child abuse and evidence of sexual abuse may present at a later date. Both the children and the adoptive families need expert advice and support to which doctors can make a major contribution.

CHILDREN IN CARE

Children are admitted to care either on a voluntary basis or through the courts. During the past decade the number of children in care has dropped from 100 000 to around 73 000; the majority are admitted on a voluntary basis. Not unexpectedly, there are more children in care in cities than elsewhere. With the growing recognition of the benefits to the child of a secure family placement there has been a steady increase in the proportion of children placed in a foster home (boarded out) or with relatives. Those children placed in local authority or voluntary homes are usually in the older age groups.

Fostering

Foster care offers a child care within a family setting. It does not provide legal permanency since parental rights remain with the natural parents, the local authority or the courts, depending on the legal circumstances. There are different types of foster care which present the foster parents with varying tasks and require different skills. Short-term fostering often involves the care of babies awaiting adoption or young children for whom the return to the care of their parents is expected. Some foster parents offer specialist care to children whose needs are such that placement in an adoptive home is not immediately appropriate. For some older children, with natural family ties, long-term fostering is the placement of choice.

Foster parents offer a variety of skills and provide an invaluable resource. They are selected by a foster panel, which is not as specifically constituted as an adoption panel, and are paid allowances which vary depending on the age and the needs of the child, and from one local authority to another.

Until recently the health status of foster parents was not taken into account. Now more attention is given to this aspect, by recognising the stresses involved and the possible effects on the children concerned. The health issue currently under debate is the wisdom or otherwise of placing babies and young children in households containing heavy smokers.

Medical aspects of children in care

Children in care are vulnerable in many different ways. In the past, consideration of the health and developmental needs of children was not given high priority. Medical care was often fragmented; communication between different health professionals was poor, so that major medical, sensory, psychological, educational and behavioural problems went unrecognised and untreated. Normally, parents monitor their children's health and progress admirably. Foster parents want to fill the same role, but are rarely given enough background information to be able to do so. Children who pass in and out of care for short periods of time, or who pass from one caregiver to another, are particularly at risk. The case for parent-held child-health records is strong for all families; but it is especially relevant to children in care, and the introduction of a health record which moves with the child would immediately transform the process of health surveillance for these children.

Particular health hazards which face children in care include failure of registration with a GP, loss of immunisation records and information about growth and essential screening procedures.

A new issue which substitute parents will have to face is the risk of HIV infection in the children being placed. Routine screening is neither possible nor desirable and the interpretation of antibody testing in the young baby difficult.

Confidentiality has to be preserved but social workers are statutorily bound to consider the child's best interests above all else.

Practical issues

Good practice should ensure that all children receive a full health and developmental assessment which will provide a basis for monitoring progress while in care. Children placed with foster parents have to be examined at 6-monthly intervals under 2 years of age, and at yearly intervals when older. Foster parents should have written information about the child's health status and needs. BAAF has produced forms allowing this to be easily recorded on entry into care; their use is strongly recommended.

Local authorities are advised to identify a health professional to interpret medical reports. In many districts, a consultant community paediatrician or a senior doctor working in the community child health service maintains oversight of all children in care and is closely involved with those less than 5 years old.

Consent to medical examination and treatment for children in care or placed for adoption has to be specified each time a child moves to new care-givers; BAAF have produced a useful practice note which helps to clarify this area.

Child care law

All doctors working with children should have some knowledge of child care law. Useful summa-ries of the law in England and Wales, and Scotland, are produced by BAAF.

Place of safety order

A social worker can apply to a magistrate to put a child in a place of safety, such as a foster home or hospital. The order lasts up to 28 days.

A police officer can remove a child to a place of safety without a magistrate's order for up to 8 days.

The law on child care is being changed and the Place of Safety Order will be replaced by an Emergency Protection Order with different time intervals.

Care order

An application to a juvenile court for a care order is most frequently sought by a local authority, often because of child abuse or neglect. Responsibility for the child passes to the local authority and continues until the child is 18 years old unless the order is revoked.

Wardship

Wardship proceedings are heard by the High Court. Once a child is made a ward the High Court becomes the legal parent. Wardship can be terminated and automatically ceases when the child becomes 18 years old.

FURTHER READING

BAAF 1984 Consent to medical treatment for children in care or placed for adoption. Practice Note No. 3 BAAF, London
BAAF 1985 Using BAAF medical forms. Practice Note No. 10. BAAF, London
BAAF 1986 Child care law in England and Wales. Practice series. BAAF, London
BAAF 1987 Child care law in Scotland. Practice series. BAAF, London
BAAF 1987 The implications of AIDS for children in care. BAAF, London
Department of Health and Social Security 1983 Health circular guidance on adoption agencies regulations. HC(84)1. HMSO, London

8. Child abuse

J. Wynne

The 1924 Geneva Convention says 'the child deserves the best mankind has to give'.

From Roman times children have been regarded as parental, usually paternal, property and only in the last 100 years or so has there been recognition in the UK of the need to protect children from exploitation, neglect and abuse. The UK is a signatory to the United Nations Convention defining the Rights of the Child; this is based on the principles that the child should be protected, ideally within a nurturing family setting and that adults (including governments) should be committed to acting in the best interests of children.

Only in a society where child mortality is low is child abuse widely recognized. In a world context, children die unnecessarily because of undernutrition, infection, poor living conditions, inadequate health care and, increasingly, the additional hazards of urban squalor and impoverishment. High rates of malnutrition and infant mortality were typical in the UK in the last century but success in terms of public health measures, improved nutrition and immunisation of children has resulted in a generation who now expect their child to live. With this expectation the quality of the child's life is examined and there is an increasing recognition of the child as an individual in his own right. In the UK the concept of children's rights is slowly emerging, but children do not enjoy the position that many would wish. Adults often have difficulty in accepting that a child's interests may conflict with those of his parents, and that children are individuals in a societal sense.

As Lord Justice Butler-Sloss commented: 'there is a danger that in looking to the welfare of the children believed to be the victims of [sexual] abuse the children themselves may be overlooked. The child is a person and not an object of concern' (Butler-Sloss Report 1987).

The diagnosis of child abuse, the risk of further abuse, to that child and others within the household, the needs of the child(ren) are initially tested by a multidisciplinary group of professionals and are not the task of a single individual. Decisions are checked at case conferences and a minority ultimately tested in court. Social services carry the statutory responsibility for the care and protection of children, but other professionals have responsibility too. It is only 40 years since the first papers were written on 'battered babies' and whilst much has been learned, particularly in the recognition of abuse, there is much still to learn, especially in evaluation and management.

Henry Kempe, an American paediatrician said in 1979 that a society went through various stages in the recognition of abuse (Kempe & Kempe 1978). Battered babies would be recognized initially, then less severely physically abused children, and later neglect, emotional abuse, and child sexual abuse. It would be recognized that 'ordinary' people may abuse. It is not just mad people, drug or alcohol abusers, but also people who have been in no previous difficulty; and this is a lesson currently being learned in child sexual abuse.

The rate of registration of children who are thought to have been abused has doubled according to the NSPCC figures (Creighton 1988) from 1984 to 1987. Much of the recent increase has been due to the increased recognition of child sexual abuse, a 21% increase from 1986 to 1987. This does not mean an absolute increase of sexual abuse within society but reflects how little was reported before the mid-1980s in the UK, which contrasts with the USA where the increase started some 10 years earlier. Similar increases in reporting have been shown in Canada, Northern Europe and Australia and New Zealand. The NSPCC has recorded a recent fall in the number of children physically abused, but an increase in severe physical injury and death from abuse. This fall may again be apparent due to under-reporting as social work and health professionals have been overwhelmed by the rise in reported sexual abuse.

The rate of physical abuse in 1987 was 0.85 per thousand children (0–14 years) and the number of fatal and seriously injured children accounted for 14% of these. The NSPCC estimate in England and Wales was that over 8000 children aged 0–14 years were physically abused in 1987 and over 7000 children were sexually abused. Deaths from child abuse are estimated at 1–2 per week in the UK and this is likely to be an underestimate.

Neglect, failure to thrive and emotional abuse are all under-recognized. Other abuses such as poisoning and Münchausen's syndrome by proxy have been increasingly diagnosed over the last 10 years. The DHSS definition of categories of abuse have been published (DHSS 1988a) (Table 8.1).

Table 8.1 Categories of abuse (DHSS 1988b)

Neglect	The persistent or severe neglect of a child which results in serious impairment of the child's health or development, including non-organic failure to thrive
Physical abuse	Physical injury to a child, including deliberate poisoning where there is definite knowledge or a reasonable suspicion, that the injury was inflicted or knowingly not prevented
Sexual abuse	The involvement of dependent/developmentally immature children and adolescents in sexual activities they do not truly comprehend, to which they are unable to give informed consent or that violate the social taboos of family rules
Emotional abuse	The severe adverse effect on the behaviour and emotional development of a child caused by persistent or severe emotional ill-treatment or rejection. All abuse involves some emotional ill-treatment . . .

It is clear that the long-term outlook for children who have been seriously abused is often poor, particularly if the abuse is longstanding, there are multiple abuses, and especially if there is neglect or intrafamilial sexual abuse. Physical injuries usually heal but psychological abuse may damage the child's whole personality and development, his learning capacity, his social skills and his capacity as a parent later (Lynch & Roberts 1988). A recent study of the outcome of abused children (Taitz & King 1988) showed that physically abused children had the best outlook, but neglected, deprived children and children who failed to thrive did badly. Even those who appeared to do well in the short term, when followed up were shown to do worse, especially in general social adjustment, and by the age of 6 years over half were thought to have a serious emotional or behavioural problem. Studies of the long-term effects of child sexual abuse, particularly within the immediate family, show it also to have a very damaging effect on many of the victims (Frend 1981).

The medical diagnosis of abuse

This is always in the context of a full paediatric examination but also a social work assessment and sometimes a police investigation. In some cases it is necessary to have a psychological or psychiatric assessment too. The diagnosis may appear highly probable from the initial examination, for instance, a badly bruised infant with several broken bones. Where the child is neglected, emotionally or sexually abused an assessment over a longer period is often needed.

Confidentiality

Doctors are anxious about issues of confidentiality but the General Medical Council in 1987 gave unequivocal advice in cases of child abuse and child sexual abuse.

'. . . . if a doctor has reason for believing that a child is being physically or sexually abused, not only is it permissible for the doctor to disclose information to a third party but it is a duty of the doctor to do so'.

Doctors may feel a responsibility towards the whole family and when there is a conflict of interest between the child and parents what should he do? The advice again is clear (DHSS 1988b) '. . . the rights of the child should prevail'.

No professional should work in isolation in this field, and inexperienced doctors should all have access to more senior colleagues for advice. The professional secretariat of the medical defence societies are always available for advice.

In the USA there is a mandatory reporting of possible child abuse cases. All professionals are required to tell the child protection agencies if they have concerns about possible abuse. There are advantages for professionals in that they are obliged to report and the balance is towards early reporting. In the UK doctors will hesitate: can they justify their actions, is enough known, is it really serious? If there are good interagency links with respect between professionals, a doctor may feel able to ring the local social services office, discuss with the child abuse co-ordinator the case of possible abuse and work out a plan of investigation. Doctors should share appropriate information since building up a diagnosis of abuse is putting the pieces of the jigsaw together and other professionals often have information which clarifies the clinical picture. The police too have a legitimate interest in child abuse, and as part of a team will usually work in conjunction with other professionals.

Confidentiality at case conferences. This is also a legitimate concern. It should be the responsibility of local trainers under the auspices of the Area Child Protection Committee to ensure that there is a common ethical code. Information must be shared but members of the case conference need to be confident that confidentiality will be respected.

Increasingly, written reports are laid before case conferences, and medical reports should be factual remembering that later they may be used in Court.

If parents attend part or the entirety of a case conference care should be taken not to infringe a third party's confidentiality.

Consent. A child may not ordinarily be examined by a doctor without the consent of his parent, guardian or other adult with parental rights. The Children Act (1989) enables the Court to give directions as to medical or psychiatric examinations

and override parents' rights when emergency protection orders and interim care and supervision orders are made. Emergency protection orders will be available quickly if needed.

Although 16 years is the usual age of consent, a younger teenager may also give consent as long as it is informed, that is, he understands to what he is consenting and the possible consequences (Gillick principle).

Consent should be freely given and without threat, fear or coercion.

It is part of good clinical practice for the doctor to ask all children, from around 3 years onwards, if 'it's alright to have a look'.

It should also be evident that children should not be restrained during examination, apart from the very young. If a child is unable to co-operate, discussions should take place about the importance of the examination to the child. Often at a follow-up appointment a child will be more confident and the examination is completed. Occasionally sedation or a short general anaesthetic is needed and written consent is required and the reasons as to why sedation was used should be noted.

For other examinations the consent is implied, that is, the presence of the parent gives permission to the doctor to proceed.

Parents only occasionally refuse permission. The Children Act will assist in these difficult cases as the Court is able to give directions as to medical or psychiatric examinations when emergency protection orders and interim care or supervision orders are made. The direction will be to a specified medical practitioner and direct as to whether the child is to be seen as an in-patient or outpatient.

The examining doctor

This may initially be a GP, or a clinical medical officer but there should be, in each health district, a consultant paediatrician with a special interest in abuse who will accept referrals, although some injured children may be brought directly to hospital by their parents. Children should be seen in a child-centred environment, not a busy accident and emergency department, and never in a police station.

The history

It is the history that makes a doctor concerned that this may be abuse, and he should ask himself:

1. Does it make sense?
2. Does it change?
3. Has there been a delay in seeking help?
4. Has the child been to the accident and emergency department before?
5. Have there been previous health problems — failure to thrive, scalds, unexplained fractures?
6. What does the child say?

Also certain injuries should alert the doctor to the possibility of abuse:

1. Fractures at <2 years of age and especially at <1 year.
2. Multiple fractures.
3. Rib fractures.
4. Skull fractures (multiple, depressed, wide, growing, long).
5. ANY BRUISING IN INFANCY.
6. Bruises on cheek, ears, jaw, chest.
7. Scalds, burns (a minority are inflicted injuries).

The whole picture needs assessing both from the physical examination (Table 8.2) and ultimately the wider investigation (Table 8.3). There are certain medical conditions which need to be ruled out as a cause for excessive bruising. A platelet count as part of a full blood count and a clotting screen will rule out most bleeding or clotting disorders, but occasionally further haematological investigations are needed (Table 8.4).

Certain patterns of bruising

These may be recognizable; for example, a hard slap with four parallel linear bruises, or grip marks around the lower jaw with a thumb print on side and several fingertip bruises on the other. The site where bruises are usually found in normal children and children found to have non-accidental injuries have been described (Robertson et al 1982). In non-accidental injury, bruises to the face predominate, and although there is overlap, bruises due to accidental trauma, such as a toddler tripping, will tend to be on the forehead, nose or chin. Bruising of the ears, sides of the face or around the lower jaw or neck are usually due to abuse.

Table 8.2 Medical examination of the child who may have been abused

General examination	Full physical examination	(See Table 8.8 for signs of child sexual abuse)
	Assess growth, weight	Note parental height, weight gain in care or hospital. Use centile charts
	Developmental screen	Language and social skills are most often retarded. Aquisition of skills accelerate in care
Signs of neglect (photograph the child)	Hair — thin, alopecia Skin — infections, dry Abdomen — distended Nails — thickened, yellow Behaviour — apathetic, listless	General care poor, dirty clothes. Infestations. Neglected squint. Deafness or other medical conditions not adequately treated. Immunisation status
Physical injury (photograph the child)	Describe bruises (colour, size, position) (especially ears, jaw, cheeks), pattern	Blood film, platelet count Clotting studies *Recognisable patterns* of hand print, fingertip, two black eyes
Behaviour 1. During examination	Overactive, angry, sad, passive, clingy, attention seeking, indiscriminate affection, eye avoidance.	
2. .Reported (parents, health visitor, teacher, etc.)	Wetting, soiling, headbanging, rocking, crying, feeding or sleeping problems, aggressive, withdrawal, overactivity, disobedience, school failure, truancy, stealing, lying, running away, solvent and drug abuse, sexually explicit play, sexually precocious behaviour	

Table 8.3   Making a diagnosis (it's a jigsaw)

1. *History* — including what the child says, behavioural indicators

2. *Physical examination*

3. *Investigations* — skeletal survey (most bruised children <two years — but also some older too)
   — copper studies (infancy)
   — clotting studies
   — screen for sexually transmitted disease } (in cases or suspected sexual abuse)
   — forensic tests
   — pregnancy

4. What do the health visitor, school nurse, clinical medical officer and GP say?

5. Is the child on the Child Protection Register?

6. Is the child known to social services?

7. Social work investigation

8. Police investigation

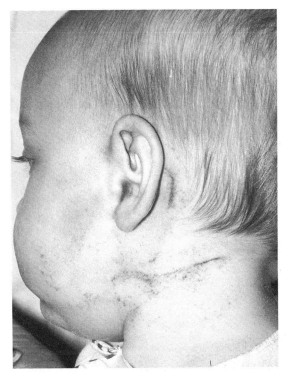

Fig. 8.2   Hand slap showing bruising of cheek, neck and behind ear in child aged 10 months.

Examples are given in Figures 8.1–8.7. Ageing of bruising is difficult and can only be estimated, not assessed with any degree of accuracy. The police may try to ask for a definition of timing which is not possible (Table 8.5). Timing of a fracture is also difficult, but Table 8.6 gives an estimate. With bony injury, particularly multiple fractures in infancy, both osteogenesis imperfecta and copper deficiency must be considered, but recent work has aided the clinical assessment of these cases (Carty 1988, Shaw 1988, Taitz 1988). Work has also been done in looking at the patterns of fractures in abuse versus non-abuse (Worlock et al 1986).

Fractures in abuse

These are often multiple (hence the need for a skeletal survey). In particular, fractured ribs, oblique or spiral fractures of long bones and periosteal new bone formation (from twisting and gripping injuries) are suspicious. Metaphyseal chip fractures are not common. Skull fractures may be difficult to assess, again there is overlap between accidents and abuse but multiple fractures, long fractures crossing suture lines, depressed fractures and 'growing' fractures are all suggestive of abuse (Hobbs 1984). It has been assessed that one child in eight under 18 months who sustains a fracture has been the victim of child abuse (Worlock et al 1986). However, child abuse cannot be diagnosed

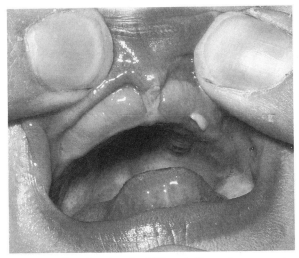

Fig. 8.1   Torn frenulum in child aged 12 months.

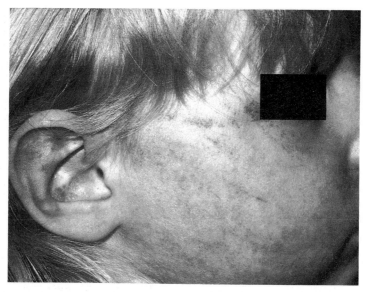

Fig. 8.3   Typical hand slap and bruised ear in 3-year-old child who has also been sexually abused.

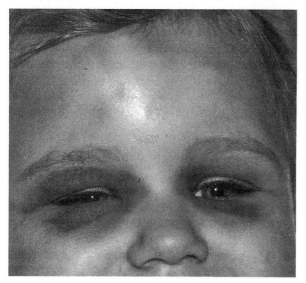

Fig. 8.4   Two black eyes in a child of 4 years, head banged against wall.

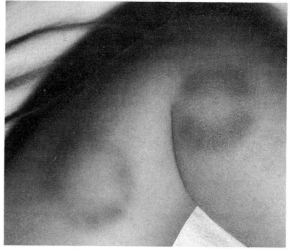

Fig. 8.5   Child bites.

from the pattern of fractures alone, this must be part of a full investigation.

In osteogenesis imperfecta there is usually a family history, blue sclerae and other radiological abnormalities such as Wormian bones in the child, and relatives with hypermobile joints, deafness and abnormal teeth or blue sclerae. Type I osteogenesis imperfecta can usually be excluded on these

features. Types II and III are severe conditions and Type IV may very rarely give cause for problems — on one estimate, in Sheffield, about once every 300 years (Taitz 1988).

Copper deficiency

This should be excluded in the preterm or babies that have been intravenously fed over prolonged

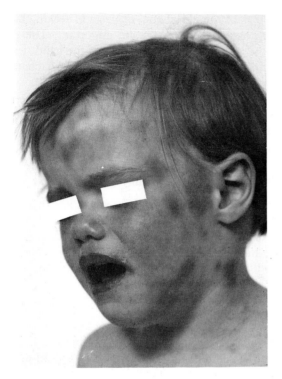

Fig. 8.6 Multiple bruises.

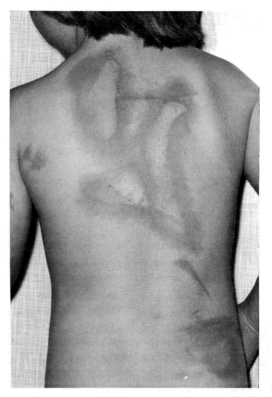

Fig. 8.7 Weals from a lashing.

Table 8.4 A child with bruises: is it a haematological disorder?

	Platelet count	Bleeding time	PTT	PT	Factor VIII level	Factor IX level
Idiopathic thrombocytopenic purpura	Low	N	N	N	N	N
Haemophilia	Normal	N	Prolonged	N	Low	N
von Willebrand's disease	Normal (defective platelet aggregation)	Prolonged	N or prolonged	N	Low	N
Factor IX deficiency	Normal	N	Prolonged	N	N	Low

N = normal; PTT = partial thromboplastin time; PT = prothrombin time.

periods, or fed copper-deficient milk. Babies with this disorder would usually have a hypochromic, microcytic anaemia, a low serum copper level and a low serum concentration of caeruloplasmin. The bony changes are usually a late manifestation; they are symmetrical with osteoporosis, metaphyseal cupping and spurs.

Scalds and burns

These are now increasingly being recognized as part of the pattern of physical abuse (Hobbs 1986) (Figs 8.8, 8.9). They may result from accidents due to lapses in protection of the child, from neglect, or from deliberate injury — often as a

Table 8.5   Rough estimate of age of bruises

Age	Bruise appearance
< 24 hours	Red or reddish-purple, swollen
1–2 days	Purple, swollen
3–5 days	Starting to yellow
5–7 days	Yellow, fading
> 1 week	Yellow, brown, have faded

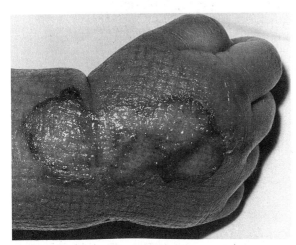

Fig. 8.8   Unexplained burn in a 3-month-old child, said to have 'burned hand on cooker'.

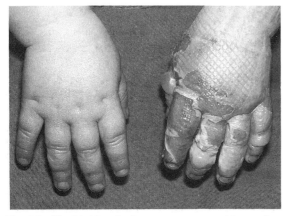

Fig. 8.9   Hand held under hot water tap as punishment for spilling cup of tea — 18-month-old child.

form of punishment. Earlier reports suggested 1–2% of children admitted with burns had been abused, but this is an underestimate. In the history, repeated burns or an incompatible history, such as blaming a sibling, or delay in seeking help and changes in the story are important. The site of the burn, especially the back of the hand, legs, buttocks and feet are worrying, as are contact burns in unusual sites and scalds with clear-cut edges in a glove or stocking distribution. There is an apparent association between sexual abuse and burns, and this probably reflects the sadistic nature of the abuse.

Other disorders may mimic physical abuse

These include mongolian blue spots, impetigo and haemangioma which may mimic common skin disorders, and idiopathic thrombocytopenic purpura as the commonest blood disorder which may be misdiagnosed (Wheeler & Hobbs 1988).

Failure to thrive

The majority of children who are failing to thrive, that is gain weight adequately, are not consuming enough calories. To grow optimally a child needs an adequate diet, but also to be loved and cherished. The interaction of relevant factors is complex, but given food most children will grow, as seen by the rapid weight gain often observed when such children are admitted to hospital. Growth charts which demonstrate the rapid acceleration of growth when the child is well cared for followed by poor or no growth at home make the diagnosis clear. Obviously, organic conditions such as coeliac disease or cystic fibrosis need to be considered, but extensive medical investigations are not indicated in most cases. There is considerable overlap between children who are neglected, fail to thrive and are emotionally deprived. *Signs of neglect* may be evident (Table 8.2 Fig. 8.10) but also failure to learn, and particularly develop skills which need parental input such as language or social skills. Neglectful parents may also fail to protect against accidents, to ensure their child is immunised, or to keep hospital appointments for treatment of squint or hearing problems; so the disadvantaged child becomes even further disabled.

Emotional deprivation

This has lasting effects as a child may grow up

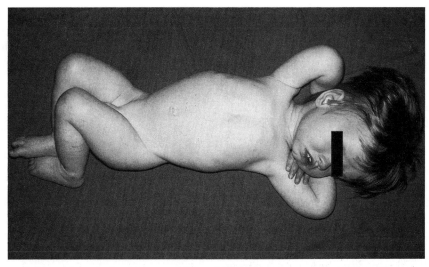

Fig. 8.10 Failure to thrive, with marked passivity — child aged 15 months.

Table 8.6 Healing of fractures in children

Fracture appearance	Timing (average)
Swelling of soft tissues resolves	2–10 days
Periosteal new bone	10+ days
Loss of fracture line definition	14+ days
Soft callus	14+ days
Hard callus	21+ days
Remodelling	3 months +

feeling unloved, unwanted, under-achieving with a poor self-image and ultimately may become an adult who has difficulty in giving love, or, and most unfortunately, having a baby at a young age so the baby will 'love' them. Cycles of deprivation are evident in depriving and deprived families; but emotional abuse occurs in all social classes with the same recurrent pattern.

Münchausen's syndrome by proxy

This is the label applied to anyone who persistently fabricates symptoms on behalf of another, so causing that person to be regarded as ill (Meadow 1977, 1985). Fictitious illness may be recognized by unexplained, prolonged illness or symptoms which are inappropriate, incongruous or only there when the mother is present. The doctor may be manipulated into performing increasingly complex investigations and prescribe drugs which are ineffective or even harmful yet do not help the 'disorder'. The management is difficult but includes confronting the parents — the mother is the usual abuser — but always involving the usual statutory agencies.

Social factors

Factors which are important in abuse, are those which add to the stress of living or detract from the quality of life for the family. Poverty is the most important stress; it is often coupled with poor housing, and financially disadvantaged parents are often the least able in society. Young mothers and single-parent families often live in circumstances which mean that their children grow up in poverty and so have all the additional problems of social disadvantage. In assessing the social aspects of a case, a social worker will also look at the nature of the incident, the vulnerability of the child and the history of any siblings, the marital history as well as the extended family and other support systems available to help the family. Practical issues of housing and finance are also assessed. The NSPCC briefing (Creighton 1988) quotes the factors which commonly precipitated physical abuse as marital problems, unemployment, inability to meet child's needs and poor parental esteem, in order of frequency.

CHILD SEXUAL ABUSE (CSA)
(Figs 8.11–8.18)

Child sexual abuse is defined in Table 8.1. Wider recognition of CSA in the UK, beyond stranger abuse or the 'stepdaughter/stepfather' story, is only recent. The medical literature is not extensive and practitioners are currently learning new skills as our predecessors developed skills in the assessment of 'battered babies' in the 1960s. That CSA does occur is evident; however abhorrent it may be, doctors will have to come to terms with the clear conclusion in the Cleveland Report (Butler-Sloss Report 1987) that: 'we have learned during the Inquiry that sexual abuse occurs in children of all ages, including the very young, to boys as well as girls, in all classes of society and frequently within the privacy of the family. The sexual abuse can be serious and on occasions includes vaginal, anal and oral intercourse . . . .'

How do children present with CSA? (Table 8.7). Clearly the evaluation of a child's story on occasion needs the expertise of an experienced psychologist or child psychiatrist, but frequently the assessment is within the skills of a paediatrician or experienced social worker or police officer. Anatomically correct (or complete) dolls may be used with young, inarticulate or intellectually slow children to 'look and say'. Drawings are also useful with children of 6 years and older (MacFarlane 1985).

The physical signs associated with CSA must be taken within the context of the whole paediatric and ultimately the complete investigation (Table 8.3; Figs 8.11–8.13). The signs seen are those of trauma and, in some, infection. As such healing takes place over days or months so there is a need for careful documentation including sketches, and in some children clinical photography. The physical signs *associated* with sexual abuse are shown in Table 8.8; Figs 8.14–8.17). It must be underlined that: 'it cannot be emphasised too strongly that no physical sign can at this time be regarded as being uniquely diagnostic of child sexual abuse' (DHSS 1988b).

The evaluation of physical signs is difficult

Table 8.7   Presentation of child sexual abuse (Frend 1981, Porter 1984, MacFarlane 1985, Jones and McQuiston 1988)

1. Disclosure	By child or third party
2. Physical indicators	Rectal or vaginal bleeding
	Sexually transmitted disease (STD)
	Vulvovaginitis/vaginal discharge
	Dysuria and frequency (possible urinary infection)
	Physical abuse
	Pregnancy
	HIV infection
3. Psychosomatic indicators	Recurrent abdominal pain
	Headache, migraine
	Anorexia or other eating disorders
	Encopresis
	Enuresis
4. Behavioural indicators	Sexually explicit play, 'excessive' masturbation, insertion of foreign bodies (girls)
a. Preschool	Withdrawal, poor appetite, sleep disturbance
	Clingy, delayed development, aggression
b. Middle years	Sexualized play or sexual precocity
	Anxiety, depression, poor school performance
c. Teenagers	Sexually precocious, prostitution, anxiety, depression, truancy, running away, solvent, alcohol or drug abuse, self-destructive behaviour, overdose or drugs, self-mutilating behaviour, anorexia
5. Social indicators	Concern by parent or third party, sibling, relative or friend of abused child
	Schedule 1 offender in close contact with child

(Butler-Sloss Report 1987, DHSS 1988b) and the place of the physical examination is widely misunderstood. Over 50% of children who have been sexually abused have *no* abnormality on examination; this does not mean that there has been no abuse. If the abuse has been oral sex, this is a serious abuse but usually leaves no signs, and similarly in masturbation or pornographic photography. Associated physical abuse is important; up to 20% of physically abused boys, and rather fewer girls, have been sexually abused. Certain patterns of bruising are more common in sexual

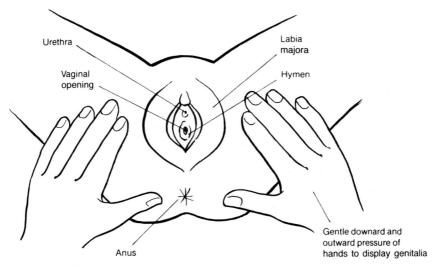

Fig. 8.11 Normal female genitalia

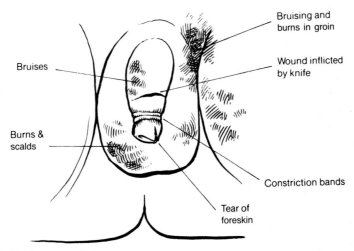

Fig. 8.12 Male genitalia showing types of abuse.

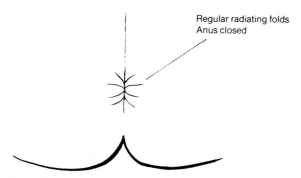

Fig. 8.13 Normal anus.

abuse (Table 8.8), and deliberate burning is also seen.

Vulvovaginitis is common in young girls and reddening of the vulva is a non-specific response. It is common in children with infantile eczema and may also be caused by rubbing, infection or contact sensitivity, for example from a bubble bath. If there is a story of forcible rubbing by an adult of the genitalia, reddening would be a consistent finding and, whilst non-specific, a contributory finding.

Table 8.8 Examination of the sexually abused child (Hobbs and Wynne 1986, Paul and Chaple 1986, Hobbs and Wynne 1987a, b, Bulter-Sloss Report 1987, DHSS 1988b, Independent Second Opinion Panel 1988)

Place	Quiet, child-centred room. Facilities need to be private to enable adequate examination, and microbiological and forensic tests. Clinical photograph
Doctor	Older children may prefer doctor of same gender Seek consent of child as well as parent or guardin Never restrain. Rarely need sedation
Equipment	Bright light source. Auriscope minus speculum. Tape measure. Swabs for screen for sexually transmitted disease. Forensic pack for use if last assault within 72 hours.
General examination	As Table 10.1. Remember to check the abdomen for signs of severe constipation
Genitalia 1. Position	Examine young child lying on mother's knee. Older child on couch, girls in 'frog leg position'

2. Signs	Girls
	  Labia: reddening, bruises, lacerations, burns
	  Perineum: reddening, bruises, laceration
	  Vulva: reddening, bruising, lacerations, swelling
	  Discharge (colour, amount)
	  Hymenal opening: size (mm), margin, tears, scars
	  Posterior fourchette: laceration, scar
	  Vaginal examination ONLY in older girls where indicated
	Boys
	  Penis: bruising, laceration, scars, burns
	  Perineum: reddening, bruising
	  Scrotum: bruising, reddening, burns

Anus 1. Position	Examine young children on mother's knee, older children, left lateral, part buttocks and observe for 30 seconds. In anal dilatation the external and internal sphincters relax and contract intermittently, usually to >1 cm
2. Signs	Inspection is the usual method, rectal examinations are unpleasant for the child and do not usually yield helpful information
a. Acute	Anal margin: swelling, reddening, bruising, haematoma laceration or tears (extend across perineum and up anal canal)
	Anal sphincter: spasm, laxity, dilatation Perianal veins: dilated
b. Chronic	Anal margin: smooth, thickened shiny skin, chronic and acute fissures, scars (rare) Anal sphincter: laxity, dilatation Perianal veins: dilated
Microbiology	Gonorrhoea, trichomonas, chlamydia, herpes, genital warts
Forensic test	As indicated: use forensic pack provided by police — tests include swabs to look for spermatozoa, semen, grouping of semen (ABO grouping etc.) saliva

Masturbation in small children is universal and usually in girls involves rubbing around the clitoris. This does not usually cause any abnormal physical signs. Masturbation is pleasurable and the child does not cause him or herself discomfort. Girls uncommonly insert their own fingers in their vagina at this age, and do not cause hymenal tears which are extremely painful.

'Excessive' masturbation or insertion of foreign bodies (which is very uncommon) needs considering as some of these children have been abused. Infection giving a mild vulvovaginitis is common and usually no organisms are grown, but the group β-haemolytic streptococcus is sometimes found. Threadworm infestation may not only cause perianal irritation, but also a vulvitis secondary to scratching. If there is a possibility of sexually transmitted infection, the child should have a careful screen for infection, usually done in conjunction with the department of genitourinary medicine. The apparent excess reporting of vulvovaginitis in abused girls is probably due to the superficial infection of small lacerations caused by rough handling.

The size of the hymenal opening in young girls is remarkably constant in the prepubertal years, it is uncommonly greater than 0.5 cm at 5 years and by the onset of puberty is still less than 0.75 cm — 1.0 cm being very uncommon. It is interesting that the size of the opening may diminish markedly if abuse ceases and healing takes place. However, some signs are of greater significance than others (Table 8.9).

A clear, spontaneous description by the child is

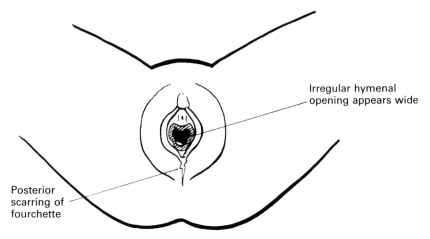

Fig. 8.14 Dilated hymenal opening and posterior scarring of fourchette.

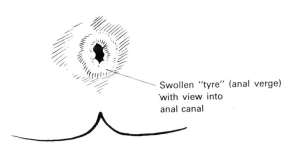

Fig. 8.15 Anus of three year old with signs following acute penetration

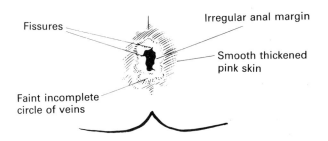

Fig. 8.16 Anus of 10 year old with signs of chronic abuse.

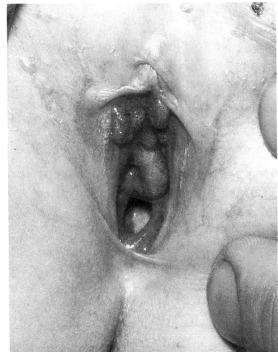

Fig. 8.17 Genital warts.

the ideal, but children are often fearful, having received many threats as to the consequences of disclosures; the skill in the management of CSA is to work out with colleagues a plan of investigation which is neither too precipitate or leaves the child unprotected. The reality is that children who are the victims of CSA often go unprotected throughout their childhood. Intervention by professionals

Table 8.9 Significance of physical signs in child sexual abuse (CSA)

Low likelihood of CSA	
	Redness of genitalia
	Single anal fissure
	Recurrent vaginal discharge
Increasing Probability	Hymenal opening 0.5 cm (prepubertal)
	Dilated perianal veins
	Anal warts
	Anal dilatation, laxity
	Multiple anal tears
Higher likelihood of CSA	Hymenal opening 1.0 cm (prepubertal)
	Vaginal tears
	Gonorrhoea
	Pregnancy
	HIV infection
Highly probable CSA	Positive forensic tests (sperm in vagina)

is difficult without a clear disclosure or corroboration from other sources or investigations. Physical examination with few exceptions will never give a short cut to management, and single physical signs, as in other disorders in medicine, do not make a diagnosis although they may raise the examiner's index of suspicion.

THE MANAGEMENT OF CHILD ABUSE

Working Together (DHSS 1988a) suggests that there are three stages in management:

1. Recognition and investigation.
2. Assessment and planning.
3. Implementation and review.

All professionals who work with children have a responsibility to recognise child abuse, even if it is only to refer the child immediately. Most districts have developed networks of skilled professionals who come together in 'teams' to work with individual children and their families. Clearly there must be a pool of doctors, social workers and police who are available; increasingly, community paediatricians are involved in this work although all paediatricians must have a greater or lesser responsibility. The district's procedures are monitored by a multidisciplinary child protection committee. Here is an example of a typical referral:

Because of bruising a child was referred from a day nursery to a consultant community paediatrician. What should she do? The plan would be to:

1. Arrange an appointment for the same day (unless there is history of a recent assault, cases of possible sexual abuse can often be seen at a later date at the convenience of all concerned).
2. Examine the child fully and arrange any investigations, and consider hospital admission.
3. Discuss with the social worker the initial clinical impression which will assist the social services department (SSD) in decisions about placement of the child, the need to see other children of the family, and whenever an Emergency Protection Order should be obtained or the police involved.
4. Write a short, concise medical report which must include a brief history, examination and opinion. It should be sent to the SSD, the GP, and the child health service. Supply police statement on request.
5. Attend a case conference.
6. Give evidence in court. (This should not be done by very junior staff below the level of senior registrar.)
7. Refer on for appropriate child or adolescent psychiatric support.
8. Arrange paediatric follow-up.

Case conference

This is important because it is a formal gathering of professionals with a legitimate interest in the child and family, and usually each has knowledge of the case. The conference allows pooling of information and a forum where opinion can be tested.

Ideally, it produces checks and balances at an early stage in the management of a case. Professionals, including doctors, should be questioned as to their views and asked to explain them. The usual participants are the SSD, paediatricians, GP, the health visitor, and the police. Parents may be invited for part of the case conference (DHSS 1988a). Other professionals such as teachers may give invaluable help, as do legal advisers.

The case conference should 'maintain a focus on the child as the primary client whose interests must transcend those of the parent where there is any conflict' (DHSS 1988a).

In summary the tasks include:

1. An exchange of relevant information.

2. A decision as to whether abuse has taken place and the need to place the child's name on the Child Protection Register.

3. An action plan for protecting the child and helping the family (including statutory proceedings).

4. Identifying a key worker and core group who are to implement the plan.

At present, the Child Care Law is being reviewed in the UK, but it is likely that the Place of Safety Order (up to 28 days) will be replaced by a shorter Emergency Protection Order.

Care proceedings are usually held in a juvenile court; the child, parents and local authority are separately represented by solicitors. The court may make no order (and therefore dismiss the case), a supervision order (where the child is supervised in his own home), or a care order. Even on a care order a child will usually be rehabilitated at home. In more complex cases wardship procedures are used. This is done in a higher court, where the matter is heard by a judge. Criminal proceedings are heard in magistrate's or Crown courts. These courts differ in the standard of proof required. The rules of evidence are very strict in criminal courts, where proof has 'to be beyond all reasonable doubt' and the rules of hearsay are strictly applied. In care courts, it is the protection of the child and what is in the child's best interest that is at stake, and evidence is assessed on the 'balance of probability'. The standard of proof, however, is still high and this depends on all witnesses, including doctors, giving clear, cogent evidence.

Whether or not care proceedings are initiated, an *action plan* for the child and family is drawn up. This will involve social work support, but may also require regular medical input. If the child has failed to thrive, regular paediatric assessments are needed to look at growth, development and so to give an objective view on progress. A paediatrician may also give advice as to continuing behavioural or management problems. Ideally, parents are able to acknowledge that there are problems and admit the abuse. This is difficult, when, as at present, a move towards more police prosecutions is now almost invariable in CSA. Unless there are more non-custodial sentences, many abusers will be discouraged from taking any responsibility for the

abuse and this makes rehabilitation very difficult. In CSA, denial by an alleged abuser (if he is indeed the abuser) makes the child take all the responsibility and indeed may ensure the child returns home unless the child is extremely convincing in the allegations. Responsibility should begin with the adult; the child should be protected but ideally should remain at home and not be made a double victim.

THE CHILDREN ACT 1989 (HMSO 1989, White et al 1989)

The Children Act 1989 is a comprehensive piece of legislation which integrates and simplifies the law regarding children. It will gradually be implemented from October 1991.

The Act is based on the principle that the welfare of the child is paramount. It also acknowledges that children are generally best looked after within the family with both parents playing a full part. The Act seeks to achieve a balance between the protection of children and undue intervention in family life.

A summary of points of the Act which are relevant to issues of child protection are given in Table 8.10 and a flow chart showing the organization of the procedure in Figure 8.18.

Criminal proceedings

A minority of child abuse cases reach criminal trial. Rules of evidence are adhered to strictly in

Table 8.10 Child protection and the Children Act

1. The Act consolidates earlier law concerning children

2. The upbringing of children is primarily the responsibility of parents, but the wishes of the child should be sought

3. A balance between child protection and undue interference in family is sought

4. In court hearings 'the child's welfare is paramount'

5. Child assessment orders are introduced

6. Emergency protection orders may be challenged in court by parents after 72 hours

7. A timetable will be set by the Court to avoid undue delay

8. A court order should not be made unless it is better for the child than not making an order

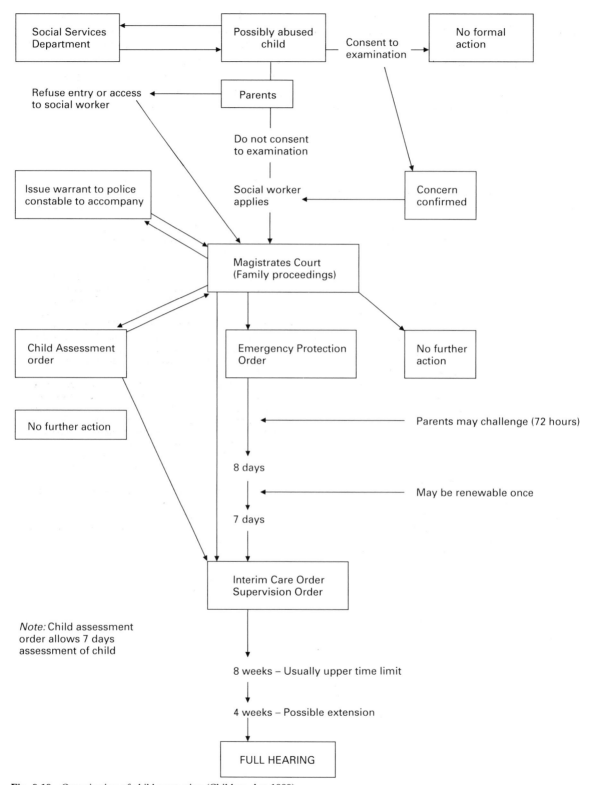

Fig. 8.18 Organisation of child protection (Children Act 1989).

criminal courts and no hearsay evidence, that is information learned from a third party, may be given. In other courts looking at the welfare of the child, hearsay evidence is admissible. In criminal courts the standard of proof is high and a case should be proved 'beyond reasonable doubt' as compared with 'the balance of probabilities' in 'case' courts. In criminal courts a doctor will therefore be asked to describe his examination and what he may deduce from that but not allowed to say what the child may have told him. The Court may hear from the child, and by the use of screens and contemporaneous videoing this has become a more practical proposition.

REFERENCES

Butler-Sloss Report 1987 Report of the inquiry into child abuse in Cleveland. HMSO, London, pp 183–203, 245

Carty H 1988 Brittle or battered. Archives of Disease in Childhood 63: 350–352

Creighton S J 1988 NSPCC research briefing no 9 child abuse in 1987 — initial findings from the NSPCC's Register Research. NSPCC, London

DHSS 1988a Working together. HMSO, London, pp 26, 29

DHSS 1988b Diagnosis of child sexual abuse: guidance for doctors. HMSO, London, p 20

Frend A 1981 A psychoanalyst's view of sexual abuse by parents. In: Mrazek P B, Kempe C H (eds) Sexually abused children and their families. Pergamon, Oxford

HMSO 1989 An introduction to The Children Act. HMSO, London

Hobbs C J 1984 Skull fracture and diagnosis of abuse. Archives of Disease in Childhood 59: 246

Hobbs C J 1986 When are burns non-accidental? Archives of Disease in Childhood 61: 357

Hobbs C J, Wynne J M 1986 Buggery in childhood: a common syndrome of child abuse. Lancet ii: 792

Hobbs C J, Wynne J M 1987a Child sexual abuse: an increasing rate of diagnosis. Lancet ii: 837

Hobbs C J, Wynne J M 1987b Management of sexual abuse. Archives of Disease in Childhood 62: 1182

Independent Second Opinion Panel 1988 Chaired Kolvin I. Child sexual abuse: principles of good practice. British Journal Hospital Medicine 39: 54

Jones D P H, McQuiston M G 1988 Interviewing the sexually abused child. Gaskell: Royal College of Psychiatrists, London

Kempe R S, Kempe C H 1978 Child abuse. Fontana, London

Lynch M A, Roberts J 1982 Consequences of child abuse. Academic Press, London

MacFarlane K (ed) 1985 Sexual abuse of young children. Holt, Rinehart and Winston, New York

Meadow R 1977 Munchausen syndrome by proxy — the hinterland of child abuse. Lancet ii: 343

Meadow R 1985 Management of Munchausen syndrome by proxy. Archives of Disease in Childhood 60: 385

Paul D 1986 Medico-legal examination of the living. In: Mant A K (ed) Taylor's principles and practice of medical jurisprudence. Churchill Livingstone, Edinburgh

Porter R (ed) 1984 Child sexual abuse within the family. The Ciba Foundation. Tavistock Publications, London

Roberton D N, Barbor P, Hull D 1982 Unusual injury?: recent injury in normal children and children with suspected non-accidental injury. British Medical Journal 285: 1299

Shaw J C L 1988 Copper deficiency and non-accidental injury. Archives of Disease in Childhood 63: 488–455

Taitz L S, King J M 1988 Growth patterns in child abuse. Acta Paediatrica Scandinavica Supplement 343: 62–72

Taitz L S 1988 Child abuse and osteogenesis imperfecta. British Medical Journal 296: 292

Wheeler D M, Hobbs C J 1988 Mistakes in the diagnosis of non-accidental injury: 10 years experience. British Medical Journal 296: 1233

Worlock et al 1986 Patterns of fractures in accidental and non-accidental injury in children: a comparative study. British Medical Journal 292: 100

White R, Carr P, Love N 1990 The guide to The Children Act 1989. Butterworth, London.

9. Accidents

J. Wynne

Accidents are a major child health problem in the UK, and inadequate consideration is given to their prevention. There are relatively simple measures, for example, the wearing of seat-belts by children in cars (Mason 1988) or helmets by pedal cyclists (Simpson et al 1988, Lancet 1988) which would have an immediate beneficial effect. The Child Accident Prevention Trust (Jackson et al 1988) has recently reviewed and continues to highlight the need for education and a multidisciplinary approach to the problem of accidents in children. Figure 9.1 outlines how doctors might be involved in accident prevention in a co-ordinated way within a health district. Table 9.1 shows examples of some successful preventative measures already employed.

How big is the problem? The morbidity and mortality resulting from accidents form the largest single health problem of childhood beyond the first year of life. Half of the deaths in children aged 1–15 years are due to accidents and over half of these are clearly caused by road traffic accidents. Deaths from accidents outnumber all deaths from other causes, including malignancy, congenital malformation and respiratory disease.

Over 900 children die each year from accidents; the order being road accidents followed by choking, burns and drowning. About one in six children attend an accident and emergency department each year and one in 80 is admitted (of the general child population). By the age of 5 years 44% of children have received medical attention as a result of an accident (Butler 1980). Over 60% of accidents occur in the home and less than 5% on the roads. However it is the road traffic accidents which account for more than half the deaths and much of the serious morbidity. In half of the fatal road accidents the child was a pedestrian.

Accidents kill and hurt children who were previously fit and healthy, in epidemic proportions. They result in much suffering to the child and his family which may be lifelong. They may cause a child to lose his childhood through disability. The incidence of serious injuries is much higher in lower social classes and so disability is added to

Table 9.1 Successful accident prevention methods

Method	Effect
1. Child-resistant containers — salicylate ingestion	85% decrease in hospital admission since introduction
2. Non-flammable nightwear legislation	80% decrease in burns injury in USA
3. Hard helmets for cyclists	90% decrease in deaths in Australia
4. Infant restraints in cars	89% unrestrained in UK

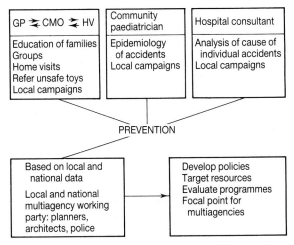

Fig. 9.1 Co-ordinated accident prevention within a health district. GP = general practitioner, CMO = clinical medical officer, HV = health visitor.

social disadvantages (Alwash & McCarthy 1988). Accidents are expensive too and consume 1% of the GNP in the UK (Vipulendran 1988). Twenty per cent of the admissions to hospital of children over the age of 12 months are due to trauma, and even for those children admitted overnight only for 'observation' there are sequelae for the child and his family.

A child's environment, whether in the home or outside, is still largely planned with the needs of adults in mind.

Children need to be able to explore, run and climb, but lack discretion and judgement, so it is the task of responsible adults (parents, planners, architects) to consider their needs and to protect them. Planners may not understand a young child's limited abilities and the need for a multi-disciplinary approach to prevention is the main theme in a recent monograph (Constantinides 1987). There is however a need for a detailed epidemiological study of accidents — where, when, how many, of what type, the means of injury and their severity, in a local as well as national context to give a scientific basis for prevention and evaluation of pilot schemes (Fig. 9.1).

From the available data it is not surprising that children from the poorest homes have the greatest risk of having serious accidents. Children from deprived inner cities are more likely to play in the street, near the railway line or on the canal bank. Boys in social class VI have almost five times the risk of being involved in fatal accidents as boys in social class I.

As children grow older bicycle accidents and motorbike accidents are important. The number of injuries to cyclists is increasing. Research shows pedal cyclists sustain more severe head injuries, and motorcyclists more severe injuries to the body. The case for pedal cyclists to wear helmets and the introduction of more cycle lanes has been made (Simpson et al 1988, Lancet 1988). A recent study from California has also highlighted the dangers of carrying young children as passengers on bicycles; in general children aged less than 12 months or weighing more than 20 kg should not be carried, the child should wear a helmet and be strapped in.

Certain sports, for example horse-riding and rugby, have recently been reviewed. The wearing of riding helmets, with chin strap fastened, and the prevention of neck injury in rugby (at least in New Zealand) by minor alterations in the rules, are welcome. Again, if each serious injury in sport is investigated by a local accident prevention team, progress should be made.

In 1986, 3090 children under 5 years were killed or injured as pedestrians (Gloag 1988). Most accidents are not around 'black-spots' but wherever children are, and it is the young unprotected child's perceptual and cognitive limitations which make him so vulnerable to fast-moving traffic. Parents too show an extraordinary lack of understanding; in one Nottingham survey, 20% of the mothers of 2-year-olds thought their children safe on the local roads and 30% of the mothers of 3-year-olds! The Government is still considering the possibility of a national preschool road safety club. In Scandinavia for some years there have been such schemes and the 'Streetwise Kids' pilot in London from 1985 suggests a favourable effect.

Home accidents are most likely to occur at times of stress. Studies show relevant factors include a young, depressed, tired mother on tranquillizers with two or more preschool children. The children are often under 5 years and described as overactive. Once again home accidents occur more commonly in socially deprived households. Poorly designed and maintained homes, open balconies and stairs are often implicated. Where are the children to play? Play areas and equipment need careful design and regular maintenance. Young children in parks need supervision, with separate facilities from older children. Children may drown in canals, ornamental ponds or paddling pools as well as the sea and rivers. There is a widespread programme to teach children to swim, but usually those older than 5 years.

SCALDS AND BURNS

Scalds and burns whilst accounting for relatively few deaths (around 8% of trauma deaths) cause terrible morbidity in some children because of scarring deformity, disability and psychological upset for the child and his family.

The chief causes of scalds are spilt hot fluids from kettles, teapots and saucepans. Children aged

15 months to 3 years are often involved as they may pull down tablecloths, flexes or cups from work surfaces.

Housefires and deaths from the effects of smoke are more common in multi-occupied, poor dwellings with poorly maintained or inappropriatly used heating.

Management

The management of a severely burned child is complex. The immediate treatment at home is to remove any clothes over which hot fluid has been spilled. Small scalds and burns may be cooled under cold running water. Any larger injury should be covered by a clean towel or sheet and the child taken to hospital.

If a child has burns of the eyes, face, neck, hands or perineum he should probably be admitted to hospital. If the burns involve more than 7% of the skin the child should also be admitted, as should children who have been in a smoke-filled room as they may later develop respiratory symptoms. Child abuse should be considered (see Ch. 8).

The management of a severely burned child includes assessing his airway, need for immediate analgesia and extent of the burns. Intravenous fluids will be needed if the child has more than 10% of his surface area burned. Charts are available to assess the area damaged. The child may be shocked from hypovolaemia and plasma and saline are used initially. If the child continues to lose large volumes of fluid, blood and protein the fluid balance and replacement fluids must be assessed carefully. A tetanus toxoid booster is given.

Children with severe burns should be seen by a specialist team and the subsequent plastic surgery often involves the child in long and complex hospital treatment.

Prevention

The prevention of burns and scalds involves better education including the use of appropriate guards around cookers, fires and care with electric flexes. Inflammable or fire-retardant materials would ideally be used for all childrens' clothes, but especially nightwear including dressing gowns. The heating of homes, use of paraffin heaters, foam-filled furniture and cigarette smoking are all causes of house fires.

CHOKING

Choking is the cause of over 100 child deaths each year, and inhaled peanuts in particular cause serious pulmonary damage. Children may choke on food such as crispy bacon or a foreign body, for example a small plastic toy, button or coin. There may be a history of choking or a sudden attack of coughing but the event may not have been witnessed and the child is seen with severe stridor, or if the obstruction is severe an increasingly cyanosed child making silent but violent respiratory effort. Large objects will tend to impact proximally whilst small fragments will tend to lodge distally and cause less dramatic symptoms.

Management

Management of the choking child is urgent. The first aid recommendation is to place the child face down and give four blows to the back. The child is placed across the adult's knee or an infant over an arm. If this fails compress the chest four times as in external cardiac massage.

The Heimlich manoeuvre in which sudden compression of the upper abdomen forces the diaphragm upward and propels the object out of the airway has been used. However in children damage to viscera may occur.

Direct laryngoscopy may be used, but if this is difficult an emergency airway can be established using a wide-bore cannula through the cricothyroid membrane until definitive treatment under anaesthetic is available.

Lower airways' obstructions present less acutely, usually involve the right main bronchus, and bronchoscopy should be arranged.

DROWNING

Drowning still accounts for over 100 deaths each year and many deaths are preventable. Ornamental ponds and the absence of supervision in bathtubs may prove lethal to toddlers. Most children now receive swimming lessons at school from around the age of 7–8 years. Children (and adults) frequently go out in boats without life-jackets, and each year children are swept out to sea in dinghies. More boys than girls are drowned and again drowning occurs more in socially disadvantaged families. Death from drowning may be because of laryngeal spasm or inhalation of water to the lungs, both of which lead to cerebral anoxia.

Management

Management involves ensuring a clear airway and usual cardiorespiratory resuscitation. In particular, if the water is cold, children have been known to survive even after prolonged periods of submersion so attempts at resuscitation should be prolonged.

Complications such as pulmonary oedema and infection should be treated as they arise.

HEAD INJURIES

Many children after even a relatively minor head injury go pale and vomit. Loss of consciousness, even briefly, is often used as an indiction for admission, if the vomiting persists or the child becomes drowsy or unwell always admit to hospital. In a younger child with an unexplained skull fracture consider the possibility of physical abuse (see Ch. 8).

If the child has not lost consciousness and appears well, give the parents oral and written instructions about observation and allow the child home.

If there is a severe injury, e.g. a fracture, especially crossing the groove of the meningeal artery, CSF rhinorrhoea, bleeding from the ear or nose or if the child has lost consciousness or shows altered consciousness, admit to hospital. Observations should include measurement of heart rate and blood pressure, pupil size and reactivity and conscious level.

The Glasgow coma scale is an objective scale which allows observers to assess changes in the level of consciousness. The responses are graded from a fully orientated patient obeying commands to a deeply unconscious one with no verbal response, no eye opening and extensor plantar responses.

The signs of an increasing intracranial pressure are a diminishing level of consciousness, a falling heart rate and a rising blood pressure, with alteration in the size and reactivity of the pupils. This may be due to cerebral oedema (without necessarily skull fracture) or intracranial bleeding. Bleeding may be extradural, usually from the middle meningeal artery, and causes early signs of increased pressure or subdural bleeding from cerebral veins which tend to be a later complication.

The immediate assessment of the child will determine the need for immediate ventilation and increasingly continuous intracranial pressure measurements. A CT (computerized tomography) scan will differentiate between bleeding and cerebral oedema or cerebral contusion.

Neurosurgery is necessary if there is compression from a clot. Bleeding may also be stopped.

Cerebral oedema is treated by intravenous mannitol, dexamethasone and hyperventilation.

The prognosis after a head injury is difficult to assess initially. Some children after even weeks of coma do surprisingly well but conversely other children unconscious for as little as 24 hours may suffer serious sequelae.

The long-term problems include learning difficulties, which may amount to severe mental handicap, motor deficits, epilepsy, behaviour problems and personality changes. 'Post-concussional syndrome' also occurs in children — often for several months after a head injury — with complaints of headache, poor concentration, anxiety, irritability and so on as in adults. Although the most significant progress following a severe head injury is in the first 12 months after the accident, a child will continue to improve, particularly in terms of motor deficit, for years. However, learning difficulties and personality problems may persist.

Many neurosurgeons use prophylactic antibiotics immediately after an open head injury and anticonvulsants for 1–2 years after the injury.

INGESTION

A large multicentre study (Wiseman et al 1987) was set up to look at the causes of accidental poisoning, their outcome, and to investigate the role of the type of packaging. As in other studies the children are young, 2–3 years, adult supervision was faulty, the ingestion took place at home with the drug in its usual storage place only 40% of the time, and 63% of substances were not in child-resistant containers. Of the children seen at hospital 22% were admitted and less than 1% needed intensive care. There were no deaths.

The range of substances taken is given in Table 9.2.

Research shows that child-resistant containers, strips, sachets and opaque blister packs are all relatively safe. *But* whilst safe packaging is needed so is safe storage. There is no child-resistant container which will fit on a standard liquid medicine bottle, although such containers exist for some over-the-counter liquid medicines, e.g. Calpol. Clearly this is a major concern given the effectiveness in reducing salicylate poisoning in the late 1970s and the knowledge that liquids accounted for 42% of the poisoning episodes in the quoted study (Wiseman et al 1987).

Continuing publicity campaigns are needed to educate the public and also further studies of the use of local telephone advice services for parents.

Management

The management begins with identification of the ingested substance, and assessment of the maximum dose which has possibly been ingested. The National Poisons Information Service Centres (Table 9.3) will give information on constituent and toxicity of different household products,

Table 9.2 Substances ingested in accidental poisoning incidents

Substance ingested	% of incidents
Drug	59
Analgesic	
Anxiolytic	
Cough medicine	
Oral contraceptive	
Household substance	37
Bleach	
Detergent	
Petroleum product	
Plants	3

Table 9.3 National Poisons Information Centres telephone numbers

Belfast	0232–30503
Cardiff	0222–492233
Edinburgh	031–229–2477
London	071–407–7600
Leeds	0532–432799
Manchester	061–740–2254

plants, and the expected consequences of ingestion of the named substances.

In general terms, after an immediate assessment of the child and the need for resuscitation, the poison is removed from the stomach unless there are contraindications. There are specific antidotes and therapy for a minority of poisonings.

Emesis is induced with 15 ml of ipecacuanha in orange juice unless the child is not fully conscious or has ingested corrosives, turpentine or paraffin.

Salicylates and tricyclic antidepressants are the most toxic of the substances commonly ingested. Corrosive household materials like bleach are potentially harmful and cause stricture but children usually take a taste and spit it out. Paraffin, turpentine and other volatile liquids may cause signs and symptoms of pneumonitis after an apparently small ingestion. Toxic fluids, e.g. weed killer, may have been decanted into lemonade bottles and drunk accidentally.

It is clear that in the very young, children may be accidentally poisoned by parents; accidental self-poisoning occurs from 2 to 9 years; from 10 years upwards intentional poisoning becomes a major problem. All these older children and their families should be assessed by the child and family psychiatric services, whereas the health visitor has a clear educational role in younger children. Older children also begin to experiment with drink, solvents and drugs. Excessive drinking is widespread in society and the adverse effects on health of alcohol abuse are much underestimated by the public in general.

LEAD POISONING

Lead poisoning is uncommonly diagnosed in the UK but there is continuing concern about the lead children inhale in inner cities and the possible effect this has on learning and behaviour.

Sources of lead:

1. Ingested lead-based paint.
2. Lead water-pipes.
3. Burning of car batteries.
4. Surma and other lead-based cosmetics.
5. Atmospheric pollution from exhaust fumes from more vehicles and industry.

Clinically children may be pale, lethargic and constipated, with pica, but many are asymptomatic. Severe poisoning may lead to an encephalopathy with seizures and coma due to cerebral oedema. The diagnosis may be made on the basis of a plain abdominal X-ray to look for evidence of lead in the GI tract, and lead lines in the long bones, the serum free erythrocyte protoporphyrin (FEP) level, serum lead level and anaemia.

Management involves removing the source of lead from the child, and in some cases chelating agents are used. If the child has an encephalopathy chelating agents are used as well as treatment of the cerebral oedema and general support.

A full family and social as well an an environmental investigation is needed.

CIGARETTE SMOKING

Cigarette smoking is gradually decreasing in society as a whole but there are worrying trends, especially in the teenage population. They are a difficult group to deter, many adolescents do not see the longer term as a problem, being unable to perceive of themselves as old as 40 years and beyond.

Education of potential parents may be more successful. Babies born to smokers are lighter and tend to be born early. Children brought up in households where the adults smoke have more recurrent respiratory problems as well as the currently described problems of 'passive smoking'. They are also ultimately more likely to smoke themselves.

ALCOHOL ABUSE

Abuse of alcohol is of increasing concern. Of the children seen in hospital most have acquired their alcohol from home. Spirits and wines are the least well tolerated. Sometimes children play dangerous games with alcohol, and many crimes in the 15–25 years' age group are performed under the influence of alcohol. From the fetal-alcohol syndrome, through neglect due to parental alcoholism and emotional and other abuse, children from homes where a parent is alcoholic often have a difficult, unrewarding childhood.

SOLVENT ABUSE

Volatile, organic chemicals are sniffed and the list is long, but adhesives, lighter fuel and nail polish remover are commonly used. There is a mortality from direct toxicity or intoxication leading to serious accidents. Children who sniff tend to come from emotionally deprived homes and there is an overlap with other abuses, for example alcohol and cigarettes, and an association with other socially unacceptable behaviour.

Teenagers often sniff in groups of children aged from 12 to 16 years, but younger children may join in too. A minority of children appear to become psychologically addicted and may sniff alone and with great regularity. The child describes effects similar to alcohol, with euphoria but subsequent depression. Long-term deleterious effects on the kidneys and neuropathic damage have been described in chronic sniffers. The habitual sniffer may be recognized by spots or reddening about the mouth but the other symptoms of fatigue, listlessness and poor school performance are common in other depressed teenagers.

SUMMARY

Doctors working in child health do have a role in the prevention of accidents (Jackson 1988). Many may feel they have a responsibility but feel uncertain about what to do (Fig. 9.1).

Armed with information of the accidents and injuries occurring, child health doctors can then take a reasoned case to the planners, designers and others responsible for making the environment safe for children. Other issues such as drunken driving, lead-free petrol and irradiation will need national action. But the main predictor of accidents in children continues to be social disadvantage.

REFERENCES

Alwash R, McCarthy M 1988 Measuring severity of injuries to children from home accidents. Archives of Disease in Childhood 63: 635–638

Butler N 1980 Child health and education in the seventies: some results on the first five years follow up of the 1970 British Birth Cohort. Health Visitor 53: 81–2

Constantinides P 1987 The management response to childhood accident. Kings Fund Centre, London

Craft A W 1988 Accidental poisoning. Archives of Disease in Childhood 63: 584–586

Gloag D 1988 Games to play and accidents to prevent. British Medical Journal 296: 378

Jackson R H 1988 The doctor's role in the prevention of accident. Archives of Disease in Childhood 63: 235–237

Jackson R H, Cooper S, Hayes H R M 1988 The work of the Child Accident Prevention Trust. Archives of Disease in Childhood 63: 318–320

Lancet 1988 When are cyclists going to wear helmets? i: 159

Mason M A 1988 Restraining infants in cars. British Medical Journal 296: 1345

Simpson A H R W, Unwin P S, Nelson I W 1988 Head injuries, helmets, cycle lanes and cyclists. British Medical Journal 296: 1161

Vipulendran V 1988 Cost of NHS accidents to children in the West Midlands. British Medical Journal 296: 611

Wiseman H M, Guest V S G, Volans G N 1987 Accidental poisoning in childhood: a multicentre survey 1. General epidemiology 2. The role of packaging in accidents involving medications. Human Toxicology 6: 293–314

10. The newborn baby

A. Whitelaw

The state of health of a fetus and newborn baby is influenced by the quality of the intrauterine environment and by the mechanics of delivery. Maternal mortality is very low in Western countries, but the mother's physical health, nutrition and social habits are important to fetal welfare; maternal morbidity may influence fetal outcome. Maternal factors associated with impaired fetal growth and increased perinatal mortality are:

1. Severe undernutrition.
2. Adverse social state.
3. Smoking.
4. Severe and prolonged hypertension in pregnancy.
5. Chronic renal disease.
6. Opiate drug dependence.
7. Alcoholism.
8. High altitude.
9. Cyanotic heart disease.

Maternal diabetes must be well controlled in pregnancy, or preterm delivery of a large fetus with subsequent respiratory distress syndrome and hypoglycaemia may result. Thyroid disorders, anaemia, urinary tract infection and cardiac disease also require careful treatment in pregnancy.

ASSESSMENT OF FETAL WELL-BEING

Regular palpation of a growing uterus and maternal perception of vigorous fetal movements are reassuring in the antenatal clinic. If there is concern about the fetus, measurements of the biparietal diameter of the head or abdominal circumference can be carried out using ultrasound. Serial measurements can reveal the rate of growth of the fetus. Doppler measurement of blood velocity in the umbilical artery and fetal aorta is increasingly used to assess the health of the fetus. Decreasing diastolic flow is associated with fetal hypoxia. Real-time ultrasound can also show abnormal positions of the placenta, anomalies of the heart, gastrointestinal tract, urinary tract, spine and brain.

The term 'fetal distress' is used to describe a fetus suffering from hypoxia. The causes are:

1. Obliterative vascular lesions in the placental bed.
2. Longstanding placental insufficiency.
3. Placental separation and haemorrhage.
4. Acute compression of the umbilical cord.
5. Fetal anaemia or haemorrhage.
6. Maternal shock or hypoxia.
7. Uterine spasm.

Fetal distress occurs most commonly during labour but may occur before. It may be suggested by the passage of meconium in utero, or by the presence of fetal heart decelerations, measured by scalp electrode or externally, persisting after a uterine contraction has relaxed (late dips or type-II dips), by a persistent tachycardia over 160 per minute with little variation, or by fetal scalp blood pH below 7.2.

RESUSCITATION OF THE NEWBORN

The need for resuscitation of an asphyxiated newborn can arise at any time and quite unexpectedly. Many hypoxic infants can, however, be predicted and in these cases a trained member of staff and resuscitation equipment should be present in the following circumstances:

1. Fetal distress.
2. Caesarean section.
3. Breech presentation.
4. Multiple pregnancy.
5. Gestation below 37 weeks.
6. Intrauterine growth retardation.
7. Maternal diabetes mellitus.
8. Rhesus iso-immunisation.
9. Use of large doses of sedatives or analgesic drugs.

The Apgar score is the most common way of recording the degree of hypoxia at birth (Table 10.1).

The Apgar score at 1 minute is useful in indicating the need for resuscitation and the 5 minute score is an indication of long-term prognosis. Those infants with a score of 3 or below are more likely to have cerebral palsy later. The most important items are heart rate and respiratory effort. Because of the risk of virus infection from maternal blood, it is now recommended that gloves and eye protection be worn by staff resuscitating an infant at a delivery. If an infant remains blue after delivery and does not cry, the pharynx should be aspirated. If the infant does not breathe within 10 seconds, place the infant supine on a flat surface, preferably under a radiant heater. Apply an infant face-mask and ventilate the baby using 100% oxygen and a Penlon or Ambu bag at 40–50 breaths per minute. Make sure the mask fits tightly over the nose and mouth and that the chest is expanding. Face-mask ventilation produces adequate lung expansion and gas exchange in many babies that are mildly asphyxiated or sedated.

Well conducted face-mask ventilation is more effective than a prolonged attempt at intubation even in the preterm infant. However, if the infant remains bradycardic (heart rate <100/min), apnoeic, cyanosed and motionless despite face-mask ventilation, endotracheal intubation is essential. If the heart rate remains below 40 per minute external cardiac massage with two fingers on the mid-sternum at 120 per minute should be started. If the mother has received pethidine or morphine within 4 hours of delivery, it is always worthwhile giving naloxone — an opiate antagonist with no sedative properties of its own — 0.2 mg can be given intramuscularly by a nurse while the doctor ventilates the baby.

Most babies requiring ventilation by face-mask or endotracheal tube are pink, active and breathing within 5 minutes. The endotracheal tube can be removed after suctioning and the baby observed. If he remains active and well, after a quick general examination he can be wrapped up and given to his mother or father to hold. If the baby develops grunting, cyanosis, indrawing or appears floppy or inactive, he needs to be transferred to a special baby care unit.

ROUTINE EXAMINATION OF THE NEWBORN

Each baby should be examined soon after birth as the parents will want to know if he is normal. The examiner should search for serious congenital abnormalities, adverse effects of intrauterine life or delivery, and should make an estimate of gestational age to see if the baby's growth is appropriate. A final examination before discharge home is necessary to look for congenital abnormalities that might have been hidden at birth, acquired disease, such as jaundice or infection, and to discuss problems such as sleeping, feeding and growth with the mother. It is best to examine the baby with the parents. Gentleness and thoroughness are required: before you handle the baby, observe posture, breathing and colour; is the respiratory rate raised above 60 per minute?; does the baby appear excessively pale, blue, red

Table 10.1 Apgar score

Sign	Score		
	0	1	2
Heart rate	Absent	<100	<100
Respiration	Absent	Weak Gasping Irregular	Good Crying Regular
Muscle tone	Completely flaccid	Some flexion of extremities	Well flexed
Reflex irritability (response to nasal catheter)	No response	Grimace	Cough Sneeze Gasp
Colour of trunk	White	Blue	Pink

or yellow? Cyanosis of the extremities is very common in newborns, but the lips and tongue should be pink.

Parents are naturally very concerned about skin blemishes and you may do a great service by explaining these. Milia are small cysts in the epidermis; they are white or pale yellow papules usually less than 1 mm in diameter around the nose and resolve during the first month. Stork bites (macular haemangioma) are flat salmon-pink or red blotches most commonly over the bridge of the nose, the eyelids and the nape of the neck. They are extremely common, but the marks on the face usually disappear within a few months. The marks on the nape of the neck may persist longer, but are covered by hair. A strawberry naevus is usually not visible at birth, but appears and grows rapidly in the first few weeks after birth. The lesions are raised, red and bumpy. They may grow rapidly in the first 6–9 months and may produce an alarming appearance if they are near the eyes. These lesions are capillary cavernous haemangiomas and are extremely vascular. They nearly always begin to regress by the end of the first year, the earliest sign is the development of pale patches in the centre, and spontaneous resolution is very likely before the child is 5 years old. Plastic surgery is extremely difficult because of the vascular nature of these lesions and should not be recommended because of the good prognosis. A port-wine stain is flat and is due to persistent dilatation of capillaries. The lesion may be extensive and, unfortunately, is usually permanent. Neonatal urticaria (erythema toxicum) affects many babies within the first 2–4 days. It usually starts on the trunk as erythematous patches with a white papule in the centre. The rash may be extensive and shows a tendency to vary from hour to hour. The cause is not known but you can confidently reassure the mother that it will disappear without any treatment. Septic spots may occur in small groups, particularly in the axillae, the groins and around the neck. The lesions are pustules and may or may not have surrounding erythema. Petechiae are small purple spots which do not blanch when pressed. They may be a normal finding around the head because of trauma during delivery. However, they are not a normal finding on the rest of the

body after vertex deliveries and their presence suggests a bleeding disorder, particularly thrombocytopenia.

The occipito-frontal head circumference should be measured carefully and compared with the range for the baby's gestational age. A cephalhaematoma is a swelling produced by bleeding under the periosteum of one of the cranial bones. This is most common on the parietal bones. The swelling is limited by the suture lines and the lesion usually increases during the first few days after birth. The haematoma leads to jaundice and the swelling may persist for months. A caput succedaneum is oedema of the part of the head presenting through the cervix, there is no limitation to particular bones of the skull and the swelling disappears in a few days.

The face should be examined. A cleft lip is obvious but the palate should also be inspected and felt to exclude a cleft. Note any purulent discharge from the eyes. Turn the overhead lighting down, support the baby's head up and, if he is awake, he is likely to open his eyes. Inspect the eyes with an ophthalmoscope noting any opacity in the red reflex filling the pupil. It is important to diagnose congenital cataract particularly if bilateral as early treatment improves the prognosis for vision. Subconjunctival haemorrhages are harmless and disappear in 1–2 weeks. Down's syndrome is suggested not only by slanting eyes and epicanthic folds but also obvious hypotonia, single transverse palmar creases, short incurved little fingers, a flat occiput, small head circumference, simple ears and abnormal dermal ridge patterns.

If the baby's breathing and colour are normal do not waste time listening to the lungs. Auscultate the heart, and if you hear an ejection systolic murmur in an otherwise well baby re-examine the heart in a few days' time. The murmur may disappear during these few days. Significant cardiac signs include the presence of a pansystolic murmur loud in intensity, a gallop rhythm, absent femoral pulses, central cyanosis not relieved by oxygen and congestive cardiac failure with rapid respiration, rapid heart rate and a large liver. The abdomen should be observed for distension. Gently feel each side of the abdomen for enlargement of the liver, spleen, kidneys or any other mass. Feel for a hernia in the groin, scrotum or labia. Note whether both the testes are in the scrotum. Small hydroceles usually resolve without treatment. Note the position of the urethra and make sure that there is a normal anal opening. In a girl make sure that the urethra and vagina are normally situated. Enlargement of the clitoris or fusion of the labia may be due to masculinisation by adrenal hyperplasia. Turn the baby over and examine the whole length of the spine for openings. Examine all four limbs and make sure that the normal number of digits is present. You will not impress the mother with your competence if you have omitted to notice that the baby has an extra finger.

It is best to leave the examination of the hips until last because this is the one part of the examination where it is legitimate to produce some temporary discomfort in the baby. This must be explained to the mother before you test for congenital dislocation of the hips. Hold the baby's legs as shown in Figure 10.1; test one hip at a time. Adduct the hip pressing downwards along the line of the femur; a dislocatable hip will slip over the posterior edge of the acetabulum with this manoeuvre. Then abduct the femur pressing medial with the middle finger on the greater trochanter. If the head of the femur re-enters the acetabulum a clunk is also felt.

The hip joint may be in place at rest but dislocatable on adduction or it may be dislocated at rest and reducible into the acetabulum on abduction. Management involves maintaining abduction with a suitable splint for 2–3 months, and taking a radiograph at 6 months to confirm normal joint development. Congenital dislocation of the hip, if untreated in the neonatal period, may be difficult to cure later even with multiple surgical operations and prolonged hospitalisation.

LOW BIRTHWEIGHT INFANTS

Babies born at less than 37 completed weeks from the last menstrual period are termed preterm and babies with birthweights below the 10th centile for gestational age are small for dates. If the mother is certain of the date of her last menstrual period and was not on the contraceptive pill, her estimated date of delivery is likely to be accurate. However, this is not the case with many mothers and the expected date of delivery may have been estimated by palpation of the uterus or ultrasound measurements of the fetus early in pregnancy. The most widely used method of assessing gestational age in the newborn is that compiled by Dubowitz et al (1970). This uses external physical characteristics and neurological characteristics, particularly tone. In babies that are ill at the time of examination, tone may be reduced and this will depress the neurological part of the score.

Preterm infants

Cervical incompetence, pre-eclamptic toxaemia, infection, placental abruption and placenta praevia are causes of preterm delivery but, in many, the aetiology is unknown. Preterm babies may develop a number of serious complications after birth due to their immaturity.

1. Hyaline membrane disease

(Respiratory distress syndrome)

2. Feeding difficulties

Babies of less than 35 weeks' gestation are usually unable to suck adequately their own nutritional requirements. Nasogastric feeding of milk may be required in small volumes at frequent intervals.

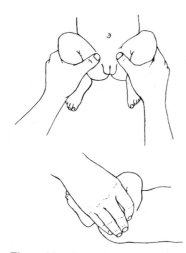

Fig. 10.1 The position for testing the stability of a baby's hips (from Brown & Valman (1979) with permission of the authors and publishers).

The capacity of the stomach may be very small and regurgitation and aspiration are possible hazards.

3. Hypothermia

The preterm baby has little insulating subcutaneous fat, an increased surface to weight ratio compared with term babies and reduced energy stores. Because of his other medical problems he is likely to be more exposed when being handled and treated. Cold stress has been shown to increase oxygen requirements, calorie requirements and mortality. Low birthweight babies require a thermoneutral environment. For most babies under 1800 g a closed incubator is the best way of achieving this. The ranges of temperature for thermoneutrality have been determined for different birthweights and at different ages after birth (Hey 1971).

4. Apnoea

Infants of less than 32 weeks' gestation are prone to periods of stopping breathing with bradycardia. These may be short lived and self limiting but in some cases obvious hypoxia occurs. Although apnoea may be a symptom of almost any underlying disease in preterm infants, it may occur purely as a result of immaturity. Infants of less than 34 weeks' gestation need to be on a respiration or heart rate monitor so that apnoea or bradycardia can be automatically detected and stimulation or resuscitation given as required.

5. Sepsis

6. Hyperbilirubinaemia

7. Maternal deprivation

Because of the factors listed above, babies who are significantly preterm tend to spend a number of weeks, if not months, in special care nurseries before they are able to be looked after at home. It may be difficult for a young mother, particularly with her first baby, to feel emotionally close to her tiny infant in a perspex incubator. Besides the physical separation and the difficulties of travelling from home to the special care nursery, the mother

may have a feeling of inadequacy because she cannot provide all the care that the baby needs. Emotional difficulties between mother and child, and child abuse have been reported as being more common in infants who have been in special care nurseries.

8. Cerebral lesions

Infants under 32 weeks' gestation are vulnerable to two types of brain lesion, both of which can be readily diagnosed in the neonatal unit by cranial ultrasound. Periventricular haemorrhage (PVH) arises in the germinal matrix under the ventricular ependyma. Haemorrhage may rupture into the lumen of the ventricle (intraventricular haemorrhage) and multiple small blood clots may obstruct the drainage and reabsorption of cerebrospinal fluid, thus causing hydrocephalus. Sometimes the haemorrhage extends into the cerebral parenchyma laterally, producing haemorrhagic infarction which subsequently necroses to a porencephalic cyst communicating with the lateral ventricle. In such cases a contralateral hemiplegia will almost certainly follow. The pathogenesis of PVH is related to immaturity, respiratory distress syndrome and its complications. Reperfusion following shock (Miall-Allen et al 1987) and fluctuating cerebral blood flow (Perlman et al 1985) have been put forward as mechanisms.

Periventricular leukomalacia (PVL) is non-haemorrhagic infarction of the periventricular brain tissue. Unlike PVH, PVL is not most common in the extremely immature infants of 26 weeks, but rather tends to be found in infants of 28–32 weeks. Risk factors include antepartum haemorrhage, multiple pregnancy and shock. The lesions are nearly always bilateral and spastic diplegia is the commonest consequence. If the lesions are extensive, quadriplegia, mental retardation and cortical blindness are likely (De vries et al 1985).

SMALL-FOR-GESTATIONAL-AGE INFANTS

The first list on p. 95 shows factors which may produce fetal growth retardation with delivery of a small-for-gestational-age infant. In severe pre-eclamptic toxaemia, intrauterine growth may come to a halt and there may be shrinking of the abdominal circumference on ultrasound. Such a fetus is in a state of starvation and is in danger of total asphyxiation with intrauterine death before or during labour. The obstetrician may well decide to deliver the baby by Caesarian section, arguing that the environment in the uterus is more hostile than the environment outside. Such a baby often requires resuscitation at birth but, if this is successfully managed, most of these babies do well with modern techniques. They are prone to hypoglycaemia having very small energy stores of glycogen and fat. They are also likely to develop hypothermia. Less commonly, small-for-gestational-age babies have polycythaemia; this is thought to result from chronic intrauterine hypoxia. If the venous haematocrit is above 70% the viscosity of the blood may be excessive and tissue perfusion may be impaired. A successfully delivered small-for-gestational-age baby of 1000 g with a gestational age of 35 weeks is likely to have a much smoother postnatal course than a 1000 g infant of 27 weeks' gestation. The prognosis for small-for-gestational-age babies depends very much on the underlying reasons for their small size. If a baby has suffered from intrauterine rubella or has a multiple congenital malformation syndrome the outlook is poor. On the other hand, a successfully managed pre-eclampsia or multiple pregnancy with careful monitoring postnatally of blood glucose and body temperature should result in a healthy infant. Babies who have had a brief period of intrauterine growth retardation have the capacity to catch up in their somatic growth if they are well nourished. However, babies who have had a prolonged period of intrauterine growth retardation (10–20 weeks) may not catch up fully in their growth later in childhood (Fancourt et al 1976).

NUTRITION

Babies require adequate calories for basal metabolism, temperature regulation, muscular activity and growth; amino acids for protein synthesis; electrolytes, minerals and vitamins. The feed should be palatable, easily digested, non-allergenic and free from infection. Breast feeding meets all the needs of full-term babies. Untreated cows'

milk is very far from being suitable for newborn babies. Pasteurisation may remove most bacteria, but cows' milk provides no added protection against infection and is capable of stimulating an allergic response. The main protein in cows' milk is casein. This tends to form a bulky curd in the baby's stomach and the proportions of amino acids in casein are not optimal for human babies. The fat in cows' milk is more saturated than that in human milk and fat absorption is reduced. The phosphate content of cows' milk is very much higher than in human milk and this may result in hyperphosphataemia with hypocalcaemic tetany. The sodium content of cows' milk is considerably higher than human milk; under most conditions a healthy baby will be able to handle this increased sodium load but if the baby develops fever and diarrhoea, the water loss involved may result in hypernatraemia.

Recently, cows' milk has been highly modified in order to reduce the above disadvantages. Initially, the milk was diluted to lower the protein content and the calorie content was maintained by the addition of sucrose. It was prepared as a powder which could then be diluted with boiled water. This feed was used for many years as National Dried Milk in the UK. However, the milk was unsatisfactory and further modifications have now been made to cows' milk. The casein content has been greatly reduced and most modern milks are based on demineralised whey. The sodium content of the modern baby milk is approximately the same as in human milk. Polyunsaturated fats have replaced much of the butter fat resulting in improved fat absorption. The phosphate content has been substantially reduced. Vitamins A, B group, C, D, E, iron, copper and zinc have been added.

Although modern baby milks are a great improvement on their predecessors, breast milk still has a number of advantages. The physical closeness involved in breast feeding helps the emotional attachment between mother and baby. Human breast milk contains its own lipase and thus helps its own digestion at a time when the baby's own pancreatic lipase secretion may be inefficient. Human breast milk contains 5 mg per 100 ml of taurine but cows' milk and artificial formula feeds contain less than 0.3 mg per 100 ml; newborn kittens have developed retinal degeneration on taurine-deficient diets but no deficiency syndrome has yet been defined in humans. Breast milk also has a number of protective factors including IgA, lactoferrin, lysozyme, an antiviral substance, white blood cells and produces a low stool pH which favours the growth of *Lactobacillus acidophilus* rather than *Escherichia coli*. Matthew et al (1977) reported that infants of allergic parents had significantly less eczema in the first 6 months of life if they were purely breast fed or received only soya bean milk when compared with babies fed with a cows' milk formula and supplemented with cereal and animal solid foods after 3 months.

NEONATAL JAUNDICE

Neonatal jaundice may need investigation and treatment because of the possibility of bilirubin encephalopathy (kernicterus) and because the jaundice may be due to an underlying disease which is dangerous in its own right. Approximately one-third of all newborn infants become clinically jaundiced during the first week. In what is often called physiological jaundice no kernicterus occurs and the jaundice fades by 10 days of age. This jaundice is due to the normal breakdown of red cells and is exacerbated by a transient deficiency of glucuronyl transferase and by reabsorption of bilirubin from the gut. Unconjugated bilirubin has a high lipid solubility and at high concentrations may saturate the bilirubin-binding capacity of plasma albumin thus allowing free unconjugated bilirubin to circulate in the plasma and enter nervous tissue. Bilirubin glucuronide (conjugated bilirubin) is poorly soluble in lipid and being water soluble can be excreted in bile and urine. Kernicterus affects the brain stem nuclei and basal ganglia particularly. Nerve deafness and choreoathetoid cerebral palsy are the commonest long-term effects but, if the condition is very severe, mental retardation and death may occur. There is a risk of kernicterus if the unconjugated plasma bilirubin rises above 400 μmol/l (24 mg/100 ml) in a full-term baby.

Preterm infants and hypoxic or acidotic infants may have a lower bilirubin-binding capacity and thus kernicterus may occur at unconjugated bilirubin levels much lower than 340 μmol/l (20 mg/100 ml). Neonatal jaundice should be con-

sidered abnormal if jaundice appears before 24 hours; the plasma unconjugated bilirubin is greater than 255 μmol/l (15 mg/100 ml); the jaundice persists beyond 10 days; or the conjugated bilirubin is greater than 34 μmol/l (2 mg/100 ml) (Table 10.2).

Treatment

If no underlying cause demands treatment, the main objective is to prevent kernicterus. If the plasma bilirubin is rising rapidly and may approach toxic levels, the baby should be treated with phototherapy. Light at a wavelength of 450 nm photo-isomerises unconjugated bilirubin to water-soluble forms which are not toxic and can be excreted without glucuronyl transferase. If, despite phototherapy, the plasma bilirubin approaches

Table 10.2 Causes of neonatal jaundice

	Causes

Neonatal jaundice before 24 hours	Haemolytic disease
	  Rhesus incompatibility
	  ABO incompatibility
	  Red cell defects
	Haematoma
	  Cephalhaematoma
	  Bruising to breech
	Polycythaemia
	  Small for gestational age
	  Twin–twin transformation

Unconjugated hyperbilirubinaemia after 24 hours	Haemolytic disease Haematoma Polycythaemia Prematurity Sepsis Dehydration Slow intestinal transit
Prolonged unconjugated jaundice	Haemolytic disease Breast milk jaundice, a diagnosis of exclusion in a well, breast-fed baby Hypothyroidism Sepsis, e.g. urinary tract infection
Prolonged conjugated jaundice (cholestasis)	Severe haemolytic disease Urinary tract infection Neonatal hepatitis Biliary atresia Galactosaemia Cystic fibrosis Tyrosinaemia

toxic levels, exchange transfusion provides a reliable way of lowering the bilirubin level. In many neonatal units, the exchange level for term infants is 400 μmol/l unconjugated bilirubin.

NEONATAL RESPIRATORY DISTRESS

The clinical signs of respiratory distress are tachypnoea (rate over 60/min), expiratory grunting, nasal flaring, cyanosis in air, and sternal, subcostal, intercostal or supraclavicular recession on inspiration. There are numerous possible causes, as detailed below:

1. Pulmonary causes:
   a. Hyaline membrane disease (respiratory distress syndrome).
   b. Retained lung fluid (transient tachypnoea).
   c. Meconium aspiration.
   d. Pneumonia.
   e. Pneumothorax.
   f. Diaphragmatic hernia.
   g. Hypoplastic lungs.
   h. Tracheo-oesophageal fistula.
   i. Congenital lobar emphysema.
   j. Lung cyst.
2. Cardiac failure.
3. Upper airway obstruction.
4. Overheating.
5. Anaemia or blood loss.
6. Neurological damage (in the brain stem respiratory control centre).
7. Polycythaemia.
8. Metabolic acidosis.

Hyaline membrane disease

In hyaline membrane disease (HMD) there is a deficiency of surfactant, a complex phospholipid which reduces surface tension and thus prevents collapse of small airways. HMD is associated with preterm delivery and asphyxia. In affected babies, progressive collapse of small airways occurs and the lungs are very stiff requiring increased work for breathing. Ventilation-perfusion mismatching and decreased alveolar ventilation results in progressive hypoxaemia and hypercapnoea. Chest X-ray shows a diffuse granularity throughout the lungs and an air bronchogram. Management con-

sists of maintaining arterial P_{O_2} at 6.7–12.0 kPa (50–90 mmHg) and nutritional support until the lungs recover after about 1 week. Some babies can maintain an adequate arterial P_{O_2} by breathing a humidified air-oxygen mixture in a head box. In more severe cases, continuous positive airway pressure (CPAP) is required to keep small airways open. This can be delivered by face-mask, twin nasal cannulae, nasopharyngeal tube or endotracheal tube. Mechanical ventilation with positive end-expiratory pressure becomes necessary if CPAP fails to maintain adequate blood gases, if respiratory acidosis allows the pH to fall below 7.2 and if the baby becomes apnoeic. Frequent or continuous monitoring of arterial P_{O_2} or transcutaneous P_{O_2} is necessary to avoid brain damage from hypoxia or retrolental fibroplasia from hyperoxia.

Retained lung fluid

This can affect term or preterm infants particularly after Caesarean section. The chest X-ray shows fluid streaks radiating out from the hila and fluid in the lung fissures. Although oxygen may be required, the prognosis is good.

Asphyxiation

Asphyxiated fetuses may pass meconium and then gasp, thus inhaling meconium. Meconium is irritating to the lungs and may obstruct airways causing collapse or a ball-valve effect with distal air trapping and the risk of pneumomediastinum. If a baby is born with meconium in the mouth, the larynx should be inspected and any meconium sucked out with as large a tube as possible. Chest X-ray shows coarse shadowing with overinflation, often with a pneumomediastinum.

Pneumonia

Group B streptococcal pneumonia may present a similar clinical and radiological picture to hyaline membrane disease. Death may occur within 12 hours. Factors favouring pneumonia would be a term infant, prolonged rupture of the membranes, maternal fever, foul-smelling liquor or a low neutrophil count (below 1500/μl). If this diagnosis is suspected, blood and a gastric aspirate should be taken for culture and ampicillin and gentamicin should be given.

INFECTION IN A NEONATE

Intrapartum and postnatal infection

Newborn infants are more vulnerable to infection than are older children because they lack IgM and IgA, have reduced complement factors and reduced chemotaxis by polymorphs. Preterm infants are even more immunodeficient as their levels of IgG are lower. Infants with sepsis in the first 48 hours usually present with respiratory distress, may have early apnoea and often develop profound neutropenia with exhaustion of the neutrophil storage pool. The organisms have come from the mother's genital tract. Group B streptococcus and *E. coli* are the commonest in most series, but *Haemophilus influenzae*, *Streptococcus pneumoniae* and *Listeria monocytogenes* are all major pathogens. Because the clinical presentation is so similar to respiratory distress syndrome, it is common practice to treat all infants with respiratory distress with ampicillin 100 mg/kg/12 hours intravenously (i.v.) and gentamicin 2.5 mg/kg/12 hours (i.v.) or intramuscularly (i.m.) (Nelson & McCracken 1983). Bacterial cultures results may take 48 hours and infants with early septicaemia may die within 12 hours. A blood culture and culture of respiratory secretions, ear or gastric aspirate should always be done prior to antibiotic treatment but lumbar puncture can be used selectively in infants with neurological abnormality or known positive blood culture.

Sepsis after 48 hours of age is usually from the infant's environment and not from the mother's genital tract. The presentation and spectrum of organisms are different. The presenting clinical features of late sepsis are:

1. Nurses' concern about baby.
2. 'Going off feeds'.
3. Fever (>37.5°C rectal) or hypothermia.
4. Vomiting.
5. Apnoea.
6. Tachypnoea.
7. Jaundice.
8. Lethargy.
9. Convulsions.
10. Purpura.
11. Palpable spleen or kidneys.

Late sepsis is often the result of invasive procedures and the commonest organism is *Staphylococcus epidermidis*. Other major late pathogens are *E. coli*, *Klebsiella aerogenes*, *Pseudomonas aeruginosa* and *Staphylococcus aureus*. Blood, urine and cerebrospinal fluid should be cultured before starting treatment. Flucloxacillin 50 mg/kg/12 hours i.v. and gentamicin is logical blind treatment but local sensitivity patterns may dictate a different choice.

Purulent conjunctivitis

This may be due to *Neisseria gonorrhoeae*. Gram stain of pus can confirm this diagnosis. Treatment is urgent to prevent corneal damage and penicillin eye drops should be given every 15 minutes until the pus clears. Intramuscular penicillin 50 000 units 12 hourly is also necessary.

Urinary tract infection

UTI may be very insidious in neonates producing only poor weight gain or prolonged jaundice. Because of the difficulties in collecting uncontaminated urine, diagnosis of UTI should be made on suprapubic aspiration.

Gastroenteritis

Epidemics of diarrhoea and vomiting are fortunately rate in neonatal units but salmonella, shigella, enteropathogenic *E. coli* and rotavirus can all spread easily from one baby to another. Management should be maintenance of fluid and electrolyte balance and isolation.

HYPOGLYCAEMIA

Hypoglycaemia (blood glucose below 2.0 mmol/l (36 mg/100 ml), is a potential cause of brain damage in infants. Infants at risk of hypoglycaemia are in the following categories:

1. Small-for-gestational-age infants (particularly if fed only from the breast).

2. Infants of diabetic mothers.
3. Preterm infants not absorbing milk feeds.
4. Infants with severe haemolytic disease.
5. Asphyxiated infants.
6. Hypothermia.
7. Septicaemia.

The brain may be able to compensate temporarily for a low blood glucose if there is plenty of oxygen and alternative substrate, such as lactate or ketone bodies but, eventually, neurological abnormalities such as convulsions are likely. There is a high incidence (up to 50%) of permanent neurological damage in babies with symptomatic hypoglycaemia.

All at-risk babies should have regular blood glucose screening with a testing strip (e.g. BM stix). If the reading is 2.0 mmol/l (36 mg/dl) or below, the blood glucose must be measured in the laboratory. If the baby appears neurologically abnormal or is unwell, 1 g/kg of glucose should be given intravenously immediately, followed by a continuous intravenous infusion of 10% glucose starting at 100 ml/kg daily. The rate and concentration of the intravenous glucose can then be adjusted in the light of repeated blood glucose estimations. Asymptomatic hypoglycaemia may be treated initially with frequent intragastric milk feeds, but if the blood glucose does not rise above 2.0 mmol/l intravenous glucose should be used.

VOMITING

Nearly all babies regurgitate some milk at some time. Vomiting is abnormal if it is bile stained, blood stained or persistent. Bile-stained vomit (i.e. greenish) is likely to be due to intestinal obstruction at any level below the sphincter of Oddi. There may be atresia, stenosis or malrotation with volvulus of the small intestine or aganglionosis of the large gut (Hirschsprung's disease). Erect and supine X-rays of the abdomen may confirm obstruction by showing dilated loops of intestine with fluid levels.

Blood-stained vomit may be due to haemorrhagic disease but this should be preventable by the injection of all newborns with 1 mg vitamin K in the delivery room. An acute gastric erosion may cause a haematemesis. Swallowed maternal blood may be vomited by the baby but the adult haemoglobin can be distinguished because sodium hydroxide denatures maternal but not fetal haemoglobin. Persistent vomiting may be due to sepsis, neurological damage, hiatus hernia and, later in the neonatal period, adrenal hyperplasia and pyloric stenosis.

DIARRHOEA

Breast-fed infants may pass rather loose stools up to four to six times a day. In spite of this the babies look well and thrive. Diarrhoea is only a problem if watery stools are copious, frequent and cause weight loss. Gastroenteritis is the most likely cause. If the diarrhoea is bloody, then necrotising enterocolitis and a bleeding tendency are also possible. Green stools often worry parents but do not signify disease.

NEUROLOGICAL ABNORMALITIES

Spina bifida

Spina bifida may result in an open lesion of the spinal cord with disorganised nervous tissue and meninges forming a swelling in the lumbar area (myelomeningocele) or a closed lesion with a swelling of the meninges containing CSF overlying the spine (meningocele). In the case of myelomeningocele, spinal cord function is often absent at and below the lesion whereas it may be intact at and below a meningocele. A paediatric surgeon can close an open defect and remove a swelling but this does not restore spinal cord function, although further damage from infection and drying is prevented. In a severe lower thoracolumbar myelomeningocele, there may be total paralysis below the umbilicus with resulting dislocation of the hips and talipes equinovarus deformities of the feet. There may be dilatation of the bladder and ureteric reflux. Even with successful surgery, the patient is paralysed below the waist and incontinent of urine and stool. Spina bifida is often associated with a downward displacement of the medulla resulting in defective circulation and reabsorption of CSF. This causes CSF to accumulate inside the cerebral ventricles with resulting hydrocephalus. This can be treated by insertion of a ventricular catheter connected to a one-way valve and leading to the right atrium or peritoneal cavity. Many experienced paediatricians feel that babies with extensive spina bifida and hydrocephalus have no chance of an independent happy life even with multiple surgical procedures. For a review of these issues see Lorber (1972).

Focal paralysis

The commonest lesion is Erb's palsy caused by traction on the upper nerve trunk in the brachial plexus (C5/6). The deltoid, biceps and supinator muscles are weak and the arm lies pronated by the side of the trunk. The grasp is normal. Muscle strength usually returns over 1–3 weeks unless the nerve trunks have been avulsed.

Convulsions

(See Ch. 24). The causes of convulsions in the newborn are:

1. Birth asphyxia.
2. Intracranial haemorrhage.
3. Hypoglycaemia.
4. Hypocalcaemia + hypomagnesaemia.
5. Hyponatraemia or hypernatraemia.
6. Meningitis.
7. Maternal opiate withdrawal.
8. Pyridoxine dependence.
9. Cerebral malformations.
10. Hyperammonaemia.

EEG studies have shown that subtle changes in eye movements and apnoea may be manifestations of seizure activity. However, a clinical diagnosis of convulsions in practical terms, means repetitive clonic movements with or without altered consciousness, respiratory changes or extensor rigidity.

The immediate management of convulsions is to clear the airway and give oxygen if required. Exclude hypoglycaemia as a possible cause and investigate the other possibilities as indicated. Phenobarbitone 20 mg/kg i.v. is the initial anticonvulsant treatment. If necessary, this is followed by paraldehyde 0.1 mg/kg rectally or 5% paraldehyde solution i.v. at 1 ml/kg/hour. Phenytoin 20 mg/kg i.v. should be given over 20 minutes. Diazepam i.v. may give rapid anticonvulsant effect but the dose required and the duration of action are very unpredictable.

Hypotonia

A full-term infant has a considerable degree of flexor tone, will resist extension of all limbs and will not let the head flop backwards more than about 45 degrees when lifted forwards from supine. Hypotonia with loss of antigravity power in the limbs, and postural abnormalities such as talipes would suggest a neuromuscular disease. As the prognosis and inheritance vary, it is important to support the infant with mechanical ventilation, if necessary, until a definite diagnosis is reached. A careful family history and examination of the mother are important.

Hypertonia

The neonatal brain reacts to various types of insult by producing extensor hypertonus. The neck extensors override neck flexion producing head retraction.

The limbs tend to be extended and adducted with feet crossed. The extensor tendon reflexes, such as the knee and ankle jerks, may be exaggerated and with sustained clonus. There may also be pathological irritability. Extensor hypertonus may occur with birth asphyxia, subarachnoid haemorrhage, hypoglycaemia, hypocalcaemia and raised intracranial pressure.

THE OBJECTIVES OF GOOD PERINATAL MEDICINE

Modern obstetrics and neonatal paediatrics has been strikingly successful in improving survival of babies and each year's mortality rate is usually lower than the last. There is now much emphasis on the prevention of handicap. The majority of children with cerebral palsy have had a perinatal mishap, most commonly birth asphyxia, periventricular leukomalacia or periventricular haemorrhage. Some children with mental retardation, epilepsy, deafness or blindness have perinatal causes for their handicap, such as hypoxia, hypoglycaemia, intraventricular haemorrhage, meningitis, kernicterus, gonococcal ophthalmia and retrolental fibroplasia. Good perinatal care may reduce these handicaps. Newborn infants in the UK are screened at 1 week for elevated blood levels of phenylalanine (phenylketonuria), tyrosine (tyrosinaemia) and, in some cities, thyroid stimulating hormone (hypothyroidism). Further handicap is prevented by the early treatment of these serious biochemical disorders.

The final objective of perinatal medicine is a happy and healthy family. Modern medicine need not drive a wedge between mother and baby. In the past, measures to prevent infection caused much separation of mothers and newborn infants and, in a few cases, made bonding difficult. Sensitive staff can promote the natural physical and emotional closeness of mother and baby even if the baby requires observation, investigation and treatment.

REFERENCES

Brown R J K, Valman H B 1979 Practical neonatal paediatrics, 4th edn. Blackwell, Oxford, pp 14, 29

De Vries L, Dubowitz L, Dubowitz V et al 1985 Predictive value of cranial ultrasound in the new born baby: a reappraisal. Lancet ii: 137–140

Dubowitz L M S, Dubowitz V, Goldberg C 1970 Clinical assessment of gestational age in the newborn infant. Pediatrics 77: 1–10

Fancourt R, Campbell S, Harvey D, Norman A P 1976 Follow-up study of small-for-dates babies. British Medical Journal 1: 1435–1437

Hey E 1971 The care of babies in incubators. In: Hull D, Gairdner D (eds) Recent advances in paediatrics. Churchill Livingstone, Edinburgh, p 171

Lorber J 1972 Spina bifida cystica. Archives of Disease in Childhood 47: 854–873

Matthew D J, Norman A P, Taylor B, Turner M W, Soothill J F 1977 Prevention of eczema. Lancet i: 321–324

McCracken G H, Nelson J D 1978 Antimicrobial therapy for newborns. Grune & Stratton, New York

Miall-Allen V, de Vries L, Whitelaw A 1987 Mean arterial pressure and neonatal cerebral lesions. Archives of Disease in Childhood 62: 1068–1069

Perlman J, Goodman S, Kreusser K, Volpe J 1985 Reduction in intraventricular haemorrhage by elimination of fluctuating cerebral blood flow velocity in preterm infants with respiratory distress syndrome. New England Journal of Medicine 312: 1353–1357

11. Infant feeding and nutrition

M. J. Brueton

A sound nutritional intake forms the basis of normal health, growth and development in childhood. As understanding of infant nutrition has increased, the technology required to manufacture sophisticated artificial milks has progressed rapidly. The range of formulations currently available reflects both the demand and the industry's continuing aim to match the elusive subtleties of human breast milk.

NUTRITIONAL REQUIREMENTS

The nutritional demands of the infant are unique. They are related to the requirements for growth, homeostasis, and the maintenance of a high metabolic rate. A balanced diet is essential and must include water, protein, fats and carbohydrates with their associated energy, vitamins and minerals. The requirements necessary in infancy are given in Tables 11.1 and 11.2. They should be regarded as guidelines, since individuals vary in their efficiency of food utilisation, and the values given were calculated theoretically on the basis of the intake found necessary to avoid deficiencies and promote normal growth in healthy children.

Fats

Most fat is ingested in the form of triglycerides (triacylglycerols), that is glycerol molecules in which three hydroxyl groups have each been esterified with fatty acids. These fatty acids may be long, medium or short chain according to the number of carbon atoms contained in each molecule. One-half of the fatty acids in human milk are long chain (more than 12 carbon atoms); medium chain fatty acids (8–12 carbon atoms) are of

Table 11.1 Daily requirements for young healthy infants (0–6 months) for energy, protein and water/kg bodyweight

Water	125–180 ml
Protein	2.2 g
Energy	115 kcal (0.48 MJ)

Energy values of nutrients as kcal/g = protein 4, carbohydrate 4, fat 7 (1 kcal 4.2 kJ, 1 MJ 240 kcal)

Table 11.2 Advisable vitamin and mineral intakes per kg bodyweight/day in healthy infants (0–6 months)

Vitamins		Minerals	
A(retinol)	420 μg	Sodium	1.5–2.5 mmol
D	10 μg	Potassium	2–3.5 mmol
C	35 mg	Iron	5–10 mg
Thiamine	0.3 mg	Calcium	350 mg
Riboflavin	0.4 mg	Magnesium	50 mg
Nicotinic acid	6.0 mg	Phosphorus	150 mg
E	3 mg	Iodine	35–45 μg
K	15 μg	Copper	60 μg
Folic acid	50 μg	Zinc	3 mg

interest since they are absorbed from the gut more readily. Fatty acids are also classified according to the number of unsaturated or double-bond linkages between the carbon atoms. Some of the polyunsaturated acids are not synthesised by the body and are essential in the diet, notably for prostaglandin production. These fatty acids include linoleic (18:2) arachidonic (20:4) and linolenic acids (18:3), vegetable fats are particularly rich sources. Other important constituents of fat are cholesterol and phospholipids. Cholesterol is the precursor of steroid hormones and bile acids, phospholipids are essential components of cell membranes and various other cellular components, and they play a part in the absorption and transfer of fatty acids.

Fat absorption is a multistep process. In the intraluminal phase, lipolysis and emulsification of triglycerides occurs in the duodenum secondary to the action of pancreatic lipase which requires colipase and bile salts for optimum activity. Monoglycerides, free fatty acids, and glycerol are released and interact with bile salts to form micelles. Micelles are water soluble and are able to diffuse through the microvillous membranes of the intestinal epithelial cells to enter the mucosal phase of fat absorption. Fatty acid uptake is facilitated by a binding protein which is concerned with transport to the endoplasmic reticulum of the cells. Triglycerides are resynthesised there and chylomicrons are formed in association with apoproteins. The final phase of absorption is the passage of these chylomicrons into the mesenteric lymphatics and to the portal venous system.

Carbohydrates

Carbohydrates provide the major source and bulk of calories in the diet. The disaccharide, lactose, containing the monosaccharides glucose and galactose, forms the major carbohydrate in milk. Cereals contain sucrose (glucose and fructose) and the starches, which are complex carbohydrates consisting of glucose units linked into dextrins and amylopectin. Carbohydrates also constitute an energy store in the form of glycogen, another polysaccharide of glucose. It should be noted that the major sites of glycogen storage are the liver and muscle which, in the infant, represent only a fraction of the adult reserves.

The intraluminal phase of carbohydrate digestion commences in the mouth with the action of salivary amylase on starch. Amylase is also secreted by the pancreas. Enterocyte brush border disaccharidases are then responsible for the mucosal digestion of lactose, maltose and sucrose. Glucose and galactose are absorbed by active transport systems, some of which are sodium dependent; fructose does not share the same mechanisms.

Proteins

Proteins provide nitrogen as well as calories. They contain amino acids linked by CO–NH bonds into long peptide chains. Eleven amino acids, at least, cannot be synthesised by the newborn and are essential in the diet. These include histidine, tyrosine and cystine, in addition to those necessary to avoid a negative nitrogen balance in adults, which are isoleucine, leucine, lysine, methionine, phenylalanine, threonine, tryptophan and valine. The structural proteins of the body can only be formed when the correct balance of amino acids is available. A high quality protein is one which supplies all the essential amino acids in sufficient amounts to fulfil the requirements for body maintenance and growth. Such proteins are said to have a high biological value. The balance between grams of amino acid nitrogen in the diet and non-protein calories is also critical, since the energy supply available forms a limiting factor to their efficient metabolism.

Protein digestion is initiated in the stomach by a group of proteases which are activated from precursor pepsinogens. The polypeptides released stimulate cholecystokinin and secretin which promote pancreatic enzyme secretion, and also enterokinase activity from the intestinal brush border membrane. The enzymes released include trypsin, chymotrypsin, elastase, the carboxypeptidases and aminopeptidases. There are several different transport mechanisms for the products of intestinal hydrolysis. Uptake of dipeptides and tripeptides occurs and is quite distinct from amino acid transport systems.

Water, minerals and vitamins

Water is second only to oxygen as a necessity for life and is even more important to babies than to older children. It represents 70–75% of their bodyweight; the intake volumes required are high and are also related to caloric consumption and the kidney's limited ability to conserve water in infancy.

The major minerals necessary include sodium, potassium, calcium, iron, phosphorus and magnesium. Many trace elements are also recognised to be essential, these include iodine, copper manganese, zinc, cobalt, molybdenum, selenium, chromium, tin, vanadium, fluorine, silicon and nickel. Vitamins A, D and C are of particular importance since supplementation is required. The vitamin B complex, vitamin E and folic acid must also be available.

GASTROINTESTINAL FUNCTION DURING INFANCY

Many aspects of gastrointestinal function are less well developed in the newborn than in the older infant and child. Gastric acid and pepsin activity are reduced in preterm neonates. Tryptic activity in duodenal juice and pancreatic lipase levels are low and increase rapidly after birth. Bile acid concentrations in the duodenum are often below the level required for micelle formation; this may be an important factor in the newborn's lesser ability to absorb fats. The activities of brush border sucrase and maltase increase during gestation and reach maximal activity by the eighth month, whereas lactase concentration increases close to term.

MILK FEEDING

Human milk

Most of the normal nutritional requirements for the young infant are provided in breast milk. The advantages of human milk over cows' milk mean that whenever possible mothers should be encouraged to breast feed. Even a period as brief as 2 weeks has been shown to be valuable, although ideally breast feeding should be continued for the first 4–6 months of life.

The advantages of breast milk include:

1. Its chemical composition. This differs from cows' milk (See Table 11.4 and below).

2. It is sterile, cheap and attractively packaged.

3. It does not contain proteins which will provoke allergic reactions.

4. It encourages a bowel flora favouring lactobacilli and discouraging *Escherichia coli*.

5. It contains antibodies and immunocompetent cells which are important in the development of the infant's immune system.

6. The intimacy of breast feeding promotes bonding with the infant.

7. Metabolic disorders in the newborn such as hypocalcaemia and hypernatraemia are less common.

8. Certain conditions such as gastroenteritis, eczema and cot death occur less frequently.

There are few contraindications to breast feeding; these are essentially confined to serious health problems in the mother. Acute or chronic maternal illess may impair the supply of milk, in which case supplementary feeds will be required to achieve satisfactory growth. A breast abscess may infect the milk with staphylococci or other organisms and is an indication for at least temporary artificial feeding. Active open tuberculosis is a contraindication until the infant is immunised; this is often done with isoniazid-resistant BCG and the baby is also given a protective course of isoniazid. Nearly all drugs ingested by the mother can be assumed to be excreted into the milk to some extent. Most antibiotics, salicylates, antihistamines and barbiturates are clinically insignificant to the infant in the concentrations commonly found. Breast feeding should be discouraged if the mother needs to take phenindione, lithium, antithyroid or antimitotic drugs. Specific information should be sought about new or unusual drugs.

In the baby, immaturity, illness or anatomical abnormalities such as cleft palate may impair sucking, necessitating the administration of expressed breast milk. Infants with certain metabolic disorders, such as phenylketonuria or galactosaemia will deteriorate if dietary modifications are not carried out. Neonatal jaundice associated with an icterogenic factor in breast milk has been described, its existence is, however, controversial and breast milk jaundice must be regarded as rare. Even when it is suspected, only a temporary period of artificial feeding will be required.

Artificial milks

Cows' milk contains more curd protein and the mineral content is higher, while the levels of polyunsaturated fatty acids and the lactose concentration are lower. Ordinary pasteurised cows' milk (doorstep milk) is thus unsuitable for feeding newborn infants. Evaporated milk has the advantage that if unopened it will keep for months in liquid form without refrigeration. During processing the fat globules have been homogenised and this contributes to a reduction in casein curd formation. The sugar content is unchanged and dilution must be carried out before use. This preparation is however little used in this country. Condensed milk has a high concentration of sucrose added to it and is generally unsuitable for infants.

Early approaches to modifying cows' milk included reducing the protein content by simple dilution with water, increasing the carbohydrate concentration by adding sucrose, or removing the fat as in skimmed milk, a by-product of butter manufacture. Iron and vitamins were then added.

There are currently two major groups of modified cows' milk formulae available. In the first group the animal fat is substituted with vegetable oils, and in some cases some of the lactose is replaced by the maltidextrins. In the second group the protein source is demineralized whey (Table 11.3). Any one of these milks is suitable for infant feeding.

The addition of carbohydrate dilutes the protein content and reduces the concentration of phosphate, sodium and other minerals, which would otherwise represent a high solute load and predispose the infant to hypocalcaemia or hyperosmolar states. The maltidextrin added reduces the increased osmolar load on the gut caused by supplementary lactose or sucrose, alternatively, fat and lactose may be added.

The substituted fat or filled milks substitute a mixture of vegetable and animal fats for cows' milk fat and aim to mimic the polyunsaturated fatty acid composition of human milk. The theoretical advantages of this approach have yet to be confirmed in infants and their use necessitates various other manipulations to the formulations, such as the addition of vitamin E, during manufacture.

Demineralised whey formulae contain much lower concentrations of the less well digested curd protein, casein. Whey is demineralised by electrodialysis and then minerals, vegetable oils, lactose and a small amount of skimmed milk are added. It is, therefore, a highly modified preparation.

Specially modified milk formulae are also available for low birthweight babies.

The choice of an artificial formula for a normal baby can be any of the milks shown in Table 11.3. The final decision will depend on availability and price as much as on nutritional factors.

Special milk formulae

Most infants thrive well on breast milk or the commercially available artificial milks. Despite this, there are many parents who become dissatisfied with some aspect of their baby's behaviour, such as his mood, stool character or sleeping pattern, and then attribute the problem to the milk given. There is a temptation to change the formula used quite empirically. This practice should be discouraged and replaced by appropriate counselling of the parents. Specialised milk feeds should only be used to treat specific conditions. The use of elimination diets may lead to an inadequate nutritional intake if care is not taken. Cows' milk protein allergy is unusual although often suspected; lactose intolerance is more common but is usually shortlived and it is seen if brush border damage to the small bowel mucosa has occurred such as after gastroenteritis. These conditions and the use of special formulae are discussed in Chapter 15. The formulations available are shown in Tables 11.4–11.7. The changes involve the replacement of lactose with other carbohydrates, the replacement of cows' milk protein with casein hydrolysates to render the milk hypo-allergenic, the use of soya protein, and the modification of the fat content to include medium chain triglycerides. The latter milks are readily absorbed in the absence of pancreatic enzymes and bile salts.

Table 11.3   Infant formulae available in the UK

Modified milk formulae	Demineralized whey formulae
Ostermilk Complete Formula	Osterfeed
Ostermilk-2	Cow & Gate Premium
Cow & Gate Plus	SMA Gold Cap
SMA White Cap	Aptamil
Milumil	

Table 11.4 Artificial feeds for infants: comparison of infant formulae with breast milk and cows' milk (breast feeding should normally be encouraged; if formula feeding is necessary infants should be given a modified artificial milk which is nutritionally similar to human milk. These milks are sometimes known as 'low solute' or 'humanised' milks. It may be beneficial to continue with a modified formula up to 1 year rather than change to cows' milk)

Composition per 100 ml*	Kcal	Protein (g)	CHO (g)	Fat (g)	K+ (mmol)	Na+ (mmol)	Ca+ (mg)	P (mg)	Fe (mg)	
Cow's milk	65	3.3	3.8	4.1	3.83	2.17	120	95	0.05	
Human milk	67	2.0	3.7	6.9	1.74	2.1	25	16	0.07	
Transitional										
Mature	69	1.3	4.1	7.2	1.49	0.6	34	14	0.07	
Modified artificial milks										
Gold Cap (Wyeth)	65	1.5	3.65	7.2	1.44	0.65	45	33	0.67	These milks have
SMA/S₂₆Nan (Nestlé)	66	1.6	3.4	7.3			50	34	0.8	a correlated
Osterfeed (Farley Health)	68	1.45	3.82	6.97	1.46	0.83	46	31	0.65	casein–whey ratio
Premium (Cow & Gate)										such that the amino acid
Ready to feed										composition is
Reconstituted	65	1.8	3.45	6.9	1.5	1.0	48	31	0.65	nearer to human
from powder	68	1.5	3.8	7.2	1.54	0.78	40	27	0.65	milk. The milks
Similac PM 60/40 (Ross)	68	1.57	3.54	7.57	1.49	0.69	40	20	0.26	contain mainly
Nenatal										blends of butter,
(Rousell)	76	1.8	4.5	7.2	1.54	0.87	100	50	0.8	fat and vegetable
Premature formula										oils with lactose
Prematalac (Cow & Gate)										as the source of
Premature formula	79	2.4	5.0	6.6	2.4	2.6	67	53	0.65	CHO. The milks
Improved formula	62	1.8	2.4	8.3	2.03	1.3	65	65	0.65	are fortified with
Ostermilk — 2 (Farley Health)										vitamins and minerals, except
Milumil (Milupa)	68	1.9	3.1	8.4	2.21	1.17	71	55	0.7	Similac PM 60/40
Ostermilk Complete (Farley Health)	65	1.7	2.6	8.6	1.79	1.3	61	49	0.65	which requires iron
Plus (Cow & Gate)	65	1.9	3.5	6.9	2.28	1.22	66	53	0.65	supplement.
SMA (Wyeth)	65	1.5	3.6	7.0	1.9	1.1	56	44.5	0.67	
Similac with Iron (Ross)	68	1.55	3.61	7.23			51	39	1.2	
Similac (Ross)	68	1.55	3.61	7.23			51	39	Trace	

* Figures from Paul & Southgate 1978

Some of these milks require the addition of mineral and vitamin mixtures. It is important to note that the use of these formulae may, in fact, mean several changes in the diet, for instance, many of the cows' milk protein-free products are also lactose free. If goat's milk is given, folic acid supplements are required.

FEEDING PRACTICES

Breast feeding

The success of lactation depends on both physical and emotional preparation, generally begun in pregnancy. Cracked or inverted nipples reduce the chances of success, while the physiology of lac-

Table 11.5 Specialised infant formulae and products used in paediatrics (These products should only be used as directed by specialist medical and dietetic advisers)

Name	Manufacturer	Source of nutrients	Supplements needed especially when used as only source of nutrition	Indications for use and further considerations
Lactose-free formulae				
A1 110	Nestlé	Purified casein, cream, corn oil, glucose, vitamins and minerals	Complete formula	Lactose intolerance/ galactosaemia. As an unmodified formula, a special dilution and additives are advisable for infants under 6 months to meet individual requirements
Galactomin 17 and Galactomin 18 (reduced fat)	Cow & Gate	Partially demineralised casein, coconut and maize oils, glucose, some vitamins and minerals	Cow & Gate vitamin and mineral tablets (contain trace of sucrose) + source of vitamins A and D	
Galactomin 19 (fructose formula)	Cow & Gate	Partially demineralised casein, coconut and maize oils, fructose, some vitamins and minerals	Sucrose free complete vitamin and trace element supplement	Glucose-galactose intolerance. Unmodified formula for feeding special dilution/additives for infants under 6 months to meet individual requirements
Isomil	Ross	Soya protein isolate, methionine, coconut and soy oil, corn syrup, sucrose, vitamins and minerals	Iron	Cows' milk protein for lactose intolerance/ galactosaemia
Formula S	Cow & Gate	Soya protein isolate and methionine, glucose syrup, vegetable oil, vitamins and minerals	Complete formula	As above. Also sucrose free
Prosobee powder	Mead Johnson	Soya protein isolate and methionine, corn syrup solids, coconut and corn oils, vitamins and minerals	Complete formula	Cows' milk protein intolerance +/or lactose intolerance. Galactosaemia, sucrose free
Prosobee liquid	Mead Johnson	Soya protein isolate and methionine, corn syrup solids, soya and coconut oils, vitamins and minerals	Complete formula	As above
Wysoy	Wyeth	Soya protein isolate and methionine, taurine, carnitine, vegetable and animal fat	Complete formula	As above
Pregestimil*	Mead Johnson	Enzymically hydrolysed casein, + tyrosine, cystine and tryptophan, corn syrup solids, modified tapioca starch, corn oil, MCT oil, soya lecithin, vitamins and minerals	Complete formula unless severe steatorrhoea or other malabsorption exists	'Elemental' formula used in malabsorption problems including intractable diarrhoea, steatorrhoea intestinal resection, sensitivity to instant protein, lactose +/or sucrose intolerance. Pancreatic insufficiency (cystic fibrosis)

Table 11.5   (continued)

Name	Manufacturer	Source of nutrients	Supplements needed especially when used as only source of nutrition	Indications for use and further consideration
Neocate*	Scientific Hospital Supplies	Synthetic amino acids, coconut fat, groundnut oil, animal fats, vitamins and minerals	Complete formula	As above
Peptide 0–2*	Scientific Hospital Supplies	Hydrolysed pork, beef, soya, coconut fat, groundnut oil, animal fats, vitamins and minerals	Complete formula	As above
Nutramigen*	Mead Johnson	Enzymically hydrolysed casein (low in cystine), sucrose, modified tapioca starch, corn oil, vitamins and minerals	Complete formula	Unmodified formula for use in malabsorption problems, including biliary obstruction, pancreatic insufficiency, intestinal resection, lactose intolerance
MCT (1)*	Cow & Gate	Partially washed casein, glucose syrup, MCT oil, some vitamins and minerals	Cow & Gate vitamin and mineral tablets (contain trace sucrose) + source of vitamins A and D	Unmodified formula, very low in cystine and devoid of essential fatty acids and may require sodium supplement. More suited for older infants with fat absorption abnormalities and can be used in treatment of intestinal lymphangiectasis and chylothorax
MBF (meat base formula)*	Gerber	Beef heart, cane sugar, sesame oil, modified tapioca starch, vitamins and minerals	Complete formula unless severe malabsorption exists	Hypo-allergenic liquid formula used in treatment of cows' milk intolerance.
Comminuted chicken meat*	Cow & Gate	A dispersion in water of finely ground chicken meat	Requires added CHO and fat of choice with complete vitamin and mineral supplements	A modified infant formula can be prepared by appropriate dilution and additives for use in malabsorption states including intractable diarrhoea, cows' milk protein intolerance, CHO intolerances according to CHO added, steatorrhoea, intestinal resection
Albumaid hydrolysate complete	Scientific Hospital Supplies	Hydrolysed beef serum with some added vitamins and minerals	Requires source of CHO, fat, vitamins and minerals according to individual requirements	Adaptable for use in malabsorption syndromes particularly where there is failure to absorb whole protein

* These formulae can, theoretically, be used for infants with lactose intolerance, but it would be more appropriate to use a modified lactose-free formula based on cows' milk protein or a soya-based formula as these are less expensive

Table 11.6 Products used in mineral abnormalities

Product	Manufacturer	Source of nutrients	Supplements needed especially when used as only source of nutrition	Indications for use and further considerations
Edosol — minimal sodium formula	Cow & Gate	Partially demineralised casein, lactose, coconut and maize oils, some vitamins	Cow & Gate vitamin and mineral tablets and source of vitamins A and D	Development of low solute artificial feeds has mainly replaced occasion to use such a low sodium feed. As unmodified milk special dilution/additives advisable for young infant and used with extreme care with constant biochemical follow up of infant sodium levels.
Locasol — low calcium formula	Cow & Gate	Partially demineralised casein, whey, lactose, coconut and maize oils, vitamins and minerals	Complete except for calcium and vitamin D	Used in treatment of hypercalcaemia

Table 11.7 Products used in disorders of amino acid metabolism

Disorder	Product	Manufacturer	Amino acid(s) lowered in product
Phenylketonuria	Minafen	Cow & Gate	Phenylalanine
	Albumaid XP	Scientific Hospital Supplies (SHS)	
	Lofenalac	Mead Johnson	
	Aminogram	Allen & Hanbury	
	Cymogram	Allen & Hanbury	
	PKU Aid	SHS	
	Maxamaid XP	SHS	
Maple syrup urine disease	MSUD Aid	SHS	Branched chain amino acids
Homocystinuria	Albumaid (methionine low)	SHS	Methionine
Cystinosis	Albumaid (cystine low)	SHS	Cystine
Histidinaemia	Albumaid (histidine low)	SHS	Histidine
	Formula HF (2)	Cow & Gate	
Tyrosinosis	Maxamaid XP	SHS	Phenylalanine, tyrosine

All products require supplements of natural protein or amino acids and most require suitable sources of energy with vitamin and mineral supplements. Specification of all products and nutritional guidelines vary from country to country

tation can be affected by the mother's emotions. An actively sucking infant enhances both the secretion and ejection of milk; the hormone prolactin promotes secretion of milk and oxytocin the ejection of milk by the let-down reflex.

Breast feeding should begin at birth or shortly after. The breast should subsequently be offered on demand and at least every 3–4 hours with suckling at both breasts for as long as the mother wishes. Advice which suggests restricting the time or frequency of suckling reduces the chances of successful breast feeding. A newborn baby at about 6 days may often feed 12–14 times a day. A normal newborn baby does not need routine supplements of water or artificial milk.

Attention must be paid to maternal hygiene and nutrition, and the advice and encouragement given regarding details of technique and expected newborn behaviour.

Bottle feeding and introduction of solids

Milk powders must be reconstituted in a sterile fashion according to the manufacturer's instructions. The total volume of milk offered per day is calculated from the infant's expected weight. An average amount is 150 ml/kg divided into five or six feeds, giving an energy intake of 462 kJ/kg. As the infant gets older the calorie requirement falls to 420 kJ/kg. After the age of 4 months the nutritional requirements for optimal growth cannot be supplied by milk alone; as the infant becomes heavier the volume of milk that would be required become less manageable. The first solid food to be introduced is usually a cereal, which in Europe is usually wheat or rice based with added iron and vitamin D. By the age of 6 months or so most children are developmentally ready to chew solids as distinct from taking thickened feeds. They begin to start drinking from a cup and various diluted fruit juices may be introduced. The variety of solids soon needs to be increased to provide the essential components of the diet. Most babies take to a new food readily if it is given in teaspoon amounts initially.

New food additions should be made gradually. Many manufacturers produce strained foods for the younger infant and less finely divided foods for the older child. When mixed feeding is well established doorstep milk may replace powdered milk. At around 1 year a liquidised mixed adult diet is usually adequate; this is given three to four times a day with up to 600 ml of milk daily. Providing the child is thriving, accurate dietary assessments are usually not necessary. By 18 months most children are anxious to feed themselves and puréed meals have given way to cut-up and minced foods. Most parents start introducing finely chopped foods from about 9 months.

Vitamin and mineral supplements

Vitamin supplements are recommended for breast-fed infants. The British DHSS vitamin drops contain vitamins A, C and D (0.2 ml or 7 drops, contain 300 μg of vitamin A, 30 mg of vitamin C and 10 μg of vitamin D). Supplementation is not usually essential for babies given formula feeds since these are fortified, but become necessary when doorstep milk is given. Additional folic acid may be required in some preterm infants. Deficiency of the B complex vitamins is rarely encountered in Europe and specific supplemen-

tation is not given. Vitamin E and K deficiencies are occasionally seen in neonates.

It is uncommon to encounter deficiencies of minerals other than iron. Calcium, phosphorus and magnesium are well provided for in most milks. The normal child does not require trace element supplements, although their importance has been emphasised following the use of synthetic diets for the treatment of inborn errors of metabolism, the development of intravenous nutrition, and the recognition of the hazards of environmental pollution.

FEEDING PROBLEMS

Refusal to suck, slow weight gain, continual crying, vomiting and colic are all common problems in infants and often cause great anxiety to their parents. In the vast majority of cases there is no underlying infection, metabolic, cardiac or respiratory abnormality, although these should always be considered. The first observation must be to watch the mother feeding her baby. Simple mechanical problems such as a small or blocked teat, or engorged breasts may be corrected, while errors of technique such as allowing the baby to swallow excessive amounts of air may become obvious. Under-feeding and over-feeding must be recognised, the former being more common in breast-fed, and the latter in bottle-fed babies. Test feeding the breast-fed baby and then weighing him before and after may not give an answer, since individual feeds are so variable in quantity. Monitoring for a 24-hour period may be necessary. The effect of a mother's anxiety or depression on her baby's behaviour should not be underestimated. Sympathetic discussion and follow-up is often fruitful.

Food refusal is a normal phase in many toddlers. Ignoring it is the treatment of choice lest it becomes an attention-seeking device thereby provoking anger, bribery or even violence in the parents. The paediatrician should demonstrate that, despite the most alarming history, the child is pursuing a relentless course along the appropriate height and weight centile lines.

The older preschool child who has a small appetite may also cause concern. It should be appreciated that the rapid growth rate of infancy declines in the 3–5-year-old with a proportionate decrease in calorie requirements and hence appetite. If the parents have an unrealistic demand for food intake and their child takes the offensive, meal times may be transformed into a battleground of opposing wills. Parents should be aware that the pre-school child's appetite will reduce, and the child should be encouraged into an active lifestyle avoiding an excessive intake of milk, carbohydrates, and between-meal snack foods.

WEIGHT GAIN

The underweight child

Weight gain normally averages 20 g per day for the first 5 months of life, and approximately 15 g per day for the remainder of the first year. The full-term infant will thus usually have doubled the birthweight by 5 months and tripled it by 1 year of age. The small or thin child is not necessarily failing to grow. Birthweight and genetic factors must be taken into account. Weight loss or failure to gain weight consistently should be taken seriously and investigated thoroughly if the cause is not immediately obvious. The commoner causes are discussed in detail elsewhere but will broadly fall into those listed in Table 11.8.

The overweight child

Obesity is the commonest nutritional disorder of children in wealthy countries. It is a matter of concern because of the high proportion of overweight children who become obese adults, and the high morbidity of the condition in later life. The definitions used are arbitrary, but clearly, any infant whose rate of weight gain greatly exceeds height velocity is at risk, particularly if the parents are also overweight.

The pathogenesis is multifactorial, involving both genetic, environmental and psychological factors. Endocrine disturbances are unusual. The evidence that early nutritional experiences in man affect cellularity and hence bodyweight is still debated. Recently, it has been found that obese people show an unusually small increase in metabolic rate in response to many stimuli such as food, cold and thyroxine. It is suggested that they store ingested fat as triglyceride in their expanding fat stores, rather than dissipating it as heat. The tissue responsible for the thermogenesis induced by dietary fat is thought to be brown adipose tissue, which is found not only in babies, but also in the para-aortic, renal and perirenal fat depots of adults.

There is no doubt that the fat infant is at a disadvantage. He suffers more respiratory infections and is less mobile than his normal weight contemporary. Feeding practices should limit bland carbohydrates and desserts and other high calorie infant foods. It may be necessary to ask the whole family to change its eating habits and become involved in energy-expending activities if the recalcitrant 5 year old is to successfully lose weight.

NUTRITIONAL DEFICIENCIES

Vitamin D deficiency (rickets)

Nutritional rickets is a disorder of adequate mineralisation of bones during rapid growth. It may be prevented by ensuring an appropriate intake of vitamin D (10 μg or 400 iu per day) and of calcium. Pathogenesis depends on altered or decreased endocrine action of 1,25 dihydroxycholecalciferol ($1,25(OH)_2D$) on the gut, bone and kidneys. The long-recognised association of lack of sunlight with rickets is explained by the poor synthesis of cholecalciferol (vitamin D_3) in the skin together with decreased ingested ergocalciferol (vitamin D_2). Vitamin D_2 and D_3 undergo 25-hydroxylation ($25(OH)D$) in the liver, and a

Table 11.8 General causes of failure to thrive in infancy

Deficiency in energy intake	Increased catabolism
Inadequate feeds	Infections
Feeding difficulties	(urinary,
Faulty preparation	respiratory)
Poverty	Malignancy
Poor parent-child relationship	
Local, oral or upper respiratory abnormalities	
Mental retardation	
Excess energy loss	**Miscellaneous**
Vomiting	Metabolic disorders
Hiatus hernia	Congenital abnormalities
Malabsorption	Emotional deprivation
Coeliac disease	

further hydroxylation in the kidney to give the active form $1,25(OH)_2D$. Studies of nutritional rickets in pigmented ethnic groups, who have a higher incidence of nutritional rickets in the UK than do the indigenous population, have suggested that the skin is probably a more important source of $25(OH)D$ than the diet.

Clinical features

Rickets is characterised clinically by abnormalities in those bones which are undergoing active growth. In the infant, the skull vault bones become thin and softened (craniotabes), and later thickened (bossed), while the long bones and rib ends become broadened; the wrists are swollen and the costochondral junctions show a rickety rosary. As the child sits up the spine and pelvis become deformed and as he starts to walk the tibiae begin to bow and short stature becomes apparent. Motor development may be delayed as a result of generalised muscle hypotonia.

Investigation and management

Radiological changes include demineralisation of the long shafts and cupping and fraying of the ends of long bones with widening of the epiphyseal plate. The biochemical changes depend on the extent of vitamin deficiency and the degree of secondary hyperparathyroidism. There is, in general, a rise in plasma alkaline phosphatase and a fall in phosphorus with normal or low serum calcium concentrations.

Neither human nor cows' milk contains sufficient vitamin D_2, so most artificial milks are fortified. Breast-fed and older infants established on doorstep milk should begin oral vitamin supplements. Rickets may be treated with 250 μg of vitamin D_2 daily. If healing is not initiated within 1 month, further investigation of renal and gastrointestinal function is required. An excessive intake of vitamin D_2 produces toxic effects such as vomiting, anorexia and failure to thrive with associated hypercalcaemia. This was a particular problem before the levels of vitamin D fortification of cows' milk were reduced; some patients, however, appear to be unduly sensitive to the vitamin.

Scurvy

The fact that scurvy is extremely rare in the UK should not obscure the importance of an adequate dietary intake of vitamin C (ascorbic acid) of 10 mg per day. Breast milk usually contains sufficient for the newborn unless the mother is on an inadequate diet. Cows' milk contains much less and a large proportion is destroyed on heating. The artificial milks now have adequate supplements. In the past daily fresh fruit juice was advised as a main source. In scurvy there is defective formation of mesenchymal intercellular ground substance. Fibroblasts, osteoblasts and odontoblasts are all affected.

Clinical features

Petechiae are seen, while bruising occurs readily, and pseudoparalysis results from subperiosteal haemorrhage and fractures. Symptoms appear between 6 and 12 months of age; the infants are pale, fretful, anorexic and feverish. The gum changes are similar to those seen in adults but are confined to areas where teeth have erupted. A hypochromic anaemia frequently develops.

Investigation and management

The radiological features are characteristic, and include decalcification and atrophy of the bony trabeculae while leaving the denser cortical bone unaffected. The corners of the long bone ends pull away, epiphyseal displacement occurs and subperiosteal haematomas calcify. Measurement of plasma levels of ascorbic acid is often unhelpful, since there is a considerable normal variation. Daily treatment with oral vitamin C, 200 mg, gives rapid improvement.

Vitamin A deficiency

The major sources of vitamin A (retinol) are animal tissues (e.g. liver) and milk. Precursors of the vitamin occur in carrots, dark green leaves, red palm oil, and wheat, but not rice. The minimum requirement varies with age, being up to 500 μg (1700 iu) per day in the child under 4 years of age. Its absorption is promoted by fats so that in situations where animal fat is rarely consumed deficiency is common. This is particularly seen in those rice-eating areas of the world which are nutritionally deprived. The main function of retinol is for the synthesis of visual purple (rhodopsin) in the retina. It is also essential for the integrity of epithelial tissues.

Clinical features and management

The earliest sign of vitamin A deficiency is night blindness, but this is rarely clinically evident in young children. More severe deficiency causes xerosis of the conjunctiva and Bitot's spots. These consist of grey, raised plaques of desquamated epithelial cells on the temporal conjunctiva. Xerosis causes haziness, thickness and drying of the eyes and leads to corneal scarring. It is the major preventable cause of blindness in the world. Keratomalacia requires urgent treatment with intramuscular water-miscible vitamin A (3000 μg/kg bodyweight) followed by an equivalent oral dose for 5 days, and then 1500 μg daily until the eyes are normal. Associated protein energy malnutrition is common in such children.

Vitamin B complex deficiency

Thiamine (B_1)

Thiamine is a coenzyme involved in the hexose-monophosphate shunt and in the decarboxylation of alpha-ketoacids. Deficiency particularly occurs in communities who eat parboiled rice. Its presentation is protean, beri-beri in infants can cause cardiac failure, pseudomeningitis or hoarseness due to laryngeal oedema or laryngeal nerve paralysis. Emergency treatment involves parenteral thiamine 50–100 mg, followed by maintenance 5–10 mg daily.

Nicotinic acid (niacin)

Nicotinic acid in the form of phosphorylated nicotinamide adenosine dinucleotide (NADP) is an essential coenzyme in many oxidation-reduction reactions. Deficiency is seen in maize-eating communities where it causes pellagra. This dermatosis is symmetrical and appears on exposed parts of the body. Mucocutaneous junctions are often fissured and sore while the tongue becomes red, swollen and painful. Diarrhoea and neurological changes may also be seen. Treatment with 20 mg/day oral niacin should be accompanied by a diet containing adequate tryptophan from milk, meat and eggs.

Riboflavin (B_2)

Riboflavin also forms part of coenzymes involved in oxidation-reduction reactions. It rarely causes an isolated deficiency but its absence is characterised by angular stomatitis, cheilosis and the appearance of a magenta colouration of the tongue. The usual dose used in treatment is 20 mg orally.

Iron deficiency

Neither breast milk nor cows' milk contains sufficient iron to meet nutritional needs after the age of 4–6 months. In the fetus, the greatest accumulation of iron occurs at the end of intrauterine life. During the first 2 months after birth there is a minimal requirement for iron due to the physiological decreases in the circulating red cell mass. From the second to sixth month, active haemoglobin synthesis begins. Preterm and low birthweight infants are, therefore, liable to develop iron deficiency later in infancy. Many milk formulae and infant cereals contain added iron and other important dietary sources include meat and green leaf vegetables such as spinach. It should be noted that the iron content of food does not correlate well with the iron available for absorption. Inorganic iron is absorbed better than food iron and ferrous salts more efficiently than ferric. Dietary phosphate and phytate reduce iron absorption.

The clinical features of iron deficiency are those of anaemia and are discussed in Chapter 23. Pallor is the most common sign and splenomegaly may occur. Cardiac failure complicates extreme cases. Haematological features include hypochromic microcytic red cells and a low ferritin concentration. Investigation must also exclude the possibility of blood loss, particularly from the gut. Treatment should be given using oral ferrous salts in a daily dose of 6 mg of elemental iron/kg.

MALNUTRITION

A prolonged period of inadequate nutritional intake, interacting with infection, may precipitate protein energy malnutrition (PEM). The clinical presentation varies with the degree and duration of deprivation, the age of the individual concerned, and the effects of associated vitamin and mineral deficiencies. The spectrum of growth failure extends from marasmus to kwashiorkor, with mixed features of both extremes in some children. The onset is most common after weaning, between the ages of 9 months and 2 years. Recognition of current and past malnutrition is based on measurements of weight, height, mid-arm circumference, head circumference and skin fold thickness. Classification is related to the weight for age, weight for height and height for age. The clinical features of marasmus and kwashiorkor are discussed in Chapter 28.

Children with protein-energy malnutrition experience profound changes in both body composition and organ function. The total body water is increased with a proportionate rise in extracellular fluid. Protein catabolism is regulated independently of anabolism, the total body protein and especially muscle mass is reduced. Lipid accumulation occurs in the liver, probably as a result of decreased synthesis of transport proteins, and the release of fatty acids from adipose tissue. The total body fat is reduced unless the carbohydrate content of the diet has been high. Potassium is depleted more than other minerals with a disproportionate loss occurring in those patients with diarrhoea. Secondary changes in cellular metabolism are thus widespread. Gastrointestinal function is impaired as a result of reduced exocrine secretions, functional and morphological mucosal changes, and infection. Many of the endocrine glands are atrophic; concentrations of cortisol, growth hormone and thyroid stimulating hormone, however, are usually maintained or increased, although plasma insulin responses to glucose are low. Immune function, particularly cell-mediated immunity, is usually compromised. Gram-negative bacteria and viral infections are common but may exhibit few typical clinical signs on presentation.

Management

This requires more than just nutritional rehabilitation. Electrolyte disturbances, dehydration, hypoglycaemia, infections, anaemia and hypothermia must all be corrected. Dehydration may be difficult to assess because of muscle wasting or oedema. Fluid overload may lead to cardiac failure in the presence of a low reserve in myocardial function, anaemia, hypokalaemia, and a diminished glomerular filtration rate. In the absence of renal failure additional potassium is required as well as calcium and magnesium. Hypoglycaemia and hypothermia are easily overlooked and are often associated with a septicaemia which should be suspected and treated. Dietary treatment is complicated by the presence of diarrhoea and vomiting. Long-term intravenous therapy is rarely practical, oral/water and electrolyte solutions should be given and within 2 or 3 days increasing concentrations of milk administered. If carbohydrate intolerance is confirmed by finding that the stool water has a pH less than 6 and contains glucose, a lactose-free feed may be necessary. Vitamins A and D must be given and a mixed diet appropriate to the locality gradually introduced. Vitamin K should be given parenterally. Early iron supplementation has been shown to be associated with an increased incidence of infection and is, therefore, usually commenced only when the general condition of the patient has started to improve.

In severe PEM normal vigour and growth may not be regained for many months. The long-term effects on growth and brain development are debated since the interaction between malnutrition and other environmental factors is complex. The unfavourable social circumstances which frequently accompany an inability to provide an adequate diet contribute materially to morbidity. On the other hand, there is no doubt that a foundation of good nutrition in the preschool years enables a child to make the most of his environment and fulfil his potential for both physical and intellectual growth.

FURTHER READING

Arneil G C, Stroud C E 1984 Infant feeding. In: Forfar J O, Arneil G C (eds) Textbook of paediatrics, 2nd edn. Churchill Livingstone, Edinburgh, Ch 6, p 259

Bentley D, Lawson M 1988 Clinical nutrition in paediatric disorders. Ballière Trindall, London

Department of Health and Social Security 1988 Present day practice in infant feeding — third report (Reports on Health and Social Subjects: No 32). HMSO, London

McLaren D S, Burman D (eds) 1982 Textbook of paediatric nutrition. Churchill Livingstone, Edinburgh

Paul A A, Southgate D A T (eds) 1978 McCance & Widdowson's composition of foods, 4th edn. HMSO, London

12. The handicapped child

A. Butterfill

Defect, disability and handicap

These terms are not synonymous. A defect such as poor vision or a hemiplegia will normally result in a functional disability. Whether or not this disability constitutes a handicap by preventing a person from achieving his or her full potential or from leading a full life depends upon many factors other than the disability itself, although the nature and degree of the disability are, of course, central.

The word 'handicapped' is acquiring derogatory overtones and 'disabled' is often preferred by those affected and their families.

Associated abnormalities

In this chapter handicapping conditions are considered singly, but it must be remembered that handicaps are often multiple. The presence of additional disabilities, which should be carefully sought, complicates management, and even relatively minor additional disabilities can have a significant effect on overall function and progress.

The multidisciplinary team

The range of problems presented by handicapped children is wide, covering many disciplines including paediatrics, orthopaedics, neurology, psychology, psychiatry, speech and physical therapies and social work. The needs of most handicapped children go beyond the limits of any one person's expertise, and it has become common practice to adopt a team multidisciplinary approach.

Early diagnosis

The earlier particular handicaps are recognised, and corrected or circumvented, the less severe will be the developmental consequences. In addition to the immediate effects of a handicapping condition, secondary defects can develop if appropriate help is not given. For example a child with impaired speech, having repeatedly experienced failure in communication, may become withdrawn. These secondary effects can profoundly influence the child's behaviour, and may become as detrimental as the original handicap.

Emotional and behaviour disturbance

In view of the difficulties faced by handicapped children and their families, the higher incidence of behavioural and emotional disturbance is not surprising. Emotional disturbance among the mentally handicapped is common, and may be difficult to recognise.

Disturbances of behaviour including immaturity, sleep and feeding, demanding behaviour, aggression and simple disobedience are common, and may cause greater problems than the underlying handicap. Children of low intelligence will tend to behave in a way more appropriate to their mental age and their low intelligence may contribute to their slowness in learning acceptable behaviour, although this is usually not the only factor.

Supporting the family

Handicap is a family problem. The need for special consideration of one member of a family, time spent in hospital clinics and therapy, the expense of adaptations to the home and family car can affect all the family. People rarely embarrass their doctors by telling them just how difficult life is, but doctors need to bear this in mind when planning treatment programmes.

Relief (or respite) care can be vital. A holiday for the child or a short admission, preferably to a purpose-run unit, short stays with friends or relatives or just baby-sitting may give the rest of the family the break without which they could not go on caring for the handicapped child.

The need for full and sympathetic explanation of the implications of a child's handicaps is obvious. The issues may be complex, requiring more than one session.

Explanation from a doctor is often not enough. Parents are likely to experience shock, denial and anger of a grief reaction when the news of their child's handicap is first given. Therapists, who may spend a lot of time with parents while treating the child, can play a vital role in helping parents to work through and understand their feelings. A social worker or counsellor may help. Help and support from other parents or support groups (e.g. Mencap) may be of great value.

Various allowances are available to help families of handicapped children (Table 12.1). Help may also be available from the Family Fund and local charitable sources. Parents should be made aware of the allowances to which they might be entitled.

Genetic counselling

The possibility of having another handicapped child is a vital issue for most parents. Where the exact cause of the handicap is known an informed recurrence risk and information about the possibility of prenatal diagnosis can be given; indeed this is one of the main values of an exact diagnosis. When the diagnosis remains imprecise (e.g. cerebral palsy, non-specific mental retardation) after reasonable attempts to discover the aetiology, an empirical recurrence risk can be given.

Progressive disorders

The majority of handicapped children have suffered some specific insult damaging the brain or the body, but once caused the damage does not progress. Despite their impairments all except the most profoundly affected of these children will be able to make developmental progress. There is a much smaller group of children who have not had one major insult, but who suffer progressive impairment (e.g. muscular dystrophy, Tay–Sach's disease), eventually leading to death. These children are usually managed by a paediatric neurologist, but it is important for doctors dealing with the handicapped to recognise such conditions if they present to him.

The management of these disorders aims at preserving function for as long as possible. The development of contractures is prevented or delayed by physiotherapy; calipers and splints can prolong the period of ambulation. Various splints may improve hand function. Immobility, for example during intercurrent illness, must be minimised as rapid loss of function can occur during these times.

Although in the later stages walking may be very restricted, with inability to cope with steps, slopes or rough ground, persisting with walking is worthwhile because once the child becomes chairbound scoliosis, which may become gross, joint contractures, respiratory problems and constipation will inevitably develop.

Special education

Following the Warnock Report which showed that up to 15% of all children have special educational needs at some time in their school career, the Education Act 1981 introduced changes in the way

Table 12.1 Allowances — qualification criteria (outline)

Attendance	Child over 2 years of age who requires either frequent attention or continual supervision as a result of severe physical or mental handicap
Mobility	Child over 5 years of age who is 'unable or virtually unable to walk'
Vaccine damage	Severe disability as a result of vaccination
Invalid care	Either man or woman who cares 'regularly and substantially' for a person who receives the attendance allowance (i.e who is disabled)
Severe disablement	Disabled person over the age of 16 years who is incapable of work

education authorities provide for handicapped children. The act requires a detailed assessment of a child's special educational needs, leading to the drawing up of a Statement of Special Educational Needs, which must be met, adapting the education to the child if necessary, and not vice versa as had previously been the case. The assessment is detailed and multidisciplinary, involving input from medicine, education and psychology and from other disciplines if relevant.

The main provisions of the act are:

1. Children having special educational needs should be provided for in normal schools if possible.

2. Education authorities are required to assess the special educational needs of a handicapped child (section 5) and to draw up a Statement of Special Educational Needs.

3. The education authority must inform parents that their child is to be assessed, and that they have the right to submit their own evidence.

4. When the Statement has been drawn up the parents have the right to comment on it and to appeal against it.

5. Parents may request the education authority to perform an assessment (section 9), which the authority must do unless the request is unreasonable.

6. Special education must be provided for handicapped children from 2 years of age if it is required.

7. Health authorities have a duty to notify the education authority of a child of under 5 years of age who has, or may have, special educational needs, having first informed the child's parents.

VISUAL HANDICAP

The figures usually quoted for blindness (an acuity of 6/60 or less in the better eye) and partial sight (6/24 or less in the better eye) are arbitrary and not entirely suitable when dealing with children. Even with an acuity of 6/60 a child may have useful residual vision, but the use he is able to make of it depends as much upon eye movements, visual fields and cortical processing of the visual input, as upon the measured acuity. The approximate prevalence of visual handicaps is shown in Table 12.2 and the causes of severe visual handicaps in Table 12.3.

Table 12.2 Prevalence of visual handicaps among children

Visual handicap	Prevalence (per 1000)
Squint	30
Refractive error	50
Registered blind	0.25
Registered partially sighted	0.3
Attending school for the blind or partially sighted	0.4

Table 12.3 Causes of severe visual handicap in children

Optic atrophy	Secondary to perinatal insult Inherited
Inherited retinal degenerations	
Ocular malformation	Anophthalmia Microphthalmia Coloboma Aniridia
Cataract	Genetic Prenatal rubella Metabolic
Postnatally acquired	Infection Trauma Other } to either eye or brain
Cortical blindness	Perinatal insult Postencephalopathy
Retinoblastoma	Prenatal infection
Glaucoma	
Severe refractive error	
Albinism	
Other	

Developmental effects of severe visual impairment

Many severely visually handicapped children have developmental delay due to associated handicaps (Table 12.4). Vision is one of the main avenues for learning about the world for a young child and among those who are otherwise normal their visual handicap may have profound effects upon their development. Mobility is often delayed because of impaired awareness of space. Social and language development may also be affected. The development of manual exploration, the concept of object permanence and sound localisation may also be

Table 12.4   Severe visual impairment — associated handicaps

Visual impairment	% of cases
Severe subnormality	30
Epilepsy	15
Behavioural/emotional problems	13
Deafness	10
Cerebral palsy	6

delayed. Feeding problems are common in blind children.

The presence of severely impaired vision in a young child may be suspected on the grounds of obvious ocular abnormality, a lack of visual fixation, abnormal eye movements (roving), gross nystagmus, and the absence of opto-kinetic nystagmus.

Squints do not impair vision greatly, but good binocular vision is not likely to develop, and subtle perceptual problems have been noted. Refractive errors can usually be substantially corrected.

Cataracts, although eminently treatable surgically in the elderly, have severe and continuing effects on vision if they are present from birth. By obscuring vision in the early weeks of life essential neural development in response to visual input is prevented. Once the cataract is removed refractive errors and lack of accommodation continue to adversely affect visual development and moderately severe impairment will inevitably remain. Early detection, either by ophthalmoscopic screening of all newborns or by detecting babies with poor visual fixation at the 6-week screening examination, and early treatment gives the best chances for later visual function.

Registration of blindness and partial sight (form BD8, normally completed by an ophthalmologist) is optional, but helps in obtaining certain benefits and services.

Management

Correction of refractive errors is important. Children with congenital visual handicaps may appear to improve over the first year, sometimes dramatically, presumably because of the child's increasing ability to make sense of his defective visual input. Training of residual vision may further capitalise on this.

Non-visual awareness

The child with congenitally severely impaired vision often uses other senses poorly, at least initially, because vision normally plays such an important part in the development of these senses. Touch, sound and smell give only an incomplete picture of the world, unless the information is coordinated by vision. The use of other senses can, nevertheless, be encouraged, and this will improve the child's ability to learn from his surroundings.

Education

Most children with visual handicaps cope in normal school, perhaps with some specialised teaching support and low vision aids. Placement in a school catering specifically for children with visual handicaps will depend upon a number of factors including intelligence and the presence of other handicaps in addition to visual function. Very severe visual impairment renders reading of print impossible, or at least inefficient, and a tactile code (Braille) is used.

PRENATAL RUBELLA AND DEAF-BLINDNESS

The probability of congenital abnormalities following rubella infection in pregnancy is high, about 25% if the infection occurs within the first month of pregnancy. Multiple abnormalities are common, and prenatal rubella is the commonest cause of severe combined deafness and blindness in children (Table 12.5), although deafness or cataracts can occur singly.

Management of the deaf-blind child

Impairment of both vision and hearing is an uncommon but devastating handicap. With impairment of the two main routes of learning development will inevitably be interfered with, even without the mental handicap which may be present. If the child's awareness of the world is sufficiently impaired he is unlikely ever to es-

Table 12.5 Causes of severe deafness and visual handicap

Prenatal rubella

Other prenatal infections, e.g. cytomegalovirus

| Insults affecting optic and acoustic nerves (or organ of Corti) | Prematurity
Meningitis
Trauma |
| Inherited conditions affecting both senses | Usher's syndrome (deafness with retinitis pigmentosa) |

tablish meaningful contact with his parents or surroundings, and may withdraw into a self-centered state similar to autism.

Maximising residual vision and hearing with appropriate aids is important. It is often difficult to assess the degree of residual function and a period of training is worthwhile even if it appears initially that no useful function remains.

Developmental training attempts to establish an awareness of self as an individual within the world, to enlarge experience of the world and to promote communication through touch and movement, using residual vision and hearing where possible.

DEAFNESS

The approximate prevalence of hearing impairment is shown in Table 12.6. The causes of severe hearing impairment are:

1. Inherited:
   a. Recessive:
      i. Pendred's syndrome (deafness with goitre)

Table 12.6 Prevalence of hearing impairments in children

Hearing impairment	Sound level (dB)	Prevalence (per 1000)
Mild	35–50 dB	13
Moderate	50–70 dB	2
Severe	more than 70 dB	1

Normal average threshold at each frequency is designated zero decibels (dB). Other sound levels are related to this: decibel no. = $10 \times \log_{10}$ sound pressure level − threshold SPL. Thus 20 dB represents a sound pressure level 100 times greater than the threshold. Thresholds up to 20 dB are accepted as normal.

      ii. Usher's syndrome (deafness with retinitis pigmentosa)
      iii. Other (many different disorders)
   b. Dominant:
      i. Waadenburg syndrome (deafness with white forelock)
      ii. Other
   c. X-linked
2. Inner ear malformation.
3. Malformations of the face involving the middle ear cleft:
   a. Cleft palate
   b. Treacher Collins syndrome
   c. Other
4. Meningitis.
5. Prenatal infections:
   a. Rubella
6. Perinatal:
   a. Asphyxia
   b. Jaundice
   c. Drugs
7. Other

Testing hearing in the early months of life is difficult because of the lack of clear-cut responses to sound. The auditory response cradle detects behavioural responses to sound in neonates, and has been used for population screening in some areas. Brain stem auditory evoked responses (BSER) have been used for screening high-risk neonates and can be used in older children when the results of clinical tests are unsatisfactory. An alternative is to identify children at high risk of deafness and to follow them with regular hearing tests. Risk factors for deafness are:

1. Family history of hereditary childhood deafness.
2. Rubella or other prenatal non-bacterial infection.
3. Physical malformations around the ear.
4. Low birthweight.
5. Severe neonatal jaundice.

About 8% of children will fall within these criteria including 70–80% of those with early deafness. A disadvantage of this method is that a sizeable minority of children with severe hearing problems are not identified by risk factors. Parents are often the first to recognise their child's deafness. A parent's concern should always be taken seriously.

Deafness due to chronic secretory otitis media (CSOM) is common. Conductive loss, of mild or moderate degree, fluctuates, and tends to get better as the child gets older. However, there may be a significant effect on language development. High and low frequencies are affected more or less equally. Sensorineural deafness tends to be more severe and to affect the high frequencies more severely, and thus tends to have a more severe effect on language development.

Developmental effects of severe hearing loss

Severe deafness during the first years of life prevents a child from hearing speech, and thus his language development will be delayed. When deafness is profound (90 dB or more) speech development is likely to be prevented altogether. However, the deaf child will learn to communicate using strategies such as gesture and facial expression.

Management of severe deafness

Aids are used to make optimum use of residual hearing. Few children have no perception of sound at all, and a trial period of aids and auditory training is almost always worthwhile. A teacher of the deaf is involved at an early stage to encourage the use of residual hearing and communication. The use of gesture or even a sign language helps communication and is generally believed to promote rather than hinder speech development. Reduced auditory feedback tends to impair speech production; speech training to overcome this is usually required.

The language training of the early years is vital. At school age most children with useful residual hearing will be integrated into the normal school system, often in units for the hearing-impaired in normal schools. Those without useful hearing are more likely to require separate education, and have continuing difficulties with understanding and production of speech which may contribute to poor educational progress.

Mild hearing impairment

Mild transient hearing loss following ear infections is usual. Failure of resolution of an ear infection resulting in CSOM is the commonest cause of mild and moderate hearing loss in children, affecting up to 7% of children at some time or another, and being commonest between 6 months and 7 years. Typically the tympanic membrane looks dull and retracted, and the finding of low middle ear pressure with reduced compliance on impedance audiometry are diagnostic. Decongestants sometimes clear the condition, but aspiration of the middle ear is often required, sometimes with the insertion of grommets or more permanent tympanostomy tubes to ensure middle ear ventilation.

Although the handicap of CSOM may not be severe, it may contribute a significant additional handicap to a child who already has language or other problems.

LANGUAGE DELAY

It must be remembered that language includes comprehension as well as speech and covers communication by methods (e.g. sign language) other than speech. Language disorders may affect areas other than speech, but speech is nearly always the most severely affected language function. Speech makes greater demands on motor co-ordination and intellect than any other activity of the young child, and it is not surprising that speech delay is common (Table 12.7).

The causes of speech delay are:

1. Constitutional.
2. Understimulation.
3. Mental retardation.
4. Deafness.

Table 12.7 Prevalence of speech delay

Speech delay	%
Unintelligible at school entry (poor articulation)	5
Reduced speech content at school entry	1
Severe language difficulty (not due to deafness or mental retardation)	0.1

5. Abnormalities of the speech apparatus:
   a. Neurological:
      i. Cerebral palsy
      ii. Cranial nerve abnormalities
   b. Physical.
      i. Cleft palate
   c. Lip and tongue dyspraxia
6. Specific language disorder.
7. Psychiatric:
   a. Autism
   b. Elective mutism

Most preschool children with language delay not due to deafness or retardation will have caught up within a few years. This developmental pattern is known as constitutional speech delay.

Understimulation or social deprivation is the commonest cause of minor language delay. Improving the child's language environment by nursery attendance may be all that is required. Children with more severe language disorders may not benefit from the unstructured language environment of an ordinary nursery, and to progress they may need more specific and individual attention.

The speech delay of the retarded child is part of the overall picture of developmental delay, although it is not uncommon for speech to be more delayed than other areas of development.

The deaf child does not hear speech and so his learning of language is impaired. However he will communicate in other ways, for example by gesture.

Abnormalities of the speech apparatus impair a child's speech production (articulation), but not the sense he is trying to convey (content), except when the disorder is severe. The majority of young children with poor articulation do not have any obvious physical or neurological abnormality and their abnormality of speech will generally resolve in time, although some have a more severe or persisting disorder.

In contrast to constitutional speech disorder, specific language disorders are more severe and persisting. The disorder may involve expression alone, or both expression and comprehension.

A child with any sort of language problem should be followed up to detect as early as possible those who have a more serious or persisting disorder.

There is an increased incidence of reading and writing disorders in children who have had language disorders.

Management

A child of under 2 years who has normal comprehension and a problem only with expression has a good outlook for language development, and little intervention is required. When there is a problem of articulation speech training may be required, but this often has to wait until the child is old enough to 'understand' and is sufficiently motivated.

When there is impaired comprehension the outlook is less good. Developmental help, often provided in units for language-delayed children, may be required.

Alternative methods of communication

Where a child's language abilities are grossly impaired, sign language may improve communication, possibly assisting speech development at the same time. A simple pictorial system may assist communication of basic needs. 'Bliss-symbols' is a further development of this, in which a board with up to 400 symbols is used to communicate by pointing to the required symbols. Wordprocessors and typewriters, some simplified and made portable, may be of great value to those who can use them.

MENTAL RETARDATION

The normal range of intelligence is taken to extend down to an IQ of approximately 70 (corresponding to -2 standard deviations below the mean). About 3% of the population fall below this level. For educational purposes mental retardation is divided into moderate (IQ approximately 50–70; prevalence 30 per 1000) and severe (IQ less than 50; prevalence 3 per 1000) learning difficulty. Psychologists are reluctant to give an overall IQ figure as it gives little information and can misrepresent the child. The figures quoted here are given as a rough guide only.

The degree of mental handicap depends upon a variety of factors in addition to the insult primarily responsible for the retardation (Table 12.8). Deprivation and the presence of additional handicaps can increase the deficit, while an optimum environment maximises developmental potential.

Screening for phenylketonuria and hypothyroidism has practically eliminated retardation due to these causes.

Investigations

Where the history and clinical examination do not suggest a diagnosis, the following investigations should be considered; urine for amino acids and organic acids; plasma electrolytes; serology for prenatal infections; chromosomes and thyroid function. If clinically indicated further investigations such as skull, CT head scan, and electroradiograph encephalogram may be done. The results of these tests are often abnormal, but less often clearly diagnostic. There are few remediable causes of mental retardation, and investigations should be kept to a reasonable minimum. Often the main value of a diagnosis is that it enables more informed genetic counselling to be given.

Table 12.8 Causes of mental retardation

Prenatal (75%)
  Genetic
    Chromosomal — Down's syndrome commonest
    Single gene
    a. Biochemical disorders — phenylketonuria, etc.
    b. Neurocutaneous syndromes
      i. Tuberous sclerosis
      ii. Sturge–Weber syndrome
  Recognisable syndromes (and those with dysmorphic features, but not falling into a recognised category)
  Prenatal infections

Perinatal (15%)
  Prematurity
  Birth asphyxia
  Birth trauma
  Severe jaundice
  Hypoglycaemia

Postnatal (15%)
  Trauma
  CNS infections
  Severe metabolic disturbances

Management

Early management consists of optimising opportunities for learning after having attended to remediable problems such as hearing loss. Starting from the child's present developmental level further skills are taught. A finely graded system of developmental stimulation activities known as Portage (after the town in North America where it was developed) is often used. The therapist, usually a health visitor, teacher or nursery nurse, instructs the parent in how to encourage the desired behaviour or activity, and the parent works with the child. The same system can be used in a nursery class for children with developmental problems.

The school placement of the retarded child is not made on the basis of intelligence alone, but also on motivation, behaviour and attainments, especially in borderline cases. While schools for children with moderate learning difficulties pursue the normal curriculum, albeit at a much slower pace, those for children with severe learning difficulties tend to concentrate on behaviour, communication and independence and social skills.

Prognosis

One can never be confident about the future of a child with delayed development; in general, the existing pace of development is likely to continue in the absence of significant additional external changes (such as the discovery and correction of a hearing loss). There may be early levelling off of developmental progress, especially in the more severely retarded.

DOWN'S SYNDROME

This is the commonest single cause of severe mental retardation with an approximate incidence of one per thousand births. The common clinical features are:

1. (Present in three-quarters of Down's children):
    a. Upslanting palpebral fissures
    b. Flat facies
    c. Flat occiput
    d. Loose skin on the neck
2. (Present in about half of Down's children):
    a. Broad hands

b. Short fingers
c. Incurved fifth fingers (clinodactyly)
d. Single transverse palmar crease
e. Malformed auricles
f. Epicanthic folds
g. Speckled iris (Brushfield's spots)
h. Protruding tongue
i. Hypotonia
j. Broad space between great and second toe

Associated abnormalities of Down's syndrome are:

1. Cardiac defects:
   a. Atrioventricular canal defect
   b. Ventricular septal defect
2. Intestinal malformations:
   a. Duodenal atresia
3. Strabismus.
4. Convulsions — although less frequent than in other conditions causing severe mental retardation, convulsions are more common than among the general population.
5. Deafness — mainly conductive.
6. Endocrine:
   a. Hypothyroidism
   b. Diabetes mellitus
7. Coeliac disease.

Aetiology (see Ch. 13)

The underlying defect is an autosomal trisomy. In 95% of cases there is a simple trisomy of chromosome 21. In the remainder there is an unbalanced translocation, with the additional chromosomal material translocated onto chromosome 14, or occasionally 15.

The chances of non-disjunction (producing simple trisomy) increase with maternal age, reaching about 1% of live births by a maternal age of 40 years. This accounts for about half of all babies with Down's syndrome.

Intelligence

Early development is delayed, but not grossly so, with average performance being about two-thirds of chronological age in the first 2 years. In later years progress is slower, and the average IQ is around 50, with most Down's children falling in the range 20–70.

Life expectancy

The life expectancy of Down's children has increased during this century. There is a high early mortality of about 25% in the first 2 years, with cardiac defects the commonest cause of death. Thereafter infection is the commonest cause of death. The overall life expectancy is about 30 years.

PHYSICAL DISABILITIES

Approximately 25 children in every 10 000 suffer from a significant physical handicap. Half of them require special education because of their handicap. The common causes of physical handicap are:

1. Cerebral palsy.
2. Congenital heart disease — the handicap is usually relatively mild.
3. Spina bifida.
4. Congenital limb deformities.
5. Muscular dystrophy.
6. Polio — now rare.
7. Haemophilia.
8. Juvenile chronic arthritis.
9. Arthrogryposis.
10. Other.

Cerebral palsy

Cerebral palsy is a non-progressive disorder of movement and posture caused by an insult to the immature brain. The incidence is two to three per thousand births. Various patterns of cerebral palsy are seen (Table 12.9). Many cases show features of more than one type. For example, there may be athetoid features in the movement disorder of the predominantly spastic child, or vice versa, and ataxia will be a feature in most cases to some degree.

Features of cerebral palsy

Posture. There are many typical postures. Adduction and internal rotation of the legs with

Table 12.9 Patterns of cerebral palsy

Patterns	%
Spastic	
Generalised (quadriplegia)	15
Hemiplegia	30
Diplegia	5
Athetoid	20
Hypotonic	5
Ataxic	5
Mixed	20

Table 12.10 Cerebral palsy — associated problems

Associated problem	%
Epilepsy	40
Squint	30
Severe visual handicap	10
Speech delay	
Not speaking at 5 years	20
Poor articulation at 5 years	50
Deafness	15
Subnormal intelligence	50

equinus at the ankles is common, as is adduction and internal rotation at the shoulders with flexion of the wrists and elbows.

Responses. Primitive responses, Moro, grasp and asymmetric tonic neck are late disappearing, and the secondary responses, parachute and propping reactions are late developing.

Movement. Weakness, inco-ordination, involuntary movements and poor control are all common.

Tone. Muscle tone varies with time, state and posture, and is different in different muscle groups. The spine and neck are often hypotonic, even in the predominantly spastic child.

The manifestations of cerebral palsy may evolve with time. Most children are initially hypotonic, with spasticity or athetosis developing later. The earlier onset of spasticity or athetosis tends to indicate a better prognosis, while the persistence of generalised hypotonia into the second year of life is a poor prognostic sign. Apparent neurological deterioration may occur in adolescence when a rapid spurt in growth of height and weight may exacerbate problems of weakness and poor co-ordination.

In addition to the movement disorder, children with cerebral palsy often have other problems (Table 12.10). Only about one-third of children with cerebral palsy will be able to cope in normal schools.

Management

The presence of associated problems will complicate management, and in some children with very complex handicaps, integrating the various aspects of management will itself be a major task. The mainstay of management of cerebral palsy is physiotherapy which will include seating, control of posture and everyday handling as well as specific physical exercises to increase movement and prevent contractures. There are many 'schools' of thought in physiotherapy. Bobath therapy attempts to correct the abnormal patterns of movement and posture which are often secondary to the underlying neurological deficit, and tend to become self-perpetuating. The Peto approach covers all areas of development and concentrates more on encouraging the child to perform tasks, with less emphasis on the method of execution. Surgery can correct some deformities, but elongating tendons and muscles lead to further weakening of already weak muscles, and a period of immobilisation following surgery may be detrimental to the programme of education and therapy. The selection and timing of cases for surgery is critical. There are a variety of non-surgical methods of reducing hypertonia. Nerve or muscle infiltration with alcohol produces an effect analogous to the surgical release of the muscle, but which is temporary. Its main use is to assess the likely benefits of surgery. Baclofen and diazepam reduce spasticity. These are not often beneficial as the child frequently suffers greater disability from the weakening of muscles that he can use than benefits from inhibiting spasticity.

Spina bifida

This is becoming less of a problem with antenatal diagnosis and termination. The problems associated with spina bifida include infection, spinal cord damage, weakness of the legs (which may require braces to control weakness and surgical tendon transfer to prevent deformity), sensory loss, incontinence (managed by regular bladder expression, penile appliance, intermittent self-catheterisation or occasionally urinary diversion), constipation, hydrocephalus, kyphosis and scoliosis, renal problems (reflux, infection), squint, emotional and behavioural problems and intellectual impairment (typically non-verbal skills more impaired than verbal).

13. Genetic disorders

S. Bundey

Genetic disease is now relatively more common as infections and perinatal trauma have decreased. Among livebirths, single gene disorders occur in 1% (0.7% autosomal dominant, 0.05% X-linked recessive and 0.25% autosomal recessive), chromosome disorders in 0.4% and polygenic malformations in around 2%. These are population figures and the proportions of disease that are wholly or partly determined genetically are much greater in medical practice (Table 13.1). Genetic diseases often give rise to longer and more frequent admissions to hospital and to more outpatient visits than other problems. In 1959, 26% of institutional beds in Northern Ireland were occupied by patients with genetically determined illnesses, and in British Columbia in 1964 about three-quarters of children registered as handicapped had a condition that was entirely or partially genetically determined.

It helps families with genetic problems to give them the risks of recurrence and an understanding of basic genetics is required by any doctor caring for children.

SINGLE GENE DISORDERS

These conditions are the simplest to understand; they are caused by an abnormal mutation in one or both members of a single pair of genes. The family patterns are logical and consistent.

Autosomal dominant diseases

Autosomal dominant conditions are those which are caused by a single mutant gene present on one of the 22 pairs of autosomes. Since a child inherits half his father's genes and half his mother's genes, he has a 1 in 2 chance of inheriting the abnormal gene from whichever parent is affected. Thus he or she has a half chance of developing the disease if one parent is affected. Some examples of autosomal dominant conditions which can affect children are achondroplasia, tuberous sclerosis, neurofibromatosis, myotonic dystrophy, and lobster-claw syndrome. A pedigree illustrating the inheritance of dominant optic atrophy is shown in Figure 13.1

Table 13.1 Genetic contribution to illhealth in childhood

Among	Single gene or chromosome disorders (%)	Malformations that are partly genetic (%)
Stillbirths and neonatal deaths	6–10	30–40
Paediatric inpatients	4–8	20–25
Severely mentally retarded children	46	10
Deaf schoolchildren	50	1–2
Blind schoolchildren	42	8

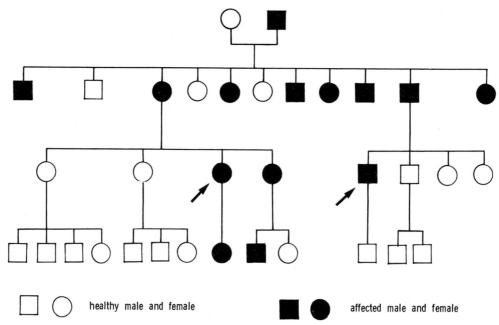

Fig. 13.1 Family showing dominant inheritance of optic atrophy (by kind permission of S. J. Crews & G. Harding).

□ ○ healthy male and female   ■ ● affected male and female

Autosomal dominant conditions are often very variable, both in severity and in age of onset. It may be difficult to decide whether a symptomless relative carries the gene (i.e. is a heterozygote). For example, while 60–70% of patients with tuberous sclerosis are mentally retarded and around 90% are epileptic, there remain 10% who are without symptoms and who only have skin or eye lesions. It is these 10% who are likely to become parents, not knowing that they run a 1 in 3 risk of having a mentally handicapped child. Thus, when counselling the parents of a child with severe tuberous sclerosis it is essential to know whether one of them is mildly affected. Each parent must have a careful examination of the skin and optic fundi. The skin and retinal features that are pathognomonic of tuberous sclerosis usually occur together, but each has been described in a parent as the only manifestation of the disorder. These features are: adenoma sebaceum, shagreen patch, subungual fibromas, pale white macules and retinal phakoma. At least one of these features should have appeared by adult life in an individual who is a heterozygote for tuberous sclerosis. If neither parent has one of these lesions, then they may be reassured that their child is affected by a new mu-

tation, and that recurrence in another sibling is most unlikely. (There is a slight caveat here, for two families have been described in which apparently normal parents have had more than one child with tuberous sclerosis. Such families are clearly extremely rare.)

This leads to the next point about dominant conditions, namely that a proportion of patients are affected by a new mutation. This mutation would have occurred during meiosis (the formation of either ovum or sperm); in this situation, the parents are normal and therefore there is little chance of the disorder occurring again in another child. In dominant disorders, the proportion of patients affected by new mutations is directly related to the overall fertility of patients. For example, in achondroplasia, the average number of children born to patients is about one-fifth of the average number of children born to unaffected individuals. This is partly due to failure to marry as dwarfism is a social handicap, and partly due to the patients' knowledge of the genetic risks. The proportion of achondroplasts who are new mutations and who have healthy parents is four-fifths, in neuro-fibromatosis the proportion is one-half, and in tuberous sclerosis, about four-fifths.

If two individuals with the same dominant condition marry, there is a 1 in 4 chance that a child could be homozygous abnormal, that is, possess two similar dominant genes. This has been observed with achondroplasia, Thomsen's disease or myotonia congenita, and distal myopathy as well as in other disorders. In each case the homozygous child was more severely affected than the parents.

Autosomal recessive conditions

These conditions occur when a child possesses two abnormal members of a gene pair, one inherited from the mother and one from the father. The parents are both symptomless carriers (or heterozygotes) and are not usually identified as such until they have had an affected child. Once this has happened, it is clear that there is a 1 in 4 risk of recurrence and the parents should be told this. The risk of recurrence is very small for half-siblings, or for a sibling conceived by donor artifical insemination (AID). Autosomal recessive diseases, in contrast to autosomal dominant ones, are fairly consistent in age of onset and in severity. Some examples are phenylketonuria, Tay–Sachs' disease and acute spinal muscular atrophy (Werdnig-Hoffmann disease).

The recessive diseases are thought to be caused by specific enzyme abnormalities, either an enzyme deficiency, or a structural change in an enzyme which impairs its activity. In some cases, a specific enzyme abnormality has been identified and, moreover, may be demonstrable in amniotic cells or fluid, thus making prenatal diagnosis possible. The list of conditions that can be diagnosed prenatally is growing, and an up-to-date authority should be consulted when one comes across a family at risk. In addition, there are tests for the carrier (or heterozygote) in certain recessive disorders, and these are useful if the condition is common. For example, the carrier state for Tay–Sachs' disease (hexosaminidase A deficiency) can be recognised. Since the carrier state for this condition in Ashkenazi Jews lies between 1 in 20 and 1 in 30, it is worthwhile testing Jewish couples on marriage, and certainly worthwhile testing the siblings of patients and their spouses. The healthy sibling of a child with an autosomal recessive disease has a 2 in 3 chance of being a carrier.

Table 13.2 lists the frequencies of some commoner autosomal recessive diseases. Most, however, are less frequent, and perhaps the average frequency of the carrier state of a particular recessive disease is 1 in 100. This means that if a man or woman is a carrier (and probably everyone is a carrier for at least one recessive gene), then the chance of marrying someone who carries the same gene is about 1 in 100 and, therefore, the chance of having an affected child is about 1 in 400. Of course, the chance of marrying a carrier is increased in marriages between relatives. A carrier who marries a first cousin, for example, has a 1 in 8 chance of marrying another carrier, since cousins have one-eighth of their genes in common. This is why there is an excess of cousin marriages among the parents of children with less common recessive diseases. On the other hand, the empirical risk for married first cousins having a child with a recessive disease is relatively small, about 1 in 30.

In autosomal recessive diseases genetic counselling is easy, for there is, inevitably, a 1 in 4 risk of recurrence for further children of a couple who are carriers for the same disorder. Since recessive conditions are often serious it is important to recognise a condition as being recessive after the first

Table 13.2 Frequencies of some commoner autosomal recessive conditions

Disease	Frequency of disease	Frequency of carrier state
Cystic fibrosis in Europeans	1 in 2000	1 in 22
Tay–Sachs' disease in Ashkenazi Jews	1 in 2000	1 in 22
Thalassaemia in Cypriots	1 in 150	1 in 6
Sickle-cell disease in West Africans	1 in 900	1 in 15
Phenylketonuria in UK	1 in 12 000	1 in 55
Werdnig–Hoffmann disease in UK	1 in 25 000	1 in 80

case in the family. Diagnosis must depend upon clinical features, and not upon the presence of an affected relative.

Finally, here is a warning about phenylketonuric women who are leading normal lives as a result of treatment or because they have a mild form of the disease. It is now clear that women with serum phenylalanine levels that are over 15 mg/100 ml during early pregnancy, have a high risk (almost 100%) of having children who are retarded in growth, microcephalic and mentally retarded and some of them also have congenital heart disease or other malformations. It is important that such women are placed on a low phenylalanine diet before pregnancy occurs.

X-linked recessive diseases

X-linked diseases are those produced by a gene on the X chromosome. Although the X chromosome in a woman is paired, that in a man is not, for he has a small Y chromosome in place of the second X. Thus, a recessive gene on one of a woman's X chromosomes will usually show no ill-effects. A recessive gene, however, on the X-chromosome of a male will manifest itself fully since there is no normal homologue.

The family patterns obtained are very characteristic. If a man is affected, all his sons will be normal (for in order to be sons they will have inherited their father's Y chromosome) and all his daughters will be carriers. If a woman is a carrier, half her sons will be affected and half her daughters will be carriers. A family tree showing the inheritance of X-linked retinitis pigmentosa is given in Figure 13.2. The propositus in this family had visual problems from an early age and was registered partially sighted at the age of 7. His mother had not previously been given genetic advice, but now says that she certainly would have liked it. Examples of other X-linked conditions are Duchenne and Becker muscular dystrophy, haemophilia, Lesch–Nyhan disease, Menkes' disease, adrenoleucodystrophy, and certain types of mental retardation.

Some of these diseases are serious and affected males never reproduce. Since the diseases are not disappearing, this means that some new cases arise because of new mutations, in the same way that some patients with severe autosomal dominant conditions are affected by new mutations. The relationship between severity of disease and the proportion of X-linked mutants is not straightforward as with the dominant conditions, since a

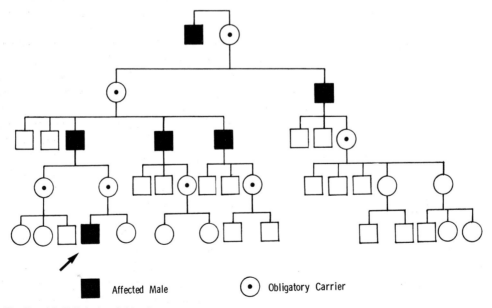

Fig. 13.2 Family with X-linked retinitis pigmentosa.

mutation occurring in a female is not immediately apparent: with lethal conditions such as Duchenne muscular dystrophy, the proportion of boys who are affected by new mutations and who have mothers who are not carriers, can be calculated as one-third. Looking at it differently, the mother of an isolated male with a lethal X-linked disorder has a two-thirds chance of being a carrier. (These are useful working figures but, in fact, the calculations are only correct if the mutation rate is equal in the two sexes, which is not always so.)

From the point of view of genetic counselling, it is important to know precisely whether a female relative is a carrier. For some diseases, for instance, Menkes' disease and Lesch–Nyhan disease, there are accurate carrier tests, although these are often tedious to carry out. The basis for these tests is the phenomenon described by Dr Mary Lyon in the early 1960s, namely that only one X chromosome is active in each cell of a female, and that inactivation of the second occurs early in development and at random. This means that a woman is composed of two populations of cells, in one of which the maternal X is active, while in the other it is the paternal X that is active. If cells from skin are cultured in vitro and then cloned, so that each clone is derived from a single skin cell, then some of the clones will demonstrate the activity of one X chromosome and some the other. In Lesch-Nyhan disease and Menkes' disease, a specific metabolic abnormality can be demonstrated, not only in patients, but also in clones from carrier females, and in amniotic cells from an affected fetus. However, in some other X-linked disorders, a precise biochemical abnormality has not been demonstrated and accurate carrier tests are less reliable. In many instances, DNA investigations are helpful (see pp. 138).

X-linked dominant inheritance

Examples of conditions showing X-linked dominant inheritance are vitamin D-resistant rickets and Albright's syndrome of pseudohypoparathyroidism. The characteristics of this type of inheritance are that more females are affected than males; females are usually less severely affected; all the daughters but none of the sons of affected males are affected; and one-half of the offspring of affected females are affected.

There are three disorders thought to be due to X-linked dominant inheritance, with lethality in males. These are incontinentia pigmenti, Rett's syndrome and the Aicardi syndrome. All patients with the Aicardi syndrome have been females; there has been no recurrence in siblings and the sex ratio is equal in unaffected siblings. It has been suggested that all female patients are new mutations, and that the mutations in male fetuses lead to intrauterine death. In incontinentia pigmenti about two-thirds of patients are new mutations, since some females are mildly affected and become mothers. Occasional male cases have been reported.

Fragile-X syndrome

This is an X-linked mental retardation syndrome which has some odd features about the way it is inherited. Its importance lies in the fact that it is the commonest cause of mental retardation after Down's syndrome. It affects males and females in equal numbers and accounts for about 10% of all mentally retarded children.

The syndrome consists of an association between mental retardation and a cytogenetic abnormality, a fragile site on the distal end of the long arm of the X-chromosome. Nearly all males who possess this fragile site are mentally retarded, and so are about one-third of female carriers. The retardation is usually mild rather than severe, and other clinical features are a head size above the 50th centile, large testes, protruding ears, large lower jaw and large hands and feet (Bundey 1987). The diagnosis is made cytogenetically by finding the fragile site at Xq27–28 in a proportion of lymphocytes. Although the fragile site is always present in mentally retarded patients, it cannot always be demonstrated in female carriers of normal intelligence.

Inheritance is X-linked but the mutation appears to arise in two or more stages, so that members of earlier generations, in particular grandparents, may carry the gene but be clinically and cytogenetically unaffected. One parent is always a carrier, so there is a high risk for mental

Table 13.3   Recurrence risks for all degrees of mental retardation

Type of mental retardation in proband	Recurrence in:		
	Brothers	Sisters	All sibs
Mental retardation with fragile-X	1 in 2	1 in 5	1 in 3
Severe idiopathic retardation without fragile-X	1 in 9	1 in 23	1 in 12
Mild retardation without fragile-X	1 in 4	1 in 6	1 in 5

retardation occurring in sibs (Table 13.3) and in sisters' sons. It is therefore important to recognise the condition in patients and to investigate their relatives. Prenatal diagnosis is available.

Linkage analysis using probes for DNA polymorphisms

A potentially very helpful aid to counselling in single gene disorders is the use of DNA probes to detect DNA polymorphisms and indirectly to detect genes which are located near the polymorphisms. This technique was developed because DNA can be cut into fragments by bacterial enzymes known as endonucleases or restriction enzymes, because these fragments can then be incorporated into bacterial plasmids or phages (a technique known as recombination) and reproduced or cloned in the bacterial host, and because subsequently the fragments can be made radioactive with ^{32}P. These synthesised radioactive fragments can be used to identify complementary fragments of DNA obtained from the white blood cells of individuals to be investigated. They are called probes because of their value as investigative tools.

These DNA probes are useful because they enable recognition of the polymorphic variation that exists in DNA from different individuals. These polymorphisms occur because the endonucleases (referred to above) cut DNA at specific sites. If a specific site is not present in an individual, because of a variation in DNA structure at that point, then the enzyme will cut the DNA at a later site and a fragment of DNA that is longer than usual will be formed. Thus, the polymorphisms recognised through DNA probes are different lengths of DNA that are secondary to altered DNA structure.

Figure 13.3 shows a family with an isolated case of Duchenne muscular dystrophy who has been investigated for DNA polymorphisms of the 21 region of the short arm of the X-chromosome (Xp21). The DNA of David (the affected boy) and his relatives has been isolated, and then broken into fragments by different experiments, using several restriction enzymes. For each experiment a different pERT probe has been used to identify distinct lengths of DNA (restriction fragment length polymorphisms or RFLPs). In Figure 13.3 the RFLPs have been named according to their lengths in kilobases.

The mother, Carol, possesses several RFLPs and it is only possible to arrange them on her two X chromosomes because the RFLPs in her father are known. Since a man has only one X chromosome there can be no X chromosomal cross-over between him and his daughter, who will receive his X chromosome unchanged. The chromosome in Carol which bears the RFLPs 3.1, 2.2, 7.5,

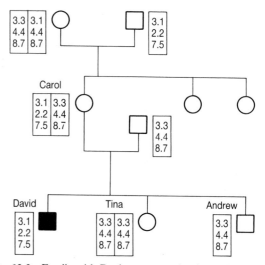

Fig. 13.3   Family with Duchenne muscular dystrophy.

has been transmitted to David, but not to the unaffected son (Andrew) nor to her daughter (Tina). Tina is therefore unlikely to be a carrier, apart from the small chance (about 2%) of a cross-over that has not been detected by these three polymorphisms.

The second point to note is that David's X-chromosome has come from his maternal grandfather who does not have muscular dystrophy. Therefore the mutation must have arisen either in the germ cells that gave rise to Carol's conception, or alternatively in her germ cells which led to David's conception. The question may be resolved by measuring creatine kinase levels in Carol to determine her carrier status. In any case, Carol's sisters are unlikely to be carriers, since it is improbable that more than one mutation will have occurred in their father's germ cells.

Let us now suppose that Tina received the X chromosome bearing the RFLPs 3.1, 2.2, 7.5, from her mother, and let us suppose also that Carol had high creatine kinase levels indicating that she was a carrier. These facts would indicate that Tina is almost certainly a carrier. Fortunately she could be offered prenatal diagnosis of an affected male fetus, since her paternal X chromosome can now be distinguished from the maternal one. The RFLPs can be identified on chorionic villus biopsy at 10 weeks of pregnancy.

Similar methods can be used to investigate other single gene disorders. For example, in cystic fibrosis it is often possible, using RFLPs that are linked to the cystic fibrosis locus, to identify a sib of a patient as being affected, or a carrier. Thus, prenatal diagnosis can be offered to parents who already have an affected child. In some patients with single gene disorders a specific gene deletion can be recognised using intragenic DNA probes. Such deletions are more useful for genetic counselling than linked RFLPs since assessment of carrier or presymptomatic status does not depend on testing relatives.

POLYGENIC INHERITANCE

In this type of inheritance many genes are involved; each are of little individual effect, but they act together to produce an additive predisposition to disease. Usually some factors in the environment act upon this genetic predisposition.

This type of inheritance was first used to explain those characteristics, such as height, which show a continuous variation in the population; it was then applied to human diseases by C. O. Carter. The distribution of height in the population has a normal or Gaussian shape, which can theoretically be caused by the action of many discrete factors, such as genes. Family studies show that adult height is almost entirely genetically caused, and the patterns in relatives fit the expectations from polygenic inheritance with a few exceptions due to assortative mating and the presence of at least one pair of dominant genes for shortness. Similarly, studies on relatives, twins, and adopted children demonstrate that the genetic component of the normal range of intelligence is also due to polygenic inheritance. With both height and intelligence there are individuals at each extreme who do not conform to the Gaussian distribution, and whose deviance has different causes. These are the dwarves and the giants; the imbeciles and the geniuses.

With diseases it is not possible to measure the underlying genetic predisposition, and this has to be inferred from observations in patients and their relatives. In polygenic inheritance it is assumed that there is an underlying genetic liability to a particular disease, which is normal or Gaussian in shape, and that patients are at one extreme of this distribution. One assumes a threshold beyond which individuals are susceptible to environmental factors. On such a polygenic model, the following family patterns would be expected and are in fact observed.

If the patients represent one extreme of a polygenic predisposition, their relatives must share some of this predisposition to an extent related to the proportion of genes shared with the patient. Thus, relatives must have an increased risk of disease; the incidence of disease in first-degree relatives approximates to the square root of the population incidence and, therefore, is absolutely greater, but proportionately less increased as the population incidence increases.

The incidence in second- and third-degree relatives falls off sharply and some illustrative risk figures for neural tube malformations are given in Table 13.4.

Furthermore, the polygenic model predicts that those patients who are the greatest deviants from the underlying genetic predisposition will need fewer environmental triggers than the less genetically predisposed patients. If such patients can be identified, their relatives should show a higher incidence of disease than the relatives of patients with less genetic predisposition. Sometimes a particularly severe malformation indicates extreme genetic predisposition, and this is seen for example with bilateral cleft lip and palate, following which the recurrence risk is 1 in 16, whereas the recurrence risk after unilateral cleft lip plus or minus palate is only 1 in 40. On the other hand, an extensive neural tube defect does not mean that the patient is particularly genetically predisposed; on the contrary, individuals who have multiple vertebral abnormalities but no overt spinal lesion have the same risk of having a child with a neural tube malformation as if they had overt spina bifida.

A second way by which a patient can be identified as being particularly genetically predisposed, is by being the unusual sex for that malformation. For example, it is five times more common to find pyloric stenosis in a boy than in a girl; the risk of recurrence after a boy with pyloric stenosis is 1 in 30 but after a girl it is 1 in 16. Finally, families of increased genetic susceptibility may be recognised when they have had more than one affected individual; in South-east England the recurrence risk after one sibling with a neural tube malformation is 1 in 22, but after two affected siblings the risk increases to 1 in 10. In Northern Ireland the risk of recurrence after one affected sibling is 1 in 12, but after two it rises 1 in 5. Risks of recurrence after the other polygenically inherited malformations are given in Table 13.5.

The important point about these polygenically inherited malformations is that environmental factors usually play some part in their development and, therefore, there is hope for preventing the condition if the environmental triggers can be recognised and controlled.

It has been known for some time that environmental factors are important in the aetiology of neural tube defects, for there is a seasonal variation consisting of an excess of February, March and April conceptions, and there is a marked and consistent social class effect with a greater incidence in social classes IV and V. These observations, together with the finding of a low red cell folate level and low leucocyte ascorbic acid level in early pregnancy in women who later gave birth to babies with neural tube defects, led to the suggestion that poor nutrition with vitamin deficiencies could be causative factors in some women at risk. In a prospective controlled study of pregnancies at risk because the woman had at least one previous baby with a neural tube defect, a lower risk of neural tube defects has been found if the woman had received vitamin and iron supplements for 1 month prior to conception and for 6 weeks afterwards. This observation gives rise to optimism that neural tube defects may be prevented in some women at risk. In the meantime, tests on amniotic fluid (that is, the levels of α-fetoprotein and acetylcholinesterase) and ultrasound examination can detect all cases of anencephaly and the great majority of babies with spina bifida. Women at higher than usual risk, who should be offered these prenatal tests, can be recognised by a family history of neural tube malformation or by a high level of α-fetoprotein in their serum.

CHROMOSOME DISORDERS

Techniques

The 22 pairs of autosomes, and the X and Y chro-

Table 13.4 Risks of neural tube malformation* in South-east England

Random population risk	1 in 340
If one sibling is affected[†]	1 in 22
If two siblings are affected	1 in 10
If a half-sibling is affected	1 in 50
If a parent is affected[†]	1 in 22
If an aunt, uncle, nephew or niece is affected	1 in 70
If a cousin is affected[‡]	1 in 148

* Term includes anencephaly, iniencephaly, encephalocele, myelomeningocele and meningocele
[†] Similar risks are found if the affected relative has spinal dysraphism or multiple vertebral anomalies
[‡] This risk figure refers to the incidence in mother's sisters' children, where knowledge of abnormalities is likely to be greatest

Table 13.5 Risks of recurrence in those congenital malformations that are polygenically inherited (after *British Medical Bulletin* 1976)

Malformation	Population incidence (per 1000 total births)	Risks of recurrence	
		After one affected child	After two affected children
Club foot	2.0	1 in 35	?
Persistent dislocation of the hip	1.0	1 in 22	1 in 12
Cleft lip ± cleft palate	1.0	1 in 28	1 in 12
Congenital heart defects	6.0	1 in 25*	1 in 10
Pyloric stenosis			
In males	5.0	1 in 30	1 in 7
In females	1.0	1 in 16	1 in 4
Neural tube defects in South-east England	2.9	1 in 22	1 in 10

* For the same heart malformation as in the index patient

mosomes, can be unambiguously distinguished from each other, during mitosis, by their lengths and banding patterns. There are many methods available for staining chromosomes. For example, chromosomes can be treated beforehand, by a proteinase, or a lipase, or by a hot salt solution, or by alteration of pH, and then stained with Giemsa, revealing G, C, or R bands according to the specific pretreatment given. The G bands are those most often seen in photographs of chromosomes; the C bands are particularly useful in demonstrating those areas near the centromeres which contain highly reiterative DNA. Another method is to use fluorescent quinacrine derivatives, which give rise to a characteristic Q banding pattern; the bright Q bands correspond to the dark G bands. Using a variety of staining methods it may be possible to distinguish the individual chromosomes of each pair for 1, 9, 13, 14, 15, 16, 21, 22, and occasionally for pairs 6, 11, 17, 18.

There is also a technique which reduces the amount of folic acid in the medium in which the chromosomes are cultured, either directly, or by using folic acid antagonists. This method allows fragile sites to develop, in particular the fragile site at Xq27–28, which is a marker for X-linked mental retardation. The chromosomes are then stained in the ways outlined above, in order to assign any fragile sites to the correct chromosomes.

Frequency of chromosome abnormalities

The frequency of overt disease due to a recognisable chromosomal abnormality is about 4.1 per 1000 livebirths. Only around 5% of patients with a chromosome abnormality have inherited it from a parent; the remainder are due to a recent error of meiosis or of postzygotic development. The incidence of chromosome abnormalities in abortuses and in stillbirths is much higher than the incidence in livebirths (Table 13.6), and is greatest in the early abortuses. The incidence of chromosome

Table 13.6 Incidence of chromosomal abnormalities

	Frequency (%)				
	Abortuses		Stillbirths		
	Early	Late	Macerated	Fresh	Livebirths
Autosomal trisomies	50	20	13	5	0.12
Unbalanced structural rearrangements	3.5		0.25		0.05
Sex chromosome abnormalities	10.0*		1.25		0.24

* Mainly 45, X

abnormalities in conceptuses of women over 40 could be as high as 1 in 2.

Clinical features of chromosome abnormalities

Numerical abnormalities of the autosomes always give rise to clinical disease, and some distinguishing clinical features are listed in Table 13.7. The clinical features that are common in a baby with a chromosome abnormality are low birthweight, poor feeding and failure to thrive, an abnormality of tone, an odd appearance with or without specific malformations, and developmental delay.

Structural abnormalities of the autosomes (such as a translocation or an inversion) only give rise to clinical signs if they are unbalanced; that is, if a segment of a chromosome is actually lost or duplicated. However, for carriers of balanced translocations there is a risk of producing unbalanced gametes and thereby abnormal offspring. One danger here is that an abnormality which appears to be 'balanced' may in fact be unbalanced and a small deletion may be unnoticed. The empirical risk of clinical abnormality for the possessor of a de novo apparently balanced structural abnor-

mality (for example, one found in cultured amniotic cells) is about 1 in 10.

Numerical abnormalities of the sex chromosomes give rise to less morbidity, and often only after puberty; the 45, X condition or Turner's syndrome is the only chromosome abnormality which often produces clinical signs at birth.

Down's syndrome

This autosomal disorder is the one that is of greatest significance in older children and in adult life, because most of the other autosomal disorders are associated with a short lifespan; it accounts for around one-third of all mentally retarded children. The commonest cause of Down's syndrome is trisomy 21, due to non-disjunction occurring in either maternal or paternal meiosis. The 21 chromosome shows several normal variations in its staining pattern, and in around 25% of patients the paternally derived chromosome 21 can be distinguished from that derived maternally and, therefore, the source of the non-disjunction can be identified. Usually the non-disjunction is maternal in origin.

Table 13.7   The most distinctive features of some chromosome disorders which are present in a baby

Trisomy 21 (Down's syndrome) Low to normal birthweight Hypotonia Brachycephaly Oblique palpebral fissures Small flat nose, rosebud mouth, darting tongue Congenital heart malformation Duodenal atresia	45, X (Turner's syndrome) (This is often not recognisable at birth) Slightly low birthweight Loose folds of skin of neck Oedema of hands and feet Hypoplastic, hyperconvex nails
Trisomy 13 (Patau's syndrome) Low to normal birthweight Microphthalmia, coloboma Deformed ears Post-axial polydactyly Cleft palate and lip Exomphalos VSD Hydronephrosis	Trisomy 18 (Edwards' syndrome) Low birthweight Long narrow skull Prominent occiput, small chin Low-set faun-like ears Finger flexion, small nails VSD Hips limited in adduction Rocker-bottom feet, short big toe
4p- (Wolf syndrome) Microcephaly Frontal bossing, high forehead Ocular malformation Harelip ± cleft palate Vertebral malformations Hypospadias	5p- (cri-du-chat sydrome) High-pitched mewing cry Micrcephaly Anti-monogoloid slant to eyes Widely set eyes Moon face

Less commonly, Down's syndrome is due to an unbalanced translocation where an additional chromosome 21 is attached to a chromosome 13, 14, 15, 22 or to another 21. This may arise de novo or it may have been inherited from a parent whose translocation was balanced. Recurrence risks for the different forms of Down's syndrome are shown in Table 13.8. With the inherited translocations the risk to offspring varies according to whether the mother or the father is the carrier, probably due to selection against the translocation-bearing sperm.

Two factors appear to be concerned with the aetiology of Down's syndrome. One is advanced maternal age, and the other is therapeutic radiation to the mother many years previously. The relationship with radiation is not firmly substantiated as it is based on retrospective studies, but the relationship with increased age is very clear (Table 13.9).

There is a smaller but definite association of other trisomies with advanced maternal age. Because of these associations, 'elderly' pregnant women are offered prenatal diagnosis by karyotyping cells from amniotic fluid or chorionic villus sample. As a result of this practice it has been observed that the incidence of chromosome abnormalities in amniotic cells at 16 weeks' gestation is nearly twice the incidence in livebirths. This may be partly due to the condition in stillbirths not being recognised, but there may also have been an increase in the incidence of Down's syndrome during the last decade.

Indications for chromosome studies

First, chromosome studies on the blood of a patient should be requested if there are definite indications of a known chromosome syndrome, if there are suspicious features of such (for example, low birthweight, failure to thrive and odd appearance) or if several malformations are present in either a still- or livebirth. Other indications include ambiguous or incongruous genitalia, primary amenorrhoea, secondary amenorrhoea, short stature, infertility in a man, a couple who have had three or more spontaneous abortions, or a mentally retarded male who is thought to have the fragile syndrome. In all these instances the chance of finding a chromosome abnormality is at least 5%.

Second, chromosome studies on amniotic (fetal) cells should be offered if the mother is aged 35 or over (depending upon local resources), if one parent carries a balanced structural abnormality, if there has been a previous trisomic child, or if there is a high risk of an X-linked disorder in a son, for which prenatal diagnosis is not available.

GENETIC COUNSELLING

Genetic counselling is essentially a service to patients or to their families. It is provided for those who ask for advice, and should be offered to those who do not, if there is a high risk of a serious disease or a lower risk for a disease that can be detected prenatally. Genetic counselling should also be available for those women who know of no disease in their family, but who find themselves in a high-risk category; such as those with a high serum α-fetoprotein level in the second trimester of pregnancy, or those women who have an increased risk of having a chromosomally abnormal child because they are elderly.

The first aim of genetic counselling is to give

Table 13.8 Recurrence risks for Down's syndrome

Abnormality	Relative frequency (%)	Recurrence risks for sibs
Trisomy 21	93	1 in 100
Mosaicism	2	Small
De novo translocation	2	Random risk
inherited translocation		
14/21; 13/21; 15/21	1	1 in 6* 1 in 100*
21/22	1	1 in 10 1 in 20
21/21	1	100%

* First risk is when mother is the carrier, the second when father is the carrier

Table 13.9   Maternal age and trisomy 21

Maternal age group	Incidence of liveborn mongols	Incidence of trisomy 21 at amniocentesis
Under 20	1 in 2000	These age groups
20–24	1 in 1600	are not screened
25–29	1 in 1000	by amniocentesis
30–34	1 in 760	
35–36	1 in 390	1 in 196
37–38	1 in 225	1 in 122
39–40	1 in 120	1 in 72
41–45	1 in 60	1 in 37

Table 13.10   Some empirical risks used in genetic counselling

Condition in child	Recurrence in sibs
Unexplained microcephaly	1 in 6 to 1 in 8
Asymmetrical cerebral palsy	<1 in 100
Unexplained cerebral palsy which is symmetrical	1 in 9
Congenital deafness	1 in 8
Hypospadias	1 in 10
Petit mal epilepsy	1 in 14
Febrile convulsions	1 in 5 to 1 in 10
Generalised idiopathic epilepsy	1 in 12 to 1 in 15
Insulin-dependent diabetes mellitus	1 in 10 to 1 in 15
Renal agenesis	1 in 12
Asthma	1 in 5 to 1 in 10

accurate risks of recurrence to couples, and to put those risks into perspective. Some indications of the risks in genetic or part genetic disorders have already been given. The counsellor should explain to couples the range of severity likely if another child is affected, and whether treatment of the condition, or prenatal detection of it, is possible now or likely to become so in the future.

The second aim is to alert the obstetrician, paediatrician or GP to the risk of a particular disease developing in a neonate. Some diseases should be treated promptly to prevent complications, e.g. galactosaemia, to prevent cataract formation, and congenital adrenal hyperplasia (21-hydroxylase deficiency, which may be difficult to recognise in a male) in order to prevent collapse and death during intercurrent illness.

The third aim of genetic counselling is to reduce the birth frequency of severely handicapped children in the population. This is a general aim, for on an individual basis there is no pressure by the genetic counsellor to persuade couples to behave in a certain way. The decision is left to them once they know the accurate risks on which to base it.

It is often not easy to give accurate risks of recurrence for those conditions where the aetiology is mixed or is not clear. In an undiagnosed but possibly genetic condition in a male, one should always think 'could this be X-linked?' for the genetic advice given to mother and sisters in such a case is very different from that given for an autosomal recessive condition. Table 13.10 lists the empirical recurrence risks for some clinical disease categories.

Malformation syndromes

These may present a difficult problem in diagnosis. In assessing a child with dysmorphic features it is useful first to consider whether they could be explained by an event during pregnancy. Examples would be maternal ingestion of drugs or alcohol, an intra-uterine infection or pressure, or the formation of amniotic bands. Secondly one should consider whether the features might be secondary to a single malformation, such as glossoptis and cleft palate occurring in the Pierre Robin syndrome, all secondary to mandibular hypoplasia. If there are several unrelated and unexplained signs, it is useful to list them, taking measurements where appropriate, and comparing these to the normal ranges (Smith 1982). It is then helpful to choose the most unusual feature, and to seek its presence in particular syndromes, using the index of abnormal signs given in Smith (1982).

So many genetic syndromes are now delineated that it is not possible for one person to remember even a majority of them. In order to help with accurate diagnosis, a computerised dysmorphology data base has been assembled at the Institute of Child Health in London, to which clinical geneticists have access. It is therefore worth seeking a genetic opinion. Chromosome studies are indicated in a dysmorphic child if several abnormal features are present, together with low birthweight, altered tone, and developmental delay. However some syndromes are associated with such small chromosomal deletions that they are difficult for a cytogeneticist to recognise unless the clinician can suggest which chromosome should be studied closely (Schinzel 1984). If no single gene nor chromosomal syndrome can be identified, then the recurrence risk for non-specific malformation syndromes is 1–2%.

It has recently become clear that only 15–20% of couples who have a recognisable risk for having a severely handicapped child actually receive genetic counselling. This is largely a failure of doctors, either to appreciate the risk, or to explain it to the couple concerned, or to search out other relatives who might be at high risk. A population study in Birmingham on the heterogenous condition of retinitis pigmentosa, demonstrated that almost all couples who had symptoms by the time of marriage would have liked to have known the genetic implications of their condition. In autosomal dominant disorders and X-linked disorders there are often high risks for relatives outside the nuclear family and some follow-up system, like that provided by genetic registers, is needed. The conclusion is, inevitably, that many more people than receive it at present would like to have, and should be offered, genetic counselling.

FURTHER READING

British Medical Bulletin 1976 Human malformations. 32: 1
Bundey S 1987 The fragile X syndrome. The Practitioner 231: 910–914
Carter C O 1969 An ABC of medical genetics. Lancet, London
Emery A E H 1986 Methodology in human genetics, 2nd edn. Churchill Livingstone, Edinburgh
Roberts D F, Chavez J, Court S D M 1970 The genetic component in child mortality. Archives of Disease in Childhood 45: 33–38
Schinzel A 1984 Catalogue of unbalanced chromosome aberrations in man. Walter de Gruyter, Berlin
Smith D W 1982 Recognizable patterns of human malformation, 3rd edn. W B Saunders, Philadelphia
Weatherall D J 1985 The new genetics and clinical practice, 2nd edn. The Oxford University Press, Oxford

14. Behaviour disorders and child psychiatry

E. Earle

INTRODUCTION

Children with disturbance in their behaviour usually cause problems to others more than themselves and it is parents or teachers who seek help rather than the child himself. Some children do suffer from anxiety or depression and the symptoms cause them enough distress to ask for help.

Few children will admit that they are disturbed by their thoughts and feelings; they show their upset by disturbed behaviour. The Isle of Wight survey showed that 6% of 10–11 year olds had a psychiatric disorder requiring treatment or further assessment; one-third of these children had problems at home and at school; of the remainder, one-half showed problems only at school and the other half only at home.

Disturbed behaviour in a child must be assessed in relation to the stage of development, if it is to be understood; the child who shows his frustration by lying on the floor and kicking may be considered normal at 2 years of age, but disturbed at 12 years old. The preverbal child has few outlets for his feelings and any upset is usually shown by some disturbance in sleep, eating habits or bowel and urinary function. Older children may be able to discuss their feelings; but an objective description from parents and teachers is important.

Once a child can speak he may show disturbance by negative behaviour such as refusal to speak, refusal to go to bed alone, or separate from mother. Habits may develop such as nail biting or withholding of faeces. This negative behaviour is part of the usual behaviour of toddlers, often described as the 'terrible twos'. Parents who are worried about their child's behaviour, can be re-assured that it may be a passing phase, but should it persist treatment may be required.

Children over the age of 3 may show these symptoms mentioned above or, more commonly, failure in toilet training, enuresis or encopresis. Problems are common in children of this age; if the symptom becomes incapacitating, it requires treatment. Somatic symptoms in the form of headaches, abdominal pain or vague aches and pains, may also develop. If a positive medical diagnosis cannot be made, then a positive psychiatric diagnosis should be sought, but these symptoms should not be over-investigated. Adolescence poses its own problems.

Common problems in childhood are outlined in Table 14.1.

Table 14.1 Common problems in childhood

Birth–1 year	Difficulty in going to sleep or waking
	Poor feeding or vomiting
	Restlessness
1–3 years	Refusal to separate from mother
	Refusal to go to bed alone
	Nightmares
	Constipation
	Nail biting
Over 3 years	Clinging behaviour
	Encopresis
	Phobias
	Abdominal pain or headaches
	Delayed or incoherent speech

PSYCHOLOGICAL ASSESSMENT IN CHILDREN

This should be based on school reports, a detailed

history from the parents or guardians, and interview with the child and psychological tests if indicated.

A school report gives an indication of whether the child shows disturbance in relationships with adults or children, or whether there is any learning difficulty.

The history

Both parents should be seen if possible, as they may have different views of the child. It also allows the interviewer to make some assessment of the marital interaction. Questions should be asked concerning the following matters:

1. Current problem. The parents will describe this and some questions can be asked as to possible precipitating factors such as separation or illness.

2. The pregnancy and birth. Was this baby planned and how did the mother feel during the pregnancy? Was there any separation following delivery?

3. Feeding. Was the baby breast or bottle fed and was this easily established. Were solids accepted? Has there been any feeding disturbance or food fads?

4. Toilet training. How was this introduced and established? Have there been any relapses?

5. Sleep. What has been the child's sleep pattern and has this altered in any way? Does the child have nightmares or talk about dreams?

6. Speech development. Has speech developed appropriately or is it delayed?

7. Habit disorders. Does the child have any mannerisms or tics or disorders such as thumb sucking, nail biting or head banging?

8. Motor development. When did the child start to walk and to draw and write.

Interview with the child

This must be geared to the age and stage of development of the child. It is important to reassure the child that you are not going to give him an injection or hurt him, and some explanation that you are there to listen to any worries he may have will be reassuring. Younger children will want to use toys. They will also be able to draw and give you associations to the pictures.

If a child has difficulty in talking then questions may help, but may only produce monosyllabic answers. A child's three wishes will also give insight into his areas of anxiety.

The child should be seen together with his parents and also separately.

Information gained from interviewing the child alone includes: appearance; motor development; attention span; speech; manner of relating; emotional state; attitudes to home, school, parents; and feelings about his problems.

Psychological tests

These are used to measure IQ and levels of achievement, while projective tests will highlight areas of difficulty. It is important to know whether school failure is due to low IQ or to anxiety, as the treatment differs. Educational psychologists or clinical psychologists attached to the Child Guidance Clinics will be qualified to adminster these tests.

Diagnosis

The careful history taking and collating of reports from other professionals allows a diagnosis to be made. Child psychiatric diagnoses must take account of five different elements or axes:

1. The first axis is *clinical psychiatric syndrome*: this may range from no obvious disorder, through to a simple emotional disorder, and/or conduct disorder.

2. The second axis is *specific delay in development*: this includes speech disorders, reading retardation, learning disorders.

3. The third axis is the *level of intelligence*: this is measured with appropriate tests and the child may fall anywhere on the normal distribution curve from severely subnormal to highly intelligent.

4. The fourth axis is a prevailing *medical condition*: e.g. asthma, eczema, cerebral palsy.

5. The fifth axis is the *psychosocial situation* which may range from accepted normal, to family discord, to abuse of the child.

CHILDREN IN HOSPITAL

Inevitably some young children have to be admitted to hospital either for short- or long-term treatment. The effects on the child may be two-fold:

1. Separation from mother and his familiar surroundings.
2. The effects of pain and medical and surgical interventions.

Separation

Children under the age of 4 years are entirely dependent on their parents and have an especially close relationship with their mother, or primary caretaker. Separation from mother should be gradual and only for a few hours in the beginning; children may start at a half-day playgroup or nursery from the age of 3 years. If the child has to go into hospital it is best that his mother stays with him and, if this is not possible, that she is allowed free visiting during the day in order to minimise the effects of separation, such as the feeling of deprivation of love and security. Children under 4 years of age are too young to understand that they are ill or have to be separated from their parents. Despite preparation for admission, and the presence of the mother, many children still show sleep disturbance, temper tantrums and may be insecure even 6 months after a stay in hospital.

Prolonged hospital admission may lead to serious impoverishment of the personality. Children who are in hospital for a long time may be 'promiscuous' in their behaviour and latch on to any adult in their search for affection.

Effects of medical and surgical treatment

Although the taking of blood by venepuncture may seem relatively insignificant to doctors, children perceive it as extremely traumatic. It may be viewed as an assault and the 'stealing' of something important. Children in hospital have to passively accept ministrations of nurses and to hand over ownership of their own body. Thus, a child who is toilet trained and proud of it, may suddenly be required to urinate or defaecate in front of a strange adult — if he complies this may lead to a regression once he returns home and an inability to maintain bowel and bladder control. Children may make more fuss over apparently minor interventions than over major surgery, and may even deny it is going to happen.

Before any procedure, an age-appropriate explanation should be given to the child. This may simply be that the prick of the needle will hurt for a second, but there will be no lasting pain. It is not worth trying to pretend to, or deceive a child that a procedure will be painless because he will never believe you again.

Chronic illness and death

Children who are subjected to chemotherapy will develop coping strategies, but these do not always meet with medical and nursing approval. It is natural for a child to be angry when he is ill and it is healthy to express this anger. The anger however, is often directed towards adults who are trying to help the child and they may find it hard to accept. From the child's point of view it is worse to turn the anger inwards and become depressed, but from the parent's and staff's viewpoint it may be easier to manage. No child should be forced to acknowledge that he is dying if he does not want to know; sensitive handling of questions will often allow parents, staff, siblings and the dying child to share feelings which allow the child to die peacefully instead of fighting and struggling.

It is remarkable that children frequently choose the most junior nurse or medical student to ask 'will I ever get better?' or 'am I going to die?' Perhaps they sense that the inexperienced will be more honest. These questions, however, need not be answered directly nor avoided, but the subject can be opened up by replying 'what has made you think that?' The child can then share his experiences and understanding of the treatment and perhaps make more realistic plans for the future.

DEVELOPMENTAL AND HABIT DISORDERS

In these conditions there is a delay in acquiring

control of a function or functions or the body, or there is a regression to earlier modes of behaviour.

Enuresis (see Ch. 20)

Rutter, in the Isle of Wight study, found that 15% of 7-year-old boys are wet at night less often than once a week, and only 7% wet more frequently than this. At the age of 5 as many girls are wetting as boys but by the age of 10 it is 1.6 boys to 1 girl and at 14 years of age 1.77 boys to 1 girl.

The cause may be physical or emotional; emotional disturbance is usually seen as regressive behaviour after bladder control has been established. Stresses leading to regression may be a death in the family, including death of a pet, birth of a sibling, or separation due to parental or the child's own illness, and hospitalisation.

Treatment

1. Exclude a physical cause.
2. An active interest in the child is important; the family may be very angry with the child, but often the mother is surprisingly compliant with the child's symptom. A carrot, not a stick, is the basis of treatment but it is unrealistic for the mother to wash sheets daily with no comment and possibly the child and mother should change the bedding together.
3. Reward systems may be valuable. A simple star chart or payment for a dry night may encourage the child.
4. Explanations may also be important to the child and parents, particularly if bedwetting is associated with nightmares. It usually occurs in stage 4 sleep, but may have a meaning to the child, if this is explored in an interview.
5. Drug treatment: tricyclic antidepressants.
6. Conditioning with a pad and buzzer. The child's bed is made with two aire gauze sheets separated by a cotton sheet and connected to a bell or buzzer. As the child starts to wet the bed he completes the electric circuit and the buzzer wakes him. Gradually he wakes before the alarm goes off, as the feeling of a full bladder is associated with waking. This is not suitable under the age of 8 years.

7. Psychotherapy may be indicated if there are clear emotional precipitants. Depending on the clinical assessment, this may be aimed individually at the child, or in a family setting to elucidate the interactions. Formal psychotherapy should be with a trained therapist.

Encopresis

This usually presents as soiling the underclothes on the way to or from school, although occasionally soiling occurs at night. It may also be associated with smearing of faeces or defaecating in unusual places. Soiling is more frequently seen in boys than girls.

1. Continuous soiling may be due to lack of toilet training and may occur in children who are generally ill cared for.
2. Regressive soiling may be associated with secondary enuresis and the precipitating factors are similar.
3. Aggressive soiling. This is seen in children who feel oppressed by parental demands to be clean and tidy and to perform well at school.

Treatment depends on the cause, but retraining and removal of impacted faeces may be necessary. In regressive and aggressive soiling, psychotherapy or family therapy may be indicated.

Nightmares and pavor nocturnus

Many children recount their dreams and will talk freely about nightmares, these are usually related to anxiety or wishes which they know are unacceptable in the daytime. Nightmares often have a precipitant, such as the birth of a sibling, and if the child can talk about his anger and feelings of displacement, the nightmares will disappear. Where nightmares occur in REM sleep, pavor nocturnus occurs in stage 4 sleep and children have no memory of the disturbance. Parents describe the child as calling out in his sleep, sitting bolt upright and staring. The child does not appear to hear the parents' calming words but within a few minutes he lies down and continues to sleep.

Reassurance is usually sufficient for both parents and children. If pavor nocturnus persists the child might need a small dose of a tricyclic anti-depressant at night to make sleep lighter, and break the pattern.

Other habit disorders

These include feeding disorders, nail biting, speech defects and sleep disorders. All of these may reflect poor training and poor mother–child interaction. Treatment is aimed at helping the child to develop normally and helping the parents to be consistent in their handling of the child.

CONDUCT DISORDERS

By definition these disorders cover the group of children whose behaviour is antisocial. It is usually society and not parents who complain about the child, and juvenile courts, probation officers or social workers are often involved. Although parents may complain of the child's behaviour, the parents themselves are often antisocial. They may be inconsistent and rejecting towards the child. Symptoms include lying, stealing, truancy, physical aggression and vandalism.

It is difficult to give figures for the prevalence of these disorders because methods of assessment and categorization vary. The Isle of Wight study showed conduct disorders to be present in 4% of 10–11 year olds and non-delinquent conduct disorders accounted for 1% overall. Boys are more affected than girls; in inner city areas the prevalence is much greater in both groups.

Truancy

As with other conduct disorders, this is more common in boys than girls. There may be a family history of truancy, although the parents are not aware that the child is truanting. He will leave for school in the morning and return home at the appropriate time in the evening, but during the day he will be involved in petty crime. These children are usually not highly intelligent and find school unrewarding. Truancy is more common in the older age groups.

Treatment must be aimed at both the family and the individual and may involve social change. Some children have to be removed from home to boarding school or residential placements. Other children can be helped via the parents, who receive social help, or encouragement to set consistent limits.

NEUROTIC DISORDERS

Neurotic children suffer from their symptoms. The symptoms are persistent and incapacitating in some areas of life.

Common symptoms are depression, anxiety, obsessional rituals and somatic symptoms. Although some anxiety is common in response to new situations, neurotic children respond out of all proportion to the stimulus.

School refusal

This is an extremely common condition, although it may not always be obvious to the general practitioner, paediatrician or even school as such. The child may appear physically ill, or present with complaints of headache, stomachache, or general malaise. There may be a genuine physical illness initially, from which the child fails to return to school. Sometimes lengthy physical investigations reveal no illness and it is only then that anxiety and panic are recognised.

The Isle of Wight study showed on overall prevalence of less than 3% of 10–11 year old children with a psychiatric disorder. In other studies the figure has varied from 1% to 8%. The variation probably reflects the differing diagnostic criteria between doctors in the community and in Child Guidance Clinics.

The child often expresses the wish to go to school but is unable to leave home, or if he does he cannot enter the classroom. However, once he returns home he appears perfectly well. Girls outnumber boys in primary school age, but in adolescence this disorder becomes more of a problem for boys. Although the child may say a specific teacher or subject is what he is trying to avoid, this is usually a rationalisation and the real problem is that of leaving mother. Mothers of these children often have phobic symptoms or excessive anxiety and the mother and child become locked into a mutually clinging relationship.

The symptom of school refusal can have two

possible sources, the second being truancy where the parents are unaware of the problem (Table 14.2).

Treatment

The child must be given a date to return to school and the father or educational welfare officer, or other outside agent should be involved in actually taking the child from home to school, this helps child and mother.

The child should not be allowed to change school or have home tuition as this colludes with his problem. Physical examination is necessary to rule out physical illness, but long investigations should not be embarked upon. The teachers will need information about the child and how to manage him when he says he feels ill. Diazepam may be helpful as a single dose on waking in the morning, but should not be used long term.

Ongoing work with the family, aimed at helping them to adjust in a more healthy manner, will be necessary if the symptom is not to recur.

Other forms of anxiety

As a child develops it is important that he develops *signal anxiety*. This means that he does not rely on the presence of adults to warn him of danger, but can recognise when he needs to avoid danger. An example of this is that children learn to judge the speed of cars when crossing the road.

As this signal anxiety is developing it may appear to be exaggerated at times, almost to phobic proportions. Thus it is common to see children who are phobic of dogs or other animals. This may be a developmental phase but if it persists it may

need full investigation, as it may represent a displacement of anxiety from a deeper irrational fear to something which seems to have a rational basis.

Depression

Children may show symptoms of depression, tearfulness, listlessness, inability to concentrate, poor appetite, excessive sleepiness and hopelessness. It may be clear that the child is reacting to a family disturbance or loss of a parent, but sometimes there seems to be no precipitating cause. The child may develop obsessional behaviour as a defence against depression. This is usually seen in ritual behaviour where the child must do things in a particular order, and he believes this will prevent his feeling sad.

Treatment

Treatment is usually based on psychotherapy for the child, to help him to understand his feelings and therefore to react differently. Family therapy may be indicated if there are tensions which are not being openly discussed.

CHILDHOOD PSYCHOSIS

Psychotic children have an altered contact with reality and are attempting to adapt to a subjectively distorted concept of the world. In young children, the diagnosis can be made from the behaviour which includes a failure to make normal emotional contact with people. It is important to try to distinguish psychotic behaviour from that of the intellectually subnormal child. It is also important to rule out any other organic pathology.

Acute toxic conditions

In these children there is a diffuse impairment of cerebral function with a state of delirium or confusion. Common causes are systemic infection, intracranial infection, metabolic disturbances, chemical intoxications including drugs, and brain injury.

Table 14.2   Non-attendance at school

	School refusal	Truancy
Age	5–11 years	Over 12 years
Parents	Collude with child over non-attendance	Unaware of problem
Achievement	High with high goals	Non-academic, with only practical goals
Treatment	Insight therapy	Structural change

Chronic organic causes

Lead encephalopathy

Lead encephalopathy may present as a behaviour disorder with symptoms of irritability, restlessness, inability to concentrate and loss of interest.

Cerebral lipidoses

The onset of symptoms is usually between 3 and 5 years of age and the child's condition deteriorates rapidly Although neurological signs are usually present the child may present as psychotic.

Psychoses of mixed aetiology

a. Infantile psychosis or autism.
b. Late-onset psychosis or childhood schizophrenia.

A distinction may be made between the two conditions (Table 14.3), and also between them and mental subnormality.

Infantile psychosis

Kanner in 1943 described three features of autistic children: a lack of awareness of people and an avoidance of contact; delay or absence of speech with abnormalities such as echolalia, where the child merely repeats what is said to him, and an obsessional desire for sameness, differences causing a catastrophic reaction. Parents may describe the baby as 'very good' and able to entertain himself. However, this usually means he is avoiding social contact and prefers objects, often a hard object, to people. The parents may also describe rituals which the child has developed, or stereotyped behaviour. Autistic withdrawal and speech delay, or absence of speech development usually lead parents to seek advice during the child's second year, but they usually describe problems from birth. The incidence is 4–5/10 000, with four boys to one girl. The incidence appears to be higher in social classes I and II but some people argue that intelligent parents push harder for action than less intelligent parents.

Treatment. All forms of treatment have been tried with mixed claims of success:

1. Institutional care. Some families are unable to care for their autistic child, either because of violence, other children or the parents suffer too much. There are a few specialised institutions offering skilled teaching and handling

2. Behaviour therapy is aimed at rewarding acceptable behaviour and punishing unacceptable behaviour. A programme must be worked out for each individual child

3. Psychotherapy is very time consuming and not always rewarding, although it can lead to breakthroughs in communication

4. Drugs may be needed to treat symptoms such as violence or sleeplessness, but are not curative.

Late-onset psychosis

Children appear to be developing normally and then after the age of 5 years the parents or teachers

Table 14.3 Comparison of early-onset and late-onset psychosis

	Early onset (autism)	Late onset (childhood schizophrenia)
Age of onset	Before 3 years	After 5 years
Speech	Delayed or echolalia	No abnormality
Schizophrenic symptoms	Absent	Auditory and bodily hallucinations, thought insertion and withdrawal and broadcast delusions
Motility	Stereotypies	Loss of volition Apathy
Incidence of schizophrenia in relatives	Lower than average	Above average
Drug treatment	Symptomatic relief only	Phenothiazines useful

notice abnormalities of behaviour and academic performance falling off. The symptoms are similar to those adult schizophrenic symptoms described by Schneider. These include hallucinations, delusions, thought withdrawal, thought insertion, and loss of volition. In talking to these children the clinician will know that the child is psychotic because of his apparent chaos and misunderstanding of the world. The parents of this group of children have a significantly higher rate of schizophrenia than the general population. They also tend to be isolated, which is attributed to their personalities. This contrasts with parents of the infantile psychosis group, whose social isolation is secondary to their child's illness.

Treatment

Treatment of children in these two groups also varies. The *infantile psychosis* group pose severe difficulties in day-to-day handling and often have to be admitted to day units or residential units for behaviour modification or long-term psychotherapy, the parents also need long-term counselling.

The *late-onset* group respond well to phenothiazine tranquillisers or haloperidol, although short-term hospital admission may be necessary. Supportive psychotherapy for the child and parents may also be beneficial and some families benefit from family therapy. The course of the illness is usually progressive and insitutional care may be necessary eventually.

ADOLESCENCE

Adolescence poses its own problems. There are often lengthy discussions about the differences between the normal adolescent process and illness requiring treatment. Adolescence is a time of turmoil and can cause distress to both the adolescent and those who have contact with him.

The task for each adolescent is to leave behind his childhood dependency on his parents and to begin to function more as an independent person. He must be able to risk parental disapproval without feeling that he must give in to parental demands. This may be in the area of sexuality, friendships or work. The parents have to allow their adolescent son or daughter to make mistakes

and to be different from parental ideals. This is not always easy and many parents, especially mothers who may be menopausal, find it hard to allow their children free expression of sexuality.

The adolescent also has to come to terms with his or her sexually maturing body. He must feel in control of his body and find acceptable outlets for sexual and aggressive feelings. This involves changes in types of relationships with friends of the same and the opposite sex. The demands and expectations of these friends will be more adult.

The problems of adolescence are numerous, but there are two serious conditions, anorexia nervosa and drug addiction.

Anorexia nervosa

The condition occurs mainly in girls although it has been described in boys. The onset is usually soon after puberty in a girl who is overweight and starts to diet. She finds herself unable to stop and becomes emaciated. Her periods cease, if they have commenced, and the girl becomes determined to keep her weight at pre-pubertal levels. These girls have an unrealistic perception of themselves and believe they are fat when, in reality, they are thin; their perception of other people is not distorted. The girl herself is often active and cheerful and it is her parents who seek help.

Once recognised this condition requires specialist help. This usually means patient treatment in a special unit with therapy available both for the adolescent and her family. Untreated these girls survive on the brink of death and may die while still denying their problem.

Drug addiction

Drug addiction is increasing in our society. In its widest definition it covers smoking, drinking, the use of diazepam, sniffing solvents through to the abuse of LSD and heroin. Adolescence is a time of experimentation and many young people test for themselves the effects of alcohol and tobacco. They may also take various tablets and cannabis without becoming dependent on them. However, the dividing line between experimenting and addiction is very narrow. The adolescent who becomes dependent on drugs is usually one who is depressed and may have had early losses in his or her life. These adolescents are disillusioned with life and may be on the fringe of criminal activity, drug addiction forces them further into crime because they have to finance the habit.

If an adolescent is suspected of drug abuse because of erratic or other changes in behaviour, clinical examination and an objective history are essential. This may reveal altered pupil size or reaction, injection sites or infected injection sites. In solvent sniffers there may be inflammation and sores around the mouth and nose. Urine can be analysed for the presence of drugs and once the diagnosis is confirmed treatment at a drug addiction clinic is usually indicated.

THE ROLE OF THE DOCTOR

It will be clear from these descriptions of both the physically ill children who respond to stress with behaviour problems, and those children under stress who have somatic symptoms, that the GP will be the first doctor whom the parents consult. In order to sort out the physical and emotional problems the doctor will have to spend time taking a history and listening carefully to the child, the family and their worries.

Once a diagnosis has been reached much of the treatment can be managed by the GP or a paediatrician. If a referral to a child or adolescent psychiatrist is made, the reasons must be carefully explained to the child and family. Too often, the family feel that the doctor has given up or become 'fed up' with them, and is therefore handing them over. Joint management of a family can be extremely rewarding.

Individual therapy must be given by a trained therapist but marital therapy and family therapy are often given by two therapists, one of whom may be a doctor and the other a psychotherapist or social worker.

Children attend school and their teachers are often concerned with day-to-day management, so that regular communication is vital if they are to complement treatment. It is also important to involve community social workers and probation officers, who already know the family, when planning a treatment programme. The multidisciplinary approach can be destructive if it is used merely to dispel anxiety of the professionals and allows no one to take responsibility for helping a child and his family. If used properly the involvement of different professionals can be most rewarding.

FURTHER READING

Barker P 1971 Basic child psychiatry. Staples Press, London
Earle E M 1979 Psychological effects of mutilating surgery in children and adolescents. Psychoanalytic Study of the Child 34: 527–546
Freud A 1973 Normality and pathology in childhood. Penguin, Harmondsworth
Graham P J 1966 Psychiatric disorders in ten to eleven year old children. Proceedings of Royal Society of Medicine 59: 382–387
Graham P 1986 Child psychiatry, a developmental approach. Oxford University Press, Oxford
Kahn J 1981 Unwillingly to school. Pergamon, Oxford

Kolvin I 1971 Studies in childhood psychoses. British Journal of Psychiatry 118: 341–419
Laufer M 1975 Adolescent disturbance and breakdown. Penguin, Harmondsworth
Robertson J 1975 Young children in hospital, 2nd edn. Tavistock, London
Rutter M L 1975 Helping troubled children. Penguin, Harmondsworth.
Rutter M, Hersov L 1985 Child and adolescent psychiatry, modern approaches. Blackwell, Oxford
Winnicott D W 1964 The child, the family and the outside world. Penguin, London

15. Infectious diseases

T. Lissauer

Infections are the commonest reason for children to be brought to their GP. Infections of the upper and lower respiratory tracts, gastrointestinal and urinary tracts, bone, joints and central nervous system are described in other chapters. This chapter will focus on some of the common infectious diseases seen in children in this country. How these infections may affect the fetus and newborn infant is also described. A guide to the clinical diagnosis of the rashes caused by the major acute infectious diseases in children is included at the end of the chapter.

COMMON INFECTIOUS DISEASES OF CHILDHOOD

In the UK there has been a dramatic reduction this century in the morbidity and mortality from infectious diseases. Many factors are responsible for this change, including improved housing conditions, sanitation and nutrition, and the introduction of vaccines. The role of medical treatment and the widespread use of antibiotics is more difficult to determine. Some of the infectious diseases are kept under surveillance (Table 15.1) and preventive measures taken in the community, when appropriate, to avoid the spread of infection. In industrialised countries many of these infectious diseases of childhood have become more of an inconvenience than serious illnesses. However, the loss of time from school for the child, and from work for their parents, both during the illness and until the child can return to school, can be significant (Table 15.2). Although they are uncommon, there are still serious complications of these infectious diseases and they have also taken on a

Table 15.1 Notifiable infectious diseases, England and Wales 1988

Acute encephalitis	Leprosy*	Relapsing fever
Acute meningitis	Leptospirosis	Rubella
Acute poliomyelitis	Malaria	Scarlet fever
Anthrax	Marburg disease	Smallpox
Cholera	Measles	Tetanus
Diphtheria	Mumps	Tuberculosis
Dysentery	Ophthalmia neonatorum	Typhoid fever
Food poisoning	Paratyphoid fever	Typhus fever
Lassa fever	Plague	Viral haemorrhagic fever
	Rabies	Viral hepatitis
		Whooping cough
		Yellow fever

* Data collected centrally in confidence by the Department of Health

renewed importance in children who are immunocompromised.

Measles

The measles virus is transmitted by direct contact or droplet spread of respiratory secretions and is highly infectious. The illness is so common in children that it tends to be regarded as a normal event of childhood. This is unfortunate as it is unpleasant, potentially serious and is preventable. After the introduction of measles immunisation, the incidence declined, but it continued to be widespread as the acceptance rate for immunisation

Table 15.2 Incubation period and period of exclusion from school of the common infectious diseases

Illness	Incubation period (days)		Minimum period of exclusion from school (assuming full clinical recovery)
	Range	Usual period	
Measles	7–14	10	4 days from onset of the rash
Chickenpox	10–24	14	6 days from onset of the rash provided all lesions are crusted
Rubella	14–21	18	4 days from onset of the rash
Mumps	12–31	18	Until swelling has subsided (7 days approximately)
Hepatitis A	15–50	28	Until clinical recovery and not before 7 days from onset of jaundice

was only 70%. Since the introduction of the combined measles, mumps, and rubella vaccine (MMR) in the UK in 1988, there has been an improvement in vaccine uptake and a reduction in the incidence of measles.

Clinical features

The incidence of measles is highest in the preschool child. Since the introduction of measles immunisation, an increasing proportion of affected children are of school age.

The incubation period of around 10 days is followed by a prodromal illness of fever and widespread congestion of the mucous membranes, with coryza, conjunctivitis and cough. The prodromal illness lasts 3–4 days, during which the child is very miserable and anorexic. Bronchitis is part of the illness as the involvement of the mucous membranes includes the epithelium of the bronchi and bronchioles and crepitations can usually be heard on auscultation of the chest. Observing Koplik's spots is helpful in making the diagnosis at this stage as they are pathognomonic of measles. They may be difficult to detect and are tiny white spots, like grains of salt, on the inflammed buccal mucosa and are best seen opposite the second molar teeth. They are visible 2–3 days before the onset of the rash and then fade when the rash appears. They are sometimes still visible a day or two after the rash has emerged. The rash starts behind the ears, and spreads to the forehead and then to the face and down the body. It is initially a dull red, maculopapular rash but becomes confluent and blotchy. The rash and fever are usually maximal a day after the onset of the rash. In the week following the disappearance of the rash staining of the skin may be quite marked in some patients. The rash starts to fade by the third day in the same sequence as it appeared.

Complications

Complications arise from extension of the inflammation caused by the virus or from superadded bacterial infection. They are most likely in those who have a severe attack and in infants and young children. The commonest complications are respiratory, especially bronchopneumonia, otitis media and laryngotracheitis, but these are seen only infrequently in well-nourished children. Children with leukaemia or who are immunocompromised may develop a severe giant-cell pneumonia which is usually fatal.

Febrile convulsions may occur during the prodromal illness and during the first 2 days of the rash. Postinfectious encephalitis has been reported to occur in up to 1 in 1000 cases. Approximately 7–10 days after the onset of the illness the child develops a headache, vomiting and drowsiness which may progress to coma and be accompanied by convulsions. The course is unpredictable; 60% recover completely, but as many as 25% have permanent brain damage and in 15% it is fatal. A rare late complication, occuring in 1 in 100 000 cases, is subacute sclerosing panencephalitis.

Treatment

There is no specific treatment. Regular paracetamol will assist in reducing the fever and may make the child feel less miserable. Antibiotics are only required for bronchopneumonia or otitis media. Children with encephalitis or significant upper airways obstructions from laryngotracheitis will need to be closely monitored in hospital.

Measles in the developing countries

Measles remains a serious illness in the developing

countries where it carries a high morbidity and mortality. This is primarily related to the socio-economic conditions and it is an especially serious illness in areas where the diet is deficient in protein. The rash in these malnourished children may be confluent and become deep red, purple or even haemorrhagic, and then desquamate. There is a high incidence of secondary bacterial infection with otitis media and bronchopneumonia. These children often have a very sore mouth and severe diarrhoea resulting in a marked loss of weight, which may take many weeks to be regained. It is important to ensure that these children do not become dehydrated and to maintain their nutrition both during and after the illness.

Chickenpox and shingles

Chickenpox (varicella) and shingles (zoster) are caused by the varicella-zoster virus. Chickenpox, the primary infection, is highly infectious and is transmitted by droplet spread or direct contact, either from lesions in the mouth and respiratory tract or, less commonly, from vesicles on the skin. Shingles cannot be contracted directly from a patient with chickenpox but results from reactivation of the virus which lies dormant in a dorsal root ganglion. It is a source of infection to those who have not had chickenpox.

Chickenpox is characteristically a mild illness in children. The incubation period usually lasts 14 days and may be followed by a short prodromal stage of malaise and a low grade fever but, more often, the onset of the illness is marked by the appearance of the rash. This begins as red macules which progress rapidly to papules and vesicles. The vesicles then dry to form crusts which form scabs and these fall off without leaving scars. The lesions are itchy and premature removal of the scabs or secondary infection may result in scar formation. The lesions appear in crops, so that all the stages are visible even over a small area. There are often two or three successive crops of lesions over the or first few days, but this varies widely from a handful of lesions to five or more successive crops. The rash starts in the hair and has a centripetal distribution, with the lesions most densely grouped on the trunk and decreasing in density on the limbs and face, although they may spread as far as the palms and soles. Lesions are usually present on the mucous membranes where they take the form of shallow ulcers as the roofs of the vesicles are removed.

Complications of chickenpox

Occasionally lesions become secondarily infected, usually with *Staphylococcus aureus* or streptococci. Other complications are very uncommon in healthy children. In chickenpox encephalitis, symptoms and signs develop 3–10 days after the appearance of the rash, and ataxia from cerebellar involvement is common. The prognosis is much better than in measles encephalitis, and most recover completely. Adults with chickenpox tend to experience a more severe form of the disease, and are more likely to develop chickenpox pneumonia. In contrast to normal children, chickenpox in an immunocompromised host may cause pneumonia and be very severe or even fatal. This includes children with leukaemia or lymphomas, and those on cytotoxic drugs or high doses of corticosteroids. When any of these children first present, the state of their immunity to varicella should be assessed so that their parents can be alerted to the potential danger of chickenpox. The patients should try to avoid contact with infected children but this is difficult and should it occur, zoster immune globulin should be given as soon as possible, preferably within 48 hours. Haemorrhagic chickenpox, which has a high mortality, is fortunately rare. Occasionally, children develop Reye's syndrome shortly after they have had chickenpox. Aspirin ingestion has been implicated in the pathogenesis of Reye's syndrome and although their true relationship is still unclear, it is recommended that aspirin should not be given to children with chickenpox or any febrile illness.

Diagnosis of chickenpox

It is seldom necessary to have laboratory confirmation of the clinical diagnosis. The virus can be demonstrated by electron microscopy of vesicular fluid, by culture or fluorescent-antibody staining. Infection can also be confirmed serologically by a four-fold rise in antibody.

Treatment of chickenpox

In most cases no specific treatment is necessary, but calamine lotion may be soothing. If the pruritus is troublesome, an oral antihistamine, such as trimeprazine tartrate (Vallergan), can be given. Acyclovir (Zovirax), an antiviral agent which acts as a competitive inhibitor of the viral DNA polymerase, is effective against varicella-zoster infections and has low toxicity. A course of acyclovir should be given in immunocompromised children and those with serious complications.

Features of shingles

Herpes zoster is much less common than chickenpox in childhood but is occasionally seen even in infants and young children. It is usually confined to the skin supplied by the sensory nerves of one or two dorsal root ganglia. Unlike adults, itching, burning or pain rarely precede the lesions, and it is usually a mild illness causing little discomfort and without postherpetic neuralgia.

Herpes simplex infections

Herpes simplex infections are caused by the viruses herpes hominis, types 1 (HSV 1) and 2 (HSV 2). HSV 1 is mainly associated with infection of the mouth and lips, eyes, skin and central nervous system, whilst HSV 2 causes mostly genital and neonatal infections.

Type 1 infection is common in childhood. Primary infection with clinical symptoms occurs in less than 10% of infections, so, in most instances, the infection is not apparent. By adulthood 70–90% of people have antibodies to the herpes simplex virus. Sometimes the virus remains latent and produces recurrent clinical symptoms.

Primary infection causes gingivostomatitis, vulvovaginitis, keratoconjunctivitis, or encephalitis. Acute gingivostomatitis (Fig. 15.1) is much the commonest. It affects children between 1 and 3 years old, who develop a high fever, irritability and sore throat resulting in refusal to eat or drink. The gums become swollen, red and friable. White plaques or shallow ulcers appear on the buccal mucosa, tongue, palate and fauces. Saliva drools from the mouth and may result in satellite skin

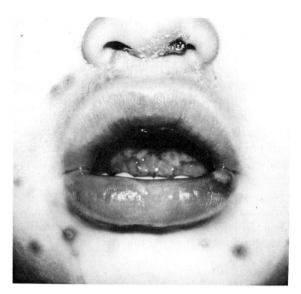

Fig. 15.1   Herpes simplex gingivostomatitis.

lesions around the mouth and anterior chest. The anterior cervical lymph nodes may be enlarged and tender. The severity of the illness varies, but in severe cases the illness lasts 10–14 days. The child may become dehydrated from refusing to eat or drink. Vulvovaginitis sometimes results from transfer of the organism from the mouth with contaminated fingers. In children with eczema, the infection may become extensive or even generalised (Fig. 15.2). Superadded bacterial infection (*Staphylococcus aureus* or streptococcal) is common. The illness may be very severe or even fatal from viraemia, septicaemia, shock from plasma loss or disseminated intravascular coagulation. Keratoconjunctivitis is uncommon, but dendritic ulcers may proceed to scarring and loss of vision. Herpes simplex encephalitis is a serious condition but is fortunately rare. Presentation is with focal neurological signs, convulsions and deteriorating level of consciousness in a febrile child.

The diagnosis is usually made from the clinical appearance. It can be confirmed, if necessary, by culture, electron microscopy of vesicular fluid, microscopic examination for inclusion bodies, or serologically.

Treatment of the gingivostomatitis is mainly supportive and the child's state of hydration must be kept under review. Painful oral lesions can be

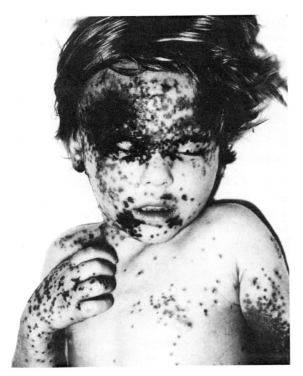

Fig. 15.2 Severe extensive herpes simplex infection in a child with eczema (Kaposi's varicelliform eruption).

children but is also seen more often in older children and adolescents than the other childhood exanthematous disease. The incubation period is about 18 days; with a range of 14–21 days. In children, it is usually a very mild illness and symptoms before the appearance of the rash are uncommon. The infection is often subclinical. The pale pink macular or maculopapular rash starts on the face and behind the ears and spreads down the body. It has usually started to disappear from the face by the second day and faded completely by the third day. It often loses its discrete appearance and can become scarlatiniform. There may be generalised lymphadenopathy especially involving the suboccipital, postauricular and cervical lymph nodes. Coryza, conjunctivitis and sore throat, if present, are minimal. In the adolescent or young adult there may be a mild prodromal illness, with a slight fever, malaise, a few swollen and sometimes tender lymph nodes and they often have arthralgia or arthritis, mainly affecting the joints of the hands and feet, 2–3 days after the onset of rash. The complications of rubella, encephalitis and thrombocytopenic purpura, are extremely rare.

treated with topical acyclovir, but most children find any interference with the lesions very unpleasant; it is usually best avoided. In severe herpes simplex infections, treatment with acyclovir is indicated. In eczema herpeticum, the topical steroids used to treat the eczema should be stopped and systemic antibiotics and antiviral therapy with acyclovir will be required. Keratoconjunctivitis should be managed by an ophthalmologist. Topical acyclovir is available for the treatment of ocular lesions. Although treatment with acyclovir has improved the prognosis of children with herpes simplex encephalitis, a high proportion suffer permanent neurological damage.

Rubella

Rubella or German measles is caused by the rubella virus and is transmitted by close and repeated contact with the respiratory secretions of an infected person. Rubella is common in young

Hepatitis

Five causes of viral hepatitis have been identified. In addition to viruses A and B, a further, relatively common, agent is virus C which causes non-A, non-B hepatitis. However, it is not yet possible to identify hepatitis C infection accurately by serological tests. A presumptive diagnosis of non-A, non-B hepatitis is made. The Epstein–Barr virus and cytomegalovirus can also cause hepatitis.

Hepatitis A virus infection

Hepatitis A is the commonest form of hepatitis seen in children. The hepatitis A virus is an enteric virus, transmitted through close contact by the faecal-oral route, often on contaminated fingers. The infection is commonest when the living conditions are overcrowded and inadequate and the standard of hygiene poor. Most children in these conditions have antibodies to the hepatitis A virus by late childhood, whereas the frequency of antibody in children of high socioeconomic status is low. There has been a marked decrease in the incidence of hepatitis A in the UK over the past few years. The virus can be identified in the stools of infected persons by electron microscopy 1–2 weeks before, and usually a few days after, the onset of jaundice, and infectivity is maximal during this period.

The incubation period is between 15 and 50 days with an average of 28–30 days. Three to 5 days before the onset of jaundice, the patient becomes anorexic with nausea, vomiting and there may be dull abdominal pain, especially over the right hypochondrium or epigastrium. There may be a fever and mild diarrhoea. Just before the icteric phase the urine may become dark from the presence of bilirubin, the right hypochondrium becomes tender on palpation and there may be mild enlargement of the spleen and lymphadenopathy. In young children the infection is mostly subclinical or mild. They often remain anicteric. If they become jaundiced it is usually only for a day or two. The vast majority of affected children recover completely.

The liver function tests are abnormal with a rise in the serum aminotransferases. The bilirubin may or may not be raised. Investigations will be required in children with hepatitis when the illness is atypical, especially severe or protracted. Other causes of jaundice will then need to be considered, especially hepatitis B, the hepatitis of infectious mononucleosis or cytomegalovirus, chronic active hepatitis and Wilson's disease. In obstructive jaundice, the alkaline phosphatase level is markedly elevated, whereas it rarely rises above one and half times normal in hepatitis A infection. A diagnosis of hepatitis A can be made by detecting anti-hepatitis A virus IgM, which indicates recent infection.

There is no specific treatment. Children who are feeling unwell will restrict their activities accordingly and bed rest need not be enforced.

No special diet is required, but dietary fat may be restricted if it is found to cause nausea. Hands must be washed diligently and a high standard of personal hygiene maintained to prevent spread of the disease to others. In hospital, these patients are isolated and nursed with enteric precautions. An injection of pooled immunoglobulin following exposure may prevent or modify the illness and is recommended as soon as possible for household and institutional contacts. Prophylactic immunoglobulin is recommended for travellers to countries where hepatitis A infection is endemic if they stay in areas where the personal hygiene and sanitation are poor.

Hepatitis B virus infection

Hepatitis B is a relatively uncommon illness in children in industrialised countries, but the incidence is much higher in countries where the carrier rate of the hepatitis B surface antigen (HBsAg) is high. In Northern Europe and North America the carrier rate is low, around 1 in 1000 adults, but it is much higher in the Far East and Africa. Children at special risk for hepatitis B are babies born to mothers who are HBsAg carriers, those who live in institutions, or are immunocompromised. Those who receive multiple blood transfusions or blood products are also at increased risk but this can be minimised by screening all blood for HBsAg.

The clinical features are similar to those of hepatitis A but the prodromal phase of malaise tends to be longer and the jaundice may be more prolonged. Adolescents and young adults may have arthralgia, usually of several small joints, and prodromal skin rashes. Most patients make a complete recovery. Some become chronic carriers of the HBsAg but are perfectly healthy, and a few develop chronic persistent hepatitis or chronic active hepatitis and cirrhosis. In countries where the carriage rate of HBsAg is high, it is associated with primary liver cancer in adult life. Special precautions must always be taken when drawing blood samples or handling the blood of these patients to avoid self-inoculation and, if it occurs, anti-hepatitis B immunoglobulin should be given immediately. Children with hepatitis B can return to school when they have recovered clinically. Those who become carriers should not be excluded from school, but this information must be provided for any dental or surgical procedures. A hepatitis B vaccine has recently been developed from fully purified formalin-inactivated HBsAg particles derived from the plasma of chronic carriers of the antigen and more recently, recombinant DNA vaccine has been introduced. With this vaccine it has become possible to offer protection to those at increased risk of infection in the UK. As well as the infants of mothers with HBsAg this includes health care and laboratory staff and patients and staff in institutions for the handicapped.

HIV infection

Although the acquired immune deficiency syndrome (AIDS) was first recognised only in 1981 it has rapidly become a major problem throughout the world. In the UK, by June 1990, 3280 cases had been reported of whom 56% have died. There were 12 370 HIV antibody positive cases reported. Although the majority are homosexual or bisexual men, about 8% are women and 3% children. Most children have become infected from perinatal transmission from their mothers, who have acquired the infection mainly from intravenous drug use or heterosexual transmission. Some children have received contaminated blood or blood products, particularly haemophiliacs from Factor VIII. As screening of blood is now possible, the transmission of infection by this route has become uncommon. There is a wide variation in the prevalence of HIV infection. In Massachussetts, USA, screening newborn infants in 1987 revealed that 2 per 1000 women giving birth must have been positive for HIV antibody, with a seropositive rate of 8 per 1000 in the inner cities. In some countries in Africa, where heterosexual transmission is particularly widespread, up to 20% of pregnant women have been found to be HIV seropositive in some urban areas. The World Health Organisation estimates that between five and ten million persons worldwide are infected with the HIV virus and AIDS will become an increasingly significant cause of morbidity and mortality in children.

The cause of HIV infection has been identified as the human immunodeficiency virus (HIV) which is a retrovirus. A second human immunodeficiency virus (HIV II) has been described from West Africa.

There is a wide range in the clinical manifestations of HIV infection. Children may be infected but asymptomatic. The majority of children who become clinically ill present with non-specific signs and symptoms, particularly failure to thrive, generalised lymphadenopathy, hepatosplenomegaly, recurrent diarrhoea and eczematous rashes within the first 2 years of life. Opportunist infections especially of the lung with *Pneumocystis carinii* pneumonia (PCP) is common. Less frequent are candida oesophagitis and disseminated cytomegalovirus infection. Severe and recalcitrant oral thrush is also common. Some children develop a chronic pneumonitis, lymphoid interstitial pneumonitis (LIP). Unlike adults, children are prone to serious bacterial infections which are a major cause of morbidity and mortality. Neurological manifestations are a prominent and distressing feature of the illness in children. There may be delay or regression of developmental milestones or the development of an encephalopathy. Impaired brain growth is accompanied by microcephaly and cortical atrophy with ventricular dilatation may be demonstrated on a CT scan (Fig. 15.3).

Testing for antibody has been available since 1984. In spite of this, diagnosing HIV infection in the first 18 months of life remains problematical. Infants born to seropositive mothers acquire maternal antibody transplacentally and initially the antibody test is positive. Approximately 25% of these infants will still have antibodies and will be considered infected at 18 months of age. In a small number of infants maternal antibody has cleared

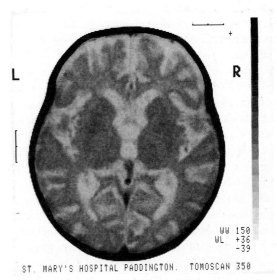

Fig. 15.3 CT scan of an infant with HIV encephalopathy showing ventricular dilatation and cortical atrophy.

but HIV antigen has been detected, indicating infection in spite of the absence of antibody. Children may develop immunological abnormalities with hypergammaglobulinaemia, reduced helper lymphocytes, reversed helper/suppressor lymphocyte ratios, and impaired humoral immunity. Lymphopenia is uncommon in children until they are terminally ill.

Medical management revolves around supportive care as no cure is available. Attention is focused on maintaining the child's nutrition and on early treatment of bacterial and opportunistic infections. In children with HIV disease, regular immunoglobulin or prophylactic antibiotics may reduce the morbidity and mortality from recurrent infection.

Zidovudine (AZT), a reverse transcriptase inhibitor which is currently widely used to treat adults with symptomatic HIV infection, is currently being assessed in children.

The family and child also need considerable support and counselling to help them understand and come to terms with the child's illness. There are often considerable difficulties in the child's home circumstances as the mother may be ill from HIV infection herself or have died. The parents may be intravenous drug abusers or socially deprived. Good communication, education and counselling are required if the child is to be cared for successfully at home, nursery or school, or if the child is fostered or adopted. Confidentiality must be respected whilst ensuring that important information is not kept from other professionals.

Scarlet fever

Scarlet fever is caused by the erythrogenic toxin of the group A haemolytic streptococcus. The severity of the illness has waned considerably and fortunately it is now a mild illness with very few complications. There have also been marked changes in the post-streptococcal diseases, rheumatic fever and glomerulonephritis. Rheumatic fever has become rare in the UK, although it remains of considerable importance in many developing countries and in certain parts of the USA. Post-streptococcal glomerulonephritis has become much less common and the illness less severe.

The incubation period is 2–4 days and starts with tonsillitis, fever, headache and malaise. In most cases the child has a sore throat and the tonsils are red and congested, usually with a white exudate. The rash develops in 12–24 hours and is a punctate erythema, with tiny pin-head size puncta against an erythematous background, which blanches on pressure. It is most profuse on the trunk and limbs, with reddish discolouration in the skin creases, especially in the antecubital fossae and groins. On the face, the skin is flushed with sparing of the area around the mouth giving circumoral pallor, but this appearance is seen in other febrile conditions, especially lobar pneumonia. There is a thick white coating of the tongue through which the inflamed papillae project, giving the white strawberry tongue. By the third to fifth day, the coating disappears leaving the papillae prominent — the strawberry tongue. The rash fades after a few days and this may be followed by desquamation, especially of the palms and soles. Although in the past this desquamation was often dramatic, it tends now to be very slight with perhaps a small area of desquamation around the nails. Occasionally, scarlet fever is seen as a complication of infected wounds and burns.

It is usually possible to identify the organism from a throat swab, or a streptococcal infection can be demonstrated from a raised antibody titre to streptolysin O (ASO), or other streptococcal antibodies. In practice, most children in whom a clinical diagnosis of scarlet fever is made do not have any investigations but are given a course of penicillin. This may modify the illness if severe, but probably has little or no effect on the mild illness seen today. In countries where rheumatic fever is prevalent, a full course of penicillin (10 days if given orally) should be given as prophylaxis against rheumatic fever.

Infectious mononucleosis

Infectious mononucleosis (glandular fever) is caused by the Epstein–Barr (EB) virus. It is transmitted by close contact. The virus is excreted in nasopharyngeal secretions during the illness whether symptomatic or asymptomatic and may continue for some months afterwards. It is also excreted intermittently by healthy individuals who are seropositive for EB virus antibody and who must often be the source of infection, as few patients are aware of recent contact with an affected person.

Clinical disease from infectious mononucleosis has a peak incidence in adolescents and young adults. It usually has a gradual onset with malaise, anorexia and a fever. Most have a sore throat and tender swollen glands. On examination of the throat, petechiae may be visible on the palate and sometimes the tonsils are enlarged and covered with a thick white exudate. Peritonsillar oedema may be severe and cause difficulty in swallowing and breathing. There may be generalised lymphadenopathy especially affecting the cervical lymph nodes and splenomegaly. Some patients have a maculopapular rash, which is especially florid if ampicillin has been taken. Only a small percentage of patients are jaundiced, although over 80% have abnormal liver function tests. Cranial nerve palsies and other central nervous system abnormalities are very rare. Infectious mononucleosis is not uncommon in young children, especially in those of lower socioeconomic circumstances, but the clinical course is often much milder with much less prominent pharyngeal symptoms.

Differential diagnosis

The differential diagnosis depends on the mode of onset. Where there is exudative tonsillitis, streptococcal tonsillitis and diphtheria need to be considered. Prominent lymphadenopathy will need to be differentiated from other causes especially leukaemia and lymphoma, cytomegalovirus and toxoplasmosis.

Diagnosis

The blood film shows atypical mononuclear cells affecting more than 10% of the total. They are not specific for infectious mononucleosis but may also be seen in other viral infections especially cytomegalovirus, adenovirus and also in toxoplasmosis. The diagnosis can be confirmed by showing heterophile antibodies with the Paul–Bunnell or 'Monospot' tests. Heterophile antibody is present in 85–90% of affected adolescents and adults but many chil-

dren do not produce heterophile antibodies at any stage of the illness. A definitive diagnosis of infectious mononucleosis in young children requires detection of antibody to EB virus.

Treatment

In virtually all cases the disease is self limiting and only symptomatic treatment is necessary. Sport is often restricted if the spleen is enlarged to reduce the small risk of splenic rupture. Very severe pharyngeal oedema causing respiratory obstruction or severe hepatitis will usually respond to a short course of corticosteriods.

Mumps

Mumps is caused by a paramyxovirus. It is transmitted by droplet spread or direct contact with the saliva of an infected person. The incidence of infection is highest in school-age children.

The incubation period is 16–18 days which ends in fever, anorexia and malaise. The next day a parotid gland may enlarge and this progresses over the next 1–3 days. The child may complain of earache which is made worse by movement of the jaw, especially eating. The gland is painful and tender, but this gradually subsides over the next 3–7 days. Within a couple of days the other parotid gland usually becomes enlarged, but in one-quarter of cases the parotid enlargement is unilateral. The submaxillary and sublingual salivary glands are occasionally involved. In around one-third of cases the infection is subclinical.

The illness is mostly localised to the parotid glands. When making the diagnosis the enlarged parotid has to be differentiated from enlarged cervical lymph nodes. If the parotid gland is enlarged the ascending ramus of the mandible cannot be palpated. Mumps is an important cause of aseptic meningitis, which usually develops 3–7 days after the parotitis, but may also precede the parotitis or the parotitis may be absent. Recovery is usually uneventful, although very occasionally the patient has a unilateral or bilateral sensorineural hearing deficit. Epididymo-orchitis is rare before puberty and pancreatitis is a well-recognised but rare complication.

Investigations are not usually required, but

infection with mumps can be identified either se-rologically or by isolating the virus from saliva, urine or cerebrospinal fluid. The serum amylase is elevated in two-thirds of cases of mumps parotitis. There is no specific treatment. The incidence of mumps in the UK has declined following the inclusion of mumps vaccine into the standard immunisation schedule.

Erythema infectiosum

Erythema infectiosum, also called 'Fifth disease', usually affects school-age children. At the onset of the illness the child is mildly ill, may have a fever and develops a distinctive rash. The rash begins on the face, producing an intensely red 'slapped cheek' appearance with circumoral pallor and spreads to the arms and trunk, where it has a lace-like pattern. The rash may recur for a couple of weeks, and varies in intensity, being particularly obvious after a bath or exposure to sunlight. Arthralgia may occur during convalescence.

Human parvovirus, a small virus containing a single strand of DNA, has been implicated as the cause. The virus cannot be grown in the laboratory and specialised tests are required to identify it. The illness may occur in epidemics and household contacts, both adults and children, may also be affected. Parvovirus has also been implicated as causing marrow aplasia in children with sickle cell disease. There is also recent evidence that human parvovirus can be transmitted from the pregnant mother to her fetus, and may result in fetal anaemia and fetal hydrops.

Roseola infantum (exanthem subitum)

The commonest cause of this disease is thought to be herpesvirus 6. Infants between 6 months and 4 years of age, particularly those around 1 year old, are most commonly affected. The infant suddenly develops a high, sustained fever which lasts for 3–4 days. During this period the infant may have a febrile convulsion, but otherwise does not seem as ill as one would expect from the high fever. There are few abnormal physical signs other than the fever, perhaps a slightly injected pharynx and some lymphadenopathy. There is a dramatic fall in the fever to normal and

simultaneously, or shortly afterwards, a wide-spread rose-pink maculopapular rash develops first on the trunk and then spreading to the face and extremities. The diagnosis can only be made after the appearance of the rash and is clinical as confirmatory tests are often not done. There is no specific treatment.

THE PERINATAL PERIOD

The fetus may be exposed to maternal infection throughout pregnancy and at delivery. Fortunately, few infections damage the fetus. Rubella and cytomegalovirus in the mother are important infections which may result in damage to the fetus. Toxoplasmosis is rare in the UK but may also cause severe fetal damage. Exposure of the fetus to herpes simplex, chickenpox, parvovirus and hepatitis B are less common, but all may cause serious disease in the newborn infant. There is no consistent evidence that mumps, the enteroviruses (coxsackie or echovirus) or influenza cause damage to the fetus.

Congenital rubella

The outcome for an individual fetus when a pregnant woman has rubella is difficult to predict. There is a risk of damage to the fetus when the mother has a primary rubella infection but not if she has reinfection. The stage of pregnancy at which the infection occurs is critical. Infection in the first 4 weeks of pregnancy may result in spontaneous abortion, whilst the risk of fetal damage in the first 8 weeks of pregnancy may be as high as 70% falling to 50% at 9–12 weeks and is more likely to lead to hearing impairment than other defects. Infection at 13–16 weeks causes damage in less than 30% of infants, usually as hearing impairment. After 18 weeks the risk of damage is minimal. Some infected babies are normal at birth but subsequently develop deafness and developmental delay later in childhood.

A wide range of defects is seen in infants and children with congenital rubella (Table 15.3). Most affected infants are small for gestational age and fail to thrive in early life. There is often damage to the eye (cataracts, glaucoma and pigmentary retinopathy), the heart (especially patent ductus

Table 15.3 Features of congenital rubella

	Type of defect
Growth	Small for gestational age, failure to thrive
Ears	Sensorineural deafness
Heart	Patent ductus arteriosus, ventricular septal defect, and peripheral pulmonary stenosis
Eyes	Cataract, glaucoma, microphthalmia, pigmentary retinopathy
CNS	Microcephaly, mental retardation, cerebral palsy
Other	Thrombocytopenic purpura, hepatitis, hepatosplenomegaly, pneumonitis, myocarditis, osteopathy, translucency of metaphyses of long bones, especially distal femur and proximal tibia

Table 15.4 Clinical history of mothers of children with congenital rubella

Clinical history	%
Clinical rubella	46
Rash (not diagnosed)	13
Contact: no illness	16
No illness or contact	25

arteriosus), the ear (perceptive deafness) and there may be damage to the central nervous system (microcephaly, mental retardation and cerebral palsy). Other manifestations in early infancy include thrombocytopenic purpura, hepatitis, hepatosplenomegaly, myocarditis and pneumonitis.

Diagnosis

The diagnosis can be made by culturing the virus in the urine or from the nasopharynx, or by demonstrating IgM-specific antibodies to rubella in the blood in the first few months of life. Affected infants may excrete virus for many months and they then have the potential to transmit infection to other susceptible individuals.

Rubella during pregnancy

The proportion of pregnant women susceptible to rubella has been reduced from 10–15% before vaccination was introduced to 2–3%. Rubella infection during pregnancy may be suspected from a rash or if the woman comes into contact with an affected person, usually a child in the family (Table 15.4). Many rubelliform rashes are caused by other virus infections, and an early and accurate diagnosis of rubella is essential if proper management of the pregnancy is to be offered to the mother. Investigation is required as soon as possible after exposure. The most widely used serological test is for haemagglutination-inhibiting (HAI) antibodies.

The diagnosis of a recent rubella infection is made in conjunction with the clinical history and, in particular, after considering the time between exposure and testing. If the first blood sample is taken within 10 days of exposure, which is well within the incubation period and shows no HAI antibody, the patient is susceptible to rubella and further antibody tests should be done after 10 and 20 days. A seroconversion on paired samples indicates a recent infection.

Antibody detected within the incubation period suggests previous exposure to rubella and that the patient is immune. This is best confirmed with a second specimen taken after the end of the incubation period, when there should not be a significant change in antibody titre. If the first specimen is taken after the incubation period and antibodies are present, the patient may be immune or have had a recent infection. A recent infection can be identified by finding rubella-specific IgM antibodies as they are detectable for only a few weeks after rubella infection.

The routine screening test for HAI antibodies performed in the antenatal clinic only indicates whether the person is susceptible or immune to rubella and whether immunisation should be recommended postnatally. If antibody is present it does not indicate the time when the infection occurred and although this is usually before pregnancy, it may have been recent. Rubella immunisation of 11–13-year-old girls began in 1971 in the UK and the incidence of congenital rubella has declined. As the virus remains in the community, any pregnant women who is susceptible to infection remains at risk. In 1986–87 there were 372 pregnant women in the UK who had laboratory-confirmed rubella infection, and about 20 children a year with congenital rubella syndrome are identified. The measles, mumps and rubella

(MMR) vaccine has been introduced for all children in the second year of life to remove the virus from the community so that pregnant women will no longer be exposed to the virus.

Women should avoid becoming pregnant within 3 months of receiving rubella immunisation. The inadvertent administration of rubella vaccine to a susceptible pregnant woman may result in fetal infection in about 20–25% of cases. No evidence of damage has been documented in these cases but the numbers are relatively small.

Cytomegalovirus

Cytomegalovirus (CMV) is the commonest known infection of the fetus. In industrialised countries it can be isolated from about 1 in 300 newborn infants.

Between 20% and 60% of pregnant women in industrialised countries do not have antibody to CMV. Almost all mothers who acquire CMV during pregnancy are asymptomatic, although occasionally an illness resembling influenza or even glandular fever occurs. Approximately 1 in 100 women who are susceptible to CMV at the beginning of pregnancy will have a primary infection during pregnancy. Congenital infection may occur after primary infection in the mother or from recurrent infection which is usually due to reactivation of latent virus.

Congenital abnormalities are seen more frequently in infants born after primary maternal infection than in those born after recurrent maternal infection. About 40% of primary infections result in infants with congenital infection. Most babies from whom CMV is isolated are asymptomatic. Only 10% or less have clinical evidence of damage at birth, but it is estimated that some form of damage is detectable during infancy or childhood in 10–15% of all babies with congenital CMV infection. Some affected babies are small for gestational age and may have hepatosplenomegaly, hepatitis, thrombocytopenic purpura and occasionally pneumonitis. Some have neurological damage with microcephaly, mental retardation and deafness. There may also be a retinopathy and cerebral calcification on a skull radiograph. Congenital CMV is a significant cause of sensorineural hearing loss.

The virus can best be identified by isolation in tissue culture, preferably from urine or from a throat swab. IgM-specific antibody to CMV in the blood is not always present in infected infants. No specific treatment is of proven benefit. Excretion of the virus by affected infants may extend for several years. Although transmission of infection to susceptible contacts is extremely rare, provided normal levels of hygiene are maintained, a seronegative pregnant woman should avoid caring for an infant known to be excreting the virus.

Chickenpox and shingles

Chickenpox infection during pregnancy is uncommon. Shingles does not affect the fetus but chickenpox may. The effect will depend on the period of pregnancy when the infection occurs. Infection during the first 4 months does not usually affect the fetus but a very few infants have been described with a characteristic pattern of malformations. This has been named the congenital varicella syndrome and includes scarring of the skin, muscular atrophy, hypoplastic extremities, atrophic digits and cerebral cortical atrophy with microcephaly and mental retardation. The babies of women who have chickenpox 1–3 weeks before delivery often have mild chickenpox. If chickenpox occurs within 4 days of delivery there it insufficient time for the fetus to receive maternal antibody and the newborn baby may develop severe generalised chickenpox (Fig. 15.4). This has a mortality of up to 30% and the infants should be given zoster immune globulin at birth. Treatment is with acyclovir.

Herpes simplex virus

Infection of the newborn infant with herpes simplex virus usually occurs from the maternal genital tract at the time of delivery. The genital type 2 (HSV 2) strain of virus is slightly more common as the pathogen than the type 1 strain (HSV 1).

Neonatal herpes may be localised or disseminated. When disseminated, the infant may be jaundiced, have purpura and develop respiratory distress and shock. The central nervous system may also be involved with meningitis and encephalitis. The mortality is extremely high, 80% of

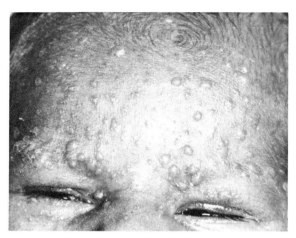

Fig. 15.4 Chickenpox in a neonate.

these infants die and one-half of the survivors have permanent damage. The infection may be confined to the central nervous system, or localised to the skin, eyes and mouth. At present infection in this country appears much less common than in the USA.

When active maternal genital herpes occurs at the time of delivery, exposure of the baby can be minimised by delivering the baby by Caesarean section, preferably before or within 4 hours of rupture of the membranes. However, in most cases of neonatal herpes infection there is no history of genital herpes in the mother. Treatment of infected infants is with acyclovir.

Hepatitis A and B

Maternal infection with hepatitis A during pregnancy has been associated with premature onset of labour, but there is no definite evidence of fetal damage. Should a pregnant woman come into contact with hepatitis A, it is generally advised that she should be given immunoglobulin.

Vertical transmission of the hepatitis B virus from mother to baby mostly occurs at delivery or within the first few weeks of life. Most pregnant women who are HBsAg positive are chronic carriers and often come from South-East Asia or Africa. Those who also carry the e antigen (an internal component of the core) in their blood are often of Chinese origin and have an increased risk of transmitting HBsAg to their babies. Other mothers with an increased risk of carrying HBsAg are those who are drug addicts, have received transfusions of blood or blood products or been tattooed. Primary clinical infection of the mother is uncommon, but when it occurs in the third trimester, the infant has a high risk of acquiring HBsAg. The baby is exposed by the ingestion of maternal blood at delivery or from inoculation through abrasions in the skin.

Most infants who acquire HBsAg are asymptomatic, but they may well become chronic carriers and a few may develop serious liver disease and be at increased risk of primary liver cancer in adult life.

The management of babies born to mothers who are HBsAg carriers is still controversial. Normal pooled immunoglobulin is not of any value, but there is evidence that hepatitis-B immunoglobulin administered within 48 hours reduces the acquisition of the HBsAg. This should be combined with a course of hepatitis B vaccine for long-term protection.

HIV infection

Perinatal transmission occurs transplacentally from an infected mother to her fetus. Other potential routes of infection are from exposure to blood and cervical secretions during birth or postnatally via breast milk. 25–30% of infants born to HIV seropositive mothers show evidence of infection with the virus at 18 months of age.

HIV has been identified in breast milk and there are a few case reports where a breast-fed infant is thought to have acquired HIV infection postnatally in mothers who received HIV seropositive blood in the postpartum period. The Department of Health has recommended that to avoid possible added risk to the infant all mothers known to be HIV infected should be discouraged from breast feeding. This advice has been extended to include not only mothers known to be HIV infected but also those at high risk, although the vast majority of these women will not be infected. Whilst these guidelines apply to the UK, they need to be reassessed in developing countries where bottle feeding may not be safely achieved and the risk from abandoning breast feeding may exceed the potential risk of acquiring HIV infection.

Toxoplasmosis

Toxoplasmosis is caused by the protozoon *Toxoplasma gondii*. Infection in pregnant women is almost always asymptomatic, but sometimes is similar to mild flu or glandular fever. The incidence of primary infection during pregnancy varies widely in different countries. In the UK it is uncommon, with an incidence of congenital infection of only 1 in 2000 live births. At birth, most babies with congenital toxoplasmosis are asymptomatic but up to 10% have clinically recognisable damage. The severely affected infant may be small for gestational age and have jaundice, hepatosplenomegaly, anaemia, thrombocytopenia, convulsions and hydrocephalus or microcephaly. There is a characteristic chorioretinitis and there may also be intracranial calcification.

The most widely used diagnostic test is the toxoplasma dye test. The diagnosis can be confirmed by demonstrating a persistently raised or rising titre. IgM antibodies to toxoplasma can also be detected using immunofluorescence.

Drugs used to treat a pregnant woman or affected infant include pyrimethamine, sulphadiazine or spiramycin.

RASHES

There is considerable overlap in the rashes caused by different infections. In arriving at a diagnosis, additional information is needed. A particular infection may be prevalent at the time within a community, the organism may have been identified and the natural history of the illness known. There may be a history of contact with an infected person. The patient's past history of infection needs to be known, although this is notoriously unreliable for some infections, e.g. rubella. The immunisation history may be more helpful, although it should be remembered that inoculation is not synonymous with immunity. Other factors are the length and clinical features of the prodromal period. In addition to the appearance of the rash, there is its distribution and the sequence in which it appeared and disappeared. Associated symptoms and signs are often helpful. A definite diagnosis may not be possible from the clinical features when the child is first seen, but may become apparent from the subsequent course of the illness. Laboratory investigations are sometimes required to identify the cause of the illness.

Petechial and purpuric rashes

It is important to identify petechiae or purpura in an unwell child as they may be caused by meningococcal septicaemia, which is likely to be fatal within hours unless treated. Initially, there may be only a few petechiae, sometimes only evident on the conjunctivae in a febrile and unwell child. The lesions may become widespread, variable in shape and size and may subsequently develop a necrotic centre (Fig. 15.5). The septicaemia may progress so rapidly that the meninges remain unaffected. The child becomes shocked and in severe cases there is disseminated intravascular coagulation. Similar skin lesions are also seen, although much less frequently, in *Haemophilus influenzae* and pneumococcal infections, and in Rocky Mountain spotted fever and arbovirus infections in endemic areas.

Any child in the community who develops a petechial or purpuric rash and is febrile and unwell should be presumed to have meningococcal septicaemia and immediately given a large dose of penicillin parenterally. Although this may prevent the organism from being identified by culture, the antigen can still be positively identified, and it

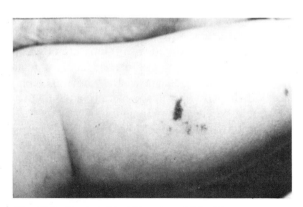

Fig. 15.5 Typical skin lesions in a child with meningococcal septicaemia.

may be life saving. The child must be transferred urgently to hospital.

Petchiae or purpura are seen in many other conditions. The cause may be thrombocytopenic or non-thrombocytopenic. They are seen in the non-thrombocytopenic vasculitis of Henoch–Schönlein purpura where the purpuric rash has a characteristic distribution over the buttocks, legs and elbows, often with arthritis, gastrointestinal pain and renal involvement. Important causes of

Table 15.5 Clinical diagnosis of the rashes seen in the major acute infectious diseases

Rash	Causes	Comments
Erythematous		
Scarlatiniform	Scarlet fever	Post group-A streptococcal infection of the throat or skin. Associated features — tonsillitis or infected skin lesion, characteristic appearance of the tongue. Punctate erythema, spreading from neck downwards avoiding the face which is flushed and has circumoral pallor. Desquamation
	Viruses	Scarlatiniform rashes are seen in a number of viral illnesses, e.g. adenovirus
	Chickenpox	Transient scarlatiniform rashes sometimes before the vesicles appear
	Drugs and other allergic reactions	Wide variety of allergens, e.g. antibiotics
	Kawasaki's disease (mucocutaneous lymph node syndrome)	First described in Japan, but seen increasingly in Europe and North America. Erythematous rash on the trunk. Other diagnostic features of the illness are: spiking fever lasting 5 or more days; bilateral conjunctivitis; dry, cracked, red lips with erythematous nasopharyngeal oedema; reddening of the palms and soles on days 3–5 with desquamation by the second or third weeks and enlarged cervical lymph nodes; 1% mortality from thrombosis and aneurysms of the coronary arteries
	Staphylococcal toxic shock syndrome	Most common in menstruating women, but also occurs in children. Associated with fever, shock, conjunctival injection, strawberry tongue and scarlatiniform rash. Desquamation during convalescence. Caused by toxin producing *Staphylococcus aureus*
Morbilliform (measles like)	Measles	Rash is dusky-red, blotchy and becomes confluent. Spreads from behind the ears and back of the neck then to the face, trunk and limbs. Staining of skin. Koplik's spots are pathognomonic but may not be visible. If conjunctivitis, coryza, or cough are not present, it is unlikely to be measles
	Adenovirus Coxsackie }	Morbilliform rashes may be seen in other viral infections
Rubelliform	Rubella	Rash, even with postauricular and occipital lymphadenopathy not specific to rubella. In a pregnant woman, diagnosis of rubella or exposure to possible rubella must always be confirmed serologically
	Adenovirus Echovirus Coxsackie }	Can all cause a rubelliform rash
	Roseola	Rose-pink rash, starts on trunk and appears when fever subsides
	Allergic reaction	Allergic reactions to drugs and many other allergens. Wide range of rashes, including scarlatiniform, morbilliform and rubelliform rashes. Extensive and sometimes confluent rash in patients with infectious mononucleosis especially after taking ampicillin
	Collagen vascular disorders	Rash in systemic juvenile chronic arthritis appears with the fever, disappears in a few hours. Often localised, mainly on the trunk and proximal limbs
Papulosquamous	Pityriasis rosea	Rose-coloured papules with white scales on the surface. Herald patch on trunk. Lesions mainly on the trunk and may assume Christmas tree-like configuration as they may follow a diagonal pattern from the spine following the ribs. May be itchy
	Psoriasis	Lesions are chronic

Table 15.5 (continued)

Rash	Causes	Comments
Vesicular	Chickenpox	Variable number of vesicles. Even if there are only a few lesions, more can usually be found on the scalp and mucous membranes. Lesions first appear on the trunk
	Shingles	Confined to sensory nerve dermatome
	Smallpox	Now eradicated
	Herpes simplex	Usually gingivostomatitis with lesions on tongue and buccal mucosa and some satellite lesions around the mouth, or vulvovaginitis or cutaneous lesions
	Eczema herpeticum	Herpes infection on eczematous skin. Lesions may become widespread (Kaposi's varicelliform eruption) and the patient may become severely ill
	Hand, foot and mouth disease	Shallow ulcers in the mouth, vesicles on the hands and feet, and on the buttocks in infants. Usually caused by coxsackie A16 virus
	Herpangina	Vesicles or ulcers on fauces and mucous membranes of posterior part of mouth. Fever, anorexia and dysphagia for 2–5 days. Mainly caused by coxsackie virus infection
	Impetigo	The vesicles are usually around the mouth and become pustular and crust. Mostly caused by *Staphylococcus aureus*, also streptococci
	Viruses	Vesicular rashes are sometimes seen in a number of viral infections, e.g. coxsackie, echovirus
Erythema multiforme	Allergy to food, drugs, etc.	Discrete circular macules, often with central clearing to form a target lesion, mostly on the upper limbs. May be a wide variety of lesions, with macules, papules, urticaria, and bullae and several different types of lesions present at once. A severe form of the disease, with mucous membrane involvement of the mouth, conjunctivae and genitalia is the Stevens–Johnson syndrome
	Viral infection — herpes simplex, coxsackie, echovirus	
	Bacterial infection — Group A streptococcus	
	Mycoplasma	
	Collagen vascular disorders	
	Cause often not identified	
Urticaria	Allergic reaction (causes as for erythema multiforme)	Raised lesions, variable size and shape. White lesions on surrounding erythematous base. Itchy and evanescent. Sometimes accompanied by angioedema of eyes and face and, rarely, tongue and upper airways which may be life threatening
Erythema marginatum	Rheumatic fever	Erythematous rash with a pale centre. The margin is sometimes raised and it migrates across the skin
Bullous	Bullous impetigo	Caused by *Staphylococcus aureus* and less commonly by streptococcal infection of the skin. Roof of a bullous lesion may be readily removed and lesions then resemble scalds (scalded-skin syndrome)
	Herpes simplex Chickenpox Erythema marginatum Stevens–Johnson syndrome	Some of the lesions in these acute illnesses may be bullous. Bullae may also be seen in ammoniacal napkin rashes, burns, and in a number of rare, chronic skin conditions

thrombocytopenic purpura include idiopathic thrombocytopenic purpura, leukaemia, the haemolytic-uraemic syndrome, disseminated intravascular coagulation and congenital infection from rubella, cytomegalovirus or toxoplasma.

A guide to the clinical diagnosis of the rashes seen in the major acute infectious diseases is given in Table 15.5.

Acknowledgements

I should like to acknowledge the contribution to this chapter of the late Dr Bill Marshall, whose untimely death occurred shortly before the first edition of this book was published. I would also like to thank Professor M. Levin for his helpful comments.

16. Respiratory diseases

R. Dinwiddie

PULMONARY FUNCTION TESTS IN CHILDREN

It is possible to perform simple lung function tests in children from the age of 5 years. The tests, which require co-operation, consist primarily of lung volume measurements such as vital capacity, forced expiratory volume (FEV) in 1 second, and peak expiratory flow rate (PEFR) (Fig. 16.1, Table 16.1). Flow–volume curves are useful in assessing small airway obstruction (Fig. 16.1). Pulmonary function testing in babies requires special complicated apparatus, usually only available in research departments.

The technique of ventilation-perfusion lung scan is very useful in evaluating lung function at all ages. Radioactive krypton (half-life 13 seconds) is inhaled and its lung distribution measured using a gamma camera; technetium-labelled microspheres (half-life 6 hours) are injected into a peripheral vein and become trapped in the pulmonary capillaries, thus outlining pulmonary perfusion.

Table 16.1 Respiratory function in children

	Age		
	5 years	10 years	15 years
Vital capacity (ml)	1200	2200	3500
FEV$_1$ (ml)	1000	2000	3300
PEFR (l/min)	140	280	400

The radiation dose is no more than that of a single chest X-ray. Apart from being a very useful diagnostic tool this technique can be used to assess progress of disease and outcome by serial scanning over a period of months or years as necessary.

Arterial blood gases reflect the final pathway of gas exchange and can be measured at any age. Inspired oxygen concentration at the time of sampling must be noted. The most common sampling site is the radial artery, but the brachial and posterior tibial vessels can also be used. The femoral arteries should be avoided if at all possible. Capillary blood gas sampling gives reliable mea-

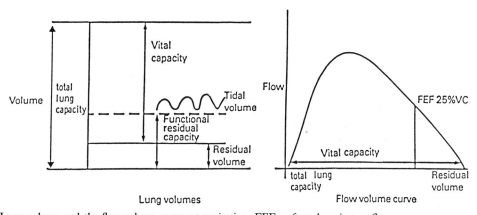

Fig. 16.1 Lung volume and the flow-volume curve on expiration. FEF = forced expiratory flow.

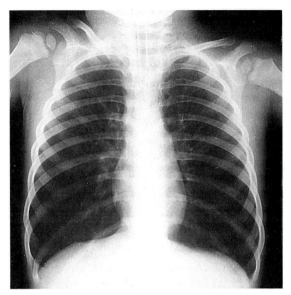

Fig. 16.2 Severe overinflation during acute asthma.

surements for acid-base and carbon dioxide concentrations but not for oxygen. The advent of oxygen saturation monitors has made continuous non-invasive oxygen monitoring extremely simple. Properly calibrated transcutaneous oxygen and carbon dixode electrodes are also useful, especially in the neonatal period.

INFECTIONS

Respiratory tract infection in infants and children is extremely common. World wide it is thought to account for some 15 million deaths under the age of 5 per annum. It is the most frequent reason for seeking medical advice in this age group, the average GP in the UK can expect to have 5–600 such consultations per year. The majority of infections affect the upper respiratory tract: approximately 20% cause significant symptoms in the lower tract. Alveolar growth principally occurs before birth and in the first 2 years of life, but the process does continue at a slower rate until the age of 7–8 years. Severe infection before this age carries the potential for permanent damage to the growing lung and long-term sequelae.

The epidemiology of respiratory tract infection in childhood is dependent on several factors including the virulence and dose of the organism, and host resistance. The host's resistance is related to age, degree of immunological development, previous experience of infection and stage of lung growth. These factors influence the environment in which the invading organism finds itself and thus its potential for causing disease. Certain physical factors are also important in determining the severity of infection; these include low birthweight, male sex, obesity, younger age groups, previous significant respiratory difficulties and the presence of congenital malformations. External environmental factors such as atmospheric pollution, overcrowding, parental smoking, exposure to active infection and seasonal variation of disease incidence are also important. The clinical pattern of disease is related to the part of the respiratory tract most affected.

Upper respiratory tract infection

Coryza (common cold)

This infection is relatively mild and is characterised by a mucoid nasal obstruction, sore throat and often cervical adenopathy. Fever may be present. Many different viruses are implicated in the aetiology, but the most common include rhinovirus, respiratory syncytial virus (RSV), influenza, parainfluenza, adenovirus and coxsackie. Management is symptomatic. Antibiotics are not indicated except where there is clear evidence of a secondary bacterial infection or a more serious underlying disease such as cystic fibrosis or bronchiectasis is present.

Acute infection of tonsils, adenoids and pharynx

Infection of the tonsils, adenoids and pharynx is common and occurs principally in the 3–8-year age group. It is characterised by fever, sore throat, malaise and occasionally vomiting. Examination of the throat reveals infection of the pharynx, peritonsillar area and the tonsils themselves. There is usually an associated enlargement of cervical lymph nodes. The tonsils are enlarged and inflamed with tiny haemorrhages and exudate. The surrounding inflammation of pharynx and adenoids frequently leads to cough and nasal obstruction and difficulty in swallowing.

A virus is the aetiological agent in approximately 90% of cases; the most frequent isolates include RSV, influenza, parainfluenza, coxsackie, echo and adenovirus. The most prominent bacterial pathogen is the group A β-haemolytic streptococcus. Infectious mononucleosis may also present with florid tonsillitis while *Corynebacterium diphtheriae*, although rare, should never be forgotten.

Tonsillitis may occasionally be epidemic, particularly in closed communities with outbreaks of streptococcal infection or pharyngo-conjunctival fever due to adenovirus.

Treatment consists of an adequate fluid intake and symptomatic measures such as the control of fever and sore throat. Penicillin should be given 6-hourly for 10 day when a streptococcal infection is suspected. If the patient is vomiting or otherwise unlikely to take the drug, intramuscular long-acting penicillin is useful. Erythromycin is a suitable alternative to penicillin if there is a history of penicillin allergy.

Complications of bacterial infection are fortunately rare, largely because of the widespread use of antibiotics. Immediate problems include peritonsillar or pharyngeal abscess and acute cervical adenitis. In peritonsillar or pharyngeal abscess there may be marked dysphagia and obvious displacement of tissues on examination. A retropharyngeal abscess may be seen on a lateral neck X-ray. The neck may be held extended in order to facilitate breathing through the partially obstructed airway. Cervical adenitis may occur in association with acute tonsillitis and occasionally leads to abscess formation. Treatment of these problems includes the appropriate antibiotic in large doses, and occasionally surgical drainage.

Late complications of streptococcal infections include rheumatic fever and acute glomerulonephritis. The early and widespread use of penicillin has probably contributed to a significant reduction of these diseases.

Chronic or recurrent infection of tonsils and adenoids

Recurrent and frequent infection of the tonsils and adenoids is common in young children. A significant increase in incidence is seen on starting play-school or nursery, followed then by a natural decrease to the adult frequency at the age of 7–8 years. With this pattern of illness in mind relatively few children should require adeno-tonsillectomy in their early years, and the current decrease in the popularity of this operation should continue (Table 16.2). It is probable that less than 1 child in 25 in the general population needs removal of tonsils and adenoids by the age of 8.

In a number of children removal of tonsils and adenoids is, however, of significant benefit; these include those who have frequent severe attacks, three to four a year, which cause significant systemic symptoms, general ill health and interfere with normal growth. In the younger age group, 1–3 years old, a small number have severe mechanical airway obstruction due to adenotonsillar hypertrophy; these children are chronic mouth breathers with persistent nasal obstruction and discharge, they usually snore at night and may have difficulty sleeping due to recurrent obstruction with short periods of sleep apnoea. Paradoxically they often demonstrate excessive daytime somnolence. In some cases, cor pulmonale will develop due to pulmonary hypertension and right heart failure. Chronic infection may also contribute to

Table 16.2 Indications for and against tonsillectomy and adenoidectomy

For
Adenoidectomy
Persistent nasal obstruction due to large adenoids
Recurrent otitis media if large adenoids are thought to block the lower end of the Eustachian tube

Adenotonsillectomy
Sleep apnoea syndrome

Tonsillectomy
Recurrent cervical adenitits or peritonsillar abscess because the tonsils are an ineffective barrier against repeated pharyngeal infection
Recurrent tonsillitis, significantly affecting growth and weight gain
Suspected tonsillar tumour

Against
Parental pressure on doctor
Large tonsils which cause no symptoms. Large tonsils are frequently wrongly assumed to be unhealthy. Parents should be reassured that lymphoid atrophy frequently reduces the size of the tonsils after about the eighth year
Any child with a submucous or frankly cleft palate or bifid uvula should not have his adenoids removed because of the risk of aggravating nasal speech due to pharyngopalatal incompetence

recurrent middle ear problems and hearing difficulties. Adenotonsillectomy in this group often produces a dramatic improvement in the child's general health, appetite and growth.

Otitis media

Otitis media or middle ear infection occurs as a result of an infecting organism travelling up the Eustachian tube, helped by forceful nose blowing or coughing. The commonest bacterial pathogens include *Streptococcus pneumoniae*, *Haemophilus influenzae*, group A β-haemolytic streptococcus, and *Staphylococcus aureus*; viruses frequently also cause the disease.

Once an infection becomes established, the mucosal lining of the middle ear produces an inflammatory exudate. If the Eustachian tube is blocked by the exudate or oedema, the exudate increases in volume, may become frankly purulent and can lead to pressure necrosis and perforation of the tympanic membrane, resulting in a discharge from the ear and subsequent relief of earache. With treatment, the exudate resorbs or drains through a patent Eustachian tube, so normal middle ear function is restored. If the exudate does not resolve, and becomes thick and gelatinous, a chronic secretory otitis, or glue ear, supervenes and there is interference with sound conduction (conductive deafness). Conditions which interfere with middle ear ventilation through the Eustachian tube, such as enlarged adenoids or vasomotor rhinitis, may predispose to recurrent otitis media.

Most children will have suffered an attack of otitis media by the age of 6 years. Older children may accurately describe symptoms of pain and hearing loss. The very young may also present with fever and hearing difficulty or with non-specific signs such as vomiting, diarrhoea, persistent crying and irritability. The ears of all fretful and febrile babies should always be examined. In early otitis, the edge of the drum may be reddened and there are commonly dilated vessels on the handle of the malleus. This effect can also be produced, to a lesser extent, by crying. The drum in addition is dull and loses its lustre. Later the drum becomes very red and the normal anatomical landmarks are no longer visible. The drum may subsequently bulge and perforate, in which case the external auditory canal will be full of debris and pus.

Management of acute otitis media:

1. Relief of pain with paracetamol which will also reduce any associated fever.
2. All children with inflamed tympanic membranes should receive a course of an appropriate antibiotic. *Haemophilus influenzae* is common in children under 5 years; amoxicillin is appropriate but if the child is allergic to penicillin, erythromycin or co-trimoxazole are also effective. In older children, penicillin is a better choice because *Streptococcus pneumoniae* and *Strept. pyogenes* are the common pathogens. If the membrane has perforated, a swab should be taken of the discharge and the antibiotic treatment changed according to the results of culture. Treatment should be continued for at least 1 week. Ear drops have no place in the treatment of acute otitis media.
3. Follow-up must continue until the doctor is satisfied that the infection has settled, that any drum perforation is healing and that hearing has returned to normal.

Complications of otitis media:

1. Glue ear with hearing loss.
2. Chronic suppurative otitis media.
3. Mastoiditis.
4. Meningitis.
5. Intracranial abscess.
6. Lateral venous sinus thrombosis.

The occurence of complications other than glue ear is now much less common, largely due to the widespread use of effective antibiotics.

Glue ear

Glue ear is not uncommon and is due to the persistence of a gelatinous exudate in the middle ear. This condition is often undetected with important consequences on hearing and learning. It is characterised by a dull bluish discolouration of the tympanic membrane, which is often retracted and immobile. A fluid level may be seen behind the ear drum.

Evidence of transient hearing loss may occur in

up to 30% of children following acute otitis media. In the older child, a tuning fork may be used to determine whether bone conduction is greater than air conduction (Rinne's test), demonstrating a conductive hearing loss in the affected ear. Simple audiometry may be used to show a loss of hearing at various frequencies and below certain levels of intensity. The testing of hearing in younger children may need to be done by the use of the Stycar miniature toy method (see Ch. 3).

Treatment

1. If a hearing loss is found, the administration of a decongestant may restore Eustachian tube function and result in 'medical' drainage of the middle ear.

2. If after 6 months, hearing is still abnormal or gets worse despite treatment, then a myringotomy may be needed. The surgeon incises the tympanic membrane under direct magnification, and then the gelatinous glue can be sucked out from the middle ear.

3. The insertion of grommets into the myringotomy incision leaves a ventilation tube in situ which will allow re-aeration of the middle ear. The grommets extrude themselves after a few months and may sometimes be found lying in the external auditory meatus. While a child has grommets in place it is necessary that a close-fitting protective hat or earplugs are used if the child goes swimming. Diving should be prohibited as water may enter the middle ear.

4. Adenoidectomy may be performed at the same time if it is thought that enlarged adenoids are causing obstruction to the lower end of the Eustachian tube.

Sinusitis

Acute infection of the sinuses is only seen in the older child, as the maxillary and ethmoid sinuses remain relatively small and the frontal sinuses do not develop until the early school years. The sphenoidal sinus appears even later. Acute sinusitis is usually viral in origin and causes fever, pain, headache and nasal discharge; bacteria include *Strep. pneumoniae* and the group A β-haemolytic streptococcus. Treatment is with penicillin for 10 days, but erythromycin is a useful alternative. Decongestants may also be useful. Chronically infected sinuses may need surgical drainage; the possibility of other diagnoses such as IgA deficiency, allergic rhinitis or cystic fibrosis should be considered.

Lower respiratory tract infection

Laryngotracheobronchitis (croup)

Laryngotracheobronchitis, or croup, is due to an acute inflammation of the upper portion of the lower respiratory tract. Acute inflammation of the epiglottis is considered separately (see below). Laryngotracheobronchitis is most commonly viral and is frequently due to parainfluenza viruses; respiratory syncytial virus and rhinoviruses are also prominent pathogens.

Croup occurs mainly in late infancy and early childhood, with a peak incidence between the ages of 6 months and 4 years. It presents with initial upper respiratory tract symptoms followed by the development of hoarseness and a barking croupy cough. Stridor commonly occurs and, if airway obstruction increases, indrawing of respiratory muscles is seen on inspiration. The rate of clinical progression is much more gradual, and the patient less toxic, than with epiglottitis. Signs of significant airway obstruction require hospitalisation for close observation, oxygen if necessary and occasionally endo- or naso-tracheal intubation to bypass the airway obstruction. General care involves minimal handling, adequate fluid intake, added humidity and oxygen if necessary. Antibiotics are not specifically indicated unless additional bacterial pathology is suspected.

Epiglottitis

Acute epiglottitis is an extremely dangerous condition; it is seen in the age range 6 months to 6 years with a peak incidence in the second year of life. Infection with *Haemophilus influenzae* type B is the commonest cause; β-haemolytic streptococci cause only a few cases.

The patient presents with a rapid onset of fever, toxicity, and sore throat; within a few hours there is respiratory obstruction, drooling of secretions at the mouth, and neck extension to ease the passage of air through the obstructed airway. Clinically, there is inspiratory stridor with indrawing of respiratory muscles and, as hypoxaemia and hypercapnia worsen, restlessness and cyanosis appear. Acute airway obstruction and respiratory arrest may occur at any time.

If epiglottitis is suspected no attempt should be made to visualise the throat and no instruments should be put into the mouth because of the risk of acute complete obstruction. The child should be taken immediately to hospital; visualisation of the epiglottis is then undertaken *only by an experienced person* who can intubate immediately or, if this fails, perform a tracheostomy to relieve obstruction. A lateral neck X-ray is not to be recommended unless the diagnosis is seriously in doubt, as the additional handling can precipitate total obstruction. In an acute emergency, the passage of a large-bore needle into the trachea below the cricoid cartilage may be life-saving. Rapid antigen screening of the blood for *H. influenzae* may give confirmation of the diagnosis within an hour or two. Supportive measures include the use of intravenous antibiotics, usually chloramphenicol nowadays (as often haemophilus is resistant to ampicillin), fluid therapy and antipyretics. Once the obstruction is bypassed, oxygen is often no longer required.

Pertussis (whooping cough)

This is a potentially serious disease in infants and young children. Pertussis epidemics have now recurred because of the recent increase in unimmunised children in the community and it has been estimated that nearly three-quarters of those who are not protected are likely to contract the illness, with varying severity, before school age. Classical pertussis is due to infection with *Bordetella pertussis*, although other organisisms such as adenovirus, *Bordetella parapertussis* and *Bordetella bronchiseptica* have been implicated in pertussis like syndromes.

The incubation period is 10–14 days. The illness begins with a mild cough and mucoid nasal discharge which is followed by a spasmodic paroxysmal cough in the second week, this can result in cyanosis, apnoea, vomiting and the production of small quantities of tenacious mucus. The cough typically lasts for several weeks and has been called the 100-day cough — its name in Chinese. It may recur again during a subsequent respiratory infection although generally in a milder form. Young infants tend to have a more severe course and may contract the illness before they are due to be immunised.

Complications include subconjunctival haemorrhage, bronchopneumonia and lobar or segmental lung collapse which can lead to respiratory failure in severe cases. A small but important mortality occurs in the order of 0.5–1 per 1000 cases.

Management is symptomatic. There is no efficient medication to stop the paroxysms. Erythromycin given to family contacts is effective in preventing spread of classical pertussis and reduces the length of time the patient is infectious, but does not otherwise modify the course of the illness. Unless specifically contraindicated all infants should be immunised against pertussis whenever possible.

Bronchiolitis

Bronchiolitis is an acute infection caused principally by respiratory syncytial virus (RSV), other viruses implicated include parainfluenza, influenza and adenovirus. It occurs commonly during the first 6 months of life but is seen throughout the first year. Seasonal epidemics occur with peak incidence in winter and early spring.

At the bronchiolar level there is a marked inflammatory response which leads to small airway obstruction with wheezing and hyperinflation. In more severe cases, there may be pneumonia with areas of lung collapse or consolidation. On examination the infant is tachypnoeic with coryzal signs, there is a low grade fever and obvious chest hyperinflation with inspiratory indrawing and expiratory wheeze. Widespread expiratory rhonchi are heard on auscultation and patchy crepitations are heard on inspiration. The liver is usually palpable below the costal margin secondary to hyperinflation, associated cardiac failure is rare. In severe cases, respiratory failure supervenes with cyanosis due to hypoxaemia and an elevated arterial carbon dioxide tension ($Pa\text{CO}_2$) on blood gas analysis.

Management is supportive with humidified oxygen given if necessary. Humidity itself may be of

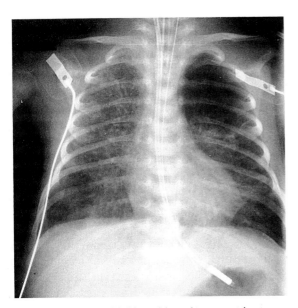

Fig. 16.3 RSV bronchiolitis and bronchopneumonia — child with underlying immune deficiency.

symptomatic value but does not modify the course of the illness. Adequate fluid intake is important but should not exceed daily requirements. Antibiotics are not indicated. Severe cases may require artificial ventilation.

Underlying conditions such as cystic fibrosis, recurrent aspiration and immunodeficiency should be considered in children with unusually severe bronchiolitis.

There remains considerable debate about the relationship of acute bronchiolitis to asthma. Up to 50% of children with acute bronchiolitis may go on to have recurrent wheezing episodes after an attack. Asthma is much more likely if there is a family history of atopic disease.

Pneumonia

Pneumonia is common at all ages, particularly in infants and young children. The commonest pathogens in the younger age group are viral, such as RSV, although the other respiratory viruses can also cause severe infection, especially adenovirus. In older children, viruses continue to be important but bacterial infection becomes increasingly common; *Streptococcus pneumoniae* is the predominant pathogen, although the incidence of *Mycoplasma*

pneumoniae infection increases towards adolescence. Infection with other bacteria is less common but can be severe; these organisms include *Staphylococcus aureus*, β-haemolytic streptococci and *Haemophilus influenzae*. Gram-negative organisms such as *E. coli*, *Klebsiella* and *Pseudomonas aeruginosa* are only seen in debilitated children or those with underlying disorders such as immune deficiency or cystic fibrosis. *Pneumocystis carinii*, adenovirus, cytomegalovirus and measles can produce serious interstitial pneumonia in immunosuppressed children.

In the young child, the infection is bronchopneumonic with signs of fever, tachypnoea, dry cough and increased work of breathing. Auscultation of the chest may reveal areas of diminished air entry and crepitations over the affected lung. X-ray confirms widespread areas of patchy consolidation, usually bilaterally.

In the older child, the infection is usually lobar in type. Air entry is diminished over the affected area and crepitations are heard. Dullness to percussion and bronchial breathing occur when more complete consolidation is present. In severe cases, respiratory failure occurs and ultimately circulatory failure due to cor pulmonale with associated hypoxaemia and acidosis.

Management is supportive; skilled nursing care is important, in hospital if necessary. Daily fluid intake should be limited to 75% of normal as inappropriate antidiuretic-hormone secretion can occur leading to hyponatraemia, cerebral oedema and convulsions. Humidified oxygen is given via head-box, oxygen tent or face-mask. Arterial blood gases should be monitored.

Antibiotics are indicated whenever bacterial infection is suspected. Trap sputum specimens or blood culture may help to identify the organism. A rapid antigen screen on blood may lead to early identification of the causative organism. Penicillin is the drug of choice with erythromycin as an alternative for the penicillin-allergic patient. If there is a likelihood of staphylococcal infection, cloxacillin and possibly gentamicin may be required. Erythromycin is the treatment of choice for infection with mycoplasma. Antibiotics which are active against Gram-negative organisms may be particularly appropriate for the child who has already been in hospital or those with other disorders. The choice of antibiotics should be confirmed by the results of bacteriological cultures. Physiotherapy is helpful in facilitating clearance of secretions and re-expansion of consolidated lobes of lung.

Empyema is a rare complication and is usually due to *Staphylococcus aureus* although anaerobic organisms also occur. Adequate antibiotic therapy and drainage are vital for proper resolution. These patients should be investigated for underlying immune deficiency or cystic fibrosis.

Tuberculosis

Tuberculosis in children is fortunately much less common now; however, it is still encountered in clinical practice and remains an important cause of morbidity and mortality.

The illness is caused by the organism *Mycobacterium tuberculosis*, although, rarely, infection due to atypical mycobacteria, particularly affecting the cervical lymph glands, is seen. The bacilli are usually acquired by airborne transmission from an infected person; the organ most frequently involved in primary infection is the lung. The organism multiplies and causes a primary focus to appear, this undergoes slow fibrosis over a period of many months and may eventually either calcify or disappear. Simultaneously, there is multiplication of the organism and tissue reaction within the regional (hilar) lymph nodes. The size of this reaction depends upon the age and nutritional state of the host. Resistance is less vigorous in the young or malnourished child.

Six weeks after infection the patient becomes sensitised to tuberculoprotein and the diagnostic delayed hypersensitivity reaction in skin becomes positive. This is the basis of the Mantoux test in which 0.1 ml (10 tuberculin units) of 1:1000 dilution of PPD (protein purified derivative) is injected intradermally. An indurated area of 5 mm diameter or greater is produced within 48 hours in those who are sensitive. If significant disease is suspected 0.1 ml of 1:10 000 solution should be used to avoid a severe or painful skin reaction. The Mantoux test is the most reliable test for diagnostic purposes. It may be falsely negative in those with severe infections, and after measles it is inhibited by steroid therapy.

Screening of larger populations may be carried out using the multiple puncture Heaf test. A spring-loaded gun produces a circle of six epidermal punctures through a tuberculin PPD solution placed on the skin surface. Positive reactions produce induration at the puncture sites, in those with vigorous reactions these may coalesce. The tuberculin tine test uses a device with four points or tines, which have been coated with tuberculin; they are pressed against the skin for 5 seconds. The Mantoux test is the most efficient.

Systemic symptoms may occur in association with the primary infection and include fever, lethargy, anorexia, weight loss, hepatosplenomegaly and rarely erythema nodosum and phlyctenular conjunctivitis. The vast majority of children with primary tuberculosis will, however, show no significant systemic upset and are only detected by routine testing for tuberculoprotein sensitivity in school screening programmes.

Late complications can affect a number of organs. Progressive primary lung infection including collapse, consolidation, bronchiectasis, pleural effusion and, rarely, empyema can occur. The central nervous system may be involved by tuberculous meningitis, usually within 6–12 months of the primary infection. This complication still carries a high morbidity and mortality. There may be involvement of bones and joints 1–3 years after initial infection and renal tuberculosis can occur several years later. The most serious complication is miliary tuberculosis with generalised haematogenous spread throughout the body.

Children who are shown to have had primary infection either by the presence of physical signs or by tuberculin conversion from negative to positive reaction, should be given antituberculous chemotherapy in order to prevent late complications (principally tuberculous meningitis and miliary tuberculosis). The most suitable combination of drugs for the treatment of TB in children is now thought to be rifampicin with isoniazid for a period of 6 months. This is supplemented with pyrazinamide for the first 2 months. Streptomycin is still occasionally used during the first two months if resistance is thought likely to be a problem.

A baby whose mother has active TB should receive isoniazid for the first 3 months of life. The infant is then tested for tuberculin sensitivity. If negative then isoniazid-resistant BCG is given. If positive and especially if the chest X-ray is abnormal then a further course of isoniazid is given in combination with rifampicin. There is no need to separate mother and baby in the neonatal period if both are known to be receiving adequate medication.

Management should also be directed towards improving the patient's general wellbeing and nutritional status in addition to chemotherapy specifically directed against the organism.

Protection may be achieved by the use of BCG vaccine. This is an attenuated bovine strain (Bacillus Calmette–Guèrin) which is given intradermally. It is currently offered to tuberculin-negative schoolchildren in late childhood (11–13 years of age) but may be given in the neonatal period to those at high risk of exposure, such as children of certain immigrant groups in the UK or those who are likely to travel abroad to countries with a high prevalence rate of tuberculosis.

STRIDOR

Stridor is noisy breathing heard on inspiration or expiration due to obstruction of airflow in large airways including the larynx and trachea. The amount of stridor will vary with the rate of breathing and the degree of obstruction present; it may be absent during quiet breathing or when obstruction is severe. Inspiratory stridor is usually associated with laryngeal or vocal cord problems, although it may also occur with a significant upper tracheal lesion. Bidirectional stridor is more typical of tracheal narrowing below the vocal cords.

Aetiology

The causes of stridor are:

1. Laryngomalacia.
2. Laryngotracheobronchitis (croup).
3. Diphtheria.
4. Acute epiglottitis.
5. Allergic oedema.
6. Vocal cord paralysis.
7. Vocal and cysts.
8. Cleft larynx.
9. Laryngeal web.
10. Subglottic haemangioma.
11. Subglottic stenosis.
12. Cystic hygroma.
13. Foreign body.
14. Tracheal stenosis.
15. Vascular ring.

By far the most common is laryngomalacia, which is a benign self-limiting condition in which inspiratory stridor occurs during the first few months of life. This varies with the baby's activity, crying and position, and is less prominent when the infant is prone. It is due to indrawing of the laryngeal tissues during inspiration in the presence of a small larynx and elongated epiglottis. The prognosis is excellent and most children will outgrow this problem by late infancy.

Stridor due to acute infections such as epiglottitis and laryngotracheobronchitis, should be treated with appropriate antibiotics and intubation to bypass the obstruction if necessary (see Ch. 28).

Investigations to establish the aetiology of stridor include a posteroanterior and lateral chest X-ray, lateral neck X-ray and barium swallow to exclude lesions pressing on the trachea such as cysts or a vascular ring. More detailed investigations involve laryngoscopy to assess vocal cord movement and to exclude supraglottic lesions and bronchoscopy to exclude tracheal pathology, such as tracheal stenosis, bronchomalacia and haemangioma. Thoracic CT scan may be useful in imaging extrinsic lesions affecting the trachea.

Clinical features and management

Stridor varies in severity according to the degree of obstruction and may be absent at rest or when lying prone depending on its aetiology. In supraglottic or vocal cord lesions it is usually inspiratory but, within the trachea, narrowing of this type usually produces bidirectional stridor. Wheezing is normally absent as this originates in smaller airways, although it can occur with significant tracheal obstruction causing retention of secretions.

Treatment is dependent on the lesion found but may include surgical correction for vascular ring, or laryngotracheoplasty to enlarge the trachea where significant permanent narrowing has occurred as in subglottic stenosis. In a number of cases, the airway obstruction cannot be relieved immediately and elective tracheostomy has to be performed until sufficient tracheal growth or resolution of the primary problem has occurred. Infants and children with a tracheostomy may be managed successfully at home. After operation the parents are instructed in the technique of tracheal toilet and suction; they are provided with a supply of catheters and a suction pump for use at home. As improvement occurs a silver, valved Alder–Mey pattern tube may be inserted which allows expiration to occur normally through the glottis and stimulates speech development.

INHALATION OF FOREIGN BODY

Inhalation of a foreign body is not uncommon in infants and young children. A peanut or other foodstuff is the commonest cause but many other objects such as small plastic toys, beads and occasionally seeds or pine needles may be inhaled. Frequently, there is an acute episode of cough, choking or wheeze at the time of inhalation or symptoms may develop gradually over the next few hours or days. In some cases, however, the diagnosis is delayed and the child may present with chronic cough and sputum production or recurrent pneumonia. It is in this situation that the risk of permanent lung damage, including the development of chronic bronchiectasis, is greatest. Most objects lodge in the bronchi, more often on the right side than the left.

Diagnosis based on an accurate history and careful physical examination which reveals diminished air entry on the affected side and hyperinflation if there is significant air trapping behind the foreign body. Alternatively there may be collapse-consolidation and bronchial breathing.

X-ray of the chest may show typical hyperinflation on the affected side especially on an expiratory film. Chest screening reveals hyperinflation with air trapping and diminished respiratory movement on inspiration. Areas of pneumonic consolidation or complete collapse may also be found depending on the duration of the condition.

Bronchoscopy is essential if foreign body inhalation is suspected. Removal of the object should be followed by adequate physiotherapy and antibiotics to clear the lung of retained secretions and aid the resolution of any secondary bacterial infection. In cases where the diagnosis is delayed, careful follow-up should be undertaken to assess lung function on the affected side. This may be permanently compromised by the presence of bronchiectasis or chronic peripheral pulmonary vascular disease.

CYSTIC FIBROSIS

Cystic fibrosis is a serious, life-long disorder affecting exocrine glandular secretions throughout the body. The incidence in caucasians in the UK is about 1 in 2000 live births; it is less common in other racial groups. Males and females are equally affected. The gene is known to lie on the long arm of chromosome number 7. The inheritance is autosomal recessive with a gene carrier rate in the normal adult population of approximately 1 in 20.

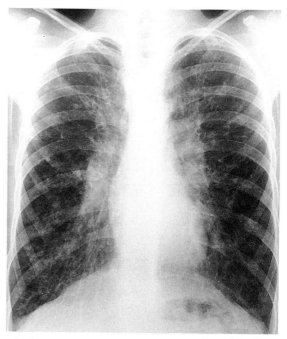

Fig. 16.4 Cystic fibrosis: generalized overinflation, bronchial wall thickening, mottled shadows indicate infection.

Adult carriers are entirely healthy and cannot be distinguished from the normal population.

Accurate prenatal diagnosis is now available utilising chorionic villous sampling at 8–10 weeks of gestation. This requires previous family studies of the transmission of the CF gene so is only available for those who already have at least one affected child.

The illness may present in a number of ways. Ten to fifteen per cent present with intestinal obstruction due to meconium ileus in the neonatal period. Most other children with cystic fibrosis present in infancy or preschool years with recurrent lower respiratory tract infection, frequent pale bulky stools and failure to thrive. Increasing numbers are now being detected at birth by screening tests such as immunoreactive trypsin measurement on blood spot taken with the Guthrie test.

Clinical features

The major clinical features affect the respiratory tree and the digestive tract. The respiratory secretions, although initially of normal viscosity, become abnormally viscid in the presence of infection. This tends to occur from an early age and causes increasing damage to the small airways leading to obstruction, sputum retention and over-inflation. Chronic bronchial wall thickening develops as infection worsens and eventually there is microabscess formation with irreversible pulmonary damage and bronchiectasis. Upper respiratory tract symptoms with chronic sinusitis and recurrent nasal polyposis are common problems in the older child.

Major digestive difficulties are seen in most cases. These are due primarily to pancreatic insufficiency with decreased trypsin, lipase and bicarbonate concentrations in duodenal juice. There may be meconium ileus in the neonatal period (see Ch. 26), or recurrent abdominal pain with partial or complete bowel obstruction in later life. The latter, called the distal intestinal obstruction syndrome or meconium ileus equivalent, is typically due to impacted faecal material in the ileo-caecal region and can be relieved by gastrografin enema. Frequently, there is also a history of poor weight gain, abdominal distension, and offensive stools which contain fat globules on microscopy. The children have an excellent appetite, unlike those with small bowel malabsorption, unless an acute respiratory infection complicates their chronic pulmonary dysfunction. In toddlers, the bulky stools can cause rectal prolapse.

A number of other clinical features may also develop including biliary cirrhosis, portal hypertension and oesophageal varices, gastric hyperacidity and diabetes mellitus due to pancreatic fibrosis. Heat exhaustion due to excess salt loss can occur in hot climates. In adult life, males are always infertile due to fibrosis of the vas deferens while females have reduced fertility and tend to have exacerbation of their chest symptoms during pregnancy. It is important to note that intellectual function is not affected.

The diagnosis is confirmed by measurement of sodium or chloride content in sweat collected by iontophoresis. A concentration of 70 mmol/l on a sample weighing more than 100 mg is diagnostic. Analysis of duodenal juice bicarbonate, trypsin and lipase concentrations following pancreatic stimulation may be helpful in difficult cases.

Management

Pulmonary

Treatment must be carried out every day. The most important aspect is care of the chest and this must be kept as clear of sputum as possible by encouraging postural drainage and physiotherapy on a regular basis every day from the time of diagnosis. Antibiotics should be used in high dosage for 2–3-week courses during intercurrent respiratory tract infections to prevent lower respiratory tract colonisation with pathogenic organisms such as *Staphylococcus aureus*, *Pseudomonas aeruginosa* and *Haemophilus influenzae*. Continuous antibiotics are indicated for prolonged periods if there is established infection. A significant number of children also develop wheeze; if this is due to reversible airway disease, as tested by peak flow measurement, then bronchodilators such as salbutamol, terbutaline or theophylline may be useful. There is some evidence that these agents may also promote mucociliary clearance. If allergy is thought to have a prominent part in symptoms then Intal may be beneficial. Mucolytic agents such as acetylcysteine are not generally recommended but do have a role in individuals with particularly viscid sputum which is difficult to clear.

Episodes of spontaneous pneumothorax or intermittent haemoptysis are other complications which become increasingly common with age. In those with the most advanced disease cor pulmonale develops and is associated with a significant worsening of prognosis. Heart–lung transplantation, although still a relatively experimental procedure, is being practised with increasing success in those with end-stage lung disease.

Nutritional

Nine out of 10 patients with cystic fibrosis have nutritional problems primarily related to pancreatic insufficency. Management is aimed at providing a high calorie, high protein, high carbohydrate and normal fat diet. Oral pancreatic enzyme replacement is given with meals using enteric-coated microspheres such as Creon or Pancrease. The dosage has to be tailored to the individual and will vary depending on the fat intake and level of pancreatic insufficiency at that time. Vitamin supplements are added to replace vitamins A, B, C, D and E. Vitamin K is given if there is hepatic dysfunction. A good salt intake is also essential and salt tablets may be indicated in hot climates where excess salt loss in sweat and heat exhaustion can occur. A significant proportion of older patients develop hepatic cirrhosis.

Social and family

Cystic fibrosis is a life-long condition with a variable prognosis; life expectancy can be from a few months or years at one extreme to the middle-forties at the other. The majority now survive to adult life. The overall management of the child and the family must include adequate counselling and support for the parents and the patient throughout childhood, adolescence and adult life. This involves the physician, physiotherapists, nurses and social workers. Most children can lead a reasonably normal life and attend normal school

if given appropriate support. In adult life they can undertake most jobs except those involving heavy physical effort or exposure to smoke and dust. Many now marry and it is important to counsel them about the management of the illness in adult life. Males with cystic fibrosis are sterile. Cystic fibrosis management is essentially hospital based; the Cystic Fibrosis Research Trust provides funding for research and also meetings and literature for affected families.

BRONCHIECTASIS

Bronchiectasis is a chronic lung condition caused by bronchial dilatation in the presence of infection and is characterised by chronic cough and purulent sputum production. It is the pathological end-result of a number of disease processes:

1. Cystic fibrosis.
2. Lower respiratory tract infection.
3. Immunodeficiency.
4. Foreign body inhalation.
5. Abnormal lung development.
6. Recurrent aspiration.

The affected child may present with dyspnoea, cough, sputum production, finger clubbing, hyperinflated chest and with diminished air entry and coarse crepitations heard over the affected area.

A number of organisms, which infect the lung, can produce these changes including *Staphylococcus aureus*, *Streptococcus pneumoniae*, *Haemophilus influenzae*, *Klebsiella aerogenes*, *Pseudomonas aeruginosa*, *Bordetella pertussis* and adenovirus. Investigation of the child with bronchiectasis should include full blood count, immunoglobulins, Mantoux test, sweat test and X-rays including a radioisotope lung scan and possibly a thoracic CT scan. A barium swallow is necessary to exclude gastro-oesophagel reflux and aspiration. Bronchography is only rarely required nowadays, although bronchoscopy is essential if initial investigation fails to reveal a cause or if a foreign body is suspected.

Treatment is similar to that in cystic fibrosis. This will include regular physiotherapy and intermittent or continuous antibiotics depending on the pathogen isolated from regular sputum cultures.

The aim is to keep the lung free of infection so that recovery and resolution may occur and further deterioration is prevented. Surgery may be indicated to deal with the primary cause, for example, removal of a foreign body or cyst or a single infected lobe. There is considerable postoperative morbidity following chest surgery in patients with bilateral disease and therefore lobar removal is rarely indicated if more than one lobe is affected. Conservative management can lead to significant improvement with age in those who do not have other underlying disease such as cystic fibrosis or immune deficiency.

17. Heart disease

A. S. Hunter   A. W. Goodwin

CONGENITAL HEART DISEASE

Major advances in the precise diagnosis of congenital heart disease have occurred in the last decade. Initially these came through the medium of angled angiographic views and subtraction angiography. More recently high-quality cross-sectional cardiac ultrasound, with colour flow mapping of intracardiac flow by Doppler ultrasound, have revolutionised the diagnostic process. Parallel with these advances a new descriptive nomenclature has been accepted in the UK and throughout Europe. This system eschews Latin and embryological terms and is used throughout this chapter.

The medical treatment of infants and children with congenital heart disease has not altered significantly. It is well described in major texts and will not be dealt with in this chapter in any detail. There have been two major therapeutic advances. The pharmacological control of the patency of the arterial duct has significantly altered mortality in the neonatal period. Indomethacin is used to close the duct and prostaglandin to maintain its patency in duct-dependent lesions such as pulmonary atresia or coarctation of the aorta. In the treatment of heart failure, vasodilators and ACE inhibitors are now in fairly widespread use with some clinical benefit.

The full spectrum of congenital heart disease is not within the scope of this chapter which is intended to give a broad overview of the subject with indications for invasive or non-invasive investigations, medical treatment and surgery.

LEFT TO RIGHT ATRIAL SHUNTS

Atrial septal defect (ASD)

Atrial septal defects represent 10% of congenital cardiac malformations. Seventy per cent of these occur centrally in the atrial septum and are known as central or secundum atrial septal defects.

Central atrial septal defect

This defect occurs in and around the area of the oval pit (foramen ovale). Although usually single, it may be multiple.

Most children with this condition are asymptomatic in childhood and the lesion is found by chance because a murmur is heard at a school or welfare clinic examination or during an incidental illness. These children are frequently slim and small. Uncorrected patients with atrial septal defects become symptomatic in the third or fourth decade of life with the development of pulmonary hypertension, pulmonary vascular disease and atrial arrhythmias.

Clinical findings include increased pulmonary flow with an ejection murmur at the pulmonary area and a mid-diastolic tricuspid flow murmur. The second heart sound is widely split and fixed because inspiration cannot further increase the volume loading of the right ventricle.

The ECG usually shows right axis deviation (although a small percentage of patients have left axis), an RSR pattern in V4 and V1 and a terminal S wave in the left chest leads. This is often loosely referred to as an 'incomplete right bundle branch block' although evidence of a block in the conducting system is slim.

The chest X-ray shows cardiomegaly of varying degree. The size of the heart on X-ray is often not well correlated with the size of the shunt measured at cardiac catheterisation. The prominence of the right atrium, right ventricle and main pulmonary artery along with plethoric lung fields demonstrate the presence of a left to right atrial shunt, and right ventricular volume overload.

On echocardiography right ventricular volume overload is demonstrated by paradoxical septal movement with right ventricular cavity enlargement. Sector scans invariably visualise the defect and localise it to the centre of the septum. Although such a defect can be recognised in scans from the apex as well as from the subcostal approach, the latter is the method of choice. From the apex the ultrasound scan runs parallel to the interatrial septum which is frequently very thin. This leads to 'artefactual' dropout in the region of the interatrial septum, suggesting the presence of a defect when it is not present. From the subcostal approach the scan hits the interatrial septum at right angles and artefactual dropout is not a problem.

The management of patients with secundum ASDs is simple. When the pulmonary flow exceeds systemic by approximately 2:1, the defect should be closed surgically to remove the possibility of the problems in later life already mentioned. Surgical closure is either by patching or stitching the defect.

Atrioventricular septal defects ('Endocardial cushion defects')

One of the main aims of the new nomenclature was to remove such terms as 'endocardial cushion defect' and 'atrioventricular canal defect' These names were neither descriptive nor embryologically correct.

Recently the existence of a third cardiac septum — the atrioventricular septum — has been demonstrated. In the normal patient this lies between the left ventricle and the right atrium. In the group of patients described as having atrioventricular defects, this structure is largely absent.

The clinical spectrum of atrioventricular septal defects includes what used to be called 'primum atrial septal defects' and 'atrioventricular canal defects'. These are all defects of the atrioventricular septum but with a considerable spectrum of severity and abnormality. All have continuity of atrioventricular valve structures from the right to the left side of the heart. The normal offsetting of septal insertion between the mitral and tricuspid valve is absent. In the complete form of the defect there is a common orifice as well as a common atrioventricular ring. It is now no longer accurate to describe any of the atrioventricular valve structures in these patients as either mitral or tricuspid. The common valve has a series of leaflets of which two are known as bridging leaflets. These pass from the body of the left ventricle across the centre of the heart into the body of the right ventricle. In the case of the partial defect these structures are linked together by this tongue of tissue to each other and to the crest of the septum. In the complete form the bridging leaflets are not attached directly to the crest of the septum and there is thus a ventricular defect under the bridging leaflets.

The presentation varies considerably according to the underlying morphology. Complete defects present in early infancy with failure to thrive and heart failure. The presence of a large obligatory left to right shunt and much atrioventricular valve regurgitation results in significant increase in pulmonary blood flow and pulmonary hypertension. The murmurs may be very unimpressive but the presence of a loud pulmonary component to the second heart sound is almost invariable. Sometimes the systolic murmurs are heard better towards the apex, suggesting that they arise from the atrioventricular valve regurgitation. The patients are not usually blue although they may become so intermittently with exercise and chest infections. An enlarged anteroposterior diameter of the chest is frequent.

The ECG shows classically an anticlockwise rotation which gives a left axis deviation. Biventricular hypertrophy is present and sometimes biatrial enlargement also.

The chest X-ray shows cardiomegaly often with four-chamber enlargement. The main pulmonary artery is enlarged and pulmonary plethora is present.

The anatomical details which differentiate the complete from the partial defect are well demonstrated on a cross-sectional echocardiogram and it is possible using Doppler ultrasound to assess AV valve regurgitation. Echo and Doppler features of pulmonary hypertension are present.

Partial atrioventricular defect is a much less severe condition, sometimes presenting later in childhood. Pulmonary systolic and tricuspid diastolic flow murmurs with fixed splitting of the second heart sound, as in the central ASD, are present. These are frequently associated with apical pan systolic murmurs associated with left-sided AV valve regurgitation. Pulmonary hypertension is much less frequent but the patients do have significant left to right shunting and the chest X-ray shows cardiomegaly with plethoric lung fields and right ventricular enlargement. The left ventricle is not usually enlarged.

The ECG shows typically left axis deviation with an incomplete right bundle branch block pattern and sometimes in the presence of significant left-sided atrioventricular valve regurgitation there is a volume overload pattern.

Echocardiogram demonstrates nicely that the partial form has two orifices and no ventricular component to the defect.

The complete defect demands an aggressive surgical approach with 'correction' probably during the first year of life. Beyond that point the incidence of pulmonary hypertension and pulmonary vascular disease becomes very high and surgery is frequently contraindicated. Total correction in the first 6 months of life although the best long-term option is associated with a very significant surgical mortality. Partial atrioventricular septal defect is very different. Although it carries a greater mortality compared with the central (secundum) atrial septal defect, the risks are much less than in the complete defect. Closure of the atrioventricular septal defect is carried out using a patch of Dacron or pericardium to which the bridging leaflets are attached. Conservative surgery of the abnormal atrioventricular valve leaflet is difficult and is limited to attempting to reduce regurgitation. It is probable that in the complete atrioventricular septal defect, valve replacement will be required in adult life.

Arterial duct (persistent ductus arteriosus)

This is the commonest congenital cardiac lesion (12%) and is twice as common in girls as in boys. It is frequently associated with prematurity, maternal rubella and there is an increased incidence in populations born at high altitude.

The timing and type of presentation is determined by the size of the duct and the amount of blood passing through it. Large ducts with large left to right shunts will cause heart failure, failure to thrive and feeding difficulties in early infancy. Smaller ducts with smaller left to right shunts may well be asymptomatic and only found at routine medical examination by the recognition of the appropriate murmur.

Clinical findings are very variable depending on the size of the lesion and the age at presentation. In the older child there is a continuous (machinery) murmur in the second left intercostal space. It is similar to and may be confused with the venous hum which normally results from blood flowing through the great veins in the neck. The venous hum goes away with compression of the neck, rotation of the head or laying the child flat. A duct murmur does not. In infancy the classical continuous murmur is frequently not heard, the diastolic component being missing. The length and characteristic of the murmur varies with pulmonary resistance and the amount of pulmonary flow. Mid-diastolic mitral flow murmurs are present when the left to right shunt is large and the second heart sound has an accentuated pulmonary component. The peripheral pulses are jerky and the pulse pressure is large, indicating an aorto-pulmonary 'run-off' of some magnitude, similar to aortic regurgitation.

The ECG in the classic presentation shows left ventricular hypertrophy with deep Q waves in the left chest leads and inferior leads. There may be biventricular hypertrophy but most of the smaller or medium sized ducts are associated with entirely normal cardiograms.

The chest X-ray shows pulmonary vascularity is increased and prominence of the main pulmonary artery is frequent. The left ventricle and left atrium, in the left anterior oblique or left lateral films, will show enlargement. The small duct may be associated with a normal chest X-ray.

Echocardiography is very useful in this condition. Left ventricular and left atrial enlargement are present with the volume overload pattern of contraction in the left ventricle. The duct is frequently visualised from the high parasternal view using cross-sectional imaging. Even if this is not possible pulsed or continuous wave Doppler directed at the main pulmonary artery and into the origin of the left pulmonary artery will demonstrate continuous flow from the aorta to the pulmonary artery. This is easily recognised on colour flow mapping and is the quickest and best way of confirming the diagnosis.

Small infants with large ducts respond well to antifailure therapy with diuretics and fluid restriction. Particularly in the preterm infant however, this should not be for a prolonged time as it will interfere with the calorie intake and growth of the child. The spontaneous closure rate is not high and intervention is frequently needed in preterm babies. Between 28 and 32 weeks ducts in preterm infants frequently close under the effect of indomethacin — a prostaglandin synthetase antagonist. Before 28 weeks and later than 32 weeks or if the child is older than 10 days the success rate drops off so dramatically that indomethacin is probably not of value. Although indomethacin may cause gastric erosion and renal disturbance, given in the right dose at the right time the drug has made a significant contribution to the treatment of arterial ducts in preterm infants.

In the term infant and older child the duct should be surgically closed at diagnosis. The operation is safe and quick. The continuing presence of a duct in later childhood and adolescence gives a recurring risk of endarteritis and there is also evidence that even quite small ducts may in later life produce ventricular decompensation.

In recent years it has become possible to close ducts at catheterisation by inserting different types of 'plug' into the duct lumen. Although gaining in popularity this technique is time consuming and difficult. For the moment it is not the treatment of choice but it might well become so in the future.

Ventricular septal defect (VSD)

This is one of the commonest congenital cardiac malformations. While the great majority of ventricular septal defects cause no problems, a small percentage cause major haemodynamic problems and require intensive therapy and surgical closure at an early age. This should be put into perspective however by noting that as many as 60% of all VSDs will close spontaneously.

The presentation and symptomatology vary greatly with the size of the defect and the size of the left to right shunt. Small defects in asymptomatic children present as incidentally discovered murmurs. The larger defects customarily present during the first 2 months of life with heart failure, failure to thrive, dyspnoea and recurrent chest infections. The late onset of these symptoms and signs is dependent on the rate of fall of pulmonary artery pressure and pulmonary resistance following birth. As the pulmonary artery pressure falls the pressure differential between left and right ventricles allows an increasing left to right shunt. In a small percentage of children the pulmonary vascular resistance never falls. In these, pulmonary vascular disease occurs at an early stage with subsequent reversal of the shunt and cyanosis. Many large VSDs have such huge pulmonary flow that they require urgent surgical correction during the first year of life to avoid failure to thrive and the development of pulmonary vascular disease.

The patient with a large left to right ventricular shunt is breathless at rest, and has an increased anteroposterior diameter of the chest with a Harrison's sulcus and sometimes indrawing of the skin over the intercostal space. A pan systolic murmur in the 4th and 5th intercostal space at the lower left sternal edge, with or without a thrill, is usually present. When the pulmonary flow is more than twice systemic, a mitral diastolic flow murmur is heard at the apex. The presence of pulmonary hypertension is suggested by an increase in loudness of the pulmonary component of the second heart sound and a right ventricular parasternal lift or heave.

The chest X-ray is frequently normal in small defects. In larger left to right shunts, significant cardiomegaly, particularly of the left ventricle and left atrium, is seen. The lung vascularity is increased and the main pulmonary artery is enlarged, particularly in the presence of pulmonary hypertension.

The ECG, although not diagnostic, is valuable

in following these patients. Biventricular hypertrophy is common in the big shunts and as pulmonary vasculature resistance increases, right ventricular hypertrophy becomes more marked. Deep Q waves in the left chest leads are seen and this with tall R waves suggests the left ventricular volume overload pattern.

Cardiac ultrasound has revolutionised the management of patients with VSDs in recent years. Cross-sectional echocardiography can demonstrate exactly in which part of the septum the VSD lies. Longitudinal studies have shown that this helps to predict which will close spontaneously. A small muscular VSD for instance has a high probability of closing, whereas a large VSD underneath the aortic valve in the membranous septum is less likely to close. VSDs have been reliably classified using ultrasound, first of all into muscular and perimembranous, and then, according to the part of the septum, into inlet, outlet, trabecular and membranous septum. Doppler ultrasound allows the investigator to measure non-invasively the pressure drop across the VSD between left ventricle and right ventricle. If the systemic systolic pressure is known then the right ventricular and therefore pulmonary artery systolic pressure can be estimated very accurately. It is doubtful whether in the future cardiac catheterisation will be necessary except in a few selected cases.

If the defect is small then conservative management with antibiotic cover for dental extractions and operations is all that is necessary. Follow-up is usually continued until the defect closes which is identified ultrasonically and by absence of a murmur.

Small infants with large defects and heart failure are treated initially with diuretics, digoxin and sometimes vasodilators. Associated lesions such as arterial ducts or coarctation are identified and dealt with initially. If the pulmonary artery pressure is low or only slightly elevated then it is acceptable to observe conservatively, as even large left to right shunts may close spontaneously. However when the pulmonary artery pressure is raised and the VSD shows no sign of getting smaller then surgery should take place during the first year of life. Mortality for surgical correction at this age is very low and no patient now should become inoperable because of pulmonary vascular disease before surgical closure.

OBSTRUCTIVE LESIONS OF THE RIGHT HEART

Pulmonary stenosis (PS)

Pulmonary valve stenosis represents 10% of all congenital heart disease. It is most commonly at valve level but may also be at subvalvar and supravalvar level. Branch artery stenosis is a rare form but is associated with William's syndrome and occasionally with tetralogy of Fallot.

Mild pulmonary valve stenosis is usually discovered at a routine medical examination in childhood. The child is asymptomatic and has a pulmonary ejection murmur with a wide split of the second heart sound and an ejection click. The presence of the click infers that the stenosis is moderate or mild.

The electrocardiogram may be normal or show mild right ventricular hypertrophy.

Chest X-ray may be within normal limits but frequently shows poststenotic dilatation of the main pulmonary artery.

The echocardiogram is frequently within normal limits but Doppler studies using continuous wave Doppler demonstrate an increased velocity with turbulent flow in the main pulmonary artery.

More severe pulmonary stenosis presents in infancy and indeed, if critical, in the neonatal period. In critical pulmonary stenosis the babies present with cyanosis, heart failure and evidence of severe tricuspid regurgitation. The right ventricle is frequently small, dysmorphic and works at a higher pressure than systemic. The difference between this and pulmonary atresia with an intact ventricular septum is a matter of degree. On auscultation the second heart sound is usually single and there is a pulmonary ejection systolic murmur. A click is not usually heard. The cyanosis can be quite severe. This condition can present prenatally and some fetuses die of the condition before term.

Chest X-ray is critical in severe pulmonary stenosis. The pulmonary vascularity is normal and the main pulmonary artery is prominent due to poststenotic dilatation. The right ventricle and right atrium are enlarged.

The echocardiogram shows considerable right ventricular hypertrophy and usually a small right ventricular cavity. The pulmonary valve can be visualised as domed and thickened and Doppler ultrasound is invaluable in demonstrating whether or not the valve is patent. By measuring the peak velocity in the pulmonary artery (elevated in any form of pulmonary stenosis), and using the modified Bernoulli equation, the pressure gradient can be inferred with great accuracy. The presence of tricuspid regurgitation and the Ebstein abnormality of the tricuspid valve is also well seen with cardiac ultrasound.

The management of pulmonary stenosis depends on the severity. Critical neonatal pulmonary stenosis (or pulmonary atresia) needs emergency surgery. Valvotomy, either open or closed, with or without an aortopulmonary shunt, is the best way of dealing with this condition. The child's prognosis depends on the size of the right ventricle and the competency of the tricuspid valve. Beyond the neonatal period it is now normal practice in most centres to carry out balloon valvotomy at the time of cardiac catheterisation. A balloon close in size to the pulmonary valve ring is introduced via the femoral vein and inflated when across the pulmonary valve. This is a safe procedure beyond the neonatal period and associated with virtually 100% success rate. There are occasional valves which resist balloon valvotomy because they are thickened and myxomatous rather than domed and fibrous. These may be found in Noonan's syndrome and are identified from the cross-sectional echo. It is usually considered that a pressure drop of over 60 across the pulmonary valve indicates the need for surgery. Pulmonary valvotomy by balloon is so safe and entails such a short period in hospital that most paediatric cardiologists now consider carrying out balloon valvotomy down to 40 mmHg pressure drop.

Tetralogy of Fallot

This is the most common form of cyanotic congenital heart disease accounting for 10% of all cardiac malformations. Although the initial description was of four features, the underlying problem is an underdevelopment of the right ventricular outflow tract and pulmonary artery. The underdeveloped outflow tract is associated with deviation of the infundibular septum producing pulmonary infundibular obstruction and right ventricular hypertrophy. The deviation of the infundibular septum also leads to the aortic override and the development of a subarterial perimembranous VSD. Underlying haemodynamics are such that the blood in the right ventricle is partially prevented from entering the pulmonary artery because of the stenosis and passes across the ventricular septal defect into the left ventricle and out into the aorta.

The degree of pulmonary outflow tract obstruction determines the mode and age of presentation. If the outflow tract is very hypoplastic and narrowed the baby will present in early infancy with cyanosis. The more classical presentation is an asymptomatic child with a murmur whose cyanosis has started to become apparent during the first year of life, probably because of increasing infundibular narrowing.

Dyspnoea in infants, especially when feeding, increases with age. Squatting is characteristic of all the children. Squatting usually follows extreme exertion and allows the child to increase his peripheral vascular resistance and to minimise the right to left shunt. Hypercyanotic spells are common when the pulmonary anatomy is severely hypoplastic and infundibular spasm has been implicated. Increasing right to left shunting occurs because of reduced pulmonary flow and the patient becomes pale, blue and may lose consciousness. These spells are an indication for early treatment.

An ejection systolic murmur is heard at the pulmonary area and conducted down the left sternal edge. The second heart sound frequently appears single although usually there is a delayed soft pulmonary component. The more severe the narrowing of the outflow tract the shorter the murmur. During a hypercyanotic spell the murmur may shorten dramatically or disappear altogether. Finger clubbing is rare in infancy and develops gradually through childhood. · Noncardiac abnormalities are common in this condition and the paediatrician should look for gastrointestinal and genitourinary tract anomalies, present in as many as one-third of cases.

The classic sign on the chest X-ray is of a tilted

apex (*coeur en sabot*), resulting from right ventricular hypertrophy. Above the apex the pulmonary artery and outflow tract are concave and underdeveloped. There is oligaemia of the lung fields and a right aortic arch is present in 25% of patients.

ECG demonstrates right ventricular hypertrophy, right axis deviation but almost never shows right atrial enlargement. The degree of right ventricular hypertrophy is never as dramatic in comparison with pulmonary stenosis and the absence of right atrial enlargement also differentiates the two conditions.

The cross-sectional echocardiogram demonstrates very nicely the anatomy of the VSD, the aortic override and the presence of right ventricular hypertrophy. Subcostally the right ventricular outflow tract, infundibular stenosis and narrowing can be demonstrated well and frequently the size and disposition of the main pulmonary artery and right and left branches are assessed. However when the pulmonary arteries are very small the echocardiogram is often an inadequate means of determining pulmonary artery anatomy. The degree of narrowing of the outflow tract and the pulmonary artery can be demonstrated using Doppler ultrasound and an accurate assessment of gradient across the outflow tract made.

It is still usually advisable to carry out cine angiocardiography in these patients to demonstrate the size and disposition of the pulmonary arteries, the presence of additional VSDs and anomalies of the coronary arteries which are fairly common in this condition.

In infancy profound cyanosis and cyanotic spells are best treated surgically by an aortopulmonary shunt. The Waterston shunt (ascending aorta to right pulmonary artery) has fallen out of favour as it produced a unilateral increase in pulmonary blood flow and deformity of the right pulmonary artery. The classic Blalock–Taussig shunt (subclavian artery to right or left pulmonary artery) remains a better and more physiological shunt but it is often technically difficult to do in tiny infants. The modified Blalock–Taussig shunts in which Gortex or similar tubing is anastomosed to the side of the subclavian artery and the corresponding pulmonary artery, is now the method of choice. The patency rate of these is higher in infants than the classic Blalock–Taussig shunt.

Hypercyanotic spells are an indication for shunting but may need to be treated acutely by medical means. These attacks usually respond to oxygen administration (which raises the systemic vascular resistance), correction of acidaemia and administration of an intravenous beta blocker such as propranolol. Occasionally a very severe shunt will not respond fully to the above therapy and the systemic vascular resistance should be increased by administration of intravenous aramine.

All cases of tetralogy of Fallot need surgical treatment at some time. Under 5 kg the normal practice is to shunt the symptomatic child. Over 5 kg if the anatomy of the pulmonary arteries is not severe, total correction is the method of choice with closure of the VSD, resection of the outflow tract and if necessary placement of either a gusset or a conduit between the right ventricle and the pulmonary artery.

The most severe form of Fallot's tetralogy is pulmonary atresia with VSD. Clinical presentation is different in that the pulmonary ejection murmur is usually absent. Presentation is also usually in infancy and the child frequently depends on an arterial duct for pulmonary blood flow. Prostaglandin is frequently needed in the neonatal period to maintain patency of the duct until palliation by aortopulmonary shunting. Oral prostaglandins have been tried over several months to gain time to allow the child and pulmonary arteries to grow. It is probably not necessary now with the advent of the modified Blalock–Taussig shunt. Shunting to both pulmonary arteries is usually indicated in this situation to promote growth of the pulmonary arteries. Reconstitution of right-sided continuity by the insertion of a valve conduit from the right ventricle to the pulmonary artery is the ultimate aim.

OBSTRUCTIVE LESIONS OF THE LEFT HEART

Aortic stenosis

Aortic stenosis constitutes 7% of congenital heart disease. There is however probably a much higher incidence of abnormality of the aortic valve in the general population. One per cent of the normal population is said to have a bicuspid aortic valve. Aortic stenosis exists at valvar, subvalvar and supravalve level, although 83% of such lesions are at valvar level. Subvalve aortic stenosis, due to a thin discrete fibrous ledge in the left ventricular outflow tract, is not as uncommon as was once thought (9%). A more extensive fibromuscular tunnel is however fortunately very rare as it is very resistant to surgical treatment. Supravalvar aortic stenosis is commonly (but not exclusively) associated with hypercalcaemia, some degree of mental retardation and the typical facies of William's syndrome. Associated lesions under these circumstances occur in the pulmonary branch arteries which are frequently the site of multiple stenoses.

Aortic stenosis may cause heart failure in infancy. Indeed there is some evidence to suggest that it may contribute to fetal loss before birth. It is associated with a severely dysplastic aortic valve, frequently unicuspid and thickened. Such infants present in gross left heart failure and despite maximal medical therapy most will die without surgical intervention. The older child very rarely presents in heart failure. Most children grow and develop normally and are asymptomatic. Referral is because of an incidently discovered murmur although occasionally, syncope, dyspnoea and even angina are present and the cause of referral to the cardiologist.

An ejection systolic murmur in the aortic area is the classic finding in the condition. The murmur is conducted to the suprasternal notch and to the carotids and frequently also down the left sternal edge. The aortic component of the second heart sound is frequently reduced and rarely reversed splitting of the second heart sound is recorded. There is an ejection click at the left sternal edge when the lesion is at valve level but this is absent in either supra- or subvalvar stenosis. The intensity of the murmur in general terms predicts the severity of stenosis and the size of the gradient. The longer and louder the murmur the more severe the stenosis. The apex is usually rather heaving in character but often is not displaced. A small volume, slow rising, peripheral pulse is common and the pulse pressure measured with the sphygmomanometer is small. Subvalve aortic stenosis is similar in many ways, although the murmur is frequently heard best down the left sternal edge and the differential diagnosis in this case is with VSD. Supravalvar aortic stenosis frequently shows a higher blood pressure in the right arm as blood flows preferentially up the right subclavian artery.

The electrocardiogram in aortic stenosis may be entirely normal even in quite severe narrowing. Left ventricular hypertrophy however based on voltage criteria is usual in severe stenosis. Left ventricular strain pattern with ST depression and T-wave inversion of the left chest leads is common in severe lesions but not invariable. It may be necessary sometimes to exercise a patient to produce such a finding. Generally the electrocardiogram is unreliable for assessing severity of aortic stenosis.

The chest X-ray may well be normal. Left ventricular and left atrial enlargement and dilatation of the aorta are seen associated with severe valvar aortic stenosis. There are no specific radiological findings for supra- or subvalvar aortic stenosis.

The echocardiogram is the method of choice for assessing the type and severity of aortic stenosis. It is able to demonstrate very accurately the level of stenosis and the presence or absence of associated aortic regurgitation. The number of leaflets in the aortic valve can be demonstrated. Doppler ultrasound using the Bernoulli equation allows the peak pressure drop across the obstruction to be determined with great reliability.

The management of aortic valve stenosis is difficult at the best of times. In view of the unreliability of the ECG the assessment of severity of aortic stenosis is probably best accomplished by frequent assessment using Doppler ultrasound to measure aortic valve gradient. As aortic stenosis in childhood after produces no symptoms, the aortic valve gradient is most frequently the reason for surgical intervention. A peak to peak systolic pressure difference measured at cardiac catheterisation of 70 mmHg has in the past been considered severe and an indication for surgical correction. More recent studies have suggested that the minimum pressure difference should now be reduced to 50 mmHg. If the aortic valve stenosis is mild, no restrictions on activity are indicated. The patient will require antibiotic prophylaxis for dental extractions and surgical procedures, as the risk of bacterial endocarditis is high. More severe stenosis liable to cause sudden death following exertion and competitive exercise is usually banned. In the past the treatment for severe aortic stenosis has always been surgical valvotomy with the mortality of 0–5% outside infancy (infant mortality may reach 30%). Recently aortic balloon valvotomy has achieved considerable vogue as a first-stage treatment for patients with severe aortic stenosis. It would appear that it is as safe as aortic valvotomy and no more likely to cause aortic regurgitation. It is not yet known whether restenosis will occur after valvotomy as may happen after surgery. Balloon valvotomy may well replace open surgical valvotomy as the first stage in the treatment of these patients. Most patients will require aortic valve replacement at some stage in the future. Subvalvar aortic stenosis if severe benefits from surgical treatment and the results in discrete fibrous lesions are very good. Abolition of the narrowing in long fibromuscular obstructions is difficult and the mortality is higher. Supravalve aortic stenosis, if severe, should be treated surgically by inserting a gusset to widen the aortic root.

Coarctation of the aorta

This accounts for 5% of all cardiac lesions and is the commonest cause of heart failure in newborn babies. There is a frequent association with other cardiac lesions. Fifty per cent of patients with coarctation have a bicuspid aortic valve. Significant aortic stenosis, VSD and arterial duct are very common.

In the older cardiological texts coarctation is divided into preductal or infantile coarctation and adult or juxta-ductal coarctation.

Juxta-ductal discreet coarctation

The juxta-ductal or localised constriction is often diaphragm like and shows an abrupt reduction in aortic size with poststenotic dilatation. Although rarer than the diffuse hypoplasia variety, it may occur in infancy with heart failure. More frequently it is an incidental finding later on in childhood which if untreated will lead in adult life to sudden aortic rupture, cerebral haemorrhage and heart failure. Collateral circulation usually develops from the subclavian artery and its branches to below the coarctation. Flow murmurs from these collaterals are easily heard over the back of the chest where there is also an ejection systolic murmur. An anteriorly placed ejection systolic murmur however in these patients suggests the presence of a bicuspid aortic valve. Isolated coarctation without aortic valve anomaly may have very little anterior murmur at all. Systemic upper limb hypertension is present with impalpable or barely palpable and delayed femoral pulses.

In mild cases the electrocardiogram is normal or has a little left ventricular hypertrophy. Marked hypertrophy and strain is seen in severe coarctation.

The chest X-ray shows varying degrees of cardiomegaly depending on the associated lesions and also the degree of stenosis. Left ventricular enlargement in the most severe cases can be quite dramatic. Rib notching appears when the arterial collaterals are large and erode into the undersurface of each rib. A visible indentation on the cardiac shadow at the site of the coarctation may also be seen.

The echocardiogram is extremely valuable in the assessment of coarctation although in older patients it is often difficult to visualise the coarctation adequately. Continuous wave Doppler from the suprasternal approach will demonstrate turbulent flow with an increased peak velocity allowing assessment of the gradient across the coarctation.

By and large surgical resection is the treatment of choice. It is not however without its problems. Long-term studies going back over 25 and 30 years have shown that systemic hypertension may persist even after successful relief of the coarctation. Total relief of the gradient does not always occur and the significance of small residual gradients is as yet unknown. In the last few years balloon angioplasty has been employed for native coarctation. Aortic aneurysm following this procedure was reported in the American literature but this appears to be related to the use of oversized balloons. The technique is extremely effective in the short run, but long-term evaluation is awaited.

Infantile type of coarctation with isthmal hypoplasia

This condition probably results from reduced aortic flow in the fetus. Several intracardiac lesions such as VSD, arterial duct and aortic stenosis are noted in association. In addition to the diffuse tubular hypoplasia of the isthmus, a localised constriction is usually seen at the site of the duct. Clinical features are protean and depend on underlying associated cardiac lesions as well as the coarctation. Hypertension in the upper limbs is often present. Femoral pulses may vary depending on the patency of the arterial duct. Heart failure is almost invariable and the patients present in the neonatal period. The electrocardiogram frequently shows right ventricular hypertrophy with diffuse ST and T wave changes. Dominant left ventricular hypertrophy is unusual at this age.

The chest X-ray shows cardiomegaly, frequently plethoric lung fields and pulmonary venous congestion. The findings here depend very largely on the associated lesions.

A complete and detailed diagnosis can be made using cross-sectional echocardiography and continuous wave Doppler.

In the past these children who were very sick at presentation deteriorated further during angiocardiography and often died at surgery with a 30–33% mortality. Nowadays most units will treat such patients with intravenous infusion of prostaglandin to open the duct. Following a period of normalisation of the acid-base anomalies the child is then sent to surgery based on echocardiographic findings alone and without the unnecessary insult of contrast medium. Surgical mortality is now under 1% for infants in most centres.

ABNORMALITIES OF CARDIAC CONNECTIONS

Hearts with univentricular connections

This heading covers a clinically disparate group of conditions, known among other things in the past as single ventricle, tricuspid atresia and mitral atresia. The common factor in all of these is that the atria drain directly or potentially into one ventricle. These hearts may be of the double-inlet type where both atrioventricular valves drain into a single ventricular cavity or the connection may be absent (right or left) coinciding with the clinical syndromes of tricuspid or mitral atresia. Any variety of ventriculo-arterial connections may be associated with these hearts including pulmonary atresia, transposition of the great arteries and persistent arterial trunk. Other common cardiac

lesions include coarctation, arterial duct and pulmonary stenosis.

Presentation and clinical features are very variable depending on the associated lesions. Most patients do present at infancy and fall roughly into two groups — those with pulmonary oligaemia who react clinically like tetralogy of Fallot, and those with pulmonary plethora and high pulmonary pressures who are in failure and have similar clinical features to large VSDs. The electrocardiogram often shows a superior or leftward axis, this being particularly common in absent right atrioventricular connection (tricuspid atresia). The chest leads however are enormously variable and may fail to show evidence of activity of more than one ventricle.

The chest X-ray varies depending on the associated lesions and whether the patient has a high pulmonary blood flow or oligaemia. Patients with heart failure and a high pulmonary blood flow will of course have enlarged hearts. The morphology and shape of the heart however is rarely diagnostic.

Echocardiogram is without doubt the way to differentiate the various types within this group. It is able to make a precise and careful diagnosis of all types and is absolutely invaluable in the investigation of such children.

Medical treatment is obviously indicated for patients in heart failure and banding will be necessary when the child persists in heart failure despite medical therapy. Aortopulmonary shunts are necessary in the oligaemic patient. There are a number of 'corrective' procedures for hearts with univentricular connections. The right atrium or the caval veins are anastomosed to the pulmonary stem directly. These seem in the short term to be very satisfactory, although what the long-term results will be is unclear.

Total anomalous pulmonary venous drainage

This represents approximately 1% of congenital heart disease. The pulmonary venous blood drains not to the left atrium but to a systemic vein either above or below the diaphragm. In the supradiaphragmatic type, a common channel forms from confluence of the pulmonary vein and drains into the right or left superior vena cava, innominate vein, coronary sinus or right atrium direct. Infradiaphragmatic drainage is usually to the portal vein via a common descending channel through the diaphragm, but may also be to the inferior vena cava. Mixed drainage may also occur.

Most cases present in the first year of life. This mode of presentation varies with the site of drainage and the degree of obstruction. The more severe the obstruction (drainage to the portal vein) the earlier the presentation and the sicker the child. Right heart failure with cyanosis in the neonatal period is usually seen with obstruction and is most likely due to drainage to the portal vein. Pulmonary hypertension is present at systemic level and the outlook is bad without urgent surgery. Anticongestive therapy helps only briefly. If obstruction is absent and there is a high flow situation, survival is possible for months or even longer with mild cyanosis, failure to thrive, signs of a large left to right atrial shunt and variable evidence of pulmonary hypertension. Auscultatory findings are then those of right ventricular volume overload with pulmonary systolic ejection and tricuspid diastolic flow murmur.

ECG shows right ventricular and right atrial enlargement, with often very little left ventricular activity and a small heart.

Chest X-ray in obstructed cases shows intense reticular mottling of the lung fields due to pulmonary venous congestion. Non-obstructive cases show pulmonary plethora, with enlargement of the right ventricle and right atrium. The anomalous ascending vein is large and dilated, and combined with a dilated innominate vein gives rise to the classic snowman appearance, a feature seen infrequently in infancy.

The echocardiogram is the best way to make the diagnosis. Right ventricular enlargement, right atrial enlargement and signs of pulmonary hypertension associated with a small left atrium and left ventricle are seen. Cross-sectional echocardiography allows recognition of the posterior confluence of the pulmonary vein and usually demonstrates the site of drainage. Cardiac catheterisation is now rarely indicated and only performed when the echocardiogram is difficult.

Surgical correction is indicated in every case to anastomose the confluence of the pulmonary veins to left atrium. The surgical mortality in infancy and in obstructed cases is high, certainly over 25% and frequently up to 50%.

TRANSPOSITION OF THE GREAT ARTERIES

By definition transposition of the great arteries exists when the aorta arises from the morphological right ventricle and the pulmonary artery from the morphological left. The spatial relationship between the aorta and the pulmonary artery, while of importance to the surgeon, is not crucial to the diagnosis. Transposition constitutes 7% of all cases of congenital heart disease; 20% of cases have an associated VSD and 5% have a VSD with pulmonary stenosis, either valvar or subvalvar. Transposition haemodynamics are found not infrequently in hearts with double outlet of the right ventricle or univentricular connections.

Presentation is usually in the first few days of life with severe cyanosis and sometimes heart failure. In the presence of a VSD cyanosis is less marked and the presentation may be delayed for several weeks or more. The differential diagnosis in the neonatal period is from lung disease or persistent fetal circulation.

Transposition usually presents in large mature full-term infants. They are usually deeply cyanosed with loud and often apparently single heart sounds and no murmurs. Children with VSDs or ducts do develop murmurs as the pulmonary artery pressure and resistance fall during the neonatal period. The children with pulmonary stenosis have systolic murmurs in the pulmonary area.

The ECG shows marked right ventricular hypertrophy with right axis deviation. Left ventricular activity is increased only in the presence of a duct or a VSD.

Chest X-ray shows prominence of the right ventricle and right atrium. If the great arteries lie one behind the other then a narrow upper mediastinal shadow gives the classic 'egg on its side appearance'. Although this is classical it is not necessarily typical. The lung fields vary in appearance according to whether there is a duct or a VSD present.

Cross-sectional echocardiography along with Doppler makes the diagnosis easily in the neonatal period by demonstrating which great artery is attached to each ventricle. Cardiac ultrasound will also demonstrate the presence and importance of VSDs, ASDs, ducts and valve stenosis. Cross-sectional echocardiography allied with continuous wave Doppler provides an ideal way of assessing the effect of interventions in children with transposition and continuing long-term follow-up of the various procedures.

Transposition requires urgent treatment in the first days of life. In the absence of a major cardiac defect effective pulmonary blood flow is minimal and the condition is incompatible with life for more than a few hours or days. Cardiac catheterisation is performed as soon as the diagnosis is suspected as delay will lead to increasing hypoxaemia, acidaemia and death. At catheterisation balloon atrial septostomy is performed by passing a catheter with a deflated balloon across the foramen ovale to the left atrium. After inflation the balloon is pulled back to rupture the flap of the foramen ovale. An ASD is thus created which has bidirectional shunting allowing significant improvement in most cases in effective pulmonary blood flow and the survival of the child in reasonable health for periods of up to and even over a year. Definitive correction during the first year of life is usually by atrial rerouting operation. Mustard's procedure has been the procedure of choice but it has been superceded by the Senning procedure which appears to have few postoperative problems in the long term. In both procedures the blood returning through the caval veins is redirected by a baffle to the mitral valve and thence to the pulmonary artery. The pulmonary venous blood flows over and round this baffle to the tricuspid valve and thence to the aorta.

As the mortality from balloon atrial septostomy is minimal and the mortality in the first few months of life from the Senning procedure is between 1% and 2%, the outlook for simple transposition of the great arteries is good. Doubt remains however about the ability of the right ventricle to fulfil its systemic role in the long term. Over the last decade so-called 'anatomical correction' has achieved acceptance. The pulmonary artery and aorta are reconnected to the appropriate ventricles during the neonatal period. This procedure has to be done early before the left ventricle involutes and loses its muscle mass as pulmonary artery pressure and resistance fall. The coronary arteries are reimplanted. Again the long-term results are uncertain. Certainly anatomical correction should be the method of choice in transposition of the great arteries and VSD. Whether left ventricular function will be adequate and coronary artery flow normal remains to be seen.

Transposition of the great arteries, VSD and pulmonary stenosis constitute a rather different surgical problem. Many of these children require shunting in infancy. In later childhood correction is by the Rastelli procedure. An angled patch is placed from the left ventricle through the VSD to the aortic root. The pulmonary valve and artery are closed and a valve conduit inserted from the right ventricle to the pulmonary artery.

ARRHYTHMIAS AND CONDUCTION DEFECTS IN CHILDHOOD

Incidence and aetiology

Clinically significant arrhythmias are much less common in paediatric cardiology than in adult medicine. However, ambulatory tape monitoring has shown that unsuspected ectopic rhythms such as ventricular or atrial ectopics, or transient bradycardias or tachycardias, are remarkably common in the normal infant and young child. The correlation between these disturbances and sudden infant cot death is as yet unconfirmed.

Association of arrhythmias with major forms of congenital heart disease is fortunately rare.

LESIONS ASSOCIATED WITH RHYTHM AND CONDUCTION ABNORMALITIES

1. Ebstein's anomaly of the tricuspid valve — Woolf–Parkinson–White syndrome and paroxysmal atrial tachycardia.

2. Congenitally corrected transposition of the great arteries — atrioventricular block, paroxysmal atrial tachycardia, atrial fibrillation or flutter.

3. Dilated cardiomyopathy and hypertrophic obstructive cardiomyopathy — supraventricular tachycardia, atrioventricular block.

Investigation of arrhythmias in childhood involves the use of 24-hour ambulatory tape monitoring, excercise testing when arrhythmias are precipitated by exertion and sometimes invasive intracardiac electrography.

PAROXYSMAL SUPRAVENTRICULAR TACHYCARDIA

This is the commonest form of arrhythmia in childhood, and presents as a rapid regular tachycardia between 150 and 300 beats per minute, depending on age. The condition shows characteristically intermittent attacks which start and stop suddenly, and last from a few beats to several days. Prolonged attacks lead to cadiac failure. There is frequent association with an abnormal conduction pathway across the atrioventricular junction, as in Woolf–Parkinson–White syndrome. Between attacks in this condition the ECG is characterised by short PR interval (less than 0.12 of a second) with slurring of the up-stoke of the R wave.

Infants under 1 year developing paroxysmal atrial tachycardia may present as failure to thrive, colic or respiratory distress. However even at very fast rates, short attacks leave the baby relatively untroubled. Listlessness and irritability accompany attacks of longer duration and heart failure may ensue with hepatomegaly, cardiac enlargement on X-ray and even pulmonary oedema. Precipitating factors may include respiratory and other infections. Identification of paroxysmal tachycardia during an attack is made by recognising the characteristic electrocardiogram with a rate of 180–300 per minute without variation in PR interval and absent P waves.

Prognosis is generally good. Some remit spontaneously during early childhood but some persist into adolescence. Woolf–Parkinson–White anomaly usually means a persistent tendency throughout life. In infancy supraventricular tachycardia is very effectively terminated by immersing the infant's head in iced water and producing a vagal effect. If this is unsuccessful DC shock may be used.

Digoxin is still the drug of choice and in most cases is a satisfactory means of controlling paroxysmal tachycardia. A few cases are resistant and disopyramide, adenosine, verapamil, or amiodarone may be used. Flecainide which was initially introduced for ventricular arrhythmias does appear also to be efficacious in resistant cases.

OTHER ARRHYTHMIAS IN CHILDHOOD

Atrial fibrillation and atrial flutter are rarely seen, except in association with cardiomyopathy or after surgery. Ventricular premature beats are common in normal children, but ventricular tachycardias are virtually unknown except with cardiomyopathy after surgery.

Atrioventricular block

Prolongation of the time taken for the depolarising impulse to travel from the sino-atrial node into the ventricular mass via the bundle of His is due to atrioventricular block. First-degree block is found in otherwise normal children, with ASD, and in Ebstein's anomaly. It is also associated with myocarditis or digoxin therapy. The PR interval is longer than the expected value for the patient's age and heart rate. Second-and third-degree block are frequently associated with congenital heart disease and myocarditis. In second degree, occasional P waves are not conducted to the ventricles, sometimes as a random phenomenon or as part of the Wenckeback phenomenon where the PR interval lengthens progressively until a complete QRS is dropped.

Third degree or complete heart block is almost always congenital in origin, except after surgical correction, particularly for tetralogy of Fallot. The diagnosis may be made prenatally. Many children are asymptomatic. Heart rate under 1 year of age may be as high as 60–70 beats per minute, but thereafter slows to rates of under 40 per minute as the child nears adult life. It is not as benign a condition as was previously thought. Patients are either asymptomatic and lead normal lives or require pacemaker insertion because of Stokes–Adams attack and syncope. Improved pacemaker design now allows patients who are asymptomatic in early childhood to be treated satisfactorily. Insertion of such units in the neonatal period, while rare, is not unknown and can be carried out successfully. There is little place for medical therapy.

Benign systolic murmurs

The majority of murmurs referred by the GP, paediatrician or school health doctor will be benign systolic murmurs. Reliable identification of a murmur as benign can be difficult as there is no characteristic auscultatory feature. Most are quiet, although venous hums in the upper chest and back can be quite loud. These hums result from flow of blood through the great veins of the neck and alter with neck movement; they will usually disappear when the child is examined lying flat.

Although benign murmurs are usually quiet, short and soft, such murmurs may also be found in congenital heart disease.

To make the diagnosis of a benign systolic murmur, the following features should be present:

1. The child must be free of cardiac symptoms.
2. A normal single first heart sound must be heard with a normal physiological splitting of the second heart sound.
3. No added clicks or diastolic murmurs are heard.
4. The murmur usually becomes loudest in the supine position and decreases in intensity when assuming the upright posture.
5. Cardiac rhythm and blood pressure must be normal
6. The ECG, chest X-ray and echocardiogram should all be within normal limits.

CARDIAC FAILURE IN INFANCY

This may be a surprisingly difficult diagnosis to make. Dyspnoea, respiratory distress, hepatomegaly, oedema, tachycardia and cardiomegaly are all important signs. Apart from the last, all these findings may result from non-cardiac illnesses.

1. Dyspnoea. This results in slowness or inability to feed in the neonate, and it frequently occurs with other problems, e.g. upper respiratory tract infection, simple nasal obstruction, pneumonia or bronchiolitis. Other features include laboured respiration and use of accessory respiratory muscles, including flaring of the alae nasi, increased anteroposterior chest diameter, the 'blown chest', which also occurs in both cardiac and severe respiratory diseases.

2. Hepatomegaly. A sensitive indicator of severity of heart failure, but it may also be the result of metabolic disorders or intrinsic liver disease. Overinflation of the lungs with bronchiolitis may result in the liver being pushed down so that it is easily palpable. Percussion of the upper edge of the liver will differentiate this from true hepatomegaly.

3. Peripheral oedema. Oedema is commonly seen in renal disease and it may be confused with lymphoedema, as in Turner's syndrome.

4. Tachycardia. This is also associated with infection or metabolic imbalance.

5. Cardiomegaly on chest X-ray. Clinical assessment of cardiomegaly can be difficult in infancy. The chest X-ray is more reliable and echocardiography can diagnose cardiac chamber enlargement. Thus the diagnosis of heart failure should not be made in the absence of radiological cardiomegaly.

In the older child the signs are those of tachycardia, dyspnoea, hepatomegaly, raised jugular venous pressure and peripheral oedema, as in the adult. Again a large heart is seen on chest X-ray.

BACTERIAL ENDOCARDITIS

Incidence and aetiology

A chronic disease which is rarely found before the age of three. Low-grade intermittent fever, rigors, anaemia, petechiae, splinter haemorrhages under the nails and generalised wasting with splenomegaly are common findings. Sudden acute haemodynamic abnormalities follow bacterial destruction of semilunar or atrioventricular valves. Vegetations are usually found on congenitally abnormal structures or following rheumatic damage. Persistent ductus arteriosus, VSD, coarctation of the aorta and aortic stenosis are lesions most commonly affected. ASDs and pulmonary stenosis are less frequently involved.

The infecting organism varies according to age.

The most common organism in childhood is still the alpha-haemolytic streptococcus following dental extraction. After cardiac surgery, staphylococcus is the most common organism.

Dental extractions, scaling and other forms of surgery should be covered in known cases of congenital heart disease by an appropriate antibiotic. Penicillin is the drug of choice for dental work or ear, nose and throat operations, but erythromycin is the alternative when there is penicillin allergy. Following cardiac surgery staphylococcal infection is well prevented by flucloxacillin. Therapy in proven blood culture-positive bacterial endocarditis should be for a minimum of 1 month, initially given intravenously until the temperature is normal. The assessment of efficacy of treatment is by clinical evaluation, temperature recording and back titration against the organism.

Regimen for guidance of dentists and family doctors

1. Standard regimen for dental surgery under local anaesthesia: 3 g amoxicillin orally as a single dose 1 hour before the procedure.
2. Standard regimen for patients allergic to penicillin or who have received penicillin in the previous month: 300 mg clindomycin orally one hour before the procedure plus 300 mg clindomycin orally two hours afterwards.
3. Dental surgery under general anaesthesia: 1 g amoxycillin i.m. (dissolved in 2.5 ml 1% lignocaine) before induction plus one dose of 500 mg orally 6 hours later. (Under 10 years, give half adult dose.)

* Under 10 years, give half adult dose; under 5 years give quarter of adult dose.

RHEUMATIC FEVER

The incidence of this disease has drastically declined in the western world and it is now rare in the UK. Aetiologically there is a relationship to previous infection with group A streptococcus. There is probably a cross-reaction with heart muscle when heart antigens resemble those of the streptococcus, causing an autoimmune reaction.

Clinical findings and presentation

It is rare before 3 years, but more common between 5 and 15 years of age; a preceding streptococcal infection (usually sore throat) is almost invariable. There is general malaise with insidious onset and joint pain affecting the large joints and flitting from joint to joint. Pallor, sweating and pyrexia are usual. Rashes of the erythema marginetum or nodosum type are found, and a small percentage will have rheumatic nodules on the extensor surfaces of the upper limbs.

The sedimentation rate is raised, a leucocytosis is present and the antistreptolysin O titre is high and rises as the disease process continues. C-reactive protein in the patient's serum indicates ongoing rheumatic activity.

RHEUMATIC CARDITIS

Occurs in approximately 15% of cases and is indicated by the following findings:

1. Development of cardiac murmurs, systolic or diastolic, and indicative of cardiac dilatation and mitral incompetence.
2. Pericardial friction rub.
3. Increasing cardiac size on chest X-ray.
4. Frank cardiac failure with peripheral oedema and other standard signs.

Treatment

1. Penicillin to eradicate any residual streptococcal infection.
2. Bed rest but not total immobility.
3. Salicylates in large doses for the arthritic symptoms.

If carditis is considered to be present, then digoxin and diuretics are prescribed when cardiac failure is recognised. Evidence has been put forward for treating a patient with carditis with corticosteroids. This evidence is not firm, although it is believed that the recovery rate is significant if cardiac involvement is improved.

Prognosis

Recovery of joints is complete and the major risks

for these patients are:

1. Further relapses (either of rheumatic fever or Sydenham's chorea, which is commoner in girls). Prophylactic penicillin should therefore be continued orally indefinitely.

2. Development of a chronic rheumatic valve disease. The mitral valve is affected three times more commonly than the aortic valve, and thus any patient with proven rheumatic fever merits long-term follow-up after recovery.

18. Allergic and other immunological disorders

J. O. Warner

Descriptions of allergic disorders appeared in many ancient texts, but it was not until 1906 that von Pirquet introduced the term allergy. However Lucretius (94–55 BC) observed that, 'one man's meat is another man's poison' which must be the most concise definition of allergy. The twentieth century can add that the reaction is immunologically mediated.

The terms allergy and hypersensitivity can be used interchangeably. Atopy is used to describe several associated disorders such as asthma, eczema, allergic rhinitis, acute urticaria and anaphylaxis, all of which are familial though the pattern of inheritance is somewhat unclear. Family studies of IgE responses to common inhaled antigens have suggested a dominant inheritance of atopy. Molecular genetic linkage analysis in a small number of families has suggested that the gene locus rests on chromosome 11.

PRINCIPLES OF ALLERGY AND IMMUNITY

The allergic state depends on prior exposure to substances known as antigens ar allergens, with an altered reactivity on subsequent exposure. The management of allergic disease in the past has therefore focused on identifying the offending agent so that either avoidance or attempts at induction of tolerance (immunotherapy) could be used. Recent immunological investigation has given clinical allergy a firmer scientific basis which has led to progress in the understanding of allergic disease and in the development of new therapeutic modalities.

The types of allergic reaction have been divided into four categories:

Type 1: immediate hypersensitivity or anaphylactic reaction. The reaction occurs within minutes of exposure to the allergen which combines with reaginic antibody (immunoglobulin E), fixed to receptors on the surface of Mast cells and basophils, resulting in the release of vasoactive amines such as histamine, prostaglandins and leukotrienes. Examples of this reaction include urticaria due to food allergy and seasonal pollen-induced rhinitis.

Type 2: cytotoxic reaction. A reaction of varying rapidity of onset, where antibody is directed towards a cell component or an antigen fixed to cells, with damage resulting from an interaction of complement and mononuclear cells resulting in cell lysis or phagocytosis. An example would be Rhesus haemolytic disease in the newborn.

Type 3: Arthus or antigen–antibody complex reaction. A reaction which develops over a few hours and is produced by soluble complexes which are a combination of antibody, antigen in excess and activated complement. Neutrophil polymorphs are also involved in the reaction. Examples of the reaction are extrinsic allergic alveolitis and serum sickness.

Type 4: delayed or cell-mediated reaction. A reaction taking at least 24 hours to develop and mediated by sensitized thymus dependent lymphocytes (T cells) which in contact with antigen release lymphokines. This results in an inflammatory reaction with cellular infiltration by lymphocytes and macrophages. Examples include contact dermatitis and a positive tuberculin reaction.

While these four subdivisions of hypersensitivity aid understanding of secondary immune response they are not mutually exclusive but an integrated and interrelating sequence of events. Furthermore it is now clear that the reactions are more complex, involving communication between various cell types by means of a range of peptide regulatory factors sometimes known as cytokines, lymphokines or interleukins. There is a far wider range of cells which possess immunoglobulin E receptors and thus the type 1 hypersensitivity response leads to activation of additional cells including eosinophils and macrophages, the former of which contain high concentrations of platelet activating factor, a mediator which is currently considered to be of importance in asthma.

Antigen handling   (Fig. 18.1)

The mechanical barrier offered by the skin and mucous membranes provides the first line of defence against antigen penetration. Mucociliary clearance mechanisms are important in the respiratory tract. Lysozymes in tears, saliva, sweat and mucus are bacteriocidal, while iron-binding proteins such as lactoferrin in breast milk are bacteriostatic by depriving bacteria of the essential substrate, iron. Once antigen has penetrated into the tissues a complex co-operation system involving T cells, complement and antigen presenting cells (APC) such as macrophages, dendritic cells and Langerhans cells results in phagocytosis of the antigen. The APC migrates to the site of antigenic penetration, a process known as chemotaxis, and is then presented with the antigen in a phagocytosable form by a process known as opsonisation. This latter process is considered to be a function of the alternative pathway of complement. In the case of micro-organisms these are then killed by various intracellular lysozymes. The antigen is then re-expressed on the surface of the APC and in association with major histocompatability complex molecules is recognised by helper and cytotoxic T lymphocytes. The interactions between these cells are mediated by a range of peptide regulatory factors. These factors are responsible for the rapid differentiation and increase in numbers of antigen-specific lymphocytes. Thus interleukin 1 (I1) is produced by APC's and causes proliferation of T helper cells. I2 is produced by T cells and induces T lymphoctye cytotoxicity as well as stimulating natural killer

cell activity. I4 is a stimulator of B-cell proliferation while I5 is a potent stimulator for growth and differentiation of eosinophils. I6 has an enormously wide range of activity with receptors distributed on a range of cell types including B lymphocytes, fibroblasts, hepatocytes, T lymphocytes and haemopoetic progenitor cells. I7 appears to be important as a developmental factor for both B and T lymphocytes and I3 may have a similar role while also affecting haemopoetic progenitor cells. The interferons (IFN) are another group of peptides with three main types labelled alpha, beta and gamma. IFN gamma has the widest range activity and is produced during an immune response by antigen-specific T-cells and by natural killer cells which have been recruited by I2. It activates macrophages to enhance phagocytosis and has activating and growth enhancing effects on cytolytic T cells and natural killer cells. It also regulates the humeral immune response by inducing immunoglobulin secretion.

The bursa-derived lymphocytes (B-cells) are induced to transform to plasma cells by I6 and IFN gamma. The plasma cells then produce specific antibodies against the antigen. Antibody production is modulated by subsets of T cells designated helper cells which trigger and suppressor cells which suppress responses. Each reste of plasma cells produces only one antibody type of the five classes of immunoglobulin.

Immunoglobulins

Immunoglobulin G (IgG) is the major class of immunoglobulin in normal serum which, because it is of relatively low molecular weight, is also present in interstitial fluids such as breast milk and is transferred across the placenta. It is the predominant antibody produced in response to secondary antigenic challenge. There are four subtypes labelled IgG 1–4. IgG_4 whilst being only 4% of the total adult IgG, has received particular attention in relation to allergy, with speculation that under some circumstances it might have an anaphylactic effect like IgE. However this has never been satisfactorily established. It is an interesting antibody in being unable to activate complement, unlike IgG_1 and IgG_3 and to a lesser extent IgG_2. Anti-

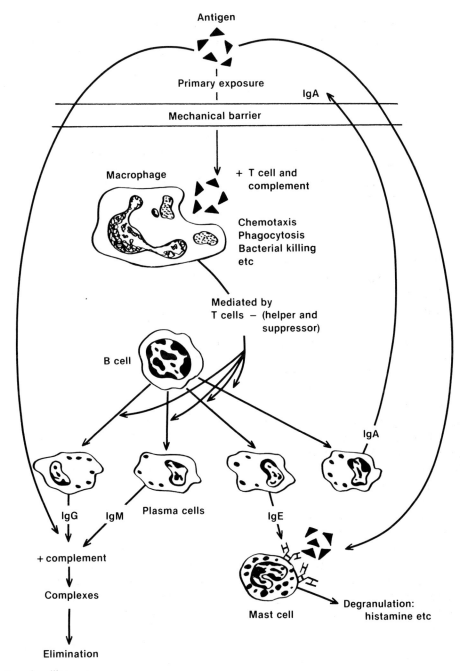

Fig. 18.1 Antigen handling.

bodies to diphtheria and tetanus toxoid are predominantly IgG_1 while antibodies to polysaccharide are predominantly IgG_2.

Immunoglobulin A (IgA) is the second most abundant antibody in the serum. It is the main antibody of secretions. It is found in significant amounts in tracheobronchial, gastrointestinal and genitourinary secretions. Thus it is particularly important in reducing the amount of free antigen absorbed through epithelial surfaces. There are two subtypes labelled IgA_1 and IgA_2.

Immunoglobulin M consists of a large molecule which is virtually restricted to the intravascular space and is synthesised largely during the primary immune response. This accounts for the need to detect IgM-specific antibodies in the diagnosis of congenital infection.

IgE is present only in trace amounts in normal serum but rises during parasitic infestation. It binds to Mast cells and basophils; and when two bound IgE molecules are linked by antigen, Mast cells degranulate releasing vasoactive amines which mediate the type 1 hypersensitivity response.

IgD exists in low concentrations in normal serum but its physiological role unclear. It may act as a B-cell antigen modulating the humoral response.

The complement system

The complement system consists of several components which when activated undergo a series of reactions, similar to the coagulation cascade, which produce cell lysis, increased vascular permeability and enhance chemotaxis and phagocytosis. Two pathways of activation are recognised: the classical which is activated by IgG and IgM when aggregated to antigen and follows a sequence involving complement components 1, 4, 2, 3, 5, 6, 7, 8, 9 sequentially, and the alternative, which is activated by surfaces of bacteria and cells expressing surface viral antigens and bypasses the early components by activating C3 directly.

Whilst type 1 hypersensitivity is not mediated by the complement system, activation products of this system may mimic the effects of anaphylaxis (such as C3A and C5A). This may be the basis for some drug-induced reactions such as those to radio-contrast materials.

IMMUNODEFICIENCY

Gross forms of immunodeficiency leading to excess infection are rare and usually obvious. Subtle and mild defects are however more common and may lead to the development of atopy which occurs in at least 15–20% of the population. Such subtle de-

fects may also predispose to the later development of autoimmune disease and lymphoreticular malignancy. Transient defects also occur. These may be due to delayed maturation in infancy or secondary phenomena such as malnutrition, some virus infections, malignant disease and drugs such as steroids. Secondary defects are much more common than primary defects. Whilst HIV infection has captured the headlines it is a relatively uncommon cause of secondary immunodeficiency by comparison with such infections as measles.

Diagnosis

A thorough history is important in the clinical assessment of a patient with a possible defect in immune function. Details of the family history and perinatal problems are important. Congenital virus infection can produce immunodeficiency; prematurity results in less maternal IgG transfer and therefore transient hypogammaglobulinaemia. Small-for-dates babies are more susceptible to infection, partly because of intrauterine undernutrition.

Most patients even with severe immunodeficiency disorders remain well for the first few months of life because of maternally derived protection. However children with DiGeorge's syndrome often have associated major congenital heart disease and neonatal hypocalcaemia which should indicate the diagnosis. Family history may highlight some of the X-linked disorders; other types of immunodeficiency are associated with a greater likelihood of relatives having autoimmune disease, lymphoreticular malignancy or atopy.

Physical examination may reveal signs of damage due to past recurrent infections, such as bronchiectasis. Failure to thrive is a common feature in immunodeficient children and therefore accurate records of weight and height plotted on standard charts will be valuable. Infants with severe immunodeficiency sometimes lack palpable lymph nodes and the tonsils may be small or absent. Characteristic defects may be seen in children with special syndromes such as ataxia telangiectasia.

A careful microbiological and viral screen is necessary as the various disorders sometimes predispose to particular infections. A lateral radiograph of the upper airway reveals the presence or absence of adenoidal tissue, whilst a chest radiograph in infancy will show a thymus and may reveal the presence or sequelae of recurrent respiratory tract infections. Specific tests of immunity include a full blood count emphasising the differential count and film, measurement of immunoglobulin concentrations and tests for the presence of specific antibodies such as isohaemagglutinin (IgM antibody), antistreptolysin 0 titre (IgG antibody) and antibodies which should have been produced by previous immunisations. Lymphocytes T- and B-cell numbers can be estimated. Skin tests using candida, trichophyton or tuberculin antigens should show the presence of a normal delayed hypersensitivity (type 4) response. Various components of the complement cascade can also be measured. The ability of the patient's serum to opsonise yeast particles for phagocytosis by polymorphs obtained from a healthy subject can also be tested. Various aspects of phagocytic function including chemotaxis, organism killing, and nitroblue tetrazolium (NBT) reduction, defective in chronic granulomatous disease, will also be indicated in certain situations. The atopic subjects can be distinguished by prick skin testing using a range of common inhalant and ingestant allergens. Table 18.1 reveals a select list of immunodeficiency disorders with their associated features.

TREATMENT OF IMMUNODEFICIENCY

Avoidance of pathogens and vigorous treatment of established infection forms the basis of much of the management of these disorders. The range of specific therapies available for primary immunodeficiency disorders is limited though its use is becoming more common. Replacement of non-antigenic specific factors by fresh blood or plasma transfusion, such as in the opsonisation defect, can sometimes be of benefit. Specific immunoglobulin replacement now preferably administered intravenously produces dramatic improvements in hypogammaglobulinaemias. Bone marrow transplantation is being increasingly used for cellular and combined immunodeficiencies.

An understanding of the peptide factors which influence immune response may well lead to a

Table 18.1 Immunodeficiency disorders

Group	Disease	Associated features and complications
Humoral defects	Panhypogammaglobulinaemia (X-linked or recessive)	Pyogenic infection: polyarthritis
	Selective IgA deficiency (1:700 population)	Asymptomatic: pyogenic infection: atopy
Predominantly cell-mediated defects	DiGeorge's syndrome	Thymic hypoplasia & absent parathyroids Hypocalcaemia; cardiovascular defects; FTT candidiasis
	Mucocutaneous candidiasis	Sometimes iron deficient: *Candida* infection
Combined defects	Severe combined immunodeficiency	Diarrhoea; FTT Infections: pyogenic; fungal; pneumocystis
	Reticular dysgenesis	Fatal in early infancy
Special syndromes	Ataxia-telangiectasia (recessive)	Low IgE and IgA Ataxia; dementia; telangiectases
	Wiskott–Aldrich syndrome (X-linked)	Combined immunodeficiency Eczema; thombocytopenia; infection
Phagocyte defects	Chronic granulomatous disease (X-linked)	Pyogenic infection; abscesses & fistulae
	Shwachmans syndrome	Pancreatic insufficiency; FTT; steatorrhoea; neutropenia; infection; short stature
Complement defects	Familial angio-oedema (dominant)	Cl-esterase inhibitor deficiency; recurrent angio-oedema
	Opsonisation defect (1:20 population)	Asymptomatic; FTT; pyogenic infection; dermatitis, atopy

range of new therapeutic options in the near future. At present only relatively non-specific immune stimulant medications have been employed. Levamisole has for instance been used with some success in patients with neutrophil chemotactic defects. Immunodeficiency patients are susceptible to infection by attenuated micro-organisms, such as those used for some immunisations and these will, therefore, be contraindicated in some of the disorders.

ATOPY

Atopy is probably the commonest manifestation of immunodeficiency. Allergic diseases affect between 15% and 20% of the child population and cause a third of all school absences due to chronic disease. A number of primary immunological defects are associated with an increased prevalence of atopy. For instance eczema is a feature of Wiskott–Aldrich syndrome and has been described in patients with X-linked hypogammaglobulinaemia. It has been noted with increased frequency in immunoglobulin A deficiency and occurs more frequently in patients with the opsonization defect and also in patients with a deficiency of C2 (second component of complement). IgG_2 subclass deficiency has been linked with severe childhood asthma. Furthermore a relative deficiency of suppressor T cells in neonates is associated with a subsequent higher incidence of eczema and allergic rhinitis. Children with cystic fibrosis have a higher prevelance of atopy and there is some suggestion that their parents might also do so.

A simple Mendelian dominant pattern of inheritance may conceivably explain the presence of atopy which has a high concordance in identical twins. However it does not explain the expression of atopy. Concordance for asthma in identical twins is between 20% and 50%. Thus subtle environmental influences must play an important role.

Much attention has focused on antigen load, particularly during susceptible periods in early infancy when maturational defects of immune response may be present. Studies have suggested that breast feeding and modification of subsequent infant feeding practices may either delay or even prevent the development of eczema (atopic dermatitis) though not asthma. Dietary manipulations during pregnancy are of no value but there may be some benefit in recommending restriction of highly allergenic foods from the mother during lactation and in delaying the introduction of those allergenic foods once the infant is weaned.

Much less information is available on the influence of early exposure to aeroallergens and the subsequent development of either allergic rhinitis or asthma. Month of birth studies would suggest that high aeroallergenic exposure in infancy, particularly to tree pollens and house dust mites, is important. Similar associations have been made in relation to exposure to cat and dog dander in early infancy and the subsequent development of cat or dog allergy.

There may be other environmental influences which affect the generation of allergic responses. Cigarette smoking may be particularly important in enhancing IgE responses, as has been demonstrated in both animals and humans. Gastrointestinal infection is associated with a subsequent development of cow's milk protein intolerance and it is possible that respiratory infections might have a similar effect. It remains to be seen whether other forms of environmental air pollution have any more than an enhancing effect on already existing respiratory disease though in animal models ozone appears to increase allergic sensitization.

So far the only attempt at prevention of atopy has focused an dietary manipulations and the development of eczema with variable success. A consensus of studies would suggest that such attempts are more likely to delay the onset of the disease rather than prevent it completely. It remains to be seen whether the same will be true of primary aeroallergen avoidance regimens.

Established atopic disease

Atopy may cause a wide spectrum of complaints including diarrhoea, vomiting, failure to thrive, urticaria, angioedema, eczema, allergic rhinitis, conjunctivitis and asthma. A wide variety of substances are known to cause reactions (Table 18.2). The type of allergy, its clinical manifestations and the allergens involved can occur in any combination making classification by allergy or disease alone confusing.

Table 18.2 Classification of allergens

Inhalants

House dust mite	*Dermatophagoides pteronyssinus*
Grass pollens	Timothy, cocksfoot etc
Tree pollens	Silver birch, plane etc
Animal danders	Cat, dog, feathers etc
Mould spores	Cladosporium, Aspergillus etc

Ingestants

Cow's milk	B lactoglobulin etc
Egg	Albumen
Fish	
Nuts	Tartrazine etc
Food colouring	

Contactants

Antibiotic creams
Rubber
Dyes

Injectants

Drugs
Antisera
Immunisations

Physical agents

Temperature
Humidity

Urticaria, angioedema and anaphylaxis all of which occur within minutes of exposure, are classical and obvious allergic disorders. Asthma, rhinitis and eczema are all recognised to be associated with and sometimes caused by allergy though sometimes timing between exposure and reaction may be more prolonged. Diarrhoea, vomiting, failure to thrive and abdominal colic are sometimes associated with food allergies though there may be many other causes. Associations between allergy and behaviour disturbances, migraine, epilepsy and various forms of arthritis remain highly contentious. It remains to be established whether these conditions are ever really caused by or are only sometimes associated with allergy. Unfortunately, all too frequently these days patients are diagnosed as having allergies without any supporting evidence, which often results in totally misplaced treatment. Thus there have been reports of frankly malnourished infants on unsupervised and unnecessary allergen avoidance diets.

Diagnosis

An accurate diagnosis of allergy must always precede any therapeutic recommendations, and clinical history with examination take precedence. The general history should be supplemented by eliciting details of possible allergenic exposure and timing in relation to the development of symptoms. Such features as infant feeding and timing of weaning may provide useful background information in relation to the onset of eczema. Specific questions on known allergen exposure such as to pets should always be asked and the association of symptoms with physical agents such as temperature, humidity, tobacco smoke, sprays and other fumes should be sought. The type of housing may influence concentration of allergens. Age of property, proximity to waterways, type of central heating, carpeting, furniture and bedding may have profound effects on the level of house dust mites. Specific dietary likes and dislikes may relate to particular food allergies. In considering the environment of the child it should be remembered that he or she will spend an appreciable time during the day at school or out of doors. Timing of symptoms in relation to such locations will be important. Reactions to drugs and immunisations may be relevant.

In eliciting information about specific disorders it should be remembered that there is a great deal of confusion among parents about such terms as dermatitis or eczema; catarrh, chronic sinusitis and rhinitis; bronchitis, chest infection and asthma.

The physical examination should be thorough. A particular note should be made of the child's facies. The allergic patient may have discolouration and swelling of the eyelids, a transverse nasal crease due to the nose being constantly rubbed up and down and evidence of mouth breathing due to rhinitis obstructing the nasal airways. The nasal mucosa can be easily examined using an auriscope and the pale swollen turbinates associated with allergic rhinitis seen. Serous otitis media with a conductive deafness is quite frequently associated with allergic rhinitis. Red runny eyes with blepharitis and a cobble-stoned conjunctiva indicate allergic conjunctivitis. Bowed sternum, spinal kyphosis and Harrison's sulci may all be signs of chronic asthma. Skin should be carefully examined, particularly in flexures and on the scalp. Hypopigmentation may indicate areas of previous skin disease.

Investigation

The presence of the atopic status can be confirmed by finding a raised blood eosinophil count, an increase of total serum IgE and positive allergy skin tests. Prick skin tests are preferred to any other technique. The skin is punctured and lifted slightly using a No 23 gauge needle held at 45° through a drop of allergen extract placed on the skin surface (usually volar surface of forearm or the back in small infants). The range of allergens used will depend on the problem but as a simple screen one might include a negative control of phenol saline and a positive control of 1% histamine, and house dust mite, cat fur and grass pollen which will give a positive yield in 85% of the atopic population. The reaction is assessed after 15 minutes and the diameter of weals recorded in millimetres. A weal of 2 mm or greater may be considered positive. It is valuable to re-examine the site of the skin test 3 to 4 hours later to see whether a late reaction with erythema and induration has developed. The latter is associated with a greater degree of allergy. Serum IgE antibody measurements can be made using the radio allergosorbent test (RAST). There are now other IgE antibody measuring tests, some of which can provide a result to a whole panel of allergens such as the chemiluminescent assay–multiple allergosorbent test (CLA–MAST).

The relative value of any allergy test as an adjunct to clinical history and examination depends on the clinical situation. In general with good allergen extracts simple prick skin testing is likely to be required to confirm the presence of a specific allergy. Rarely is it necessary to proceed to IgE antibody testing though this might be required when drastic allergen avoidance measures or immunotherapy is being recommended. Food intolerance is not easily either confirmed or excluded by any simple form of allergy testing. It is likely that much food intolerance is due to immunological mechanisms other than those mediated by IgE. Circulating immune complexes and complement consumption have sometimes been demonstrated during food-induced reactions which might aid diagnosis. Where gastrointestinal symptoms predominate small intestinal biopsy may sometimes show partial villus atrophy or cellular infiltration of the lamina propria. Where there is no objective test, double-blind challenge testing is required and even these are open to misinterpretation as other coincident events may be instrumental in causing a reaction. This has led to some authorities suggesting that a minimum of three challenges must be performed, particularly when food is involved.

ASTHMA

Asthma is the commonest chronic disease of childhood. It is eminently treatable in virtually all cases and yet remains commonly underdiagnosed and undertreated. Studies in schoolchildren have shown that less than half of those who have had recurrent wheezing in the previous year have been appropriately diagnosed as having asthma. Lack of diagnosis has usually been associated with lack of appropriate treatment which in turn leads to considerable school absence which can be reduced up to tenfold by treatment. The overall prevalence of asthma from studies done in Great Britain has ranged between 10% and 15% in mid childhood. However figures as high as 25% have been quoted in some studies. The prevalence in rural Africa and amongst Canadian Eskimos is said to be very low.

Deaths from asthma in childhood are rare but 40 to 45 children die each year in England and Wales from this disease and there has been no diminution in the death rate in the past 20 years. There was an increase in mortality in the 10- to 14-year-old age group during the mid 1960s which paralleled an increase in adult asthma deaths. The cause of this epidemic has been discussed at length and even today remains unresolved though there are strong suggestions that a relationship between inappropriate use of bronchodilator rather than anti-inflammatory prophylactic compounds such as steroids existed. The same has been suggested for the more recent epidemic of asthma deaths in New Zealand. At the same time there has been an enormous increase in hospital admissions for asthma in all age groups. It is likely that this is due to a shift in the balance in care with increasing reliance on hospital rather than primary medical care though it is also possible that there has been a real increase both in the frequency of the disease and its severity.

Childhood asthma is not a self-limiting disorder. The Melbourne Prospective Study provides the most complete data on its natural history. Mild episodic wheezing of mid childhood was predominantly self-limiting with up to 12% of the Melbourne childhood population falling into this category. Five per cent of children with more frequent earlier onset asthma were more likely to have persistent symptoms through adolescence, and the chronic severe perennial asthmatics who comprised 0.5% of the population very rarely remitted. The prognosis was less favourable with an early age of onset, frequent severe or prolonged attacks in the first year after onset and the presence of infantile eczema. The sex ratio progressed from a male:female ratio of 1:1 for mild episodic asthma to 4:1 for chronic severe perennial asthma. As the ratio for severe asthma is closer to 1:1 in adults these must be more males who improve or remit and more females who have persistent problems or develop problems for the first time in adolescence. Smoking in adolescence decreased the probability of an improvement in asthmatic symptoms among patients who had wheezed since early childhood.

Bronchial, hyperresponsiveness

The *sine qua non* of asthma is bronchial hyperresponsiveness. The definition incorporates this concept in stating that rapid variations in airflow limitation is a characterisitic feature of the condition. Furthermore this is used in diagnostic tests, with variations in either peak expiratory flow rate or forced expiratory volume in 1 second of greater than 15% being indicative of a diagnosis. This may either be demonstrated by spontaneous variation over time or by challenge such as with 6 minutes of running or by the administration of bronchodilator if the lung function is low at presentation. Only smooth muscle spasm can produce such rapid changes, but this phenomonen cannot explain the chronicity of the condition nor the intense inflammatory response, which is apparent in the airways of more persistent asthmatics and is

a typical finding post mortem. Bronchial hyperreactivity can occur in non-asthmatic conditions such as cystic fibrosis and following viral upper respiratory tract infections. Furthermore there are considerable inconsistencies in the way that nonspecific bronchial responses can be modified by drugs compared with the effect of the same drugs clinically. Thus bronchial hyperresponsivenss must not be considered synonymous with asthma though the two situations are commonly associated.

Allergy

Allergy occurs commonly in childhood asthma; 93% of asthmatic children over the age of 5 years have positive prick skin tests. Raised serum IgE and detectable IgE antibodies to allergens are commonly associated with asthma. However below the age of 5, allergy is less easily demonstrated and viral respiratory infection is a far more common precipitant of wheezing. In addition wheezing can be exacerbated by factors such as exercise, cold air and irritants such as cigarette smoke and sulphur dioxide.

House dust mite sensitivity is the commonest allergy in asthmatics in most parts of the world, followed closely by cat fur, grass and tree pollens. Foods and moulds are relatively less commonly involved.

Diagnosis

The diagnosis of asthma is usually obvious in the vast majority of children on a simple clinical history and examination. It is typical for children with this condition to have an episodic wheeze or cough which is worst at night, varies according to season or is induced by exertion or allergens. A personal or family history of other atopic disorders would also aid diagnosis. However wheezing and coughing is a feature of intrathoracic airway obstruction. There are many causes for this such as cystic fibrosis or a structural lesion in the airway; thus a diagnostic exercise must be followed by investigations which should include a chest radiograph and in dubious cases also sweat test, Mantoux test, host defence studies, and investigations for gastro-oesophageal reflux. In children who are able to do lung function, the diagnosis can be aided by demonstrating bronchial hyperreactivity with variations in lung function of 15% to 20% or greater. The presence of positive allergy skin tests may also aid diagnosis.

Treatment

The management goals common to all age groups are to reduce symptoms and optimise lifestyle with few limitations on activity at home, school and during leisure activities, utilising treatment with a low incidence of side-effects. This is achievable in all but a tiny minority of cases.

As most children with asthma over 5 years of age do have evidence of allergy, precipitating factors should be identified, and parents and children counselled on avoidance where possible. Avoidance of cigarette smoke must always be a priority. House dust mite, the commonest allergen, is difficult to remove but some environmental measures may be of value including scrupulous vacuuming, the use of plastic mattress covers and pillow cases, removal of feather bedding, bedroom carpets and soft toys from the bed. If there is convincing evidence of allergy to a family pet it should be removed though it may take several months for the dander to be eliminated from the dust. Food allergy is rare in asthma and therefore dietary manipulations are usually not indicated. Asthma may be exacerbated by emotional disturbance and asthma control can be compromised by adverse psychosocial factors. However psychotherapeutic approaches for the most part involve just simple explanation and discussion though occasionally specialist psychotherapy may be of value as an adjunct to standard drug treatment. Education of children and their parents forms an important part of the management protocol and emphasis on self management regimens will reduce the patient's reliance on hospitals.

Drug therapy follows a standard progression through a number of therapeutic options, progressing from the treatment of mild episodic asthma to that of chronic persistent and severe disease. The assessment of severity is usually based on the response to treatment. However mild asthma may be classified as discreet attacks occurring less than once a month or slightly more frequent minor episodes. All are responsive to brochodilators taken no more frequently than two or three times per week. Moderate asthma can be recognised as discreet attacks occuring no more frequently than once a week. In such circumstances sodium cromoglycate prophylaxis would be indicated with the addition of inhaled bronchodilators as required. Sodium cromoglycate must be taken at least three or four times daily for optimal effect, though the dose frequency may be reduced if control of the asthma is achieved. If despite sodium cromoglycate, a patient still requires two or three doses of bronchodilator per week on a regular basis then the prophylactic compound should be replaced with inhaled corticosteroids, usually just given twice daily. Slow-release beta-agonists and xanthine derivatives may be of value in more severe asthma, particularly for nocturnal attacks. Ipratropium bromide is a reasonable bronchodilator which may have some value in infant wheezers. Continuous oral steroids should be reserved for the very few cases who cannot be sufficiently controlled by other therapies including high-dose inhaled steroids. The lowest effective dose should be determined and used and alternate-day regimens should be preferred if at all possible as they have less growth suppressive effect. When slow-release xanthine products are employed, blood theophylline levels must be measured. Usually a dose between 16 and 24 mg per kg per day of theophylline in two or three divided doses will be required. When this treatment is prescribed it is important to be aware of possible side-effects such as gastrointestinal symptoms, sleep disturbance, poor coordination, and impaired behaviour and learning.

In general the inhaled route is preferred for the administration of all anti-asthma therapies though there are practical difficulties in the very young child. Thus, under 18 months of age only nebulised inhalation therapy will be possible. Between 18 months and 5 years of age the use of valved reservoir spacer inhalers can be recommended. Beyond 5 years either dry powder or metred dose inhalers can be employed, though with the latter there are common errors of usage which frequently compromise the control of symptoms.

Immunotherapy, sometimes known as hyposensitisation, has been advocated for the treatment of asthma for the past 70 years. However now that we have highly effective and safe pharmacotherapies, the role of immunotherapy is very much in question. Particularly in asthma, it has resulted in death from both anaphylaxis and exacerbation of asthma. Children with severe asthma do not benefit from this therapy and, even in those who respond, relapse occurs as soon as treatment is stopped. This suggest that it is little different from other prophylactic remedies and, given the frequency of complications, it currently has little place in the management of asthma.

An acute attack of asthma is a failure of prophylaxis. The use of appropriate prophylactic therapy should prevent acute episodes. Once an attack has failed to respond to standard home therapy, medical attention will be required. The initial treatment will be nebulised beta-agonists such as salbutamol or terbutaline in high dose. This will not only be therapeutic but will also provide an indication of the need for referral. Failure to respond or relapse within 4 hours of the dose will indicate the need for referral. The response may be gauged on the basis of improvement in peak flow rate and a reduction in respiration rate with improved air entry in the lung fields. Cyanosis in air and the presence of pulsus paradoxus or a peak flow rate of less than 50% of predicted after administration of bronchodilator indicates a need for hospital referral. At this stage a loading dose of aminophylline by intravenous injection slowly over 20 minutes in a dose of 5 mg per kg should be given. However if the patient is receiving oral theophylline preparations it would be safer to avoid the intravenous theophylline and to use intravenous salbutamol in a dose of 10 mcg per kg. In addition, prednisolone 1–2 mg per kg or intravenous hydrocortisone 4 mg per kg should be administered.

On admission to hospital often quite inappropriate investigations are done. The key parameters to monitor are pulse, colour, the presence of pulsus paradoxus, peak flow rate, arterial blood gases and oxygen saturation. Additional doses of nebulised beta-2-stimulants should be administered and continuous infusion of either aminophylline 0.9 mg per kg per hour or salbutamol $10–60\mu g$ per kg per hour should be maintained. Steroid therapy can be continued either as prednisolone or hydrocortisone. Oxygen administration is mandatory to maintain normal saturation. Blood gas monitoring is required in more severe cases; rapidly rising arterial carbon dioxide tension would indicate the need for admission to the intensive care unit. A small number of children require periods of paralysis and sedation for intermittent positive pressure ventilation.

Finally an acute attack must always be considered a failure of prophylaxis and before discharge regular treatment should be re-examined. It must be emphasised that it is possible to return all but a tiny minority of children to a normal life-style, which includes active participation in sports.

ALLERGIC RHINITIS

Allergic rhinitis is also a very common disorder occurring in approximately 10% of children and in up to 20% of adolescents and young adults. It occurs in 75% of children with asthma and like asthma is frequently underdiagnosed. Its importance as a cause of morbidity is grossly underestimated; school performance can be profoundly affected, with underachievement in examinations, which are usually inappropriately held during the height of the pollen season. Seasonal allergic rhinitis is estimated to occur in 5–9% of children but is quite rare under the age of 5 years. Isolated perennial rhinitis occurs in 3% of children.

Like asthma, individuals with allergic rhinitis have non-specific irritability of the affected organ. Thus symptoms of nasal congestion, sneezing, itching and rhinorrhoea can be triggered by non-specific irritants such as cigarette smoke as well as by exposure to allergens. Noisy breathing, irritating sniffing, coughing and throat clearing often lead to social isolation at school and discord at home. Itching of the pharynx and palate, hearing loss and anosmia may also occur. Particularly in seasonal allergic rhinitis an associated conjunctivitis is common. At least 20% of children also have middle ear abnormalities with hearing deficits leading to learning difficulties and speech delay.

Clinical history and timing of symptoms will provide the most useful guide to specific allergy diagnosis. Knowledge of tree pollen, grass pollen and mould spore counts may help delineate specific allergies which can then be confirmed by skin testing, IgE antibodies or nasal provocation testing. The commonest cause of perennial problems is allergy to house dust mite and here a history of profuse sneezing on arising in the morning with progressive improvement of symptoms during the day is typical. Apart from the usual diagnostic tests, examination of nasal discharge for eosinophils will aid diagnosis of nasal allergy.

The differential diagnosis includes hypertrophy of adenoids, so-called vasomotor rhinitis which is really perennial rhinitis for which no allergic cause can be found, nasal foreign body, recurrent sinus infection and nasal polyps, the latter two sometimes being associated with cystic fibrosis.

Therapy for allergic rhinitis follows similar lines to that for asthma. Allergen avoidance should be recommended if possible. It is also important to avoid non-specific irritants such as cigarette smoke. Food intolerance is a relatively rare cause of this condition. There is little to no evidence that milk or indeed any other food is a particularly common cause of rhinitis despite wide publicity to the contrary. Immunotherapy has a rather more established place in the treatment of this condition than in asthma. Pollen immunotherapy for one or more years has been associated with significant clinical improvements and reduction in requirements for other therapy. Furthermore in the absence of asthma it is likely to be a safe therapy. So far only subcutaneous immunotherapy injections have an established place with oral and sublingual immunotherapy being of dubious efficacy.

Pharmacotherapy has included nasal decongestants, antihistamines, sodium cromoglycate and topical steroids. In general, decongestants are not recommended. Antihistamines form the mainstay of treatment with the new generation of non-sedative specific-H1-receptor antagonists being preferred. They are more effective when used prophylactically rather than awaiting the development of symptoms. Indeed long-term use may even have a small anti-asthma effect. Sodium cromoglycate has been shown to be more effective than placebo provided the dose frequency of up to six times a day is maintained. However, inhaled corticosteroids have been superior in the relief of symptoms, though rather more for nasal obstruction than sneezing and rhinorrhoea. They are effective when administered only twice daily and have a good record of safety. At present the combination of a H1-specific antagonist nasal corticosteroid and ocular cromoglycate have been shown to be the best combination for the treatment of allergic rhino-conjunctivitis.

ATOPIC DERMATITIS (ECZEMA)

Children with eczema are usually atopic. Most have positive immediate skin tests and high levels of total serum IgE. Between 20% and 50% go on to develop asthma and up to 50% have allergic rhinitis. In Britain the incidence of eczema appears to be increasing; 12% of a 1970 cohort of children were reported to have eczema. This is double the incidence noted 12 years previously.

The pathogenesis of the condition, and indeed its management, is less clear than respiratory allergy. Whilst atopy is common in the condition, the role of IgE in the pathophysiology is uncertain. Allergens can be demonstrated to produce a weal and flare reaction, but they do not produce the skin lesions of eczema. Occasionally, it is possible to replicate lesions by patch testing with house dust mite in house mite-sensitive individuals. It is now well accepted that reactions to foods are important in childhood eczema, both in initiating the disease and in causing exacerbations. However positive skin tests and IgE antibody measurements do not accurately predict which foods are likely to be involved; thus the relationship between food intolerance and eczema has not been elucidated.

Eighty per cent of patients with eczema present by 1 year of age, and more than 90% by the age of 5 years; 75% of those with milder disease will clear over the first few years of life, whilst those with more severe problems are more likely to have a chronic course. The pattern changes with age. In infancy, it is characterised by dry red scaly plaques, usually appearing after 3 months; before 12 months they are confined to cheeks, abdomen and extensive surfaces of limbs. Beyond 2 years it is characterised by papules and plaques with excoriations usually in skin flexures. In late childhood and adolescence, the most common location of the rash is on the hands and feet often with pustular lesions. It is also present on the upper eyelids and skin flexures. Patients with eczema are particularly susceptible to varicelliform infections. Thus vaccinia virus can produce devastatingly severe general disease and even death. Herpes simplex virus can produce generalised lesions with eczema herpeticum, and eczematous children are particularly prone to molluscum contagiosum.

Some children with eczema do improve on dietary exclusions. This is best established in double-blind cross-over studies for dairy product and egg avoidance. Whilst the use of diets with childhood eczema has been amply justified, the long-term results are often disappointing. Diets can be nutritionally incomplete and impose an immense financial and emotional burden on children and parents. Even in highly motivated families with severe eczema associated with food intolerance, up to 20% of children under the age of 3 years, and 50% over the age of 3 will be unable to maintain the diet despite worsening of the disease. At present, it is suggested that only simple avoidance diets such as those excluding dairy products and hens egg, should be recommended for a therapeutic trial. However other allergens including contactants and inhalants may also be involved and thus avoidance of house dust mite and animal danders may also help. Local irritation by synthetic clothing, washing powders, soaps, perfumes, shampoos and other cosmetics may also be involved. The presence of lanolin (wool fat) and other skin sensitisers in creams and lotions can sometimes worsen the condition. Often a trial and error approach to topical preparations is required to establish which are acceptable.

Anti-histamine preparations, particularly those with a sedative effect, can reduce pruritus and sleep disturbance. Only corticosteroids have a dramatic effect on the condition, but they have the potential to cause skin atrophy, striae and adrenal suppression; thus low-potency preparations should be preferred avoiding the fluorinated corticosteroids. Skin sepsis should be treated with both topical and systemic antibiotics.

CONTACT DERMATITIS

Contact dermatitis is an inflammatory response on the skin due to a type 4 allergic reaction following contact with an external agent. The skin changes are very similar to atopic dermatitis but localised to areas of contact. The commonest type occuring in infancy is napkin dermatitis produced by prolonged contact with urine, faeces, antiseptics, soaps and detergents in the nappy. Other common causes include dyes for clothing, nickel compounds, rubber compounds and preservatives in various creams, medications and cosmetics. The diagnosis can be achieved by patch testing with the offending allergen held in contact with the skin for 48 hours and examined 20 minutes after removal for erythema, oedema and vesicles. Treatment consists of avoidance and a short course of topical corticosteroids to the affected area.

URTICARIA AND ANGIOEDEMA

Urticaria (hives) is a transient eruption of weal and flare reactions of varying sizes lasting from minutes to days. It occurs due to release of vasoactive substances in the superficial dermis. Angioedema is a similar reaction confined to the deeper dermis and subcutaneous tissues. Both are very common problems throughout life. Chronic urticaria persisting for months is more a problem in adults than children. Both are seen most frequently after acute illnesses such as beta-haemolytic streptococcal tonsillitis or campylobacter enteritis. Symptoms can usually be controlled with antihistamines and will resolve spontaneously within a few weeks. In some patients the condition is persistent or recurrent; the causes then include physical factors (heat, cold and exercise) or allergens, such as animal danders, drugs and sometimes foods.

Severe angioedema particularly if familial has very occasionally been associated with Cl-esterase-inhibitor deficiency. However in many patients a cause cannot be identified from clinical history or standard investigation. In such patients improvement can sometimes be obtained by employing a diet free from artificial colourings and preservatives. The mechanism of reactions to food additives is unclear. It is not associated with conventional atopy and there is no evidence of any specific antibodies. The problem is often a transient one in childhood.

In contrast, atopic urticaria and angioedema are associated with reactions to antibiotics such as penicillin or food such as dairy products, nuts or fish, and are rather more likely to be persistent. At least 50% of cases will have continuing problems through to adult life. The basic treatment is avoidance though it is sometimes possible to protect against reactions by pretreatment with oral sodium cromoglycate and antihistamines. Hereditary angioedema due to Cl-esterase-inhibitor deficiency can be treated specifically with non viralising androgen preparations such as oxymetholone, danazol or stanozolol.

OTHER FORMS OF FOOD INTOLERANCE

Food intolerance has acquired a dubious reputation and has become a highly topical subject with many lay media features. Unfortunately most genuine reactions to food cannot be identified to have an immunological basis, and thus food intolerance rather than food allergy must be employed as the descriptive title. It must be distinguished from various forms of food aversion and psychological intolerance where reactions will not be reproducible when the food is given in a disguised form.

The estimated prevalence varies widely. Up to 20% of the population perceive themselves to react to food, whereas attempts to confirm this identifies tiny numbers with genuine intolerance. Cows' milk protein intolerance has an estimated prevalence of between 0.2% and 7.5% in early childhood. Prevalence of food intolerance appears to diminish progressively and rapidly with age beyond the first few years of life. Whilst skin reactions are the most common manifestation of food intolerance, failure to thrive, diarrhoea, vomiting, gastrointestinal blood loss, asthma and allergic rhinitis can also be associated. Associations with migraine, epilepsy, infantile colic and hyperactive behaviour remain highly controversial. Some forms of Munchhausen syndrome by proxy present as apparent food intolerance and are particularly difficult to manage.

Gastrointestinal food reactions present in two forms. Some foods such as milk or eggs can produce an immediate rapid-onset reaction with vomiting, abdominal pain and shortly afterwards diarrhoea. Such patients usually have atopic manifestations with IgE-mediated reactions. The slower onset reactions which are more common take hours or even days to evolve. Such symptoms as abdominal distension, pain, diarrhoea, gastrointestinal blood loss and failure to thrive occur. Occasionally this may be associated with an enteropathy and small bowel biopsies reveal patchy villus atrophy. This condition is best described in relation to cows' milk protein intolerance, but can occur with a number of other foods. Intolerance may also lead to infantile colitis producing chronic bloody diarrhoea. In all these conditions food avoidance results in dramatic improvements. Occasionally large doses of oral sodium cromoglycate may be protective.

ANAPHYLAXIS

Anaphylaxis is a systemic reaction which is life threatening. It occurs within minutes of provocation and without treatment is rapidly progressive. Symptoms may involve virtually any system. The skin shows flushing, pruritus, urticaria and angioedema. In the respiratory tract there is stridor or hoarseness and wheezing leading to respiratory obstruction and in the cardiovascular system, a rapid weak pulse, hypotension and shock. The gastrointestinal symptoms include dysphagia, nausea and diarrhoea. There may be sweating, incontinence, and occasionally convulsions. The commonest cause is probably antibiotic allergy followed by a reaction to insect stings, foods and other drugs. It is also a very real risk during immunotherapy injections.

The key to treatment is adrenalin administered by deep subcutaneous injection in doses of 0.2–0.5 ml of a 1:1000 aqueous solution. The dose should be repeated at 10- to 15-minute intervals as required. Oxygen administration is essential and subsequently it may be appropriate to also administer intravenous antihistamines, hydrocortisone and aminophylline. Cardiovascular and respiratory support may also be necessary.

Patients known to have anaphylactic reactions to unavoidable agents such as insect stings should be supplied with emergency medication kits. They can be instructed to administer adrenalin themselves and may also use an adrenalin pressurised aerosol before reaching medical attention.

Patients who have very severe reactions to insect stings in 10–20% of occasions may have a worse reaction on subsequent stings. Measurement of specific venom IgE antibodies may aid identification of highly sensitive individuals. There is evidence that immunotherapy with venom extract is effective in reducing subsequent reactions. However the place of this therapy in paediatric practice has not been established.

FURTHER READING

Clark T J H, Godfreys (eds) 1983 Asthma, 2nd edn. Chapman & Hall, London

Kay A B (ed) 1988 Clinical immunology and allergy, vol 2, no 1. Ballière Tindall, London

Lachmann P J, Peters D K, Rosen F S, Walport M J 1989 Clinical aspects of immunology, 5th edn. Blackwell Scientific, Oxford (in press)

Lessof M H, Lee T H, Kemeny D M (eds) 1987 Allergy: an international textbook. John Wiley, Chichester

Soothill J F, Hayward A R, Wood C B S (eds) 1983 Paediatric immunology. Blackwell Scientific, Oxford

Warner J O et al 1989 Management of asthma: a concensus statement. Archives of Disease in Childhood 64: 1065–1070

19. Gastrointestinal disorders

M. J. Brueton

Gastrointestinal symptoms are common in young children. It must however be borne in mind that symptoms can be non-specific and frequently occur in association with infections and other disorders which do not primarily affect the gut. It is therefore essential to elicit a clear history, in addition taking into account that there is a great variation in the ways in which parents use such words as diarrhoea, vomiting, appetite and constipation.

VOMITING

Some of the important causes of vomiting in infancy are:

1. Feeding problems.
2. Infection:
   a. Enteral:
      i. Oral candidasis
      ii. Gastroenteritis
   b. Systemic:
      i. Respiratory
      ii. Otitis media
      iii. Urinary
      iv. Central nervous system
      v. Septicaemia
3. Gastro-oesophageal reflux:
   a. Hiatus hernia
4. Intestinal obstruction:
   a. Congenital malformations
   b. Pyloric stenosis
   c. Intussusception
5. Malabsorption:
   a. Coeliac disease
   b. Cows' milk protein intolerance
   c. Lactose intolerance
6. Cerebral
   a. Birth trauma
   b. Hydrocephalus
   c. Meningocephalitis
   d. Intracranial space-occupying lesion
7. Metabolic disorders:
   a. Galactosaemia
   b. Idiopathic hypercalcaemia
   c. Aminoacidaemias
8. Endocrine:
   a. Adrenogenital syndrome
9. Renal:
   a. Renal tubular acidosis
   b. Uraemia

The timing, frequency, volume, and content of the vomitus should all be noted, projectile vomiting must be distinguished from regurgitation or rumination.

Gastro-oesophageal reflux

Effortless regurgitation of stomach contents is often seen in healthy babies in the first few months of life. Most of these infants have a normally placed gastro-oesophageal junction and yet have a tendency to reflux gastric contents into the lower oesophagus. Present evidence suggests that effective lower oesophageal closure is brought about by the combined action of an intrinsic muscle sphincter, the presence of an intra-abdominal segment of oesophagus subject to abdominal pressures, and the mucosal arrangement at the junction which acts as a choke. In many normal babies it would appear that the integration of these factors is inadequate and reflux occurs. This causes no distress, except to the mother; weight gain is generally satisfactory, and in the majority of infants the symptoms have resolved by the age of 6 months. Simple measures that may be taken include adding a thickening agent (Nestargel, Carobel) to the feeds, reducing the volume required for each one by increasing their frequency, and posturing the young infant in a semi-prone position with the head raised.

More severe reflux may be associated with disturbances in oesophageal motility and gastric emptying, or with an abnormal position of the gastro-oesophageal junction, as in a partial thoracic stomach or hiatus hernia. Failure to thrive may occur and oesophagitis is more likely to develop, causing blood to be seen in the vomit and in some cases stricture formation. Recurrent wheezing and aspiration pneumonia may also occur. The presence of any of these features requires further investigation.

Gastro-oesophageal reflux may be quantitated using prolonged lower oesophageal pH monitoring. Motility may be studied using manometry and contrast studies, the latter will also demonstrate anatomical abnormalities. Oesophagitis is best assessed endoscopically.

The inflammatory effect of gastric acidity on the oesophageal mucosa can be reduced using preparations containing antacids and compounds which protectively coat the mucosa. In some situations histamine receptor antagonists are useful. Drugs which affect motility have been used to promote competence of the lower oesophageal sphincter and improve oesophageal clearance and gastric emptying. Children with underlying neuromuscular disorders may have particularly intractable problems which may warrant surgery.

Hypertrophic pyloric stenosis

In this condition gastric emptying is delayed as a result of hypertrophy of the pyloric musculature. It is not present at birth but develops during the neonatal period in approximately 3 infants per 1000 in the UK. The aetiology is obscure but is probably multifactorial, involving both genetic and environmental factors. It is more common in first-born children and males are affected four times more frequently than females. There is an unexplained association with unconjugated hyperbili-

rubinaemia, and various congenital abnormalities of the gut such as oesophageal and duodenal atresia and anorectal anomalies.

Clinical features

Vomiting after feeds usually commences in the second or third weeks of life. The vomit is never bile stained but it occasionally contains blood. It becomes increasingly copious and eventually projectile. The infant is hungry and will readily take another feed but, in due course, he will become wasted, dehydrated, constipated and miserable. On examination the crucial physical signs to elicit are visible gastric peristalsis and a palpable pyloric tumour. These are best observed while the infant is feeding cradled in his mother's arms with his head supported on her left. A peristaltic wave should appear as a rounded lump passing slowly from left to right across the epigastrium. Gentle and patient palpation of the right upper quadrant of the abdomen should be carried out with the tips of the fingers of the left hand. A firm smooth olive-sized mass may be felt just lateral to the right rectus muscle between the costal margin and the umbilicus. It is most easily located after a vomit and its consistency should alter as the muscle contracts and relaxes.

Management and prognosis

Imaging is not usually necessary, however, if a pyloric tumour is not definitely palpable the diagnosis may be confirmed using ultrasound, barium studies show elongation and narrowing of the pyloric canal with indentation of the antrum and duodenal cap. A hypochloraemic, hypokalaemic alkalosis accompanies the loss of gastric secretions, this together with dehydration must be corrected before surgery. Other coincidental causes of vomiting such as a urinary infection should always be considered. The treatment of choice is pyloromyotomy (Ramstedt's operation), which is curative. Postoperative complications are few, oral feeding may be resumed within 4 hours, the infant being rapidly regraded onto a full strength milk. Medical treatment with dicyclomine hydrochloride (Merbentyl) is rarely indicated.

Vomiting in older children

Some of the main causes of vomiting in older children are:

1. Infections.
2. Acute appendicitis.
3. Drug ingestion.
4. Cyclical vomiting.
5. Diabetic ketosis.
6. Migraine.
7. Motion sickness.
8. Peptic ulceration.
9. Intestinal obstruction.
10. Dietary indiscretion.

Recurrent vomiting in the absence of a recognisable pathology, and occurring in the middle years of childhood, forms part of what is known as the periodic syndrome. It may be related to emotional stress and form part of a family pattern of psychosomatic disorders. The attacks may be mild but, in some patients, there are sudden bouts of retching and vomiting often preceded by abdominal pain or headache. There may be sufficient dehydration and acidosis to necessitate the administration of intravenous fluids while intramuscular chlorpromazine helps to alleviate the vomiting. Recovery is rapid and complete. The frequency of symptoms is usually variable although often described as cyclical. The role of psychological factors remains unclear. The attacks tend to diminish with age although some children later develop migraine.

Haematemesis

Prolonged severe retching for any cause may result in blood staining of vomit. The most common source of bleeding in childhood haematemeses is the nasopharynx where a history of epistaxis and swallowed blood is relevant. More serious causes are coagulation disorders, oesophagitis, oesophageal varices, gastric erosions, duodenal ulceration and acute poisoning.

DIARRHOEA

Although many parents take a great interest in their infant's bowel function, stool gazing is an overrated occupation. The range of normality is wide, and most changes of stool frequency, colour or consistency are of no serious significance. Observations which are useful diagnostic pointers include the onset of watery diarrhoea, or the presence of blood or oil. The former is seen in gastroenteritis, carbohydrate intolerance, and in such rare disorders as ganglioneuroma or chloride-losing diarrhoea. The commonest causes of bleeding are a rectal mucosal tear or infection, a Meckel's diverticulum or colitis must also be considered. Oily stools denote gross steatorrhoea, as may be seen in pancreatic insufficiency. Small bowel malabsorption with lesser degrees of steatorrhoea may co-exist with clinically normal stools. It is important to establish the chronological development of the stool abnormality, relating it specifically to birth, infections, the dietary introduction of gluten-containing cereals, cows' milk, or sucrose, and to emotional disturbances in the family or environment.

Persistence after an acute onset should be identified. A suspicion of associated failure to thrive should ideally be confirmed by plotting the growth pattern on a centile chart. Some of the important causes of diarrhoea are discussed below, the range of possible aetiologies is detailed below:

1. Toddler diarrhoea:
   a. Irritable bowel syndrome
2. Gastrointestinal infection:
   a. Bacterial gastroenteritis
   b. Viral gastroenteritis
   c. Tuberculosis
   d. Amoebiasis
   e. Giardiasis
3. Extra-intestinal infection:
   a. Upper respiratory tract
   b. Pulmonary
   c. Urinary
4. Malabsorption syndromes:
   a. Small bowel enteropathy
   b. Carbohydrate malabsorption
   c. Pancreatic insufficiency
   d. Bile acid deficiency
5. Inflammatory bowel disorders:
   a. Ulcerative colitis
   b. Crohn's disease
6. Miscellaneous:

a. Overfeeding in infancy
b. Chronic constipation with overflow
c. Antibiotic therapy
d. Endocrine disorders
e. Gut resections

Toddler diarrhoea

Most toddlers whose mothers say that they are passing loose, frequent, bulky or offensive stools have no definable abnormality. Characteristically, they are gaining weight, developing normally and have no abdominal distension. They may well have a prominent abdomen secondary to a normal lordotic posture. Such children may be described as having non-specific diarrhoea or the irritable colon syndrome. They often pass three to six mucus-containing stools every day, undigested vegetables may be seen, but in some the stools are manifestly normal most of the time. In other children changes occur coincidentally with upper respiratory infections, or may reflect the emotional climate of the family; there may be a preceding history of an apparent gastroenteritis. The diagnosis is supported by the normal results of such simple investigations as stool and urine microscopy and culture, stool pH and reducing substance analysis, and haemoglobin and white blood cell count. The physiology of the condition continues to be studied; abnormalities in intestinal motility have been documented, and it has been noted that currently popular views on healthy eating have resulted in some parents placing their children on very high roughage and low fat diets, both of which would contribute to reduced intestinal transit times. The sensitivity of the alimentary tract to emotional factors is also well recognised, however no consistent pathogenic mechanisms have yet been identified. During management extensive investigation and dietary exclusions should be avoided, the emphasis being on explanation and reassurance that this is a benign and self-limiting disorder which usually resolves by school age.

Gastroenteritis

Infective diarrhoea and vomiting chiefly affects children under 2 years of age. Overcrowding, pov-erty and malnutrition all increase the incidence of epidemics. Symptoms follow actual invasion of the bowel wall by pathogens, or adherence of toxin-secreting organisms to the small bowel mucosa, stimulating fluid and electrolyte movement into the lumen. The major pathogenic bacteria involved include enteropathic *Escherichia coli*, salmonellae, shigellae, staphylococci, *Yersinia enterocolitica* and campylobacter. Viruses of importance are rotavirus, coronavirus and adenoviruses.

Clinical features

The illness often begins with vomiting, and progresses to watery diarrhoea within 24 hours. Blood in the stool may be seen particularly in campylobacter and shigella infections. The most important clinical features are consequent upon dehydration and electrolyte disturbances. These result in loss of skin turgor, dry mucous membranes, reduced intra-ocular tension, acidotic breathing and, in infants, a sunken fontanelle. In mild dehydration (up to 5% loss of bodyweight) these signs are minimal, but the child is symptomatic and pyrexial. In moderate dehydration (10%) the infant is drowsy and oliguric, with sunken eyes and a definite reduction in skin turgor. In severe dehydration (10–15%) the child is semiconscious, acidotic and in shock, with cold clammy and mottled skin. If, despite clear evidence of considerable fluid loss, there are no signs of circulatory collapse, hypernatraemic dehydration should be suspected; here the skin has a doughy feel to it and often neurological signs, including convulsions, occur.

Management

The cornerstone of treatment is the correction of dehydration using oral rehydration solutions containing electrolytes, glucose and water. These are commercially available in various formulations (such as Dioralyte and Rehidrat), the glucose is important since it continues to be absorbed even when the mucosa is in a secretory state, its passage across the enterocyte is accompanied by sodium and water. Most children with mild dehydration may be managed at home, the required volume of oral rehydration solution being given in small amounts at frequent intervals. Solids and milk should be discontinued temporarily, however breast feeding can often be continued only missing one or two feeds. After 12–24 hours of rehydration quarter-strength milk is reintroduced and graded up to full strength over 1–2 days. Children and particularly infants with moderate and severe dehydration require intravenous fluids.

Sometimes there is sufficient damage to the jejunal mucosal border to impair lactase activity. This temporarily causes lactose malabsorption and a recurrence of diarrhoea on reintroducing cows' milk.

Stool examination should include microscopy, microbiological culture and electronmicroscopy for virus particles. The routine use of antibiotics is not advised, there is no good evidence that they reduce mortality or morbidity and they may, in fact, cause harm by promoting a carrier state and the proliferation of resistant organisms. On the other hand, bacteraemia and septicaemia, such as in typhoid fever, should always be treated with an antibiotic to which the organism is sensitive. Drugs which reduce gut motility or which absorb fluid from the stool offer only symptomatic relief and do not alter the course of the illness.

MALABSORPTION

Malabsorption is suggested clinically by the triad of failure to thrive, abdominal distention and diarrhoea. Some of the causes in childhood are listed in Table 19.1. The major group is that which involves small bowel mucosal enteropathies. Such patients will eventually show additional signs and symptoms relating to reduced absorption of iron, folic acid and vitamins D and K, and some become hypoproteinaemic.

If malabsorption is suspected clinically, screening tests for xylose and fat absorption may be performed together with a full blood count and stool microscopy and culture. If on jejunal biopsy villous atrophy is found (Figs 19.1, 19.2), a specific diagnosis must be established. Any damage to the mucosal brush border will impair disaccharidase activity, lactase being the most vulnerable enzyme. Clinical lactose intolerance is

Table 19.1 Some causes of malabsorption

Small bowel mucosal abnormality
Morphological
  non-specific
    coeliac disease
    cows' milk protein intolerance
    giardiasis
    post-gastroenteritis
    protein energy malnutrition
    tropical sprue
    immunodeficiency states
  specific
    intestinal lymphangiectasia
    congenital microvillus atrophy
    abetalipoproteinaemia
Functional
    lactase deficiency secondary to morphological changes
    primary lactase deficiency
    sucrase-isomaltase deficiency
    glucose-galactose malabsorption
    chloride-losing diarrhoea

Intraluminal abnormalities
Exocrine pancreatic insufficiency
    cystic fibrosis
    pancreatic achylia and cyclic neutropenia
Altered bile acid enterohepatic circulation
    hepatic immaturity in preterm infant
    cholestasis
    cirrhosis
    blind loop syndrome
    ileal resection
    Crohn's disease of ileum
Anatomical
    malrotation
    insufficient length
    altered motility with 'contaminated small bowel syndrome'

a frequent secondary phenomenon which should resolve as the cause of the villous atrophy is treated.

Coeliac disease

In coeliac disease the protein alpha-gliadin, which is present in gluten in wheat and rye, causes mucosal damage characterised by complete atrophy of the villi, predominantly in the proximal small bowel. The true prevalence of coeliac disease in the UK is difficult to ascertain, but it is probably of the order of 1 in 1500–2000 with some slight family clustering. There is an association with the histocompatibility antigens HLA-DR3, DR7 and DQw2, and the disorder is commoner in girls. The aetiology remains obscure, however various immu-

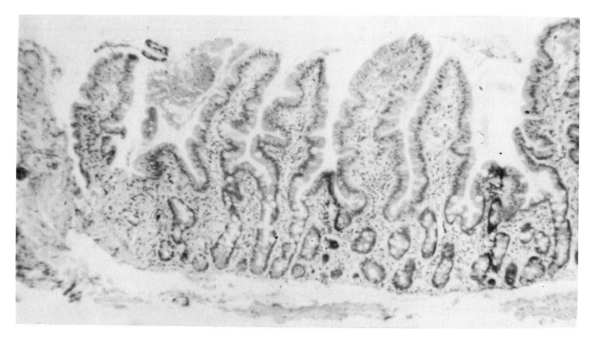

Fig. 19.1 Normal jejunal mucosa.

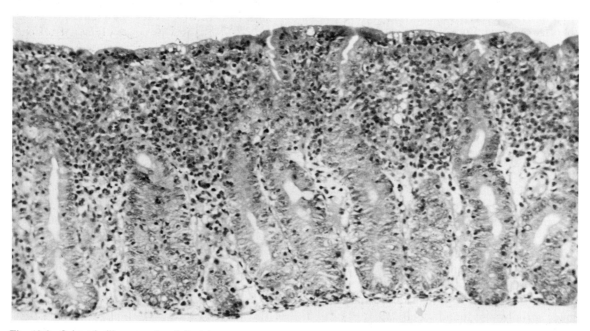

Fig. 19.2 Subtotal villous atrophy of the jejunum.

nological mechanisms have been proposed; no abnormalities of alpha-gliadin digestion have been shown.

Clinical features

The typical child with coeliac disease presents around the age of 1 year with poor weight gain, diarrhoea, abdominal distention and anorexia. Vomiting and irritability may be notable. On examination there is abdominal distension, hypotonia, and muscle wasting, with flattening of the buttocks (Figs 19.3, 19.4). An accurate dietary history relating to gluten intake must be obtained. Older children may have less obvious clinical features, growth impairment may not be marked, diarrhoea is not invariable; abdominal pain and

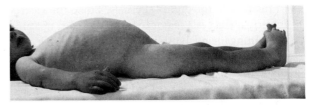

Fig. 19.4 Coeliac disease — abdominal distension still evident when child recumbent.

anaemia may be present and rickets is seen, particularly in Asian children.

Management

Withdrawal of gluten from the diet results in total clinical and histological remission. Intolerance is permanent and may be confirmed by an oral challenge carried out in relation to changes in jejunal histology. A mucosal biopsy taken on a gluten-free diet is compared with one taken 3 months later after the daily addition of 10–20 g of gluten to the diet. In children under the age of 2 years in whom it was not possible to completely exclude other causes of an enteropathy on presentation, a formal gluten challenge must subsequently be carried out. The long-term prognosis on a gluten-free diet is excellent. It is well recognised that patients whose coeliac disease has been diagnosed in adult life have an increased susceptibility to malignancy. There is no evidence to date that individuals treated from childhood are similarly at risk.

Food allergy

The normal immunological response of the gut to oral antigen is to produce a complex balance between mucosal immunity and systemic tolerance. Local IgA or circulating IgG or IgM antibodies are assumed to have a protective role; cellular responses are important but are currently poorly defined. Immunological tolerance is an active state of immunoregulation in which cellular and humoral responses are not readily demonstrable. If a situation develops in which tolerance is broken or different classes of immunoglobulin antibody such as IgE are produced in excess, hypersensitivity reactions may occur which cause local tissue damage and systemic reactions. These may be recognised

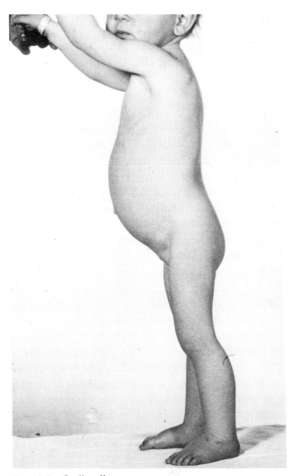

Fig. 19.3 Coeliac disease.

in relation to the gut as allergies. Since the gastro-intestinal tract is a major lymphoid organ, not only containing many lymphocytes in the lamina propria, but also being the site of extensive cell traffic involving circulating lymphocytes, immunocompetent cells may be distributed all over the body and be triggered into activity by the ingestion of oral antigen. Factors which predispose to the development of hypersensitivity reactions include luminal conditions, such as the nature of the antigen and the presence of adjuvants, and mucosal conditions which affect the presentation of antigen to lymphocytes such as maturity, nutritional status, genetic background and the presence of infection.

In the healthy gut antigen processing occurs via the Peyer's patches. If an enteropathy is present antigen will gain access to the mucosa in higher than normal concentrations and at unusual sites. The food proteins which most commonly provoke hypersensitivity reactions are contained in cows' milk, soya and eggs.

Cows' milk protein intolerance

Clinical features. Two main groups of affected children are seen. The first have an unequivocal reaction to small volumes of cows' milk which provoke immediate symptoms such as local oedema, vomiting, wheezing, rashes, or diarrhoea containing blood. In the second group of patients the onset of symptoms is more insidious with failure to thrive predominating. They may also have diarrhoea and vomiting and on examination show evidence of weight loss and, on occasion, abdominal distension.

The first group often show other features of allergy such as eczema and appear to have symptoms on their first exposure to cows' milk having previously been breast fed. The second group have often tolerated cows' milk initially and have developed their hypersensitivity following an episode of mucosal damage due to a condition such as gastroenteritis.

Management. It is very easy to assume a causal relationship if an infant's symptoms resolve on exclusion of cows' milk from the diet. Since this may be a coincidental improvement any association must be confirmed by subsequent challenge, having excluded the possibility of temporary lactose intolerance.

In the first group of patients a challenge must be carried out with care, starting with 5 ml of cows' milk and gradually increasing the volume given over 48 hours. Clinical observation remains the best way of monitoring the response since none of the various immunological parameters so far suggested have proved to be diagnostic.

The second group of infants have evidence of malabsorption and require a jejunal biopsy while on a normal diet. If an enteropathy is present it must be shown that exclusion of cows' milk is associated with histological improvement and that subsequent challenge provokes a relapse.

The most practical treatment is to replace cows' milk with soya milk or a hydrolysed cows' milk protein formula (see Ch. 11). A few patients will become sensitised to the protein which is substituted into the diet; if goat's milk is used folic acid supplements must be given.

Many, but not all, of the first group tolerate cows' milk by the age of 2 years, most children in the second group recover within a few months of diagnosis.

Lactose malabsorption

Lactose is split into its component monosaccharides, glucose and galactose, by the disaccharidase enzyme lactase. This is present in the microvillus brush border of the columnar epithelial cells which line the intestinal mucosa. When small intestinal lactase activity is deficient, lactose passes on to be metabolised in the caecum and colon by the normal gut flora. Water is drawn into the bowel due to the osmotic effect of the lactose load while the increased hydrogen ion concentration attendant on the accumulation of lactic acid impairs water absorption in the colon; the stools are fluid and the stool water is acid and contains glucose.

Lactase activity may be secondarily impaired in any disorder associated with a small bowel enteropathy. In such cases normal activity will return as the lesion resolves. Lactase levels rise to normal at or just after birth so that some newborns show a temporary deficiency. A primary lactase deficiency present from birth does occur but it is very rare and is recessively inherited. An acquired isolated lactase deficiency develops in late childhood in many non-Caucasians. Some authorities even regard the presence of lactase in Caucasian adults as abnormal, its persistence is thought to have given a genetic advantage in cattle-rearing communities.

Note that lactose malabsorption does not always result in lactose intolerance. This will depend on the lactose load given and the length of bowel in which lactase is deficient.

Clinical features and management. The passage of watery stools with a pH less than 5.5 and containing reducing substances as demonstrated by Clinitest tablets is suggestive of lactose malabsorption. The patient also experiences colicky abdominal pain, abdominal distension and increased flatus.

Lactose intolerance is confirmed if lactose exclusion from the diet relieves the symptoms and subsequent challenge using lactose, 2 g/kg body weight in a 10% solution, causes a recurrence. Normal lactose absorption may be confirmed by demonstrating a rise in blood glucose after an oral lactose load, absence of a rise may reflect malabsorption or variations in the rate of gastric emptying. If lactose has reached the colon and been metabolised by bacteria, hydrogen will be produced and may be measured in expired breath after a lactose challenge. Lactose may be measured directly in a mucosal biopsy specimen which also allows histological examination to demonstrate an enteropathy.

Treatment with a lactose-free milk in infants will control symptoms. The formulae available are discussed in Chapter 11. It is unusual to have to exclude all dairy products in older children. When lactose intolerance is secondary to acute gastroenteritis it is usually possible to reintroduce cows' milk after 2–4 weeks. Clearly, the distinction between cows' milk protein intolerance and lactose intolerance is important.

Malabsorption of other carbohydrates

Sucrose and starch are also hydrolysed by brush border disaccharidases. Sucrase, maltase and isomaltase activities are less vulnerable than lactase, and reductions are only seen in severe enteropathies. There is a rare recessively inherited deficiency of sucrase and isomaltase which causes watery stools after a sucrose or starch load. If Clinitest tablets are used to test for undigested sucrose in stool water, acid must first be added to hydrolyse the sugar. Such patients are symptomatic in early childhood and respond to a reduction in dietary sucrose and starch, but they will usually tolerate increasing amounts as they grow older. Monosaccharide intolerance may be seen in association with severe enteropathies, particularly in infancy.

Giardiasis

Giardia lamblia is a flagellated protozoan. Its distribution is world wide, humans are the main reservoir of infection and cysts are transmitted in water or food. Trophozoites are released and are found on the epithelial surface of the small bowel mucosa.

Clinical features and management

Although many children are asymptomatic, clinical disease is more common in infants and on first exposure at any age. An acute presentation resembles gastroenteritis, after a week or so the symptoms either resolve spontaneously or subside into a low-grade, chronic infection with nausea, anorexia, abdominal pain and diarrhoea, sometimes progressing to frank malabsorption with failure to thrive and the presence of a small bowel enteropathy. The stools should be examined for both trophozoites and cysts, however since excretion of the latter is often intermittent several specimens may be required. The diagnosis can only be finally excluded by microscopy of a duodenal aspirate or mucosal biopsy. Symptomatic children and asymptomatic family members should be treated using metronidazole or tinidazole (see also p. 369).

Cystic fibrosis (see Ch. 16)

CONSTIPATION

Constipation may be defined as difficulty or delay in the passage of stools. In babies the application of this definition may not be straightforward. It is wise to regard acute and chronic constipation as being different problems and to differentiate them from soiling (the passage of loose stools in clothing) and encopresis (the passage of normal stools in abnormal places).

The breast-fed baby may initially open his bowels after each feed and then quite normally pass unformed stools once a week. The bottle-fed baby's stools are usually drier and harder and may be passed with difficulty. Neither infant is necessarily constipated and an accurate history must be elicited. If there is concern, and particularly if abdominal distension is present, several disorders should be borne in mind. These include anal stenosis, a spinal abnormality, Hirschsprung's disease, hypothyroidism, hypercalcaemia or malabsorption causing such bulky stools that defaecation is difficult.

The toddler's acute problems may originate in the anxious circumstances of potty training, or following febrile illnesses, or changes in diet or environment which have resulted in a reduced food intake. If the subsequent passage of a hard stool causes a rectal mucosal abrasion or fissure, blood may be seen on the stool and defaecation may become painful and infrequent. Most acute episodes improve spontaneously, but in children who are prone to constipation a high residue diet, with or without a short course of laxatives is advisable.

Chronic constipation is associated with abdominal distension and large faecal masses are readily palpable in the abdomen. There is often a history dating back to infancy, with delay in the passage of stool lasting 3 weeks or more interspersed with intermittent leakage of faecal fluid. Physical examination should exclude obvious anal and spinal abnormalities; rectal examination reveals a ballooned rectum with stool close to the anal verge. Laxatives should not be commenced if enormous, rocky faecal masses are present, the lower bowel should first be emptied using an enema. A regular bowel habit should then be established by combining an oral intake of sufficient bulk with the use of a stimulant laxative and adequate fluid intake is also essential. Since many patients are anorexic at this stage stool bulking and softening agents such as lactulose and methylcellulose are useful initially, but it should not be necessary to repeat the enema. Relapses are common, so laxatives may be needed for several months after a normal pattern has been regained in order to cover the period during which the dilated lower bowel with its diminished sensation is returning to normal.

Behavioural problems commonly fade away as bowel control returns. Children who fail to respond to treatment or who relapse rapidly require further investigation.

Hirschsprung's disease

Hirschsprung's disease is characterised by a congenital absence from the bowel wall of the intrinsic autonomic ganglion cells which form Auerbach and Meissner's plexus. There is a concomitant hypertrophy of the extrinsic autonomic nerves supplying the affected gut. The resulting lack of propulsive activity causes chronic constipation and gross dilatation of the proximal bowel.

The original descriptions were of lower colonic and rectal involvement, however, it is now recognised that there is a wide range of abnormality from ultrashort segments to changes in the entire large and small intestine. The general population incidence is estimated to be about 1 in 5000 with familial clustering.

Clinical features

The majority of patients present in the neonatal period with delay in the passage of meconium. In some infants this rapidly progresses to complete intestinal obstruction, in others minor constipation is relieved by suppository or enema and no further major symptoms ensue for months or years. In the older child failure to thrive may be noted and the history of intractable constipation precedes potty training. Examination reveals an empty rectum while the sphincter may be tight but distensible. A serious complication of the condition is enterocolitis.

Management and prognosis

The diagnosis is confirmed by barium enema, anorectal pressure studies (manometry) and mucosal suction biopsy.

In a patient without bowel preparation the radiological appearances include a narrow aganglionic segment with dilated bowel proximal to it, tapering down to a transitional or cone zone.

Anorectal manometry shows a failure of relaxation of the internal sphincter. Rectal histology reveals absence of the submucosal ganglion plexus, hypertrophy of nerve fibres, and there is increased acetylcholinesterase activity in the lamina propria.

The principles of treatment are the relief of obstruction, usually by colostomy, with eventual excision of the aganglionic segment and anastomosis of ganglionic bowel to the anal canal. Most children thereafter eventually have satisfactory control of defaecation, while a minority continue to suffer from constipation or fail to achieve continence. The major mortality occurs in the neonatal period, particularly if enterocolitis supervenes.

ABDOMINAL PAIN

Acute abdominal pain always requires careful assessment. Recurrent abdominal pain is one of the commonest complaints in childhood. It is unusual to make an organic diagnosis in an otherwise healthy child of school age. The astute clinician can be alerted to most of the important differential diagnoses (Table 19.2) from the history and clinical examination, and by simple tests such as screening of the urine.

Recurrent abdominal pain typically makes the child stop playing and want to lie down, he often looks pale and may vomit. He points to the umbilicus or near it, when asked where it hurts. On examination there is vague tenderness but no guarding or rigidity, the descending colon may be palpable, but this is found in many normal children. Recovery is complete within an hour or two and the child returns to normal activities. It is always wise for the doctor to consider organic conditions while exploring the more likely emotional causes. It is necessary to come to an understanding of the child, and his family and school background. This takes time, but is essential if parental fears are to be explored, traumatic situations in the child's life identified and if practical advice is to be formulated and accepted. The family should not be left in a diagnostic vacuum nor should reliance be placed on placebo drug therapy. Since the diagnosis of abdominal colic is often inexact and the antispasmodic agents available have a wide range of activities, the rationale for drug treatment is suspect. Mild analgesics may be tried but there is a strong placebo effect. Drugs used to relieve spasm include mebeverine and the anticholinergics, but they have not been fully evaluated in children.

Colic

Babies are often said to have colic or wind when they draw up their legs and scream. This should never be assumed without careful consideration. Even if the interpretation is correct, no precise cause may be found. Some infants may be observed to be swallowing large quantities of air during feeding, in others, one may be led to the conclusion that they are reflecting parental anxiety or depression. Food intolerance is frequently suspected, but is difficult to prove and rarely confirmed unequivocably. Anticholinergic drugs have an atropine-like action and too many side-effects to be used routinely, nonetheless dicyclomine hydrochloride (Merbentyl) may be considered in infants over the age of 6 months in a dose of 5–10 mg three times daily, 15 minutes before feeds, and over the age of 2 years in a dose of 10 mg three times daily. Colic and sleep disturbance may be extremely disruptive in a young family, in which case placement in a well-run children's ward may result in considerable improvement. Resolution by 3 months of age is the general rule.

Table 19.2 Causes of recurrent abdominal pain of childhood

Gastrointestinal	Extragastrointestinal
Gastroenteritis	Renal infections
Appendicitis	Renal calculi
Mesenteric adenitis	Pneumonia
Henoch–Schönlein purpura	Diabetes mellitus
Intestinal obstruction	Sickle cell disease
Malabsorption syndromes	Lead poisoning
Inflammatory bowel disease	Porphyria
Peptic ulcer	Epilepsy
Pancreatitis	Migraine
Hepatitis	Referred from spine,
Tuberculosis	ovaries, testes, pelvis

Appendicitis (see Ch. 26)

RECTAL BLEEDING

Rectal bleeding is most commonly due to local lesions or infections. The latter pathogens include salmonella, shigella and campylobacter. Fissures may be associated with constipation. There is a great diversity of other causes including chronic inflammatory bowel disease, a Meckel's diverticulum, colonic polyps, which are usually benign, vascular malformations, Henoch–Schönlein purpura and haemorrhagic disorders. An intussusception may also present with rectal bleeding, as may massive upper gastrointestinal bleeding. When taking the history it must be established whether or not the blood is really coming from the rectum or the genitourinary tract. It is also important to distinguish between bright red or dark red blood mixed with the stools and streaks of blood on the outside of a stool, as would occur with a lesion in the rectal ampulla or anal canal. In the neonate rectal bleeding may also be caused by necrotising enterocolitis. In infants in the absence of a local lesion or infection, the cause often remains obscure and spontaneous resolution occurs.

INFLAMMATORY BOWEL DISEASE

Ulcerative colitis

Ulcerative colitis is characterised by diffuse inflammation and ulceration of the mucosa of the rectum and colon proximal to it. It is rare in childhood (4 in 100 000) and affects both sexes equally. The peak incidence periods are the first year of life and between 8 and 9 years of age. The aetiology is unknown but probably reflects an interaction between infective, genetic and immunological factors.

Clinical features

Most children present with bloody diarrhoea, lower abdominal pain, weight loss, lack of energy, nausea and a low-grade fever. Abdominal examination generally reveals non-specific tenderness. Extra-intestinal manifestations occur and include erythema nodosum, arthritis, mouth ulcers, and pyoderma gangrenosum. Occasionally, life-threatening fulminating toxic dilatation of the colon occurs.

Management and prognosis

Bacterial (shigella, salmonella, campylobacter, E. coli) and amoebic infections must first be excluded. A double-contrast barium enema shows proctitis and an abnormal colonic mucosal pattern, with loss of haustration, pseudopolyp formation and disordered motility. A typical X-ray is shown in Figure 19.5. Endoscopy should be done and biopsies taken to confirm the diagnosis.

Any fluid and electrolyte disturbance or anaemia needs to be corrected and the diet must contain adequate protein and calories. Opiates and anti-

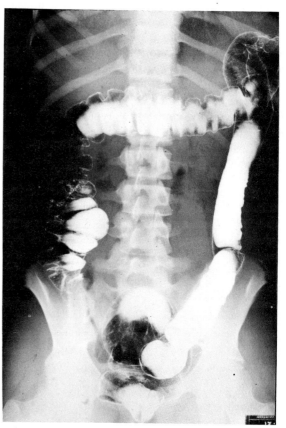

Fig. 19.5 Barium enema showing the descending colon in ulcerative colitis.

cholinergic drugs should be avoided since they predispose to the development of toxic megacolon. Specific therapy includes oral and rectal steroids, and sulphasalazine or its active component 5-aminosalicylic acid. Prednisolone is eventually given on an alternate-day regimen, gradually being withdrawn to leave the patient on daily maintenance sulphasalazine.

The clinical course is chronic with relapses and remissions. Surgery is indicated if acute symptoms do not respond to intensive medical care, if gut activity leads to chronic ill health and delay in growth or puberty, or if local complications such as perforation occur. There is an increased incidence of malignancy which is related to the duration and extent of the disease. It is of the order of 4% between 10 and 20 years from the onset of the disease.

Crohn's disease

Crohn's disease causes inflammation of the whole thickness of the bowel wall. Histologically, there is in addition granuloma and fissure formation. The terminal ileum or the colon are particularly affected, although any part of the alimentary tract may be involved, with normal bowel in between and with sparing of the rectum. It, too, is rare in childhood (1 in 100 000), but its incidence has been increasing. The aetiology is obscure.

Clinical features

The diagnosis is rarely made at an early stage. The significance of anorexia and abdominal pain is often missed; the shrewd physician is alerted by the presence of growth failure or weight loss, an abdominal mass, painless perianal fissures, anaemia, finger clubbing or an unexplained fever.

Nutritional deficiences are common and are caused by malabsorption and loss of protein and blood from the gut. Extra-intestinal lesions are less common than in ulcerative colitis.

Management and prognosis

Barium studies of both small and large bowel are necessary. Oedema, spasm and fibrosis cause narrowing ('string sign'), patchy involvement is seen (skip lesions), fistulae may be demonstrable and, in the colon, eccentric lesions and 'rose thorn' spikey ulcers are seen. A typical X-ray is shown in Figure 19.6. Endoscopy and biopsy should be performed, the classical macroscopic appearance includes aphthous ulcers and a 'cobblestone' mucosal pattern.

Unfortunately, there are no specific curative drugs available but general supportive measures, such as maintenance of nutrition, are important. Steroids, an elemental diet, sulphasalazine and azothiaprine may be effective in inducing a remission but do not prevent a subsequent relapse. If bacterial overgrowth is present metronidazole is useful.

Surgical resections of the affected bowel must be regarded as palliative since the recurrence rate in children is high. Chronic indications include growth retardation, delayed puberty, recurrent obstruction, fistulae and extra-intestinal complications. Acute indications include perforation, severe haemorrhage and acute obstruction.

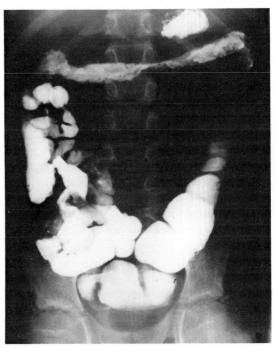

Fig. 19.6 Barium enema showing Crohn's disease of the colon.

PARASITIC INFECTIONS

Threadworms (*Enterobius vermicularis*)

Enterobius vermicularis is a common parasite in schoolchildren throughout the world. The entire lifecycle is completed in man. It is usually spread within families. The worms' habitat is the caecum and appendix from where they migrate to the lower rectum and eggs are laid on the perianal skin. Following scratching with the fingers, eggs are reingested and the cycle continues. The usual symptom is perianal irritation. The worms may be demonstrated by microscopic examination of a piece of transparent adhesive tape placed on the skin near the anus. The whole family should be treated with a drug such as mebendazole, piperazine or thiabendazole.

Roundworms (*Ascaris lumbricoides*)

Ascaris lumbricoides is principally harboured by young children both in the tropics and in areas extending well into the temperate zones. The eggs develop in moist soil contaminated with faeces. Following ingestion, larvae hatch into the small intestine, pass through the bowel wall to the liver, and thence travel to the lungs where they remain causing a local inflammatory reaction. They then move up the bronchial tree to the pharynx where they are swallowed and mature into adult worms in the small intestine.

Most patients are asymptomatic. Larval migration through the lungs causes cough, dyspnoea and wheezing. Abdominal symptoms depend on the worm load. In heavy infestations frank malnutrition may be precipitated, particularly in undernourished communities and sometimes the physical mass of parasites may cause intestinal obstruction. The treatment is piperazine, pyrantel or mebendazole.

Toxocariasis (visceral larva migrans)

Toxocara canis and *Toxocara catis* undergo a similar lifecycle in dogs and cats to that of ascaris in man. Infection is widespread. If children ingest the eggs, larvae emerge in their intestine, however, their subsequent migration is disturbed in the human environment and they lodge in various organs, becoming encysted and causing a local inflammatory response. The liver, lungs, eye, brain, kidneys, heart and muscle may all be affected. Children of preschool age are typically infected. They may show anaemia, failure to thrive, hepatosplenomegaly, eosinophilia and respiratory symptoms. Neurological and ophthalmological signs may also occur. Thiabendazole or diethylcarbamazine are used in treatment, the household pet should be dewormed using piperazine.

Taeniasis

Taenia solium and *Taenia saginatum* are tapeworms which have as their intermediate host, the pig and cow, respectively. The worms develop in the human intestine following ingestion of cysts in infected beef or pork. The symptoms include abdominal pain and diarrhoea, and segments of proglottides may be seen in the stools. *Taenia saginatum* larvae on emerging from cysts in man, lodge in various tissues causing local inflammation with calcification in muscle (cystercicosis); if in the brain, convulsions may follow. Treatment with niclosamide causes expulsion of the worms.

LIVER DISORDERS

Hepatomegaly

The liver is normally palpable in infancy and early childhood. There are numerous causes of pathological enlargement. They may be broadly classified as follows:

1. Hepatitis — acute, chronic.
2. Infiltration or deposition of fat, mucopolysaccharides, glycogen.
3. Venous congestion — right ventricular failure, tricuspid incompetence.
4. Space-occupying lesions — abscess, cyst, tumour.
5. Chronic haemolysis — thalassaemia.

The presence of splenomegaly suggests infection, a metabolic disorder or occasionally portal hypertension. Biochemical assessment of hepatic function may be followed by liver biopsy if the diagnosis remains obscure.

Jaundice

The differential diagnosis of neonatal jaundice is discussed in Chapter 10. In older children the commonest aetiology is viral hepatitis (see Ch. 15), although many other infectious agents are recognised. Other causes of jaundice include chronic active hepatitis, biliary cirrhosis and haemolysis which may due to hereditary spherocytosis, haemoglobinopathies, or G6PD deficiency.

Hepatocellular failure

Acute liver failure may complicate viral hepatitis, follow drug ingestion such as paracetamol, or represent the end stage of a chronic hepatic disorder such as cirrhosis. The syndrome provokes a complex disturbance of fluid and electrolyte balance, with a bleeding diathesis, increasing jaundice and a progressive encephalopathy terminating in coma and death. Intensive care is necessary and should be carried out in a specialised unit. Any precipitating causes should be corrected if possible. The general supportive measures include the maintenance of respiration and an adequate circulation, control of hypokalaemia, hypoglycaemia and haemorrhage, reduction of blood ammonia levels by sterilisation of the gut and control of protein intake, and provision of adequate calories and vitamins.

Reye's syndrome

This syndrome consists of an acute encephalopathy and fatty degeneration of the liver and other organs such as the kidneys and pancreas. The pathogenic mechanisms remain incompletely identified, however an association with exposure to salicylates has led to the withdrawal of their use in young children. Most patients are under the age of 2 years. After a short prodromal illness, vomiting, delirium, convulsions and coma supervene. Hepatomegaly occurs, the serum transaminases and blood ammonia are elevated, but few children are jaundiced initially. The main management problems are persistent hypoglycaemia and cerebral oedema; the mortality is high.

Chronic hepatitis

An on-going hepatitis persisting for more than 2 or 3 months may be regarded as chronic. Histological assessment is essential to distinguish between chronic persistent and chronic aggressive hepatitis. The former is characterised by inflammatory infiltrate confined to the portal tract. In aggressive or active hepatitis the hepatocytes are swollen, and there are perilobular changes with inflammatory cells spreading out from the portal tract giving the appearance of piecemeal necrosis. These changes are non-specific with respect to aetiology.

Clinically, persistent hepatitis carries a good prognosis and requires no treatment. Chronic aggressive hepatitis is more serious. Its presentation may be acute with fever, anorexia, and jaundice but, in some patients, it is insidious with arthralgia, fever, colitis or erythema nodosum. These children require treatment with steroids to which azothiaprine is added if a biochemical remission is not obtained.

Cirrhosis and portal hypertension

The histological definition of cirrhosis includes destruction of the normal lobular architecture of the liver with areas of nodular regeneration of hepatocytes surrounded by fibrous tissue. Some of the causes are:

1. Post-hepatitis:
   a. Viral hepatitis
   b. Chronic active hepatitis
   c. Hepatitis due to drugs or toxins
2. Metabolic
   a. Wilson's disease
   b. Galactosaemia
   c. Alpha-1-antitrypsin deficiency
3. Storage disease:
   a. Glycogenosis III and IV
   b. Gaucher's disease
   c. Mucopolysaccharidoses
   d. Niemann–Pick disease

4. Biliary cirrhosis:
    a. Biliary atresia
    b. Cystic fibrosis
    c. Ulcerative colitis
    d. Familial intrahepatic cholestasis
5. Indian childhood cirrhosis
6. Venous congestion:
    a. Congestive cardiac failure
    b. Constrictive pericarditis
    c. Budd–Chiari syndrome
    d. Veno-occlusive disease (Jamaica)

The clinical features vary according to the aetiology, they are minimal early in the disease but all will, in due course, show the signs of portal hypertension. Ascites, splenomegaly and hypersplenism, oesophageal varices, anaemia, finger clubbing, spider naevi and liver palms should all be looked for. Malabsorption will eventually occur.

Investigations are directed towards assessment of the degree of liver injury and to identification of the underlying pathology. Wilson's disease must always be excluded. If specific therapy is unavailable treatment is aimed at the prevention of complications. Genetic counselling may be appropriate. Steatorrhoea is lessened by giving the dietary fat as medium chain triglycerides, fat-soluble vitamin supplements may be given parenterally, and cholestyramine relieves pruritus. Ascites should be treated with diuretics including aldosterone antagonists, rather than by paracentesis. Anaemia should be corrected. Complications include haemorrhage, septicaemia and the development of hepatoma.

FURTHER READING

Anderson C M, Burke V, Gracey M 1987 Paediatric gastroenterology, 2nd edn. Blackwell Scientific, Oxford
Mowat A P 1987 Liver disorders in childhood, 2nd edn. Butterworths, London
Walker-Smith J A, Hamilton J R, Walker W A 1983 Practical paediatric gastroenterology. Butterworths, London

20. Disorders of the kidney and urinary tract

R. S. Trompeter

DEVELOPMENT OF RENAL FUNCTION

The changes that take place in renal function during the first few days and weeks of life are important in the clinical management of sick infants. In reviewing these changes, it is useful to consider the major processes in urine formation, namely:

1. Filtration (in which the major determinant is renal blood flow).
2. Tubular reabsorption.
3. Tubular secretion.

Each of these functions is an essentially independant process, but each is directed by the homeostatic requirements of the individual.

The formation of urine commences in the glomerular capillaries by a process of ultrafiltration, which results in the production of a protein-free, cell-free filtrate of blood. Renal blood flow is the major determinant of glomerular filtration and maturational changes in filtration rate are accompanied by similar changes in renal blood flow. In infancy the glomerular filtration rate (GFR) is low compared with the adult, achieving adult values at about 1 year of age. The renal fraction of cardiac output in the newborn baby is calculated as approximately 5% in the first 12 hours of life. This value reaches approximately 10% during the first week but these figures are less than the adult values of 20–25%. In addition to these haemodynamic changes, other characteristics of the immature kidney are important. One is a marked degree of heterogenicity, so that from nephron to nephron, there is more variability within the kidney both in structure and in function than one finds later in life. Another characteristic is that the kidney develops in a centrifugal fashion, so that deeper structures are the earliest formed containing the most mature glomeruli and receive the highest rate of blood flow.

The pattern in the adult kidney is of a higher rate of blood flow to the outer cortex than to other cortical areas. This is in striking contrast to the newborn in which the lowest rate of flow is to the outer cortex and the highest to the deeper cortex. During periods of hypoperfusion there is probably change in intrarenal blood flow away from the outer cortex into the inner cortex and juxtamedullary areas which could be a factor in the neonatal kidney predisposing to cortical necrosis.

The renal tubules selectively reabsorb about 98% of the glomerular filtrate. The final composition of the urine depends not only on reabsorption but on secretion as well. The transport processes involved may be active or passive. Active transport requires energy and sodium reabsorption accounts for a major proportion of the oxygen consumption by the kidney. Passive transport does not require a direct expenditure of energy and is dependent upon concentration or osmotic gradients. The fractional reabsorption of sodium in infants is comparable with that of adults (greater than 90%). Under normal conditions the infant can handle a variable salt diet. However, under conditions of salt loading the neonatal kidney may lack the capacity to excrete the excess sodium with resultant increases in extracellular fluid volume, weight gain and oedema. Possible factors that may be involved in this lack of naturiuresis may include a low intrarenal blood flow distribution. The latter would result, as described above, in the preferential perfusion of inner cortical glomeruli with long loops of Henle (salt-retaining). The newborn kidney would therefore appear to be better suited to conditions of salt deprivation than to salt loads.

Another explanation of the avidity of salt by the neonate may rest in the renin-angiotensin system. Strikingly high levels of renin and aldosterone have been demonstrated in young infants, enhancing distal tubular reabsorption of sodium and favouring vasoconstriction of the superficial cortical blood vessels.

It is recognised that the newborn kidney does not concentrate urine to the same extent as the mature kidney. The response of the adult kidney to the stimulus of dehydration is to excrete a urine with an osmolality in the range of 1000–1200 mosmol/kg water as compared with the newborn 700–800 mosmol/kg water. This led to recommendations concerning the dietary management of the infant, suggesting a need for an abundant source of water and a relatively low solute load in the diet. Another of the cortical functions of the kidney is to maintain systemic acid-base balance. In the course of metabolism, and particularly with growth, hydrogen ions are released into the extracellular fluid and must be buffered and then excreted by the kidney. Early studies suggested that the immature kidney performed this function very poorly, the kidney function being unable to acidify urine and unable to excrete much acid. This characteristic has subsequently been shown to occur only during the first few days of life and it is recognised that the infant can acidify urine in response to an acid load. Children have lower plasma bicarbonate levels up to about 1 year of age, probably due to the lowered threshold for bicarbonate reabsorption in the proximal tubules and higher plasma phosphate levels which may be in part related to the low GFR.

Renal function tests

The two most commonly used tests for making a gross estimate of glomerular function are plasma urea and creatinine concentration. Many factors will influence urea synthesis; urea production rises with an increased protein intake, gastrointestinal bleeding, infection, burns, muscle trauma or corticosteroid therapy. Production of urea falls when protein intake is reduced or the liver has been damaged. The normal range of plasma urea in children appears to be between 4.0 and 6.0 mmol/l and is somewhat less in infants.

Creatinine is formed in muscle at a relatively, constant rate from creatinine phosphate; its daily production is proportional to muscle bulk. Since mass increases faster than surface area with growth, and since GFR is proportional to surface area, the normal plasma creatinine rises with age. Normal values for plasma creatinine in relation to age are known and for children values within the range of 30–80 μmol/l are considered normal.

Measurement of GFR is the best method of assessing the amount of functioning renal tissue. Bearing in mind that the excretion of any substance found in both urine and blood can be expressed as a clearance; it follows that a substance clearance which is equal to GFR must fulfil certain requirements. These are:

1. The concentration of the substance in glomerular filtrate must be identical to that in plasma, i.e. the substance is freely filtered.

2. It must not be secreted by the tubules.

3. It must neither be reabsorped by the tubules nor leak through them.

If these requirements are met, it follows that filtrate rate and excretion rate must be identical. Since the filtration rate of any freely filtered substance is equal to the GFR multiplied by its plasma concentration (P), and the excretion rate is expressed by urinary concentration (U) multiplied by urine flow (V, urine volume/min), it follows that:

$$GFR \times P = U \times V$$

Dividing both sides by P:

$$GFR = \frac{U \times V}{P}$$

Endogenous substances such as creatinine have been used to measure GFR by clearance method. Creatinine clearance gives a somewhat overestimated GFR, due to some secretion of creatinine by the proximal tubule and is also dependent on a reliable 24-hour urine collection which is frequently difficult to obtain in children. In recent years exogenous substances such as chromium-51-labelled EDTA, have been used for measuring clearance without urine collection. This method involves analysis of the rate of disappearance of the chemical from the plasma.

Testing the kidney's ability to concentrate the urine is the simplest means of assessing tubular function. The most reliable clinical measure of concentration is given by the osmometer which measures the freezing point of urine with great accuracy. For a normal child, a simple concentration test involving no fluids for at least 12 hours, usually overnight, and eating meals without liquids, followed by the testing of an early morning urine sample (having previously emptied a full bladder if necessary), will produce a urine with a specific gravity of 1.025 or an osmolality of greater that 800 mosmol/kg water.

Tests of urinary acidification will reveal the two main causes for acidosis accompanying renal disease, which may be either an inability to excrete hydrogen ions due to reduced ammonia production (distal or type 1 renal tubular acidosis), or the inefficient reabsorption of bicarbonate ions by the proximal tubule (type 2 renal tubular acidosis). However a random urine of pH 5.5 or less suggests a normal ability to acidify urine.

URINARY TRACT INFECTION

Pathogenesis

The sequelae of urinary tract infection (UTI) in childhood are more serious than those in the adult. It is now well recognised that there is impairment of renal growth and renal scarring in children where infections are associated with vesicoureteric reflux. The scarring is seen at the site of intrarenal reflux, that is, where urine is extravasated into renal tissue by the back pressure of urine applied to the renal pelvis during micturition. Vesicoureteric reflux is found in 30–50% of children with UTI, irrespective of whether they are symptomatic and attending hospital, or asymptomatic and are found on school survey. It is, therefore, likely that reflux may cause renal damage in association with the ascent of organisms into the kidney, the presence of residual urine acting as a culture medium and the damage associated with back pressure. Apart from these situations, UTI in the absence of pyelonephritis is probably benign.

The presentation of UTI is variable but with increasing age the symptoms are similar to those in the adult (Table 20.1). In nearly 50% of children there is a history suggestive of urinary symptoms in the first year of life with dysuria, frequency and haematuria becoming common presenting features from the age of 2. Loin pain is uncommon in the very young even when renal parenchymal infection exists. Some children present with acute abdominal pain and vomiting, and appendicitis may be suspected.

The male to female ratio in the newborn is 2.5 to 1, whereas in older children UTI is 20 times more common in girls than boys. This female preponderance is usually attributed to the short urethra in the female. Bacterial invasion of the bladder is facilitated by periurethral colonisation with faecal organisms, local irritation from threadworms and from chemicals such as chlorine in swimming baths and surface tension-lowering agents such as bubble bath. Recent surveys, in normal school girls have shown that 1–2% have a urinary infection at any one time and that around one-half of these children have abnormalities on radiological examination. Up to 20% of girls with UTI will have scarred kidneys by the age of 5 but the incidence of scarring does not seem to increase much thereafter.

Diagnosis

Examination of the external genitalia is mandatory, particulary in the male to exclude balanitis. Neurological examination to include the spine should be undertaken for evidence of peripheral neuropathy or deformity. The key to the diagnosis of UTI is the microscopic and bacteriological examination of the urine. The concept of significant bacteriuria continues to be frequently misunderstood; provided the urine is properly collected, bacteria colonising the urinary tract will tend to be present in numbers of more that 10^5 organisms/ml whereas contaminants entering the urine during voiding will rarely exceed 10^3 organisms/ml. Urine

Table 20.1   Presentation of urinary tract infections in infancy and childhood (adapted from Smellie 1979)

Symptoms	Age				
	0–1 month	1 month to 2 years	2–5 years	5–12 years	Total
	$n = 45$	$n = 45$	$n = 44$	$n = 66$	$n = 200$
Failure to thrive					
Feeding problem	24	16	3		43
Screaming attacks					
Irritability					
Diarrhoea					
Vomiting	16	30		2	48
Fever	5	17	25	33	80
Convulsions	1	3	4	3	11
Haematuria		3	7	4	14
Frequency and dysuria		2			44
Abdominal or loin pain			10	37	47

microscopy is useful for early diagnosis of bacteriuria with one bacterium per high power field corresponding to 5×10^4–10^5 bacteria/ml when uncentrifuged urine is examined.

The examination of the urine for pus cells alone is of little value in the diagnosis; 90% of patients with symptomless UTI show an increased number of pus cells in the urine, but only around one-third to one-half of patients with overt infection have an increased white cell excretion.

Accurate diagnosis requires careful attention to the method of collection and storage of urine and whether or not antibiotic treatment has been commenced at the time of sampling. The demonstration that dip-slide cultures, inoculated during voiding in the home, are as reliable as carefully obtained midstream urine specimens in hospital has made an enormous contribution to the management of UTI in children. The method can be used at all ages, remembering that the preputial folds of non-circumcised boys contain large numbers of bacteria, especially proteus species, even after cleaning and must be irrigated before a urine culture is taken. Clean catch urine samples can be collected from small babies, and avoid the need for unreliable bag specimens. The mother should be taught how to collect the specimen into a sterile dish, usually about 1 hour after the feed whilst the nappy is still dry, and to inoculate both sides of the dip slide immediately (Fig. 20.1). In older children the dip slide may be held in an established stream of urine in order to wet it sufficiently. False-positive cultures and unnecessary investigation are therefore avoided. Bladder catheterisation and suprapubic urine aspiration need only be undertaken in an emergency or when equivocal results have been obtained on dip-slide culture.

Bacterial multiplication starts rapidly in vitro and after 24 hours at room temperature urines have similar bacterial numbers irrespective of the number present at voiding. It is essential, therefore, if midstream samples are to be stored before transportation that they should be kept cold from the moment of voiding. At 0–4°C the bacterial count remains unchanged for at least 48 hours.

Management

The management of UTI is based on the confirmation of infection in at least one urine sample, unless the child is clinically ill in which case parenteral antibiotics may be indicated. Preliminary investigations should include a plain X-ray of the abdomen for evidence of renal calcification, or structural abnormality of the spine; and an ultrasound scan of the renal tract pre- and postmicturition. Dilatation of the collecting systems, renal pelvis or ureters is an indication for a micturating cystourethrogram. If vesicoureteric

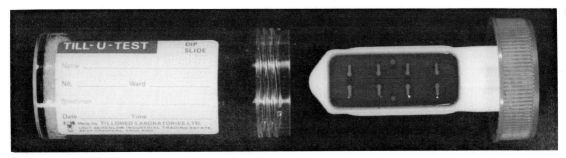

Fig. 20.1 The dip slide.

reflux is present antibiotic prophylaxis, for example low-dose co-trimoxazole, should be prescribed and followed up with regular urine culture continued for 2–3 years. The presence of renal scar formation should be evaluated by radioisotope scan using dimercaptosuccinic Acid, labelled with technetium(^{99}Tc^m-DMSA). Regular monitoring of blood pressure should also be undertaken. Recurrent infections during prophylaxis suggest the need to assess renal growth frequently and to consider surgical reimplantation of the ureter, particularly in those with grade IV–V (Fig. 20.2).

Repeat ultrasound scans of the renal tract may provide helpful information as part of a follow-up programme. Similarly repeat DMSA scans will contribute to the evaluation of new scar formation.

The reassessment of vesicoureteric reflux remains controversial as one is loath to repeat the micturating cystourethrogram. Indirect radioisotope cystography using diethylene-triamine-pentacetic acid labelled with technetium (^{99}Tc^m-DTPA) is available in only a limited number of centres and may prove to be the follow-up investigation of choice.

The natural history of UTI is poorly understood but there is evidence to suggest that in the absence of any structural abnormality the effect of treatment is negligible. Diligent management can, however, prevent the development of renal scarring in children with vesicoureteric reflux and recurrent infections.

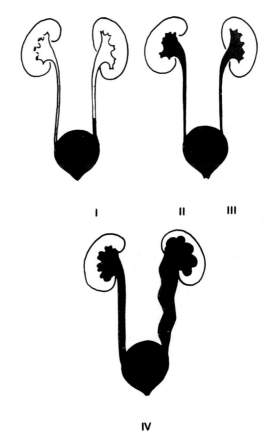

Fig. 20.2 Grades of reflux: grade I — reflux into lower end of ureter without dilatation; grade II — reflux entering up to kidney on micturition only; grade III — reflux entering up to kidney both during bladder filling and during voiding; grade IV — reflux with dilatation of ureter or renal pelvis.

ENURESIS (see also Ch. 12)

Pathogenesis

Children acquire full bladder control at different ages and most children with a continence problem are enuretic rather than incontinent. The majority of children are dry during the daytime by the age of 3 years and dry at night by 4. Ten per cent of

5 year olds wet the bed, as do 5% of 10 year olds. Nocturnal enuresis is more common than diurnal enuresis and occurs in any phase of sleep, except rapid eye movement sleep. Enuresis is classified as primary when the child has never been dry at night, but is usually dry during the day. Secondary enuresis is less common and occurs after a period of nocturnal continence and is frequently associated with emotional disturbances. Children with enuresis are probably all psychiatrically normal although emotional problems may well develop in severe, longstanding cases. Stress is more likely to influence enuresis in the 3 and 4 year olds and emotional or behavioural disturbance is more common in girls and children with diurnal enuresis. There is a strong familial association in nocturnal enuresis, if a parent was enuretic there is a 40% chance of the child being enuretic, and if a sibling is enuretic the child has a 25% chance of having the same problem. Enuresis is more frequently encountered in social classes IV and V. Decreased functional, rather than structural bladder capacity is associated with enuresis, and when the child becomes continent this is associated with an increase in functional capacity.

Management

The basis for successful management requires knowledge of the family and social history development milestones, and details of toilet training. Physical examination must include palpation of the abdomen which may reveal abnormalities of the kidneys or bladder, or evidence of constipation. Examination of the spine for evidence of spina bifida occulta or diastematomyelia, neurological examination to include gait and reflexes, and examination to exclude muscle wasting are also essential. The blood pressure should be recorded and urinalysis undertaken to exclude infection, as up to 10% of children with a continence problem have UTI. When neurological and urinary tract disease have been excluded, a plan of treatment should be embarked upon, having explained carefully to the parents that the child is normal and that the problem is one of an inappropriate physiological reflex. Parental support is essential and a positive rather than a punitive attitude is required. Simple practical measures such as cutting

down evening fluids, and encouraging voiding when awakened, can be effective, particularly when combined with a reward system such as the star charts. Around one-third of children will become dry with these measures, however, the problem must be regularly reviewed and if there is no improvement after 3 months an enuresis alarm can be tried. If used properly the bell or buzzer alarm can be used to cure up to 80% of children, and with relapsers dryness is achieved faster. Success will be more rapidly achieved if the principle of the alarm is carefully explained to the child and parents and should only be used if the child has his own bed. The child must get up after the alarm has rung and empty his bladder even if he has wet the bed. The alarm should be used until there has been a run of dry nights for 1 month.

The tricyclic antedepressant, imipramine, can be used and has been found to be more effective than placebo. A dose of 25 mg is used initially and any benefit should be noticed within 3–4 weeks, although increments in dosage may be necessary in individual cases. If there is no improvement after 2 months the drug should be discontinued. The parents must be warned to keep the drug locked away because overdose can be fatal for a young child.

Diurnal enuresis, usually associated with nocturnal enuresis is less common and more difficult to manage than nocturnal enuresis alone. The functional bladder capacity is even smaller, so frequency and urgency are commonly encountered. On urodynamic investigations many of these children are found to have unstable bladder contractions. Treatment is as for nocturnal enuresis with more emphasis on interval bladder training. The use of anticholinergic drugs is indicated in certain cases and may decrease the frequency of unstable contractions and increase bladder capacity.

Incontinence

Incontinence is the inappropriate voiding of urine as a result of neurological or urinary tract disease. It is important to diagnose surgically correctable abnormalities such as posterior urethal valves, ectopic ureters and meatal stenosis. A micturition history should suggest such an abnormality and the appropriate radiological investigation undertaken. Mental subnormality is associated with incontinence, the pattern of bladder activity being appropriate to the child's mental age. Neuropathic bladder, such as that associated with spina bifida, is a rare condition in childhood but, because of the serious implications, the diagnosis must be made early and the long-term problems and surveillance of these children managed jointly between hospital and GP.

HAEMATURIA

With the introduction of the dip-stick test the detection of blood in the urine has become very easy, although it needs to be confirmed microscopically. Establishing the cause of haematuria and its clinical significance is not so easy; Table 20.2 lists some causes of haematuria in children. How does the clinician approach the diagnostic problem of the child with blood in his urine? Inquiry may elicit a history of previous macroscopic haematuria, suggesting recovering acute nephritis, a pedigree of a familial nephritis or whether the haematuria is associated with other symptoms.

Table 20.2 Classification of haematuria in infants and children

Glomerular causes
    Acute glomerulonephritis
    Other types of glomerulonephritis (membranous, membranoproliferative)
    Henoch–Schönlein nephritis
    Systemic lupus erythematosus
    Haemolytic uraemic syndrome
    Recurrent haematuria syndromes
    (Alport's syndrome, IgA (Berger's) disease)

Non-glomerular causes
    Infections of the urinary tract (acute pyelonephritis, tuberculosis)
    Renal trauma
        direct
        indirect (shock or hypoxaemia, especially in the neonate)
    Renal stones
    Foreign bodies (urethral) and penile excoriation such as a meatal ulcer after circumcision
    Urological malformations (obstructive uropathy)
    Cysts and tumours (polycystic disease, Wilms' tumour, leukaemia)
    Haematological disorders (haemophilia, sickle cell disease)
    Drugs

Physical examination must include the genitalia and abdomen and a search for oedema. Urine microscopy is needed to confirm erythrocyturia and the finding of casts suggests a renal cause. Bacteriuria and pyuria indicate infection and the need for urine culture. Proteinuria (1+ or more by dip stick) should be quantified by timed collection and renal function estimated from the serum creatinine. If these tests are normal the child and his parents should be reassured and an annual urine check and measurement of blood pressure are all that is required. If macroscopic haematuria or proteinuria develop this will demand further assessment. Urography should be undertaken sparingly and mainly in children with symptoms in addition to haematuria. Ultrasound is an invaluable and non-invasive first-line investigation. There is hardly ever an indication for cystoscopy.

The child with glomerular disease is likely to present with an acute nephritic syndrome, nephrotic syndrome, haematuria and/or proteinuria, or acute or chronic renal failure. Unfortunately, the mode of presentation does not enable renal pathology to be predicted and the prognosis appears to be more closely related to the histological classification than to the clinical syndrome.

The ability to study glomerular disease whilst it is still evolving and the rationalisation of treatment have been simplified by undertaking a renal biopsy. Careful selection of cases, and undertaking the procedure under controlled conditions has made the technique relatively safe and it causes only minor discomfort.

ACUTE POST-STREPTOCOCCAL GLOMERULONEPHRITIS

In epidemic years acute post-streptococcal glomerulonephritis is the most common cause of haematuria in children, and is probably the most common cause of haematuria resulting from immunological injury. It is a disease with a characteristic clinical pattern, although it may present with varying degrees of clinical severity. It is generally thought to be a benign disease in children in contrast to other types of glomerulonephritis.

The disease usually follows 7–14 days after group A, beta-haemolytic streptococcal infection.

In most cases the preceding infection is localised to the upper respiratory tract, but in some cases it may follow a streptococcal skin infection. Acute glomerulonephritis occurs most commonly between the ages of 3 and 7 years and is considered rare in children under the age of 2 years. The typical syndrome comprises sudden onset of oliguria, haematuria, proteinuria, reduced glomerular filtration rate, oedema and hypertension. The disease, however, may be mild and be manifest by the presence of haematuria only. A positive throat culture for the organism is found in only 15% of cases. The anti-streptolysin O titre which rises within the first 3 weeks of the disease can be detected in more than 80% of patients, similarly the third component of serum complement (C3) is markedly reduced in up to 90% of cases. These markers usually return to normal within 3 months, however, the haematuria may persist for more than 1 year.

When the only manifestation is haematuria, all other possible causes must be excluded. A 10-day course of a suitable antibiotic, usually penicillin, is given to eradicate streptococcal infection. If there is evidence of fluid overload, oliguria, or a raised blood pressure, the child should be admitted to hospital. The salt and water retention are responsible for the hypertension which can be life threatening and associated with pulmonary oedema, hypertensive encephalopathy and cerebral haemorrhage. Long-term bed rest is not useful and does not affect the eventual outcome. Some exacerbation of haematuria after exercise or during an upper respiratory tract infection is sometimes seen during the healing phase and can be disregarded as long as it is not associated with a deterioration of renal function.

HENOCH–SCHÖNLEIN NEPHRITIS

Renal manifestations are found in from 20–100% of patients with Henoch–Schönlein purpura and tend to be more common and more severe in older children. The variable incidence of renal involvement stems from the differing criteria used to define active disease as well as by different methods used to detect microscopic haematuria. In 80% of patients with the nephropathy, urinary abnormalities will follow the onset of the typical rash within 1 month, and in most others occur within 3 months. Occasionally, urinary abnormalities may precede the onset of the rash or follow it by many months. In older patients severe alimentary system involvement, frequent relapses of skin lesions and late clinical relapses of skin lesions beyond 3 months have been particularly associated with an increased incidence of renal involvement. At presentation, microscopic haematuria with or without proteinuria occurs in from 70% to 80% of cases of Henoch–Schönlein purpura nephropathy, while 20% to 30% will have gross haematuria. The nephrotic syndrome and hypertension are uncommon initial features. A clinical presentation with a mixed nephritic-nephrotic pattern has for many years been recognised as denoting a poor prognosis and there is a small but significant mortality for renal failure (3–8%). The overal prognosis is uncertain, but a 10-year survival of approximately 95% is likely. Follow up should continue until all renal abnormalities including urine deposit have disappeared.

NEPHROTIC SYNDROME

Physiology

The nephrotic syndrome consists of a disturbance of glomerular permeability resulting in albuminuria, hypoalbuminaemia and oedema. Hypoalbuminaemia reduces the plasma colloid osmotic pressure resulting in a seepage of fluid from the intravascular to the interstitial compartment resulting in oedema. The critical plasma albumin concentration is 25 g/l. The loss of fluid from the intravascular compartment results in hypovolaemia and, as it is the plasma volume that is depleted, there is a rise in haemoglobin concentration and packed cell volume. The fall in blood volume leads to poor renal perfusion, and hypovolaemia, if prolonged, may progress to peripheral circulatory collapse, renal failure and death.

In childhood the majority of cases respond to corticosteroid therapy and have only minimal histological changes in the glomeruli evident on light microscopy. The term 'minimal change nephrotic syndrome' has gained popular usage although the expression 'steroid responsive nephrotic syndrome' has the merit of focusing on the most important objective. The condition occurs with a frequency of about 1 case per 100 000 total population per annum and is more common in boys than girls. The peak age is 3 years and it rarely presents under the age of 3 months but can occur throughout adult life. About 15% of children with nephrotic syndrome will have a more serious lesion such as focal sclerosis or membranoproliferative disease. A number of clinical and laboratory characteristics may be associated with minimal change nephrotic syndrome and are therefore viewed as favourable prognostic signs. These are:

1. Age at presentation (between 1 and 14 years).
2. No haematuria.
3. Normal blood pressure and renal function.
4. Highly selective heavy proteinuria (i.e. albumin).
5. Early response to corticosteroid therapy.
6. Normal serum complement (C3) concentration.

Relapses are often precipitated by upper respiratory tract infections.

Management

Hypovolaemia

A hypovolaemic crisis is characterised by vomiting, abdominal pain, faintness and signs of peripheral circulatory failure, and may occur early in relapse even before much oedema is clinically evident. It is a medical emergency and the child should be hospitalised and given a rapid intravenous infusion of plasma.

Diet

An adequate protein intake is necessary to compensate for urinary losses of albumin. The protein intake of a child on an ordinary western diet is probably adequate. Rigorous dietary sodium restriction is usually impractical and unnecessary in children, although excess dietary salt and high sodium-containing foods should be avoided.

Infection

The nephrotic child is prone to infection and, his-torically, the major reduction in mortality in the syndrome followed the introduction of penicillin rather than corticosteroids. Septicaemia due to Gram-negative or Gram-positive organisms and primary peritonitis due to *Streptococcus pneumoniae* should be suspected in every sick nephrotic, and there is much to be said for penicillin prophylaxis against pneumococcal infection in the oedematous child.

Corticosteroids

Prednisolone is the corticosteroid of choice and, for the induction of remission, a high dose of 2 mg/kg bodyweight every 24 hours should be given until response, i.e. freedom from proteinuria (Albustix 0 or trace) for 2 days, followed by stepwise withdrawal over a 6-week period. The same regimen should be used for the treatment of relapse. Common errors in corticosteroid therapy are to use too low a dose, to start reducing dosage before remission has been achieved and to interpret response in terms of control of oedema rather than elimination of proteinuria.

Most steroid-responsive nephrotics will go into remission within 2 weeks of therapy. Two-thirds of the responders will relapse and for the first two or three relapses the objective should be to tail off corticosteroids completely. The frequent relapser, three within 12 months, is considered steroid dependent and can be satisfactorily maintained on alternate-day prednisolone therapy. Up to 0.5 mg/kg bodyweight on alternate days as a single morning dose can be used without much toxicity, and even higher doses are possible in younger children. This regimen should be continued for at least 6 months and, if the child has been relapse-free, the dosage reduced to see if it is still necessary. Careful growth records must be maintained so that if further maintainance therapy is required the risks can be accurately assessed. The side-effects of corticosteroid therapy are well known but can be minimised with careful supervision. These side-effects are:

1. Growth retardation (less with alternate-day therapy).
2. Susceptibility to infection.
3. Hypertension and oedema.

4. Cushingoid features (obesity and striae).
5. Osteoporosis.
6. Increased protein catabolism (associated with increased appetite).
7. Diabetes mellitus.
8. Gastrointestinal complications:
   a. Perforation
   b. Haematemesis
   c. Pancreatitis
9. Intracranial hypertension (during steroid withdrawal).
10. Addisonian crisis.

Immunosupressive drugs, such as cyclophosphamide, have been established as valuable therapy in the frequently relapsing nephrotic child who has become steroid dependent and in some cases steroid resistant. However, the potential toxity of these agents is always worrying and it is generally agreed that if a nephrotic can be maintained in remission on a corticosteroid regimen that does not cause significant side-effects, then cyclophosphamide therapy is not warranted. In the long run most children stop relapsing, although a few persist beyond adolescence, and the prognosis of the steroid-responsive nephrotic child is fundamentally good.

HYPERTENSION

There has been an increasing interest in, and awareness of, systemic hypertension as a problem of childhood and adolescence. Too frequently blood pressure is measured in a hasty, casual fashion without attention to detail, the greatest errors occuring in young infants and obese children. Blood pressure should be determined with the child lying or sitting on the mother's lap and re-laxed. It is of little value if the child is crying. As a rule of thumb, a cuff containing a bladder that will cover two-thirds of the upper arm without impinging on the antecubital fossa should be used. The bladder should encircle as close to the full circumference of the arm as possible. Normal ranges for blood pressure are shown in Table 20.3 and it remains controversial at what level hypertension should be diagnosed. It is clear, however, that a single hypertensive should be rechecked and if a pattern is consistently above the normal range the child should be investigated to exclude treatable causes. Elevated blood pressures are uncommon in childhood. A careful family history for evidence of hypertension or cardiovascular disease should be taken, particularly in those who are asymptomatic. Hypertension may also be secondary and it is important to exclude other disorders such as renal disease (Table 20.4).

The most frequent symptoms include headaches, nausea, vomiting and anorexia, heart failure convulsions and other central nervous system signs such as facial palsy or hemiplegia. Renal parenchymal disease accounts for nearly 80% of sustained hypertension in children, and approximately 10% of this group will have a renovascular basis. Appropriate urography, ultrasound and isotope scanning, and arteriography may reveal the pathology, but the majority of children with chronic hypertension will not have a surgically correctable cause. This group are therefore committed to long-term drug therhapy with the associated problems of compliance adherence to dietary restrictions and regular clinic attendance for evaluation. Traditionally, the management of mild hypertension consists of using a diuretic, thiazide or frusemide, adding a beta-blocking agent such as propranolol, and a peripheral vasodilator such

Table 20.3 Blood pressure measurements in normal children

Age (years)	Mean (mmHg)		95th percentile (mmHg)	
	Systolic	Diastolic	Systolic	Diastolic
0–0.5	80	45	110	60
0.5–3	95	55	115	80
4–7	100	65	120	85
8–10	105	70	130	90
11–15	115	70	140	90

Table 20.4 Aetiology of hypertension

Renovascular	Renal artery stenosis
Parenchymal renal disease	Nephritis, reflux nephropathy, obstructive uropathy, tumours, cystic disease, dysplasia, chronic renal failure
Cardiovascular	Coarctation of the aorta
Endocrine	Adrenal cortex; congenital adrenal hyperplasia, Cushing's syndrome Adrenal medulla; phaeochromocytoma, neuroblastoma Hyperthyroidism
Metabolic	Heavy metal poisoning, hypercalcaemia, salt and water overload
CNS	Raised intracranial pressure, Guillain-Barré syndrome
Essential	

Table 20.5 Causes of acute renal failure in infancy and childhood

Perenal
  Hypovolaemia
    Acute gastroenteritis
    Nephrotic syndrome
    Post surgery
    Burns
    Salt wasting disease (renal and adrenal)

  Hypotension
    Septicaemia
    Hypothermia

Renal
  Acute glomerulonephritis
  Renal venous thrombosis
  Haemolytic uraemic syndrome
  Congenital glomerular and tubular disease
  Nephrotoxins

Postrenal
  Congenital obstructive uropathy

as hydralazine or monoxidil in the refractory or more severe cases. Children who present with a hypertensive emergency may not only demonstrate a severe elevation of blood pressure, but also acute complications such as plumonary oedema, hypertensive encephalopathy and renal failure. These patients require immediate control and maintenance of blood pressure to normal levels and in addition therapy for each complication.

ACUTE RENAL FAILURE

Acute renal failure is a syndrome characterised by sudden disruption of glomerular and tubular function. It may be transient, prolonged, reversible or irreversible. The kidneys are unable to regulate urine flow and composition as manifested by disturbances of fluid, electrolyte and acid-base balance, together with failure of elimination of the products of nitrogen metabolism. Essential for normal renal function are an adequate blood supply of healthy kidneys and a patent functioning non-obstructed urine collection and excretion system. Oliguria exists when the daily urinary output is less than 300 ml/m² surface area. Classically acute renal failure is divided into prerenal, renal and postrenal causes, aetiological factors in each of these areas being somewhat dependent on the age of the child (Table 20.5), acute renal failure is recognised by a rising blood urea and creatinine concentration.

The history and physical examination will frequently indicate the diagnosis. A history of vomiting and diarrhoea suggest salt and water depletion, and hypernatraemic dehydration is common in infants with gastroenteritis who have received high solute feeds. A poor urine stream in young infants suggests urethral valves and obstructive uropathy. A palpable bladder and enlarged kidneys indicate intravesical obstruction. Bilateral gross enlargement of the kidneys is suggestive of polycystic disease and, in acute onset of renal failure, haematuria and enlarged hard kidneys may be caused by renal venous thrombosis. The history and clinical features may be helpful in the diagnosis of nephritis, nephrotic syndrome or haemolytic uraemic syndrome. Short stature, anaemia and evidence of renal osteodystrophy are suggestive of chronic renal disease.

The management of acute renal failure in the child, especially the infant, is different from that in the adult. Treatment and diagnosis proceed concurrently. Detailed knowledge of fluid and electrolyte balance, and the nutritional requirements of the infant are necessary, as is access to the complex technology for specific investigation. The specific and frequently life-threatening problems of hyperkalaemia, hypoglycaemia, hypocalcaemia, acidosis and hypertension each require individual assessment and treatment.

CHRONIC RENAL FAILURE

Chronic renal failure is the outcome of many disease processes, but in children it is predominantly secondary to chronic glomerulonephritis or pyelonephritis (reflux nephropathy). Therapy for chronic renal failure may basically be divided into medical management, and dialysis and transplantation. Careful management of the uraemic child before dialysis or transplantation not only improves survival and prevents acute deterioration which can cause further renal failure damage, but also can ensure that affected children lead relatively normal lives. Frequent outpatient monitoring is essential and careful attention must be directed at each of the potential problems shown below:

1. Biochemical disturbances.
2. Sodium, potassium, calcium, phospate and acidaemia.
3. Nutrition.
4. Plasma proteins and urea production.
5. Infection.
6. Urinary tract and non-renal infections.
7. Renal osteodystrophy.
8. Hypertension.
9. Anaemia.
10. Growth and skeletal maturation.
11. Social development.
12. Schooling and family relationships.
13. Emotional development.

It is essential to maintain close liaison with personnel such as the paediatric dietician and pathologist so that appropriate action can be taken in the management of individual problems as they occur. It is therefore understandable that the management of children with end-stage kidney disease should be carried out in specialist paediatric nephrology units. The results of dialysis and transplantation to date undoubtedly justify considering treatment for all children. Each case must be assessed carefully by a paediatrician and the paediatric nephrology team, not forgetting the considerable stress and discipline that will face the patient and family.

FURTHER READING

Holliday M A, Barratt T M, Vernier R L 1987 Paediatric nephrology, 2nd edn. Williams & Wilkins, Baltimore
Smellie J M 1979 In: Black D, Jones B (eds) Renal disease, 4th edn. Blackwell Scientific, Oxford

21. Endocrine and metabolic disease

C. J. H. Kelnar

GROWTH

Normal growth

A healthy child grows at a normal rate. Although a normal growth rate does not always imply normal health, growth is an accurate, sensitive and useful barometer of child health. All who look after children should be familiar with the normal growth curve (Figs 21.1(a) & (b)) as only then can abnormalities be recognised.

Growth is a dynamic process and growth rate (velocity) gives much more valuable information than does a single measurement of stature. The use of decimal ages facilitates calculation of growth velocity. A slowly growing child has a current pathological disorder which requires diagnosis and, if possible, treatment; but if the condition is of recent onset the child will not have grown slowly for long enough to make him short. Many diseases will not produce obvious symptoms or signs which call attention to the diagnosis. Early diagnosis may only be achieved if all children are measured regularly in primary care.

Growth impairment is particularly likely to have long-term sequelae if it occurs when growth is normally rapid, i.e. during fetal life, infancy and puberty. Growth potential is largely genetically determined, but many differences between the heights of children of the same age depend on variations in timing — how great a proportion of their growth has already occurred. Control of the tempo of growth is probably also genetically determined but little is understood of underlying mechanisms. Assessment of skeletal maturity better estimates the percentage of growth already completed than does chronological age; but it is generally unhelpful in demonstrating presence or absence of pathology or in making specific pathological diagnoses.

Measurement of stature must be accurate. This requires apparatus which is robust, reliable and sensitive and a measurer who is interested and meticulous in attention to detail. Suitable portable apparatus for use by primary carers is now readily available. Good measuring techniques which eliminate postural drops and positional sources of error are readily learned (Fig. 21.2). As a screening test in a short child, measurement of growth velocity is cheaper, more reproducible, more acceptable to the patient and more relevant to diagnosis and treatment than is a venepuncture for the laboratory measurement of plasma growth hormone concentrations.

Unless grossly abnormal, growth velocity is best measured 3 monthly for a full year to eliminate seasonal growth variations shown by many children.

Deciding whether growth is normal necessitates reference to standard growth charts. Ideally each country and ethnic group should have its own growth standards. In practice, UK charts serve well even in developing countries or for ethnic minorities within the UK as differences in overall adult stature reflect quite minor differences in growth velocity over the whole growing period.

The genetic contribution of parents reduces the population standard deviation of height by about 30%. Thus 95% of the children will have a height within ±8.5 cm (±2 SD) of their mid-parental *centile*.

Children inherit more than genes from their parents. They frequently also acquire an adverse environment. Children's shortness, whilst superficially appropriate for their short parents, may

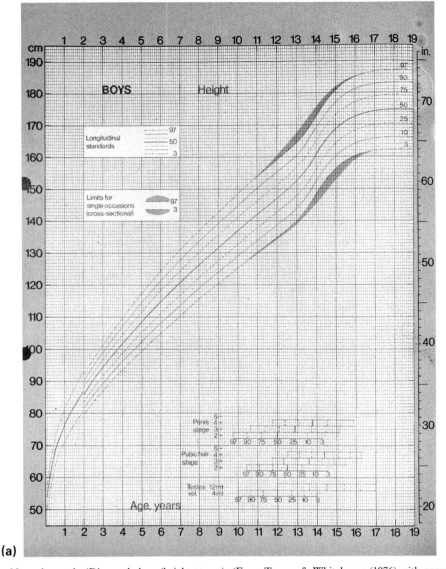

Fig. 21.1 (a)   Normal growth. 'Distance' chart (height × age). (From Tanner & Whitehouse (1976) with permission).

reflect poor nutrition or emotional deprivation continuing down the generations with no one achieving their true height potential. The mean height of children from social class IV and V families remains significantly less than that of those from social classes I and II in Britain in the 1980s as it did in the 1870s, despite the secular trend to increasing height in both groups.

It is important to exclude the possibility of an unrecognised and untreated growth disorder in one unusually short parent before attributing the child's shortness to constitutional reasons. Pathology, such as growth hormone (GH) deficiency, may also be genetically transmitted.

Weight gain is a poor guide to healthy growth (see p. 271). Even in infancy where it is of some use, as growth is very rapid, it largely reflects changes in fluid. In the older child, differences between normal and abnormal weight gain are smaller than the reproducibility of weight meas-

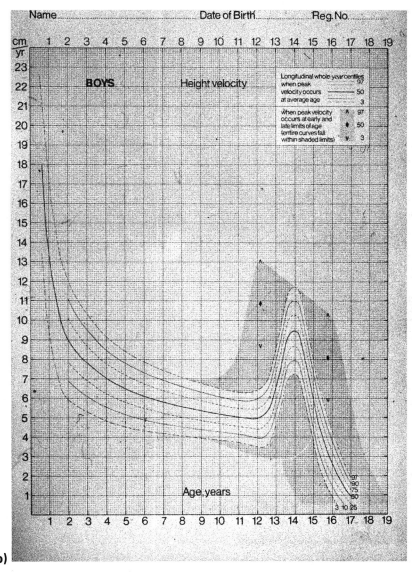

(b)

Fig. 21.1 (b) Normal growth. 'Velocity' chart (rate of growth × age). (From Tanner & Whitehouse (1976) with permission).

urements obtained even on sophisticated apparatus some months apart. Obsessional weighing at frequent intervals is valueless and causes unnecessary anxiety. The adequacy, inadequacy or overadequacy of nutrition is best assessed using skin-fold calipers (Fig. 21.3) which measure directly thickness of subcutaneous fat.

The short child

Without diagnostic clues from history or examin-

ation, the screening test for a child who presents with short stature is calculation of growth velocity. A small child who is growing normally either has small parents (constitutional short stature, but see above), growth delay, or had grown poorly in the past because of some factor no longer operative (e.g. prolonged intra-uterine growth retardation or corrected congenital heart disease) or a combination of such factors. Whatever their ultimate height prognosis (if there is significant growth delay it may be normal), many of these children

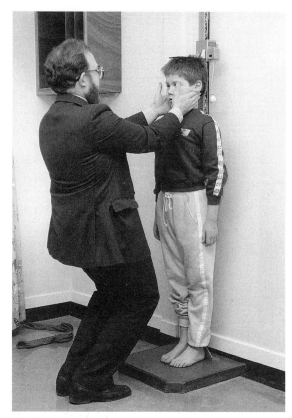

Fig. 21.2   Accurate measurement of height.

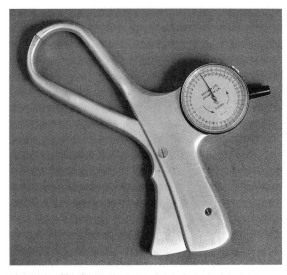

Fig. 21.3   Skinfold calipers (available from Holtain Ltd, Crymmych, Dyfed, Wales).

will be teased and bullied at school, will under-achieve and be emotionally immature. Social consequences of short stature are not dependent on the presence of underlying pathology.

Shorter people secrete less growth hormone than taller people and biosynthetic growth hormone is widely available. Social pressures are therefore increasing for treating such children with growth hormone. Research is currently aimed at answering four questions:

1. Will GH increase growth velocity in the short term?
2. Will it produce taller adults?
3. Will it produce 'better' (i.e. more socially adjusted and successful) adults?
4. What are the psychological and physical risks of treatment?

Present knowledge does not justify indiscriminate use of growth hormone in these children. Concern is most properly directed at children with inadequate growth velocity (whatever their current height) (Table 21.1).

Disproportionate short stature (short trunk or short limbs) is diagnosed from sitting height measurements (subischial leg length equals stature minus sitting height). An aetiological diagnosis requires a skeletal survey, expert radiologist and reference atlas of skeletal dysplasias. The fat short child is likely to have an endocrine cause of his short stature (and obesity).

Differential diagnosis of the child who is short and not fat covers the whole field of chronic disease. Some diseases may be suspected from history or clinical findings. Important conditions with poor growth as perhaps the only diagnostic clue include psychosocial deprivation, unrecognised asthma, malabsorption and Turner's syndrome. Clinical examination should include fundoscopy and visual fields — the earliest sign of a craniopharyngioma may be poor growth. Investigations of the slowly growing child should include skull X-ray, creatinine, urea and electrolytes, calcium, phosphate, alkaline phosphatase, haemoglobin, full blood count and ESR, but may need to include karyotype and jejunal biopsy.

Many provocation tests are available for diagnosis of severe growth hormone insufficiency. Insulin hypoglycaemia remains the best. It is a safe

Table 21.1 Differential diagnosis of short stature or slow growth

---

Short with currently normal growth velocity:
Constitutional short stature (short normal parent(s))

Previous problem affecting growth now cured or no longer operative, e.g. prolonged intrauterine growth retardation, congenital heart disease

Physiological growth delay

Growing slowly (whether already short or still of 'normal' stature):
With increased skinfold thicknesses:
endocrine disease: panhypopituitarism; severe growth hormone insufficiency, idiopathic or secondary to tumour or irradiation; hypothyroidism; pseudohypoparathyroidism; Cushing's syndrome

Disproportionate:
a. Short limbs for spine: the dyschondroplasias e.g. achondroplasia; hypochondroplasia; multiple epiphyseal dysplasia

b. Short limbs and spine (spine relatively shorter): mucopolysaccharidoses, metatrophic dwarfism

Often without other obvious signs of disease (see text). Many chronic illnesses in childhood:
a. Chromosomal: Turner's syndrome (other signs variable)
b. Unrecognised asthma (may be misdiagnosed)
c. Malabsorption due to coeliac disease, ulcerative colitis, Crohn's disease (bowel habit may be normal)
d. Psychosocial deprivation
e. Malnutrition
f. Cardiovascular or renal disease

---

test if adequately supervised by staff who perform it frequently and can be combined with other pituitary function tests. The prevalence of severe growth hormone insufficiency (maximum stimulated GH <7 mU/l) is about 1 in 5000. Such children need growth hormone therapy. An appropriate regimen is 24 units/m²/week daily subcutaneously at bedtime.

Measurement of spontaneous nocturnal pulsatile growth hormone release gives insight into secretory control mechanisms. Although there may be a relationship between the amplitude of such pulses and growth velocity, their relevance to short stature assessment remains controversial and it is impracticable to use such tests to screen large numbers of short or slowly growing children.

Treatment of short stature aims to correct the underlying problem where possible (e.g. gluten-free diet in coeliac disease, thyroxine in hypothyroidism). Treatment can only maximise growth potential available at its commencement. The sooner poor growth is recognised, its cause diagnosed and appropriate treatment started, the better the height prognosis.

Unconventional indications for growth hormone include Turner's syndrome (a 'mild' skeletal dysplasia with both poor (but variable) growth hormone secretion and poor bone response to it). Possible side-effects include hyperlipidaemia, hypertension and glucose intolerance if it is used in children already secreting significant amounts.

Anabolic steroid (e.g. oxandrolone 2.5 mg daily orally) will increase growth in girls with Turner's syndrome and in combination with growth hormone seems even more effective. The effect on final height is, as yet, unknown and clitoromegaly can be a problem. It seems effective also in increasing the (normal) slow growth of early male puberty, improving morale in those with maturational delay.

The tall child

Tall stature presents to a clinician less often than does short stature: to be tall, unless it is extreme, is socially advantageous and syndromes causing tallness are rare, whereas poor growth and ultimately short stature is a consequence of much childhood disease.

The excessively tall child may have problems whether or not he has an underlying pathological condition: because he looks older than he is, expectations are greater than he can meet and his bulk may make him both clumsy and aggressive.

Tall stature syndromes are shown in Table 21.2. Tallness with obesity is nearly always due to overeating — past or present. If overeating is continuing growth velocity will be excessive, if not it will be normal. Skeletal maturity is advanced so that final stature is not increased (see below p. 271).

Precocious puberty is a common reason for a child presenting with rapid growth and tall stature although final height will be short. Increased growth velocity without puberty or continuing overeating may, uncommonly, be due to thyrotoxicosis or, rarely, to gigantism (excessive growth hormone secretion by a pituitary tumour).

Advanced skeletal maturation may be associated

Table 21.2 Differential diagnosis of tall stature or rapid growth

---

Tall with currently normal growth velocity:
Constitutional tall stature (tall normal parent(s))

Previously rapid growth (usually due to overeating)

Physiological growth advance

Currently rapid growth (whether already tall or still of 'normal' stature):
Associated with precocious puberty (p. 254)

Not associated with signs of puberty:
a. thyrotoxicosis
b. growth hormone excess (gigantism)

With dysmorphic features or disproportion:
   Marfan's syndrome
   homocystinuria
   Sotos' syndrome (cerebral gigantism)
   Klinefelter's syndrome

With obesity: currently excessive food intake

---

with tallness in childhood (and a normal growth velocity) but this seldom results in medical help being sought, unlike growth delay.

Tall mothers sometimes worry about their daughters' heights. They remember their own adolescent problems and difficulty in finding a husband who was tall enough. Having found him they realise their daughters may become excessively tall. Height prognosis in tall stature can be computed (as with short stature) from chronological age, skeletal maturity and growth velocity. If socially unacceptable, consideration can be given to reducing it.

Unfortunately treatment, whether attempting to limit growth hormone secretion whilst allowing normal sex steroid-mediated skeletal maturation (e.g. with bromocriptine) or rapidly advancing skeletal maturation (using sex steroids), is unsatisfactory. Testosterone in boys seems successful but is seldom indicated. Oestrogen in girls causes initial increase in growth velocity and potential side-effects from the high doses necessary, both short term (headaches, nausea) and long term (diabetes mellitus, hyperlipidaemia, hypertension, endometrial carcinoma), severely limit its usefulness. It cannot be used much before the normal time of pubertal onset and treatment after the onset of the pubertal growth spurt (which occurs early in female puberty) will have only a small effect in reducing final height.

PUBERTY

Normal puberty

The Tanner–Whitehouse staging of puberty is well known (Fig. 21.4). Individual secondary sexual characteristics are the results of different hormonal events and must be assessed independently. Normal pubertal development is an harmonious process and marked discrepancies from the normal sequence of events (Fig. 21.5) should lead to suspicion of pathology.

The timing of puberty is very variable in the normal population (Fig. 21.5). There is about a 4-year difference between the earliest 3% who reach a given stage of puberty and the most delayed 3%. Social and emotional pressures on those at either end of this normal spectrum can be considerable. There are only small differences between the sexes in the average times at which nocturnal pulsatile gonadotrophin-releasing hormone activity increases sharply to induce pubertal changes. However the earliest sign of male puberty (testicular enlargement) is less obvious than breast budding in girls. Girls grow rapidly early in puberty (with increased growth velocity sometimes even preceding breast development). Boys do not reach maximal growth velocity until their testes are around 10–12 ml in volume. Girls do seem to mature earlier in emotional and psychological terms. Testicular enlargement is most simply and accurately assessed using the Prader orchidometer (Fig. 21.6).

Normal but late developing boys are growing slowly, undeveloped genitally and less broad shouldered and muscular than their peers, and can also be overtaken in height by a younger sister. Some boys worry about their small penis during early adolescence. In the plump boy it may appear buried in a fat pad. It does not enlarge until genitalia stage 3 — perhaps a year after the testes and scrotum have begun to enlarge.

Menarche in girls does not occur until after peak height velocity has been passed — the amount of growth ahead of a slowly growing girl is very different depending on whether menarche has been reached. Early periods tend to be irregular and anovular.

The greater the discrepancy between chronological age and skeletal maturity, whether due to

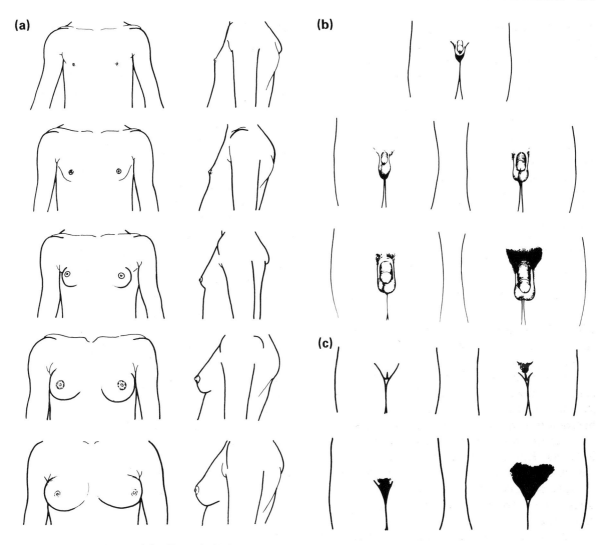

Fig. 21.4 Pubertal stages (after Tanner). (**a**) Breasts (1–5). (**b**) Genitalia in males (1–5). (**c**) Pubic hair (2–5).

pathological or physiological events, the greater the relevance of bone age to the timing of puberty. A boy with bone age of 6 years at chronological age of 9 years is *likely* to enter puberty spontaneously late and therapy to induce puberty may be appropriate.

There is no relationship between age at pubertal onset and duration of puberty. The most rapidly developing 3% of normal girls will reach stage 5 breasts within 18 months of reaching stage 2, the slowest 3% may take 9 years — the average is 4 years.

The trigger for puberty onset is unknown.

Adrenal androgens increase from about 7 years. In some children there is a coincident short-lived increase in growth velocity and steeper rises in normal blood pressure centiles occur but a causal connection between adrenarche and these events or with gonadarche (the later gonadotrophin rise) remains speculative. Adrenal androgens cause apocrine sweating, an early sign that other pubertal events are imminent.

The size of the pubertal growth spurt is much greater in boys, accounting for most of the difference in height between men and women (12.6 cm between the respective 50th centile

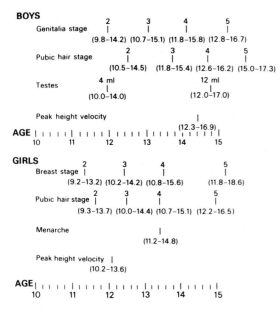

BOYS
Genitalia stage
2   3   4   5
(9.8–14.2) (10.7–15.1) (11.8–15.8) (12.8–16.7)

Pubic hair stage
2   3   4   5
(10.5–14.5) (11.8–15.4) (12.6–16.2) (15.0–17.3)

Testes
4 ml   12 ml
(10.0–14.0)   (12.0–17.0)

Peak height velocity
(12.3–16.9)

AGE   10   11   12   13   14   15

GIRLS
Breast stage
2   3   4   5
(9.2–13.2) (10.2–14.2) (10.8–15.6)   (11.8–18.6)

Pubic hair stage
2   3   4   5
(9.3–13.7) (10.0–14.4) (10.7–15.1) (12.2–16.5)

Menarche
(11.2–14.8)

Peak height velocity
(10.2–13.6)

AGE   10   11   12   13   14   15

Fig. 21.5 Sequence of pubertal events (average age at development of a characteristic plus or minus 2 SD).

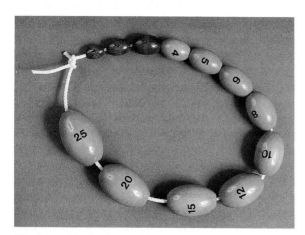

Fig. 21.6 The Prader orchidometer (available from Holtain Ltd, Crymmych, Dyfed, Wales).

heights). Growth decelerates until the pubertal stage is reached at which acceleration begins, and boys with growth delay may almost stop growing if still prepubertal at 15 or 16 years of age.

Early pubertal growth is relatively greater in the legs because of increasing growth hormone secretion — hence the gangling appearance of boys in mid-puberty. As puberty progresses testosterone secretion increases and this predominately stimulates spinal growth. Both hormones act synergistically in the context of the pubertal growth spurt as a whole. A child with early or delayed puberty may suffer just as much in emotional and psychological terms whether or not there is underlying organic pathology. Understanding the harmonious changes underlying normal pubertal development is essential if reassurance or, if appropriate, treatment is to be effective.

Early puberty

There is no specific age below which a pathological cause for pubertal development will certainly be found. It is reasonable to investigate any girl under 8 years with secondary sexual characteristics and any boy under 9 years. 'Idiopathic' early puberty seems much commoner in girls. Where a girl's development is harmonious and proceeds at a normal tempo, invasive investigations to exclude pathology are usually unnecessary. A full history and examination (including pubertal staging, height and growth velocity, central nervous system and abdomen) together with skull X-ray, pelvic and abdominal ultrasound, gonadotrophin and TSH measurements (basally and in response to thyrotrophin-releasing hormone and gonadotrophin-releasing hormone) plus basal prolactin and oestradiol measurements will normally exclude pathological causes.

Pathological causes of early puberty are:

1. Intracranial space-occupying lesions.
2. Gonadal tumours.
3. Ectopic gonadotrophin-producing tumour (e.g. hepatoblastoma).
4. Adrenal:
   a. Congenital adrenal hyperplasia:
      i. 21-hydroxylase deficiency
      ii. 11β-hydroxylase deficiency
   b. Cushing's syndrome
   c. Neoplasia
5. Oestrogen ingestion (e.g. mother's oral contraceptives).
6. Primary hypothyroidism.
7. Undefined mechanisms:

a. Birth asphyxia
b. Mental retardation including tuberous sclerosis, neurofibromatosis
c. McCune–Albright syndrome

If no underlying cause is found which itself requires treatment the need to suppress gonadotrophin secretion and further pubertal development depends on the girl's age, the rate of progression, social circumstances and family emotional relationships.

Boys present with precocious puberty less often but, as the incidence of pathological causes is greater, the likelihood of finding pathology is high — usually a cerebral lesion or pseudo-precocious puberty due to the non-salt-losing 21-hydroxylase deficiency form of congenital adrenal hyperplasia (see list above). A clue to the latter diagnosis is finding small testes — the adrenals are the androgen source.

Breast development alone sometimes occurs in a female toddler and may cause much parental anxiety. Isolated premature thelarche is unassociated with *any* other manifestation of puberty (including an increase in growth velocity); if the physical examination is otherwise normal, there may be waxing and waning in breast size but they will usually fade away. A pelvic ultrasound demonstrating normal prepubertal ovaries and uterus and a normal lateral skull X-ray will provide further grounds for reassurance.

At diagnosis of precocious puberty, sex steroid secretion has usually caused very significant bone age advance. There is no evidence that treatment will improve the very reduced height prognosis, although if optimal it will prevent it from deteriorating further. However treatment with growth hormone whilst suppressing puberty is being tried. Emotional problems may be marked in children who are initially tall and aggressive but who end up very small.

Check thyroid function (particularly TSH levels) in any child with precocious puberty even if clinically euthyroid. A failing thyroid gland causes hypothalamic release of thyrotrophin-releasing hormone (TRH). The resulting high TSH levels maintain normal thyroid function but TRH also causes prolactin and gonadotrophin release, resulting in ovarian oestradiol secretion and breast development. A goitre may be present.

Precocious puberty with delayed bone age is pathognomonic of the condition.

If normal pubertal mechanisms have become activated (for whatever reason), gonadotrophin levels will be high compared to prepuberty with a predominating luteinising hormone (LH) response to intravenous gonadotrophin-releasing hormone (GnRH) in contrast to the follicle-stimulating hormone (FSH) predominating response in prepuberty. Ovarian or other peripheral source of sex steroid will cause gonadotrophin suppression.

Vaginal bleeding unassociated with adequate breast development for this to be postmenarchal must be taken seriously. Genital tumours may present in this way as may a vaginal foreign body, sexual abuse, atrophic vulvitis and vaginitis or oestrogen ingestion.

Pathological causes of precocious puberty, such as hydrocephalus, hypothyroidism or an ovarian tumour, may require treatment in their own right. Otherwise treatment of the clinical effects by suppressing the hypothalamo-pituitary-gonadal axis may be appropriate. Cyproterone acetate, an anti-gonadotrophin which also suppresses the hypothalamo-pituitary-adrenal axis (patients need steroid cover during severe illness, infection or other stress) is being superseded by GnRH analogues which are more specific: they occupy the GnRH pituitary receptors, blocking gonadotrophin release. There is transient agonist activity before gonadotrophin secretion is turned off and development arrested. They can be given intranasally or as subcutaneous implants. Treatment ceases when the child's normal peers are at an equivalent stage of puberty, and subsequent development will progress normally.

Some children have pubic and axillary hair growth from around 7 years (premature adrenarche). Adrenal androgens (dehydroepiandrosterone, androstenedione) are usually elevated, but the hypothalamo-pituitary-gonadal axis is quiescent. No action is necessary unless follow-up indicates this to be the first sign of true early puberty.

Late puberty

Late puberty, particularly when accompanied by short stature and delayed skeletal maturation, is the commonest reason for referral to a paediatric endocrinologist. It is commoner in boys who are also more stressed by it as their growth deceleration continues until puberty is well advanced and they may become conspicuously short whilst remaining undeveloped.

Pathological causes of late puberty are listed below:

1. Hypothalamic/pituitary:
   a. GnRH deficiency
   b. Gonadotrophin deficiency including Kallmann's syndrome
   c. Panhypopituitarism
   d. Anorexia, anorexia nervosa
   e. Systemic illness
   f. Post-irradiation
   g. Craniopharyngioma, prolactinoma
2. Gonadal:
   a. Sex-steroid deficiency due to anorchia/hypoplastic testes
   b. Ovarian dysgenesis — usually Turner's syndrome
   c. Enzyme defects (also in adrenal):
      i. 20, 22-desmolase
      ii. 3β-hydroxysteroid dehydrogenase
      iii. 17α-hydroxylase
      iv. 17,20-lyase
      v. 17α-reductase
      vi. Aromatase
3. Other endocrinopathies:
   a. Hypothyroidism
   b. Congenital adrenal hypoplasia

These are much commoner in girls where gonadal dysgenesis (usually Turner's syndrome and its mosaic forms) is the cause in up to 40%. A karyotype is an important investigation in any slowly growing girl and mandatory if puberty is delayed even without any other signs of Turner's syndrome.

Assessment must include careful physical examination and measurement of height velocity. Early testicular enlargement is often overlooked by the patient and referring physician. An assessment of skeletal maturity will determine the likely delay before puberty starts spontaneously, if it will do so, but seldom distinguishes underlying pathology from physiological maturational delay.

The imminence of puberty can be assessed by measuring gonadotrophins during sleep — pulsatile nocturnal GnRH release will be observed before the clinical onset of puberty is detectable — or more practically by measuring gonadotrophins in response to a small (0.25 μg/kg) intravenous dose of GnRH. If puberty is imminent the LH response will be greater than that of FSH and a significant rise will be seen. An elevated basal level of prolactin in an unstressed child is a sensitive indicator of the presence of intracranial pathology as a cause of delayed puberty and is an indication for neuroradiological investigations. At any age normal testes will respond to stimulation by LH (given as HCG) by secreting testosterone. In hypogonadotrophic hypogonadism there is a presumed lack of LH receptors in the testis, both basal and stimulated levels of gonadotrophins will be low and the testosterone response to HCG will be absent. Absent puberty and tall stature in a boy suggest gonadotrophin deficiency or Klinefelter's syndrome. Where height and degree of skeletal maturational delay seem appropriate for the family in terms of final height prediction, the delay is probably physiological.

If pathology is suspected investigations should be carried out urgently. Treatment of the underlying lesion may be necessary and puberty induced at a normal time and tempo. Otherwise, although much can be learnt by observation of growth and for the first signs of development over a period of months, the pressures on individuals at school can be enormous and the short undeveloped and poorly qualified 16-year-old school-leaver may find it particularly difficult to obtain employment.

It is a common misconception that puberty should be induced as late as possible to maximise prepubertal growth and final stature. This is inappropriate because continuing late prepubertal growth deceleration leads to a lower point from which to accelerate and because the pubertal growth spurt magnitude in a late developer is smaller. It is also unkind to subject the child to unnecessary social and emotional pressures. With optimal treatment, puberty can be started at an average time and continued at an appropriate tempo. In practice, this is easier to achieve in girls. Oral ethinyl oestradiol 1–2 μg daily will produce some breast development and an increase in growth velocity. The dose can be doubled after 6–9 months and subsequently to reach 10 μg daily by 18 months to 2 years after starting. Breakthrough bleeding may occur on this dose and a 5-day course of progestogen followed by a week off therapy will allow a proper withdrawal bleed. A combined oestrogen/progestogen regimen should then be given cyclically. The use of Loestrin-20 (noretristerone acetate and ethinyl-oestradiol) or a similar low-dose pill has theoretical disadvantages because of the high progestogen content but the practical advantage of convenience over the use of separate preparations. An increase to 30 μg of oestrogen is sometimes necessary for full breast development.

Too large a starting dose and too rapid an escalation of the dose will reduce the magnitude of the growth spurt, produce cosmetically unattractive cyclindrical breasts and potential difficulties in the important emotional and psychological aspects of adolescent development. There are anxieties about the effects on the liver that the oral route of oestrogen administration will produce.

In boys, the situation is less satisfactory as testosterone cannot at present be given in small doses to mimic the physiological events of early puberty. A depot preparation of testosterone esters (Sustanon) can be used (100 mg i.m. once every 6 weeks and increasing to 250 mg every 3–4 weeks over a 2-year period), but the oral preparation testosterone undecanoate may be preferable (40 mg alternate days increasing to 120 mg daily over 3 years).

A boy may have 2 years or more to wait after his testes begin to enlarge before he subjectively notices growth acceleration. Oxandrolone may bring forward this increase in growth velocity without compromising final height.

INTERSEX

Gender depends on a number of features which are normally self-consistent in any one individual: genetic sex — XX for a female, XY for a male; gonadal sex — presence of ovaries or testes; phenotypic sex — the internal and external genital structures. The sex of rearing usually depends more on functional possibilities than on genetic or gonadal sex. Although later psychosexual orientation was thought to be dependent on sex of rearing, it seems likely that a fetal testis may be paramount in imprinting subsequent male orientation. The 'normal' line of fetal differentiation is female. A testis-determining gene on the short arm of the Y chromosome (at a slightly different location to the cell membrane H-Y antigen) is probably even more important than the latter in the process by which a Y chromosome directs the primitive gonad to form a testis.

Secretion of testosterone and Müllerian inhibiting hormone causes male internal accessory structures and external genitalia to develop whilst suppressing the further development of what would have become cervix, uterus and fallopian tubes. Fetal androgen deficiency in a male may lead to appearances anywhere between severe hypospadias to a 'normal female' appearance. Exposure of a female fetus to androgen may result in anything from clitoromegaly to a 'normal male' appearance. It therefore makes sense to classify disorders on an aetiological rather than descriptive basis and this is becoming increasingly possible.

The cause of ambiguous genitalia, and the sex of the infant, cannot be identified by clinical examination alone. However if both gonads are palpable in labioscrotal folds the baby is likely to be a male with XY karyotype in whom there is a defect in testosterone biosynthesis or tissue insensitivity to testosterone.

If no gonads are palpable the most likely diagnosis is congenital adrenal hyperplasia and a watch must be kept for possible salt loss in the most common form — 21-hydroxylase deficiency. Rarely hypertension will develop (11β-hydroxylase deficiency). In all cases of neonatal ambiguous genitalia an urgent karyotype must be obtained. Gender assignment should be based on all information available including ethnic background and practical possibilities.

A firm diagnosis is necessary to plan future management (e.g. the removal of intra-abdominal testes in an XY female to guard against malignant change, puberty induction) and for genetic counselling. It is essential to make a plan with a paediatric surgeon for correction of ambiguous genitalia (e.g. clitoral reduction in a girl, construction of a penile urethra in a boy). Where possible a normal appearance should be achieved by school age; however the construction of an artificial vagina is best delayed until adolescence.

UNDESCENDED TESTES

Cryptorchidism, in the context of otherwise normal external male genitalia, is less common than normally retractile prepubertal testes. Normal testes descend towards the end of fetal life because of the effects of gonadotrophin-induced testosterone secretion. They will not do so if there is gonadotrophin deficiency, if the testes do not produce testosterone or if there is an anatomical impediment in the line of descent (much more commonly a unilateral problem).

Testes may be retractile until puberty commences. A record that both testes were present in the scrotum in the newborn period or subsequently is invaluable later if testis are difficult to coax down because of an active cremasteric reflex. If doubt remains, administration of HCG for 1 week (3000 units in 3 divided intramuscular injections) will cause descent of the merely retractile testis.

An undescended testis which has not been surgically brought into the scrotum by mid-childhood is unlikely to be normally spermatogenetic. It may be atrophic or functionally inadequate (and not have descended for that reason), but for cosmetic reasons and to maximise function it should be placed in the scrotum if at all possible before school age.

Bilateral cryptorchidism is usually due to an endocrine abnormality at pituitary or testicular level, or both, and endocrine investigation (GnRH and HCG stimulation tests) and a karyotype will identify the problem and should be undertaken before surgery is contemplated. In primary gonadal failure or hypogonadotrophic hypogonadism puberty will need inducing at the appropriate time. If no functional testicular tissue is present surgery is generally not worthwhile. If there is functional testicular tissue present in an ectopic situation it should be removed if it cannot be placed in a reasonable position in the scrotum.

INBORN ERRORS

Most inborn errors of metabolism are individually rare conditions. Many have devastating consequences which can be prevented if diagnosis is early and treated appropriately. Although screening programmes have been developed for a few disorders (e.g. phenylketonuria, galactosaemia and congenital hypothyroidism), most are too rare to make screening of the whole population a practical possibility. Screening of at-risk populations may be appropriate if heterozygote detection is possible (e.g. Ashkenazi Jews for Tay–Sachs disease) or antenatal diagnosis may be possible in subsequent pregnancies following the birth of one affected infant. Sometimes an infant may die of septicaemia or respiratory failure secondary to an underlying metabolic disorder. A family history of unexplained neonatal deaths should arouse suspicion of an inherited metabolic disorder, particularly if the parents are consanguineous — many are recessively inherited.

There may be other clinical clues to a metabolic disorder: in infancy intermittent metabolic acidosis with or without coma, massive ketosis in the context of severe vomiting, persistent vomiting mimicking pyloric stenosis but with acidosis, a myoclonic seizure disorder, extensive perineal candidiasis or an unusual smell of body or urine; in later childhood, mental retardation, renal stones, coarse facial features, dislocated lenses, hypopigmentation, osteoporosis and failure to thrive.

Disorders of branched-chain amino acid metabolism (e.g. propionic or methylmalonic acidaemias in which there is intolerance of dietary isoleucine, valine, threonine and methionine) classically present with vomiting, poor feeding, acidosis, napkin candidiasis, ketonuria, failure to thrive and hypotonia. There may be associated neutropenia and thrombocytopenia.

Dietary management must provide adequate amounts of these essential amino acids to allow normal growth but not so much that toxic intermediate metabolites accumulate. Appropriate management will result in normal growth and intelligence.

Urea cycle defects (hyperammonaemias) usually present with lethargy and seizures progressing to coma in the early days of life. Secondary septicaemia may develop and death may anyway be attributed to overwhelming infection. Plasma ammonia levels will be very high. Amino acid chromatography will indicate the site of the urea cycle block. Transient hyperammonaemia of the newborn sometimes occurs in preterm babies and is self-limiting as enzyme systems mature, provided the infant survives. Mechanical ventilation may be necessary.

Phenylketonuria (PKU) is an important cause of mental retardation. Phenylalanine, another essential amino acid, is normally converted in the liver to tyrosine by the enzyme phenylalanine hydroxylase. Infants with PKU (1 in 7000 births in the UK) lack this enzyme and phenylalanine (in milk feeds) accumulates and causes brain damage. Inheritance is autosomal recessive and screening of all babies in the UK is carried out using the Guthrie test on the sixth day of life. Dietary management aims to maintain normal phenylalanine levels and thus achieve normal intellectual development. There are variants of classical PKU with biopterin (the cofactor for phenylalanine hydroxylase) deficiency, in which there is still mental retardation despite the achievement of normal phenylalanine levels. Some may respond to biopterin supplements.

Mental retardation is also common in patients with homocystinuria, probably because of intracerebral thrombotic and embolic episodes secondary to abnormal platelet function and endothelial desquamation in arteries. Pulmonary, coronary and renal thromboses may also occur. Patients are tall and thin with a *marfanoid* appearance but lenses are characteristically displaced downwards in contrast to Marfan's syndrome. Joint movement is restricted, not lax. Prenatal diagnosis is available.

Storage disorders may also cause mental retardation. The abnormal material stored may be mucopolysaccharide or lipid. In the mucopolysaccharidoses, mental retardation is common but not invariable. Each specific enzyme defect will give rise to a more or less specific clinical syndrome. There may be hepatosplenomegaly, thickened cardiac valves, corneal clouding and a coarse-featured appearance with frontal bossing, hypertelorism, a depressed nasal bridge, gum hypertrophy and a thickened tongue. Radiographic abnormalities are variable but include a J-shaped sella turcica, widening of the medial clavicles with hypoplastic distal portions, broad ribs, a hook-shaped gibbus projecting from the lower thoracic and upper lumbar

spine ('beaking') and hypoplastic ilia. Specific diagnosis is based on the nature of the mucopolysaccharide excreted in the urine, the clinical features and an examination of radioactive sulphate metabolism in cultured fibroblasts. The conditions are autosomally recessively inherited except in the case of Type II (Hunter's syndrome) which is X-linked. Treatment with bone marrow transplantation to 'provide' the missing enzyme has been used to treat affected infants.

Tay–Sachs disease is the best known variety of a large group of gangliosidoses in which a genetically determined enzyme defect of sphingolipid metabolism results in ganglioside storage in brain and viscera. Onset is in the first 6 months and 80% of cases occur in families of Ashkenazi Jewish ancestry. An early sign is the exaggerated startle (Moro) reflex to sound (hyperacusis) but otherwise there may be no abnormalities for the first 6 months of life. Subsequently hypotonia, lethargy and nystagmus develop with loss of fixation and a cherry red macular retinal spot becomes visible. Gradual deterioration occurs in developmental skills and vision and the infant becomes blind and decerebrate, usually dying by around 2 years of age. Heterozygote carriers can be identified in the at-risk population and amniocentesis in pregnancies at risk will establish the diagnosis by enzymic assay of cultured amniotic fluid (i.e. fetal) cells and the pregnancy may be terminated.

Reduction in incidence of a disease in a population cannot be achieved by intra-uterine diagnosis and selective termination. Neonatal screening is worthwhile if:

1. The disease is common.
2. It cannot be diagnosed clinically early enough to prevent serious long-term consequences in growth or neurological development.
3. Such consequences can be prevented by early appropriate treatment.
4. The screening test is reliable, simple, cheap and has a very low false positive and false negative rate.

Hypothyroidism and phenylketonuria fulfil these criteria. Most metabolic abnormalities do not.

The mapping of the human genome and development of specific gene probes is bringing closer the possibility of prevention of some metabolic defects.

HYPOGLYCAEMIA

Hypoglycaemia is not a diagnosis. It is a common but often poorly investigated and managed metabolic abnormality. If prolonged or recurrent it can lead to neuroglycopenia and potentially irreversible brain damage.

Normal metabolic consequences of starvation followed by counter-regulation are increased plasma fatty acids, glycerol, ketone bodies and branched chain amino acids associated with high levels of cortisol, growth hormone and catecholamines. Insulin levels will be low or undetectable. The marked presence of ketones excludes hyperinsulinism as causing the hypoglycaemia. Ketotic hypoglycaemia is not a diagnosis in itself but requires elucidation to find the cause.

Normal neonates and young children are less tolerant of starvation than are adults — blood glucose levels start to fall after starvation of 6–12 hours. Sepsis or birth asphyxia may make the situation more precarious, particularly in light-for-dates infants who have high glucose requirements but poor gluconeogenetic mechanisms.

Neonatal symptoms of hypoglycaemia are non-specific and include jitteriness, hypotonia, feeding difficulties, pallor, tachypnoea, convulsions and coma. In the older child symptoms are attributible to neuroglycopenia (mental confusion, bad temper, irritability, headache, visual disturbances, confused behaviour, convulsions, coma) or to the effect of counter-regulatory hormones (pallor, sweating).

Important causes of hypoglycaemia in the neonate, infants and older children are:

1. Hyperinsulinism:
   a. Nesidioblastosis (neonatal — infancy)
   b. Wiedemann–Beckwith syndrome (neonatal — infancy)
   c. Infant of diabetic mother (transient neonatal)
   d. Islet cell adenoma (childhood)
   e. Insulin administration
2. Abnormal gluconeogenesis or glycogenolysis:
   a. Enzyme deficiency (neonatal — infancy)
      e.g. glucose-6-phosphatase
         debrancher
         phosphorylase kinase
         pyruvate dehydrogenase
         glycogen synthetase
   b. Hepatitis
   c. Reye's syndrome
3. Other metabolic disorders (neonatal — infancy):
      galactosaemia
      fructose intolerance
      maple syrup urine disease
4. Hormonal disorders (any age):
      panhypopituitarism
      growth hormone deficiency
      hypothyroidism
      congenital adrenal hyperplasia
      ACTH deficiency
      glucagon deficiency
      adrenomedullary hyporesponsiveness
5. Drug ingestion:
      alcohol
      salicylates
6. 'Accelerated starvation' (see text).

Recent development of recurring hypoglycaemia in the older child is most likely due to hyperinsulinism, 'accelerated starvation', or growth hormone and/or cortisol deficiency. The accidental or non-accidental administration of hypoglycaemic agents should also be suspected and hypoglycaemia anticipated in any child who has ingested alcohol.

History and examination may provide diagnostic clues, e.g. family history of neonatal death or acidosis in an inherited metabolic disorder, short stature and small genitalia in hypopituitarism, hepatomegaly in glycogenolytic and gluconeogenic enzyme abnormalities or galactosaemia. The diagnosis can often be made from a blood sample taken *at the time of hypoglycaemia* and before treatment is started (Table 21.3).

Severe hypoglycaemia without ketonuria or inappropriately low blood ketone body levels for the glucose level is diagnostic of hyperinsulinism. Plasma insulin levels may not be elevated but will be high for the blood glucose. Hyperinsulinism due to infantile nesidioblastosis, in which there is a greatly increased number of islet cells, requires

Table 21.3 Initial investigation of hypoglycaemia (see text)

Blood sample *during hypoglycaemia* (spontaneous or induced):
  glucose
  ketone bodies
  lactate
  insulin
  growth hormone
  cortisol
  catecholamines

Urinalysis *during hypoglycaemia*:
  ketone bodies
  reducing sugars
  catecholamines

treatment with high glucose infusion rates (usually >10 mg glucose/kg/min) to maintain normoglycaemia. Treatment with diazoxide and a thiazide diuretic should be tried and other substances, e.g. somatostatin and GH, have been suggested but there are commonly side-effects with any regimen. Glucagon is valuable in acutely raising plasma glucose levels or while an intravenous glucose drip infusion is being reinserted, but is not useful in maintaining normoglycaemia. Subtotal (95%) pancreatectomy is often necessary. Diabetes mellitus may result requiring insulin treatment but control is usually good because of associated glucagon deficiency.

Hypoglycaemia is an important symptom in four inborn errors of glycogen metabolism: glucose-6-phosphatase deficiency (Type I Glycogen Storage Disease (GSD)), debrancher (Type III GSD), phosphorylase deficiency (Type IV GSD) — all associated with hepatomegaly — and glycogen synthetase deficiency. Differential diagnosis depends on responses to loading tests with oral galactose and glucagon and on hepatic biopsy, for assay of enzyme activity.

Hypoglycaemia may occur in children with congenital adrenal hyperplasia especially during intercurrent stress or infection. Cortisol deficiency may also cause hypoglycaemia in hypopituitarism and associated growth hormone deficiency may exacerbate the problem.

Some children seem particularly sensitive to periods of starvation. Symptomatic hypoglycaemia leading to convulsions may occur during intercurrent infection, particularly with vomiting, after pronounced physical activity or during preoperative starvation. Exclude other causes of ketotic hypoglycaemia before diagnosing 'accelerated starvation'.

Management consists of regular small frequent meals including a snack or sweet drink during the night and oral or intravenous glucose if ketonuria develops. Parents should be instructed in the use of monitoring sticks for hypoglycaemia and ketonuria.

The condition is almost always self-limiting by puberty. These children probably represent one end of a spectrum of tolerance to starvation but some may exemplify hitherto poorly recognised metabolic enzyme disorders, e.g. of β oxidation or medium chain acyl CoA dehydrogenase deficiency.

ADRENAL GLAND

Congenital adrenal hyperplasia (CAH)

Adrenal cortical steroidogenesis is summarised in Figure 21.7. A block due to a specific enzyme deficiency will have potential effects from hormone deficiency distal and metabolite accumulation prior to the block. The cortisol biosynthetic pathway block produces reduced feedback inhibition of ACTH secretion and increased ACTH drive. This may keep plasma cortisol levels normal as enzyme deficiency is seldom complete. An isolated cortisol result is meaningless for diagnosis. ACTH levels should be measured simultaneously; inappropriately raised levels for the cortisol characterise any variety of CAH.

Indications for suspecting the diagnosis:

1. Neonatal ambiguous genitalia.
2. Dehydration, vomiting and urinary salt wasting during the first weeks.
3. Family history of CAH.
4. Unexplained previous neonatal death particularly with consanguineous parents.
5. Collapse during stress, e.g., severe intercurrent illness or surgery.
6. Hirsutism or inappropriate virilisation.
7. Primary amenorrhoea.
8. Hypertension.

Clinical effects will suggest the specific underlying enzyme defect but definitive diagnosis is by detecting raised levels of precursors in blood by

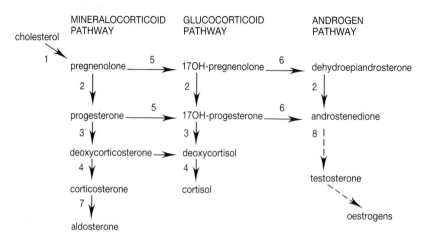

Fig. 21.7 Outline of adrenal steroidogenesis. 1, Cholesterol side chain clearing system; 2, 3β-hydroxysteroid dehydrogenase; 3, 21-hydroxylase; 4, 11β-hydroxylase; 5, 17α-hydroxylase; 6, 17, 20-lyase; 7, 18-hydroxylase and 18-hydroxysteroid dehydrogenase; 8, 17β-hydroxysteroid dehydrogenase.

radioimmunoassay and by gas liquid chromatography of urine for a steroid metabolites. Non-specific tests for classes of compounds, e.g. 17-oxosteroids for adrenal androgens or 17-oxogenic steroids for 17-hydroxylated steroids (predominantly cortisol), have been superseded by specific assays and plasma ACTH measurements.

The commonest variety of CAH is 21-hydroxylase deficiency. Males appear normal at birth but females have clitoromegaly with varying degrees of labial fusion and genital pigmentation resulting from excess androgen secretion. Salt loss may occur during the early weeks but may not present until intercurrent illness later. Only 21-hydroxylase deficiency patients with enzyme deficiency in the zona glomerulosa (affecting the mineralocorticoid biosynthetic pathway) will develop salt loss (this is usually seen in all cases in an affected family). 21-Hydroxylation in mineralocorticoid and glucocorticoid pathways is under separate genetic regulatory control. The incidence of salt loss is about 50% in Western Europe. In 11β-hydroxylase deficiency there will be ambiguity of the female's genitalia but if the enzyme is deficient in the glomerulosa deoxycorticosterone accumulation will occur and this weak mineralocorticoid will, in excess, cause hypertension.

In both these forms of CAH, puberty may be precocious (in other forms of CAH puberty may require induction) and males may not present until rapid growth and genital enlargement develop. Finding small testes with clinical signs of precocious puberty suggests the adrenals are the androgen source but growth advance can be so marked that true precocious puberty results when treatment is started. Continuing rapid growth on treatment may be due to inadequate glucocorticoid replacement, unrecognised mineralocorticoid deficiency (ACTH levels will then remain high despite appropriate glucocorticoid replacement), or the onset of true precocious puberty.

It is possible to screen newborn babies for 21-hydroxylase deficiency using the Guthrie test filter paper. Characteristic raised 17-OH progesterone levels are found. However this screen is generally considered 'uneconomical' despite the severe consequences of late diagnosis. There is significant mortality in boys who present without warning with salt loss and there are emotional problems in the non-salt-losing boy who presents in precocious puberty, large in stature but with short final height.

Urinary salt loss in the early weeks of life indicates an adrenal or renal cause. In adrenal disease, potassium levels are often high and aldosterone levels are low. Treatment is by careful rehydration with normal or even hypertonic saline intravenously — the whole body sodium deficit may be considerable. Do not give hydrocortisone — it has only limited mineralocorticoid activity and if relevant samples are not already obtained diagnosis is more difficult and will be delayed. Once sodium balance is restored start oral fludrocortisone 0.15 mg/m^2/24 h in one or two daily doses. It is possible to titrate an appropriate hydrocortisone dose against ACTH, 17-OH progesterone and adrenal androgen levels. Cortisol secretion rate is 12.5 mg/m^2/24 h and about 10–15 mg/m^2/24 h of hydrocortisone in two to three divided doses with two-thirds given in the morning is usually appropriate to normalise growth, skeletal maturation and plasma ACTH levels. A home profile of finger prick blood tests obtained by parents four times a day, once every month onto the Guthrie filter paper and posted to an appropriate laboratory for 17-OH progesterone assay provides a better guide to control than do occasional measurements in outpatients, but normal growth and skeletal maturation are the best overall guides to glucocorticoid replacement.

Inadequate hydrocortisone replacement will cause rapid growth, more rapid advance in bone age and ultimate short stature. Overadequate replacement will cause slow growth and delay, but not comparable delay, in bone age maturation again resulting in ultimate short stature. Veering from one extreme to another will cause cumulative deficits in final height.

Regular blood pressure and urinary electrolyte measurements are usually sufficient to check that mineralocorticoid replacement is appropriate; outpatient renin and aldosterone measurements are not very meaningful.

Glucocorticoid dosage must be increased two- to three-fold during stress such as severe infection or surgery which may precipitate hypoglycaemia and a Medicalert bracelet or talisman should be worn. Clitoromegaly usually requires surgical treatment which is best carried out in the first 2 years of life.

The incidence of 21-hydroxylase deficiency in Western Europe is about 1 in 5000 giving a gene frequency for heterozygosity in the population of about 1 in 35. Both heterozygote detection and antenatal diagnosis are possible, but termination of pregnancy is probably only appropriate if there is severe ambiguity of genitalia.

Adrenocortical insufficiency

Addison's disease (mineralocorticoid and glucocorticoid deficiency with raised renin and ACTH levels presenting in older children) is rare. Sexual differentiation has been normal and puberty will take place spontaneously (a contrast with congenital adrenal hypoplasia). It is commonly due to autoimmune disease and may be associated with hypoparathyroidism, pernicious anaemia, hypothyroidism, moniliasis, alopecia, diabetes mellitus or vitiligo. Diagnosis may be following sudden adrenal crisis despite the chronicity of the underlying condition. Glucocorticoid and mineralocorticoid replacement is necessary.

More commonly, adrenal crisis results from abrupt withdrawal of glucocorticoid medication when the hypothalamo-pituitary-adrenal axis is suppressed from chronic steroid medication or failure to increase glucocorticoid during intercurrent illness or to cover general anaesthesia.

Alternate-day steroid medication causes less hypothalamo-pituitary-adrenal axis suppression. The growth-sparing effect of alternate-day steroids is less well documented. ACTH treatment is associated with more rapid current growth than is high-dose steroid therapy but this probably results from additional secondary adrenal androgen secretion and if bone age advances disproportionately rapidly ultimate stature may be just as impaired.

Adrenocortical overactivity

Unlike iatrogenic Cushing's syndrome due to excessive glucocorticoid medication which is common, this is rare in children, whether due to pituitary-dependent Cushing's disease (excess ACTH secretion), adrenal tumour (benign or malignant) or ectopic tumour ACTH production. Symptoms and signs (hypertension, truncal obesity, moon face, striae, osteoporosis) are usually less clear cut than in adults and the double effect on growth of hypercortisolism and excess adrenal androgen secretion may cause growth failure or temporarily rapid growth. The former is commoner however and progressive truncal obesity the usual presenting feature. Blood pressure may not be dramatically high for age but signs of virilisation are common. Treatment depends on the cause and may be surgery (to adrenals or pituitary) or radiotherapy.

THYROID DISORDERS

Hypofunction

Congenital hypothyroidism

Few infants show diagnostic features of hypothyroidism — rounded expressionless face, small nose with depressed bridge, coarse features, low facial hairline, large tongue, jaundice, umbilical hernia and hoarse cry — at birth and, until neonatal screening programmes were introduced, over 50% were not diagnosed until after 3 months of age. Treatment started later than that age is associated with significant reduction in IQ; even by 3 months it is usually too late to preserve IQ totally. Appropriate treatment within 4 weeks leads to normal overall development and IQ, but some studies suggest that subtle motor, perceptual, speech and perhaps behaviour or personality deficits remain.

Congenital hypothyroidism can be reliably detected biochemically in the newborn period. The programme is cost effective both in financial and human terms in the prevention of long-term mental handicap.

Neonatal treatment seems effective because, although the fetal thyroid is active from mid-gestation, the major product of the gland is the relatively inactive reverse triiodothyronine whilst the level of triiodothyronine, the active mono-deiodinated thyroxine derivative, is low. Neither thyroid hormones nor TSH cross the placenta in significant amounts and thyroid hormones seem not to be essential for normal fetal somatic and brain growth in man. Following the TSH surge immediately after birth triiodothyronine levels rise markedly.

The optimal time for screening is after these postnatal changes and thus sampling can be part of the Guthrie test collection procedure.

A positive screening test leads to immediate recall of the baby for confirmatory tests and results should not be awaited before starting treatment. Because much brain growth in man is during the early postnatal period it is better to treat a baby

with transient neonatal hypothyroidism unnecessarily for a short period than to leave a case of true hypothyroidism untreated.

Measuring thyroxine alone is unsatisfactory because of overlap in levels in normal and abnormal babies. In the UK and the rest of Europe, TSH is measured; in the USA thyroxine is measured with additional TSH measurement when values are low. Both methods work satisfactorily. Measuring TSH, cases of pituitary (secondary) or hypothalamic (tertiary) hypothyroidism would be missed but these babies usually have clinical features associated with other pituitary hormone deficiencies (e.g. micropenis, hypoglycaemia) and thyroid function is usually sufficiently preserved to prevent neurological and intellectual problems even with later diagnosis.

Screening programmes demonstrate a worldwide incidence of permanent primary hypothyroidism of around 1 in 4000 births. Transient abnormalities, previously unrecognised, may be nearly as common in many countries. Preterm infants may have temporary functional thyroid disorders and clear-cut diagnosis may be more difficult to achieve in the short term.

Radioisotope thyroid scanning is not essential in the newborn period but helps to confirm whether thyroid tissue is present and whether it is ectopic. Commonly abnormal migration of the fetal gland from the back of the tongue to the neck may cause aplasia, hypoplasia or ectopia. Genetic thyroid hormone biosynthetic defects are rarer, may run in families transmitted as autosomal recessive conditions and may cause a mild goitre.

Treatment is with thyroxine, initially 10 μg/kg/day orally. Assessment is clinical and biochemical in the early months. Normal growth and development will result from thyroxine levels towards the upper end of the normal range. High TSH levels take time to fall as the previously abnormal homeostatic point of T4–TSH interaction is reset. Attempts in the first few months to suppress TSH levels into the normal range will result in overtreatment. After this, raised TSH levels represent poor compliance or undertreatment.

Except in clear-cut cases of thyroid aplasia it is important to reassess thyroid function off treatment once the critical phase of brain growth is over — after the second birthday. The time off treatment is minimised by substituting the shorter half life triiodothyronine (20 μg $\equiv$ 100 μg thyroxine) for 1 month, stopping all treatment for 14 days and then retesting.

Thyroxine dosage is less in relation to body size beyond the newborn period (see below).

Acquired hypothyroidism

Acquired childhood hypothyroidism commonly results in fall-off in school performance but this is frequently attributed to other problems. Growth slows but this too may not be recognised as few children are measured regularly and slow growth must be prolonged before a single measurement or simple observation detects conspicuous short stature. The other well-known clinical features occur late.

Enzyme deficiency in the thyroxine biosynthetic pathway may not present until this stage, usually with goitre. An organification defect (conversion of iodide to iodine) may be associated with deafness (Pendred's syndrome). Thyroid antibodies are absent. Their presence signifies autoimmune thyroiditis (Hashimoto's disease), the commonest cause of childhood-onset thyroid disease. Auto-antibodies to other organs may be associated with eventual diabetes, or adrenal failure.

Hypothalamo-pituitary disorders may present then and assessment of the whole axis clinically (visual fields, optic fundi), radiologically (skull X-ray and CT scan) and biochemically (TRH test) will be necessary if TSH levels are inappropriately low for the low thyroxine.

A recent advance is the ability to measure free (active, unbound) thyroxine levels. Compensated hypothyroidism (normal total T4 levels at the expense of raised TSH levels) — presumably an early stage in the disease process before decompensation takes place — should probably be treated with thyroxine. Prolonged oversecretion of TSH seems harmless but free T4 levels are usually low.

Mental retardation does not occur in late-onset hypothyroidism. School performance and growth will improve on thyroxine replacement. The dose is usually around 100 μg/m^2/24 hours but must be precisely tailored to the individual. TSH levels are a sensitive guide to underreplacement or non-compliance except in hypothalamo-pituitary disease. Immunoradiometric TSH assays may detect over-replacement as sensitively.

Growth and skeletal maturation assessment is vital. Good catch-up growth is characteristic of treated acquired hypothyroidism but inappropriately rapid bone age advance for that growth indicates overtreatment and will result irretrievably in stunting because of early epiphyseal fusion. Clinical signs of hypothyroidism or thyrotoxicosis indicate grossly abnormal treatment and cannot be used for monitoring.

Thyrotoxicosis

Neonatal thyrotoxicosis is rare. It may be associated with maternal Graves' disease but only about 1.5% of such mothers' babies will be affected and her disease can have been inactive for many years. There is an association with transplacental passage of maternal thyroid stimulating immunoglobulins. Often the precise aetiology is unclear.

A goitre may be present at birth and the infant may rapidly become very ill with tachycardia, congestive heart failure, weight loss (until heart failure supervenes) irritability and ravenous hunger. Treatment is with propranolol (to reduce tachycardia and treat high output cardiac failure) and antithyroid medication, e.g. carbimazole or propylthiouracil. Most infants recover spontaneously by about 6 months and can be weaned off treatment by then. Persistence suggests early-onset conventional Graves' disease as in the older child.

In children, thyrotoxicosis is much rarer than hypothyroidism and is rarer than in adults — only about 5% of patients with Graves' disease present in childhood or adolescence. As with other thyroid diseases it is commoner in girls. Hashimoto's disease can present initially with thyrotoxicosis.

Onset is often insidious with behavioural changes (emotional lability, poor concentration, temper tantrums) usually attributed to other environmental factors or adolescence.

Growth is rapid with inappropriately rapid advance in skeletal maturity. Eventually goitre, prominence of eyes, sweating, fatigue and poor co-ordination may be noticed and tachycardia, hypertension, tremor, exophthalmos and a thyroid bruit may be found. Weight loss occurs despite an enormous calorie intake.

Diagnosis is confirmed by high plasma levels of free or total T4 and T3 (the latter may be more dramatically raised).

Medical treatment aims to restore euthyroidism using carbimazole or propylthiouracil. Thyroid function may take some weeks to become normal and propranalol will reduce heart rate, nervousness and tremor and greatly improve patient well-being.

The blood count as well as thyroid function should be monitored in treated patients, as antithyroid drugs may cause significant neutropenia. Rarely, early acute agranulocytosis may occur. The dose to maintain euthyroidism may reduce and it is reasonable to attempt stopping treatment after about 2 years. Indeed autoimmune phenomena in Graves' disease may cause eventual hypothyroidism. Surgery (subtotal thyroidectomy) is considered following failure of medical management (non-remission by 2 years, difficulties of control, poor compliance) and must be in a patient who has been made euthyroid. Thyroxine will be necessary subsequently to maintain euthyroidism. Conventionally radioiodine ablative treatment is contraindicated in children because of the long-term risk of thyroid carcinoma, but the risk may have been overestimated.

Thyroid carcinoma

Thyroid carcinoma is extremely rare in childhood but functional solitary nodules in a goitre, (i.e. in the context of thyrotoxicosis) are suspicious. Medullary thyroid carcinoma (from parafollicular cells) may be an early manifestation of the multiple endocrine neoplasia syndromes, an autosomal dominant disorder. Associations are with Cushing's syndrome, hyperparathyroidism, phaeochromocytoma and gastrointestinal and oral neuromas. Diarrhoea (due to calcitonin secretion) is an early sign. Raised calcitonin levels (basally or following pentagastrin infusion) may indicate that an asymptomatic child has inherited the disease from an affected parent. Special watch must be kept for development of nodular goitre and prophylactic thyroidectomy might even be considered.

CALCIUM METABOLISM

Calcium must be accumulated by the growing child yet is important for normal endocrine and neuromuscular functioning and must remain within tightly controlled limits in extracellular fluid. Thus homeostatic control mechanisms are complex. Ionised calcium is metabolically active and its proportion of total serum calcium (including albumin-bound calcium) is controlled by vitamin D, parathyroid hormone (PTH) and calcitonin and affected by acid-base changes (acidosis increases and alkalosis reduces ionised calcium levels). In hypoproteinaemic states, total calcium may be low but ionised calcium normal.

Calcium absorption from the gut depends on vitamin D, upper intestinal pH and binding by dietary substances, e.g. phytates. Vitamin D_3 (cholecalciferol) is found in fish, eggs, butter and margarine and is synthesised by the action of sunlight on the Malpighian layer of skin. Worldwide, vitamin D dietary deficiency combined with inadequate skin synthesis is the major cause of rickets. In the UK it is a problem particularly in immigrant families of Asian origin (less so in darker-skinned families of West Indian origin, presumably for dietary reasons).

Vitamin D deficiency also occurs secondarily to malabsorption and in renal disease because 1-hydroxylation of 25-hydroxycholecalciferol is carried out in the kidney to form the most active vitamin D metabolite 1-25-dihydroxycholecalciferol. Growth hormone, prolactin and oestrogen may have roles in controlling 1-hydroxylation but calcium, PTH and phosphate are most important in its regulation.

Rickets in the toddler age group presents with poor growth, delayed anterior fontanelle closure, skull bossing, swollen wrists, rickety rosary (swelling of the costochondral junctions) and bowing of the legs. Serum calcium is normal or low and alkaline phosphatase elevated for age. X-rays of wrists and knees show widening and irregular calcification of epiphyseal cartilage (growth plate) leading to a ragged appearance with splaying out ('cupping') of long bone ends. Subperiosteal erosions (best seen on radial borders of middle phalanges of 2nd and 3rd fingers) are characteristic of secondary hyperparathyroidism. Rickets may present during rapid pubertal growth, sometimes with limb pain.

In classical 'dietary deficiency' rickets a therapeutic trial of small doses of vitamin D_3 (50 μg orally daily for 3 weeks) will confirm the diagnosis and the need for ongoing treatment by demonstrating biochemical improvement, but the dose is too small to affect metabolic forms of the disease. Precise diagnosis of these is necessary for optimal treatment as in some forms very high (and otherwise toxic) doses of vitamin D or the use of analogues (e.g. alfacalcidol) will be necessary.

Rickets can occasionally result from anticonvulsant treatment with phenytoin, primidone or carbamazepine.

Hypocalcaemia

Hypocalcaemia used to occur in full-term infants fed with high phosphate load cows' milk preparations. Finding the same problem in some babies on low phosphate milks suggests other additional factors such as low maternal dietary vitamin D intake. Affected infants are jittery, may show tetany with rhythmic focal myoclonic jerking but are otherwise well and feed normally. The problem is best prevented by giving vitamin D supplements particularly to pregnant Asian mothers and encouraging breast feeding. Oral treatment is usually safest and best: 10% calcium gluconate 100 mg/kg (about 1 ml) before each feed. It is sometimes necessary to correct hypomagnesaemia before hypocalcaemia becomes correctable.

Preterm infants, especially with perinatal problems, may have more persistant hypocalcaemia. The cause is unclear and may be multifactorial (low calcium reserves, temporary hypoparathyroidism, immaturity of end-organ responsiveness to PTH).

Chronic hypocalcaemia may be associated with dietary, malabsorption or renal rickets (see above). It may be due to PTH deficiency from absence or hypoplasia of the parathyroid glands. This may occur as an isolated developmental defect in association with thymic and thyroid aplasia (DiGeorge's syndrome), following thyroidectomy or in association with autoimmune disease. This last group may present with severe mucocutaneous candidiasis and malabsorption and hypothyroidism, Addison's disease and pernicious anaemia may develop.

In the older child, hypocalcaemia more commonly results from end-organ unresponsiveness to PTH than PTH deficiency. In pseudohypoparathyroidism, mental retardation (which may be mild) is associated with short stature, obesity and dysmorphic features, including characteristic shortening of the 4th and 5th metacarpals due to early fusion. Hypocalcaemia is not invariable, but may present with tetany or epilepsy. Depending on the presence of skeletal or renal resistance to PTH or abnormal physical features, a number of other syndromes have been identified. Clinical examination, skeletal survey, calcium and PTH measurements and (if there is hypocalcaemia) the cyclic AMP response to PTH infusion may be necessary to make a specific diagnosis.

Hypercalcaemia

Hypercalcaemia most commonly occurs in infants, is usually idiopathic but can be secondary to excess vitamin D intake or (very rarely) hyperparathyroidism. Presenting symptoms are vomiting, constipation, failure to thrive and irritability. Severe idiopathic hypercalcaemia is associated with cardiac abnormalities especially supravalvar aortic stenosis (Williams' syndrome), but many babies with other features of the syndrome (mental retardation, depressed nasal bridge, long philtrum, prominent lips, etc.) have normal calcium levels and the relationship between the connective tissue developmental abnormality and calcium remains obscure.

DIABETES MELLITUS

Incidence and aetiology

Diabetes mellitus affects about 1 in every 1500 children in the UK under the age of 15 years. Although it is the most common metabolic disorder and its incidence seems to be increasing, it is still uncommon in primary care. A UK general practitioner with an average list might look after only one insulin-dependent child diabetic. Diabetes in children and adolescents is almost invariably insulin dependent (type I diabetes is insulin-dependent diabetes irrespective of the age of onset). Rarely maturity-onset type diabetes (type II) may occur in young people.

Susceptibility to diabetes is related to HLA (histocompatability) markers and gene loci responsible for their synthesis on the short arm of chromosome 6. D and DR antigens have particularly strong associations increasing the risk of developing diabetes between three-fold (DR3) and 14-fold (DR3/DR4 heterozygosity) respectively. 90–98% of childhood-onset diabetics express DR3, DR4, antigens or both yet less than 1% of healthy subjects with such markers will ever develop diabetes.

Development depends on an environmental 'insult' such as viral infection causing continuing and irreversible pancreatic islet beta cell damage resulting in insulin deficiency.

Viral infections may account for the seasonal variation in onset. Humoral and cell-mediated antibodies against pancreatic islet cells and other endocrine organs are common in type I diabetes suggesting the importance of autoimmune mechanisms in the disease process.

The HLA identical sibling of a child with insulin-dependent diabetes mellitus (IDDM) has about a 90-fold increased risk of developing the disease before 15 years. The risk is hardly increased at all if the sibling is HLA non-identical.

Diagnosis

Although in retrospect parents may feel their newly diagnosed diabetic has not been 'right' for some time with poor appetite or malaise, onset is usually acute with increasing polyuria (due to the osmotic glucose load) and thus polydipsia with weight loss, anorexia, vomiting and abdominal pain. This may develop very rapidly in a few days or more slowly over weeks. The urine of any child who starts bedwetting having already achieved bladder control should be tested for glucose. If diabetes is suspected in a child, it is an emergency. No child should be referred by letter to an outpatient clinic; he should be seen preferably the same day and certainly within 24 hours. If diag-

nosis and treatment are not prompt increasing catabolism will cause ketosis, acidosis, coma and death. There is still significant morbidity and mortality in children who present with severe acidosis and dehydration.

Ketoacidosis

A child with ketoacidosis and severe dehydration is dangerously ill and requires emergency treatment. Symptoms include vomiting, abdominal pain and hyperventilation. There is marked dehydration and drowsiness with Kussmaul respiration. There may be circulatory collapse, oliguria and coma. Salicylate poisoning should be considered in the differential diagnosis but too often signs are misinterpreted as being due to pneumonia or an acute abdomen.

Priority in management is appropriate rehydration. This is more crucial than insulin in the early stages. The initial fluid should be 0.9% saline (150 mmol/l) or plasma if the patient is shocked or unconscious. 20 ml/kg should be given within the first 30–60 minutes. A rapid history, clinical examination and blood glucose (by indicator stick) will confirm the diagnosis and a sample for true blood glucose, urea and electrolytes, plasma osmolality and arterial blood gas estimations should be obtained as the infusion is set up. Full blood count, PCV and platelets and an infection screen (blood culture, virology, urine microscopy and culture, swabs) should be obtained and ECG monitoring set up. The patient should be weighed if at all possible and the degree of dehydration (mild, about 5%, to severe more than 12%) estimated.

A short-acting insulin is best given as a continuous intravenous infusion by syringe pump as 0.05 units/kg/hour.

Consider bicarbonate only if the child is shocked with arterial pH <7.0. The amount needed is derived from the formula:

$$\text{mmol bicarbonate (ml of 8.4\% NaHCO}_3) = \frac{\text{wt(kg)} \times \text{base deficit (mmol/l)}}{10}$$

It should be given if at all over at least 30 minutes by separate infusion. However its use increases the risk of cerebral oedema (due to the large sodium load) and of hypokalaemia (more rapid shift of potassium into the cells) and acidosis will improve with rehydration and insulin alone. After the first hour the infusion rate of saline should be reduced to give 50% of the remaining calculated deficit plus maintenance over the next 8 hours. The remaining deficit plus maintenance is given over the remainder of the first 24-hour period.

Once blood glucose levels fall below 13 mmol/l, 0.45% saline/5% dextrose should be substituted. The insulin solution should be renewed 6 hourly and its rate of infusion adjusted to maintain blood glucose levels between 7 and 13 mmol/l.

Potassium should be started at 2–3 mmol/kg/h (but not exceeding 40 mmol/l concentration) from the second hour, if urine has been passed since admission, without waiting for hypokalaemia. Antibiotics may be necessary if infection is suspected once all bacteriology specimens have been obtained. If no urine has been passed by 4 hours, the patient should be catheterised. Inappropriate ADH secretion may develop (low urine output, high urine osmolality and falling plasma osmolality) necessitating fluid restriction to prevent cerebral oedema. Apparently low plasma sodium levels may merely reflect hyperlipidaemia and plasma osmolality will be a better guide to hydration.

All urine passed should be tested for glucose and ketones. A nasogastric tube should be passed and gastric losses included in an accurate fluid balance record. Blood glucose, gases, urea and electrolytes and osmolality should be checked at 2 and 5 hours and thereafter as necessary with hourly stick blood glucose testing.

From day 2 onwards (sometimes earlier) consider allowing oral fluids (e.g. dilute diabetic squash) as tolerated and reduce the intravenous infusion rate accordingly. Solids may be started as the appetite recovers. Discontinue intravenous fluids when the child is eating and drinking a light diet and the urine is ketone free. Potassium chloride should be given orally for 4 days (1 mol/kg/24 h).

If insulin infusion is stopped before intravenous fluids are discontinued, ketonuria and anorexia will take longer to resolve and acidosis may persist. Soluble insulin should be given subcutaneously 1 unit/kg/24 h 6–8 hourly after the insulin infusion is stopped. The first subcutaneous dose should be half an hour before the intravenous infusion is stopped. Subsequently go on to a twice daily regimen (as described below). Once the child has recovered education can be started.

Initial management of the child without ketoacidosis

Many new diabetics are admitted to hospital with only mild symptoms and without ketoacidosis. Insulin is started, subcutaneously, usually twice daily. A suitable regimen is a combination of short- (soluble) and intermediate-acting (isophane) insulins 1.0–1.5 units/kg/24 h with approximately two-thirds given before breakfast (ratio of soluble to isophane <1:1) and one-third before the evening meal (ratio of soluble to isophane <1:3). After 2 or 3 days insulin requirements may reduce quite rapidly. A stay of around 1 week in hospital is usually appropriate for education of the family in basic diabetic care involving nursing and medical staff, dietitian and liaison sister. Upset, anxious or frightened parents are not receptive learners.

Long-term management

Good long-term diabetic control will delay or prevent the onset of tissue damage complications (neuropathy, nephropathy, retinopathy). The aim of management is to achieve normoglycaemia for as much of the time as possible in the context of normal family and school life and normal physical and emotional growth. Educating (instructing) the child and his family attempts to achieve this through increased understanding of the condition and self-confidence in its management. Motivation derives from encouragement and explanation, not coercion and the laying down of arbitrary rules.

Normal blood glucose levels are dependent on appropriate balance between calorie intake necessary for growth and energy expenditure and insulin. Many physical and emotional uncontrollable factors will affect blood glucose levels, e.g. growth hormone, infection, puberty, menstruation, exams, a birthday party. Exercise has major effects on glucose levels (due to increased metabolism but also by increasing mobilisation of injected insulin from injection sites because of increased blood flow and muscular activity) and in children it is variable and unpredictable in nature and intensity.

Diets should give a 'stable' carbohydrate (CHO) intake at regularly spaced intervals — breakfast, midmorning snack, lunch, mid-afternoon snack, evening meal and bedtime snack. A useful guide to CHO intake is 100 g per day for a 1 year old plus an extra 10 g per day for each additional year of age.

The carbohydrate exchange system (one exchange = 10 g CHO) is simple and allows a wide variety of foods to be eaten whilst ensuring a stable total CHO intake. CHO intake should not be restricted so that intake of saturated animal fat can be low (less-than 35% of calories should be from fat which should be polysaturated) reducing the long-term risk of cardiovascular disease. CHO type is important: concentrated rapidly absorbed sugary foods (chocolate, sweets, jam) lead to wide swings in blood glucose levels; starchy low fibre foods (white bread, cream crackers, corn flakes) are acceptable; but best, because they are gradually absorbed and metabolised, are starchy high fibre foods (wholemeal bread, brown rice, jacket potatoes, dried beans). Within these constraints, 'healthy food' is healthy for non-diabetics and diabetics alike and dietetic education involves educating the whole family's eating habits.

Insulin should balance dietary CHO intake. All insulin regimens poorly reflect normal endogenous insulin secretion. Only human or highly purified porcine insulins should be used in children to prevent lipoatrophy. Local hypertrophy can still occur if the same injection site is used repeatedly (which is less painful) and absorption will also be more variable.

The regimen must be individualised for the child and his family. Most are potentially better controlled on two daily injections (a mixture of short- and intermediate-acting insulins) than on one, but one injection may be more appropriate for a toddler. In some adolescents flexibility of lifestyle can be achieved without loss of control by using a convenient pen injector giving small amounts of short-acting insulin before main meals (which can be variable in timing and quantity) and a long-acting insulin at bedtime. Pen injectors will become increasingly popular but could lead to worse control in poorly motivated diabetics.

Many diabetic children enjoy active and healthy lives but some are poorly controlled and require frequent hospital admissions. Poor control may reflect unhappiness or instability in the family, particularly if they have never emotionally accepted the diagnosis. Control may be particularly difficult to achieve in adolescence: rapid growth necessitates a high calorie intake and must be paralleled by insulin increases; menstruation may precipitate ketoacidosis; important exams cause stress; emotional lability may cause rebelliousness against dietary restrictions, the need for monitoring control or insulin injections at all.

Assessing control

Progress is monitored in three ways: by home urine or blood glucose testing, using 3-monthly glycosylated haemoglobin ($HbA1_c$) measurements and by assessing emotional and physical growth and well-being. Haemoglobin forms a non-enzymic link with glucose and the proportion in the blood in glycosylated form provides a guide to glycaemic control over the 2–3 months preceding the test. The normal range depends on the analytical method but is commonly between 3% and 7% $HbA1_c$ measurements provide no insight into short-term blood glucose fluctuations but are useful as objective assessments of control and may confirm suspicions that test results are being 'made up' or 'improved' to keep the doctor happy.

Stick tests for urinary glucose have replaced messy and dangerously caustic Clinitest tablets. Urine tests give retrospective information (has the blood glucose been so high as to exceed the renal threshold for glucose since the bladder was last emptied?), do not warn of impending hypoglycaemia and are unsatisfactory if normoglycaemia is the therapeutic goal. Lack of glycosuria is not necessarily equivalent to normoglycaemia.

Many children find home blood glucose monitoring on capillary samples using indicator sticks more acceptable and useful. However immediate knowledge of blood glucose levels is only of major practical benefit if the family and child understand the significance and relevance of the result and are motivated to make appropriate alterations in management on the basis of consistent abnormalities. Tests done in rotation once or twice a day just before main meals, $1-1\frac{1}{2}$ hours after main meals and at bedtime, provide most information from fewest tests.

Achievement of good long-term control in the context of 'normal' lifestyle is helped by the multidisciplinary team ideally available in a children's hospital diabetic clinic. A dietitian should be present and a child psychiatrist readily available to help with the emotional impact of diabetes on diabetic control and on family dynamics. The liaison nursing sister visits families in their homes and schools, talks to diabetics, their families and their teachers, discusses practical aspects of care and provides support in sorting out specific difficulties. A consistent approach by all members of the team will do much to create an environment in which the quality of control will improve.

Hypoglycaemia

Hypoglycaemic symptoms are described on p. 260. Occasional mild hypoglycaemia – a feeling of hunger with faintness, headache or belligerency if a meal is delayed — indicates tight control. Many parents worry about hypoglycaemic episodes, particularly at night, but there is no good evidence that such episodes are harmful and it is sensible to take a positive attitude about these to try and reduce anxiety. Hypoglycaemia is usually caused by delayed or missed food, unexpected exercise or excess insulin administration (by mistake or, more rarely, deliberately). Both stress and the early stages of an intercurrent viral illness can cause hypo- rather than hyperglycaemia. Diabetics should always carry with them extra glucose or dextrose to be taken at early signs of hypoglycaemia followed by food as appropriate. A semi conscious child who cannot co-ordinate swallowing a sweet drink, should be given glucagon (1 mg intramuscularly). This will improve neuroglycopenia and the conscious level sufficiently for oral carbohydrate to be given. If it is not glucose levels will fall again. Parents should keep a glucagon kit at home. Sometimes glucagon causes vomiting but its use will often save the need for hospital admission.

The future

The long-term outlook for diabetic children has been gloomy but there is reason for optimism that current regimens and the establishment of good control will delay or prevent neuropathy, renal failure, blindness and early death in many. Screening for early detection of complications (e.g. regular retinoscopy by adolescence and blood pressure measurements) remain important. Microalbuminuria is an early sign of nephropathy. However the detection of a potential problem does not mean that its prevention is easy or even possible.

Possible future developments include modification of the molecular structure and formulation of insulin, the use of less toxic drugs to prevent continuing beta cell destruction during the initial autoimmune process, more physiological routes and methods of insulin delivery, islet cell implants and miniaturised portable closed loop infusion pumps linked to glucose sensors.

Meanwhile much more could still be achieved in many families using conventional techniques with intensified educational and emotional support from the clinic.

TOO FAT OR TOO THIN?

Weight is a poor guide to obesity and the interpretation of a high weight for the child's height as 'obesity' may be very misleading at times when growth and fatness are varying in opposite directions — a normal boy in early puberty is growing slowly but increasing body fat rapidly. Skinfold measurements are a much better guide to over- (and under-) nutrition (see p. 249).

Overeating is the commonest cause of childhood obesity. Although some fat children will remain fat, there is no necessary progression from fat baby to fat child to the fat adult who will die from hypertension, stroke or myocardial infarction. Obesity which is mild is unlikely to be associated with long-term or short-term ill health although respiratory infections are commoner in the obese infant. Advice about appropriate dieting should be given and will be successful if the child and whole family are motivated towards weight loss.

Major degrees of obesity require thought to exclude an underlying cause other than overeating. Measurement of stature is an important screening test. Virtually all hormonal disorders causing obesity (e.g. growth hormone deficiency, hypothyroidism, hypopituitarism, Cushing's syndrome, pseudohypoparathyroidism) are associated with short stature and usually with bone age delay as are such uncommon obesity syndromes as Prader–Willi.

In contrast, overeating causes an increase in growth velocity and an advance in bone age with early epiphyseal fusion and no increase in final stature. If overeating stops but there is insufficient reduction in calorie intake to lose weight, growth velocity will be normal but the child will be tall and bone age remains advanced.

In wealthy societies, eating more than is necessary for growth and energy requirements is common because eating is a social as well as nutritional activity and moderate fatness in a baby or child is seen as visible proof of mother love. Grannies are notorious for giving their grandchildren treats of high calorie foods and many parents would be surprised at how much less their child needs to eat than they are forcing down him. Fat babies tend to be placid, 'good' and little trouble. Once an individual is overweight, the calorie intake need not be excessive to maintain the obese state.

The obese child deserves dietary advice and encouragement to lose weight. Whether he does so depends on his motivation and ability to stick to what may be a very low calorie intake before weight loss will begin and be maintained. Motivation is easily undermined by lack of family support.

The regular testing of urine for ketonuria is a valuable guide to progress. If weight is being lost fatty acid breakdown will cause ketonuria and in its absence calorie intake is still too high. The short fat child is likely to have an endocrine disorder and should be investigated to make a diagnosis and provide appropriate treatment.

Obesity is a significant additional handicap in, and associated with, many mental handicap syndromes due to a variety of causes and should be treated as vigorously as possible.

In the Prader–Willi syndrome there is usually a history of reduced fetal movements, floppiness in the newborn period and early feeding problems but appetite soon becomes insatiable and gross obesity, sometimes associated with scoliosis, supervenes. Calorie restriction is sometimes impossible to achieve and may result in growth failure but gross obesity and scoliosis predispose to respiratory failure and death.

In our society more mothers worry that their child is not eating enough than that he eats too much. Skinfold measurement not weight is the best guide to thinness and undernutrition.

A healthy child who is offered appetising food in adequate amount and variety in an emotionally supportive environment will eat enough to enable him to grow normally. This may be much less than mother or granny feels he should be eating.

A child who is thin but growing normally and not getting thinner should not be investigated nor treated. The child who is getting thinner or who is growing slowly needs investigation, diagnosis and treatment. Recognisable syndromes (e.g. lipodystrophy) and malignancies are rare but unrecognised organic disease (e.g. malabsorption, asthma) may present with little overt signs at consultation and is a common cause of poor growth and thinness. Calories may be too few (worldwide the most important cause of poor growth and thinness) but some children are on inadequate diets because of ethnic or cultural customs and some mothers are so concerned that their children do not become obese and that they eat 'healthy' foods that calorie intake is deficient.

In the UK, emotional problems are a very common cause of thinness (and poor growth). Anorexia nervosa is occasionally life-threatening in an adolescent.

A battle to get a child to eat more than he needs is a battle the parent is likely to lose and can produce emotional problems in both child and parent then or later. In other situations treatment of the underlying cause is all that is necessary but this may be easier with an organic than with an emotional disorder. Reassurance that a thin child is growing normally and is healthy will often in itself defuse an emotionally strained family situation.

FURTHER READING

Aynsley-Green A, Soltesz G 1985 Hypoglycaemia in infancy and childhood. Churchill Livingstone, Edinburgh

Brook C G D 1982 Growth assessment in childhood and adolescence. Blackwell, Oxford

Brook C G D (ed) 1989 Clinical paediatric endocrinology, 2nd edn. Blackwell, Oxford

Buckler J M H 1979 A reference manual of growth and development. Blackwell, Oxford

Buckler J M H 1987 The adolescent years. Castlemead, Ware

Kelnar C J H 1989 Growth. Medicine International 64: 2632–2638

Kelnar C J H 1991 Endocrine gland disorders In: Campbell A, McIntosh N (eds) Forfar and Arneil's Textbook of paediatrics, 4th edn. Churchill Livingstone, Edinburgh (in press)

Kelnar C J H 1991 Physical growth and development — the gonads and endocrinological aspects of growth and development. In: Campbell A, McIntosh N (eds) Forfar and Arneil's Textbook of paediatrics, 4th edn. Churchill Livingstone, Edinburgh (in press)

Tanner J M 1989 Foetus into man, 2nd edn. Castlemead, Ware

Tanner J M, Whitehouse R H 1976 Clinical longitudinal standards for height, weight, height velocity, weight velocity, and stages of puberty. Archives of Diseases in Childhood 51: 170–179

Growth charts are available from:

Castlemead Publications
Swains Mill
4A Crane Mead
Ware
Herts
SG12 9PY

Measuring Equipment is available from:

Holtain Ltd
Crosswell
Crymmych
Dyfed
Wales
SA41 3UF and

The Child Growth Foundation
2 Mayfield Avenue
Chiswick
London
W4 1PW

22. Gynaecological disorders

J. Dewhurst

The gynaecological diseases which affect children reflect the endocrine background of the particular age-period. In utero a girl's genital organs are stimulated by hormones which have passed across the placenta from the mother and the appearance, of the genitalia reflect this in a newborn baby. After this, disorders characteristic of oestrogen deficiency occur, until the changes of puberty appear and a girl begins to produce her own oestrogens. The special disorders of the adolescent are mainly abnormalities of menstruation. Tumours, fortunately rare in childhood, may occur at any time.

NORMAL SIGNS IN THE NEWBORN

During the first few weeks of life the passive hormone stimulation which the baby has from the mother gives rise to several physiological manifestations. Breast swelling is seen in many babies, male and female, born at term; left alone, as it should be, this swelling usually regresses quickly and only rarely does it persist for more than 1 month. Baby girls often show congestion and swelling of the vulva and there is sometimes a prominent hymen and a white discharge which can be plentiful (Fig. 22.1); rarely the discharge may be streaked with the blood from breaking down endometrium which has also responded to maternal hormones. These changes, too, disappear quickly and call for no treatment. Hymenal tags are very common and disappear spontaneously (Fig. 22.2).

Other changes which are evident once the turgid signs of the newborn period have declined are a less prominent appearance of the labia majora and minora leaving the introitus of the vagina more ex-

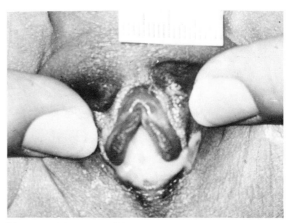

Fig. 22.1 Newborn child showing congestion and oedema of the vulva and profuse vaginal discharge (by permission of Marcel Dekker, New York).

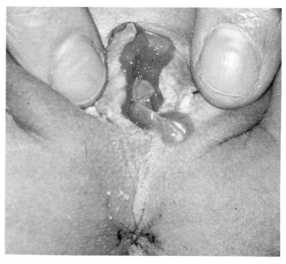

Fig. 22.2 Pronounced hymenal tag in a newborn child. This shrank and disappeared spontaneously (by permission of Marcel Dekker, New York).

275

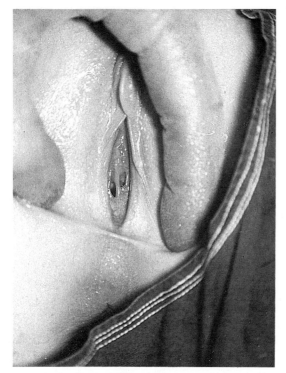

Fig. 22.3 A bifid hymen in a child. Note the thin delicate appearance of the hymen and the ease with which it can be made clearly visible by gentle retraction of the labia.

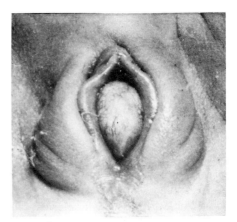

Fig. 22.4 Bulging membrane in a newborn child with hydrocolpos.

posed than at birth or when the hormone effects of puberty become noticeable later. The vulval skin has a thinner appearance and may be somewhat redder in colour than it will be later. The hymen is a thin membranous structure which is clearly visible when the labia are gently separated. Usually the diameter of the hymenal orifice will be around 0.5 cm or so during much of childhood, perhaps increasing a little as puberty approaches. Variations in the appearance of the hymen, such as a bifid one (Fig. 22.3), may occasionally be seen. With sexual abuse of the children now being given so much attention it is important to become familiar with the normal vulval appearance in the child (see Ch. 8).

VAGINAL CYSTS

Small cysts of the hymen or paraurethral glands are sometimes seen. They rarely need treatment and usually disappear spontaneously. However, one condition, hydrocolpos, is more important

since it calls for early and correct treatment. It must be differentiated from a cyst.

Hydrocolpos

Hydrocolpos is an abnormality in which there is an imperforate membrane at the lower part of the vagina behind which a quantity of milky fluid collects as a result of the hormone stimulation mentioned above. The child may be fretful due to the collection of fluid and may be unable to pass urine since the bladder neck is blocked by the large swelling. Physical signs include a lower abdominal cystic swelling — the bladder perched on top of a pelvis full of fluid — and an imperforate membrane visible when the vulva is inspected (Fig. 22.4) A rectal examination, made with a little finger, will indicate the cystic swelling anteriorly. If the diagnosis is correctly made, treatment is simple; the membrane is incised and the fluid released. It must be emphasised that the diagnosis is often made incorrectly and the abdomen may be opened with serious results.

INTERSEX

Doubt about the sex of the infant, although rare, is usually evident at birth and is discussed in Chapter 21.

VULVOVAGINITIS

After the first month or so of life the child's genital organs receive very little sex hormone stimulation and the disorders seen reflect this oestrogen lack. The most common condition is vulvovaginitis (Fig. 22.5). This arises because the vagina of the child has no protective acid secretion such as it has during the first few weeks of life and during the reproductive period.

Pathogenic organisms which are easily introduced into the child's vagina may establish themselves and cause an infection. These are usually non-specific organisms of low virulence, but may be identifiable ones, perhaps affecting the child elsewhere such as the tonsils or the middle ear; gonococcal infection is seen occasionally. Swabs from just within the introitus can be obtained, without disturbing the child, and should be placed in appropriate transport medium and sent at once for bacteriological study. This may reveal a specific organism, in which case the child may respond to an antibiotic to which that organism is susceptible. In many instances, however,

there will be no specific bacteriological findings and treatment may be carried out by the application of a little oestrogen cream to the child's vulva each night for 1–2 weeks. This improves the acidity of the vagina and allows the infection to be overcome. Treatment should not be continued for more than 2 weeks or there may be too great an oestrogen absorption and general effects. An important part of management is to ensure that the vulva is not irritated by substances applied to it. Strong antiseptic materials must be avoided, nothing should be put in the bath water, the vulva should be carefully dried with a soft towel and perhaps a little bland cream applied. Daily bathing is essential. Other possible causes of vulvovaginitis include threadworm infestations, and these should always be looked for, or rarely, a foreign body in the vagina. In the latter instance, the discharge is usually blood stained and foul smelling which should always call for careful investigation by vaginoscopy.

Not all children with vulvitis have a vaginal discharge as the cause. Some have a local skin disorder which may also be affecting other parts of the body. One lesion sometimes seen is lichen sclerosis, a vulval dystrophy in which whitish patches appear on the vulval skin and there is soreness and irritation which leads to scratching (Fig. 22.6). The condition can usually be kept under control by the hygienic measures described above or, if there is secondary infection following scratching, an antibiotic cream may be used. There is a strong tendency to improvement at puberty.

LABIAL ADHESIONS

This is also common in childhood. The labia minora adhere together in the midline leaving a tiny opening through which urine is passed. If the vulva is carefully inspected it will be seen to be flat and featureless and there is usually a vertical translucent area in the midline where the labia are joined (Fig. 22.7). This condition is often mistaken for congenital absence of the vagina; it does not resemble this since here the vulva looks otherwise normal apart from the absence of the vaginal introitus. Once it is certain that the diagnosis is labial adhesions they often separate spontaneously if a little oestrogen cream is applied

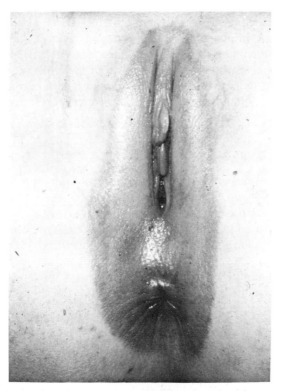

Fig. 22.5 Vulvovaginitis in a child (by permission of Marcel Dekker, New York).

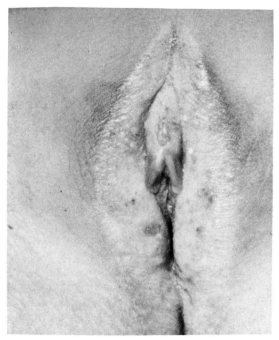

Fig. 22.6   Lichen sclerosis of the vulva in a little girl.

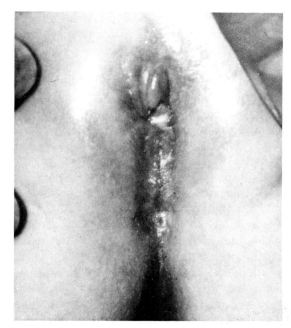

Fig. 22.7   Labial adhesions in a little girl.

nightly to the vulva for 1–2 weeks. Alternatively, the adhesions may be broken down with a blunt probe, but this can cause discomfort. Referral for advice is wise.

VAGINAL BLEEDING

This may be serious and should never be ignored. Its causes include:

1. A vaginal foreign body.
2. A malignant vaginal or cervical tumour.
3. Precocious puberty (see Ch. 21).
4. A local vulval lesion such as a prolapsed urethra or the scratching of lichen sclerosis.

In any of these conditions referral for investigation is indicated.

Around the time of puberty, girls may present irregular or heavy menstrual periods, infrequent periods or dysmenorrhoea. Irregularity is common during early menstrual life and alone calls for no treatment. Given time, the periods nearly always become more regular as the condition has a very strong tendency to spontaneous cure. Hormones must be withheld and reassurance given; iron may

be helpful to treat anaemia. If there is no significant improvement in 3–6 months referral to a special unit is indicated. Infrequent periods are relatively common at this time of life and the intervals between the periods diminish as time goes by. Should this not happen referral for further advice would again be indicated.

Painful periods

Dysmenorrhoea is often a difficult symptom to treat and it may reflect anxiety in the child's mother as much as anything else. It is usually wise to attempt to educate mother and daughter in the physiology of menstruation and to prescribe simple analgesics in the first instance; strong analgesia should be avoided if at all possible. If simple measures of this kind are not successful, the advice of a gynaecologist should be sought.

Amenorrhoea

Failure to menstruate is not an uncommon cause of concern and consultation. This symptom should never be considered in isolation, but always in association with the occurrence of the other signs of secondary sexual development. A normal girl in the UK may menstruate for the first time at any time between the ages of 10 and 16. If a girl aged 15 is seen who has not menstruated, it may therefore be tempting to think that this is not abnormal; provided the other signs of secondary sexual development are progressing normally this is likely to be so, but if there are no signs of secondary sexual development then this requires further investigation. A clue to the likely cause of failure to menstruate may be obtained by considering the other signs of secondary sexual development. Thus, if secondary development other than menstruation is good it is likely that there is an anatomical cause such as congenital absence of the vagina or an imperforate vagina; if secondary sexual development is absent or very poor, it is likely that there is a hormonal cause for this and either the ovaries are incapable of function or the hypothalamus and pituitary are not stimulating them. If there are any heterosexual changes this is a serious situation demanding urgent investigation. The other conditions, with one exception, are not urgent, but referral for gynaecological advice would usually be wise. Haematocolpos may present as an acute emergency. This condition resembles hydrocolpos, except that the fluid accumulating in the vagina and pelvis is retained menstrual blood. The patient, who is likely to be between 13 and 16, will have good secondary sexual development, but will not have menstruated although she may well have experienced intermittent pelvic pain as the blood collects. When there is enough blood to fill the pelvis she may develop acute retention of urine. The physical signs will then include a lower abdominal cystic swelling, as in hydrocolpos, a tense bluish bulging membrane of the introitus and a cystic swelling felt anteriorly on rectal examination. The patient should be sent into hospital quickly so that the membrane may be incised and the fluid released.

FURTHER READING

Edmonds D K, (ed.) 1989 Dewhurst's practical pediatric and adolescent gynecology. 2nd ed. Butterworths, London

23. Haematology

C. Haworth

RED CELL DISORDERS

The normal haemoglobin range for infants and children is shown in Table 23.1. Adult values for haemoglobin are not attained until a child is 12–14 years of age. All infants experience a drop in haemoglobin during the first weeks of life, partly due to the loss of stimulation to erythropoiesis associated with the switch to pulmonary respiration and the increasing concentration of adult haemoglobin and hence the associated increased availability of oxygen. In the preterm infant the nadir occurs earlier (6–8 weeks compared to 8–10 weeks) and is more severe; the haemoglobin may fall to 7–8 g/dl. Although this is a physiological fall in haemoglobin, in the stressed preterm infant this value may be associated with inadequate oxygen delivery to tissues and the decision to transfuse patients in this category should be made on clinical as well as laboratory grounds. Many authorities now believe that newborn babies should be trans-

Table 23.1 Red cell indices in infancy and childhood. (Reproduced with permission from Dollman and Simes (1979) and Matoth et al (1971))

	Hb (g/dl) (mean ± SD)	PCV (mean ± SD)	MCV (fl) (mean)
Day 1	19.9 ± 2.2	61 ± 7.4	119
Week 4	14.2 ± 2.1	43 ± 5.7	105
Week 9	10.7 ± 0.9	31 ± 2.5	93
Week 12	11.3 ± 0.9	33 ± 3.3	88
1 year	11.9 ± 0.6	39 ± 2	77
5 year	12.7 ± 1.0	37 ± 3	80
10 years	13.2 ± 1.0	39 ± 3	83
Normal adult			
Male	16.0 ± 2.0	47 ± 5	85
Female	14.0 ± 2.0	42 ± 5	

fused with irradiated blood to eliminate the risk of graft-versus-host disease. Others believe that the potassium leak from the cells after irradiation poses an unacceptable risk of hyperkalaemia.

ANAEMIAS

Nutritional anaemias

Iron deficiency

This is the commonest paediatric anaemia. The requirement for iron is to increase the body mass and the blood volume of the infant and is finely balanced by the iron stored from the breakdown of the initial high haemoglobin and that absorbed from the diet (0.3–0.65 mg/l human milk). Rarely, a deficiency of the iron-binding protein transferrin causes a similar picture.

Causes of iron deficiency anaemia in infants and children.
1. Low birth weight ⎤
2. Blood loss at birth ⎦ result in reduced iron stores.
3. Delayed introduction of iron-containing foods, i.e. solids
4. Malabsorption
5. Blood loss, e.g. from the gastrointestinal (GI) tract due to telangiectasia, cows' milk allergy, congenital bleeding disorders, or intestinal parasites.

Management. The majority of paediatric iron deficiency will be associated with benign cause — usually poor diet. All infants suspected of having iron deficiency should have a full history and medical examination. In the absence of features other than dietary iron deficiency, the child should be given iron supplements to raise the haemoglobin to normal levels and a further supply to replace iron stores (usually a 3-month course). Failure to maintain haemoglobin levels when iron supplements are stopped may indicate underlying pathology and should be investigated more fully.

Folate and vitamin B_{12} deficiency

Both these are necessary for DNA synthesis and their absence results in megaloblastic anaemia. The infant is never born anaemic as a consequence of this deficiency in the mother, but may have reduced stores of these haematinics which predispose to later development of anaemia.

Folate deficiency. In the preterm infant folate stores may be inadequate and deficiency may develop when there are other co-existing features, for example infection which increases the need for folate. Folate deficiency may be the presenting feature of haemolytic anaemias or malabsorption in older children. It may also be secondary to drug therapy, of which anticonvulsants are the commonest cause.

B_{12} deficiency. B_{12} deficiency may be the consequence of:

1. The adult type of pernicious anaemia.
2. Congenital intrinsic factor deficiency.
3. Failure of GI tract absorption due to a specific defect in absorption of intrinsic factor B_{12} complex (Imerslünd's syndrome).
4. Secondary to disease affecting the terminal small bowel or following small bowel resection.
5. Rarely, B_{12} deficiency anaemia may develop at 7–12 months of age in infants of B_{12}-deficient mothers who have been fed exclusively on their maternal (B_{12}-deficient) milk.

6. Congenital defects in both B_{12} and folate metabolism are rare causes of megaloblastic anaemia, as are defects in the transport protein of B_{12} — transcobalamin II (TCII).

Treatment of B_{12} and folate deficiencies. Folate deficiency, even due to malabsorption syndrome, responds to pharmacological doses of folic acid given orally. B_{12} deficiency due to failure of absorption is treated by systemic administration of hydroxycobalamin (100 μg i.m. monthly). Dietary B_{12} deficiency responds to oral B_{12}.

The routine laboratory investigations for iron, folate and B_{12} deficiency are shown in Table 23.2.

HAEMOGLOBINOPATHIES AND THALASSAEMIAS

Congenital abnormalities of haemoglobin fall into two groups:

1. Structural haemoglobinopathies in which the abnormalities, usually point mutations of protein coding regions of the gene, affect the properties of the haemoglobin.
2. The thalassaemia syndromes in which a variety of genetic abnormalities result in a reduced rate of synthesis of one of the globin chains.

The two are not always distinct and examples of structural haemoglobinopathies exist where the mutation also causes a reduced rate of production, e.g. haemoglobin E.

Structural haemoglobinopathies

Amino acid substitution can affect the properties

Table 23.2 Investigations in nutritional anaemias

Deficiency	MCV	Special investigations to confirm diagnosis	Investigations to define cause	Differential diagnosis
Iron	↓	Serum iron (↓) Iron binding capacity (↑) Ferritin (↓)	Coagulation screen Occult bloods Investigation for malabsorption	Thalassaemia Lead poisoning Atransferrinaemia
Folate	↑	Red cell and serum folates (↓) Bone marrow (megaloblastic changes)	Blood film for evidence of haemolytic anaemia Investigations for malabsorption	1 Reticulocytosis (e.g. haemolysis, haemorrhage) 2. Dyserythropoiesis 3. Macrocytosis secondary to non-haematological disease, e.g. liver, lung.
B_{12}	↑	Serum B_{12} (↓) Bone marrow megaloblastic Urinary methylmalonic acid	Intrinsic factor antibodies (serum, gastric fluid) Schilling test	

Table 23.3 Abnormal haemoglobin

Property	Associated clinical picture
Reduced solubility	e.g. sickle cell disease
High O_2 affinity	Erythrocytosis
Low O_2 affinity	Low Hb concentration
Unstable Hb	Haemolytic anaemia
Methaemoglobins	Cyanosis

of haemoglobin in a number of ways (Table 23.3). The commonest abnormalities occur in β chains and are haemoglobins S, C, D and E. Of these, haemoglobin S (β 6 glu–val) is the major clinically significant haemoglobinopathy and causes sickle cell anaemia when it is present in the homozygous state. A similar picture also occurs when HbS occurs as a double heterozygote in combination with β-thalassaemia (HbS/βthal) or haemoglobin C (HbS/C disease). The disease can be ameliorated by coexisting genetic abnormalities of haemoglobin including the presence of high levels of haemoglobin F and α-thalassaemia trait. The heterozygous state (AS-sickle cell trait) is regarded as having no clinical significance.

Haemoglobin S disease

The sickle mutation results in a haemoglobin of low solubility in the deoxy state. This results in (a) haemoglobin polymers forming which distort erythrocytes, lead to small vessel occlusion and tissue infarction, and (b) haemolysis. The following features predispose to haemoglobin precipitation:

1. Increased haemoglobin concentration within the red cells, e.g. due to dehydration.
2. Hypoxia, e.g. due to low inspired oxygen concentration, pulmonary disease, or increased oxygen demand due to activity.
3. Increased temperature.

The clinical sequelae to sickle cell disease are:

1. Chronic haemolytic anaemia — which may lead to bilirubin gallstones.
2. Veno-occlusive crises — almost all organs may be affected. Particularly common is bone infarction — infants often present with infarction of the long bones of the feet and hands (the foot-hand syndrome) but all long bones and the ribs

and pelvis may be involved. Abdominal crises may be mistaken for surgical acute abdomens and cerebrovascular occlusions may occur.

3. Sequestration crises:
a. Splenic sequestration. During childhood the spleen becomes autoinfarcted. Prior to this it may enlarge suddenly resulting in massive red cell pooling.
b. Chest syndrome — sequestration of red cells in the lung which is associated with high mortality.
4. Aplastic crises — usually due to infection with parvovirus B19.
5. Megaloblastic crises due to folate deficiency.
6. Chronic organ damage, e.g. proliferative retinopathy, aseptic necrosis of head of femur/humerus, renal impairment — concentrating defects, cardiac myopathy, and papillary necrosis.
7. Predisposition to bacterial infections; infarctions become the nidus of bacterial infection e.g. salmonella osteomyelitis; reduced splenic function; and impaired neutrophil function attributed to reduced levels of chemotactic and opsonising agents.

Methods of preventing complications of sickle cell disease. There is no therapeutic method of preventing occlusive crises although appropriate lifestyle and attention to hydration and pyrexia may help reduce the number of events. This means that everybody involved in the care of a child with sickle disease (parents, family, school, youth groups) should be educated in the problems of sickle cell anaemia and how to manage the affected child.

Children less than 3 years old are sensitive to pneumococcal infections which may be rapidly fatal. Penicillin and pneumococcal vaccine together give the maximum prophylaxis. However, if the penicillin is taken orally, scrupulous attention must be paid to its administration; missing one dose has been associated with pneumococcal infection. Antibody responses to pneumococcal vaccine are suboptimal in children less than three years old. There is no conventional wisdom as to the most appropriate age to stop penicillin therapy.

Diagnosis of sickle cell anaemia at birth may lead to parents being aware of the potentially lethal complication in young infants, resulting in more prompt medical response and possibly reduced fatalities in this age group. Neonatal screening programmes are now being established. Folic acid supplements are often given daily to reduce the risk of megaloblastic anaemia due to folate deficiency but this may be unnecessary in patients whose diet has normal folate content.

Management of occlusive crises. Mild crises may be managed at home, but patients with moderate to severe crises or those associated with pyrexia should be admitted to hospital.

Pain. The intensity of pain varies and it may be necessary to give systemic opiates continuously for analgesia. Reducing anxiety is also important and patients may respond better if they are reassured and seen and managed by the same team of individuals on each occasion.

Dehydration. Fluid balance must be maintained. Damage to the renal tubules means that patients with sickle cell anaemia often have problems concentrating urine and this may exacerbate fluid imbalances; cardiac damage leading to heart failure may also make this difficult.

Pyrexia. Painful crises may cause pyrexia in the absence of infection, however, and following routine samples of urine and blood and swabs from infected sites for microbiology, the child should be switched from penicillin to a broad-spectrum antibiotic, modified on the basis of microbiology results. Sickle cell patients are more prone than normal to infections with some bacteria including *Salmonella* spp. osteomyelitis.

Role of transfusions in sickle cell crises. Severe crises, e.g. chest syndrome, may need exchange transfusion to reduce HbS concentration and limit the crisis. (Top-up transfusion increases blood viscosity and may worsen the situation.) In splenic sequestration, transfusion is necessary to treat the shock following massive red cell pooling and splenectomy should be considered in severe cases. Following cerebral occlusion, it is considered desirable to bring the patient's haemoglobin S level down to 20–30% and to maintain it at this level by regular transfusions. Maintaining the haemoglobin at greater than 10 g/dl reduces the intrinsic stimulus to erythropoiesis and hence lowers the concentration of haemoglobin S. However, long-term transfusion is associated with iron overload.

Preoperative transfusion. If there is a risk of hypoxia during surgery, the haemoglobin S level should be reduced to less than 30% of total haemoglobin either by exchange transfusion in an emergency or by top-up transfusions during the 4–6 weeks before surgery in elective cases.

Thalassaemias

In the adult approximately 95% of haemoglobin is made up of tetramers of two α and two β chains. Gross imbalance of the α and non-α chain production results in the excess chains being precipitated, leading to intramedullary destruction of erythroid cells (ineffective erythropoiesis). In addition, the mature cells are hypochromic and microcytic and have a shortened red cell lifespan. In β-thalassaemia, the gross imbalances leading to clinical disease are only present if both the β chains are affected (homozygous β thalassaemia). The heterozygous state results in a hypochromic-microcytic picture with a low normal haemoglobin.

α-thalassaemia is much more complicated genetically and clinically. α chains are coded for by four genes, two on each chromosome 16, leading to a complicated spectrum of clinical disorders, as shown in Table 23.4.

Table 23.4 Clinical disorders seen in α-thalassaemia

Abnormal genes (no.)	Clinical picture
4	Intra-uterine death (hydrops fetalis)
3	Haemoglobin H disease — haemolytic anaemia
2	Hypochromic microcytic blood film (thalassaemia trait)
1	Asymptomatic carrier
0	Normal

β-thalassaemia

The natural sequelae of homozygous β-thalassaemia is skeletal distortion due to increased marrow activity, poor growth, delayed puberty and, commonly, death in the second decade. Regular transfusion to maintain the haemoglobin at 10.0 g/dl in combination with splenectomy at an appropriately safe age reduces these complications but must be combined with chelation therapy to reduce the risk of iron overload. At present (1989), effective chelation therapy is systemically administered desferrioxamine usually given over 12 hours subcutaneously five nights a week. (Oral agents are being studied but their toxic effects remain to be evaluated.) This can begin when the transfusion regimen is started, so that a pattern is established in the child at an early age, or it may safely be delayed until 5–7 years. The iron accumulating during this period is unlikely to be associated with tissue damage and the child is bigger and better able to tolerate the subcutaneous infusions. Anaphylaxis is a rare complication of desferrioxamine but local complications including erythema and oedema may be troublesome. Desferrioxamine has recently been implicated in damage to eyes and ears and regular assessment of patients on desferrioxamine by ophthalmologists and audiologists is recommended.

Bone marrow transplantation in haemoglobinopathies

In theory, replacing the abnormal erythropoietic system with a normal one by bone marrow transplantation is a feasible approach to these diseases. However, it can never be adopted as the main method of treatment worldwide. Nevertheless bone marrow transplantation has been carried out for thalassaemia with moderate success. Recent results show more than 80% five-year survival. In order to allow the graft to take, the recipient bone marrow has to be ablated and compatible (HLA-matched sibling) donor marrow transfused. The conditioning regimen is usually based on two cytotoxic agents — cyclophosphamide and busulphan — and it is designed to allow adequate bone marrow take without resulting in excessive drug toxicity from which the patient may die. In practice this usually results in a chimeric marrow regeneration. Several features have to be considered before advising bone marrow transplantation, including toxicity, risk of graft-versus-host disease and graft rejection. In addition, patients treated by conventional methods may live to their third or fourth decade and other treatments may become available during this period.

Haemoglobinopathies present the best theoretical opportunity for treatment by gene manipulation. The target cells (bone marrow stem cells) can easily be isolated and manipulated in vitro. However, the introduction of genes under appropriate regulator sequences leading to stable integration in the recipient cells has still to be achieved, even in experimental animals. Other approaches include studying the mechanism by which haemoglobin F synthesis can be enhanced to modify sickle cell disease and thalassaemia. Cytotoxic drugs increase haemoglobin F production but these are too toxic and inefficient for clinical use.

HAEMOLYTIC ANAEMIAS

Intrinsic

Apart from abnormal haemoglobins, congenital haemolytic anaemia can result from abnormalities of the red cell membrane or the red cell enzymes.

Hereditary spherocytosis

This disorder results from an abnormality of the red cell cytoskeleton (composed of spectrin and ankryn) leading to spherocytic red cells which are easily destroyed in the spleen. The clinical picture varies, some individuals are minimally affected and have no symptoms of anaemia, but attention may be drawn to the diagnosis if they present with evidence of increased red cell turnover, for example, gallstones or aplastic crisis due to parvovirus infection. More severely affected cases present either with the signs and symptoms of anaemia or with jaundice, either in the neonatal period or later in life, especially in association with intercurrent infections. On examination, mild to moderate splenomegaly is present.

Management. Folic acid supplements are necessary to prevent megaloblastic anaemia developing because of increased folate requirement. If the patient is symptomatic from the anaemia, e.g. poor growth, splenectomy at an appropriate age (not less than 7 years) will alleviate the anaemia, although evidence of increased red cell turnover will still be found. Prophylactic penicillin and pneumococcal vaccine should be used to reduce the risk of pneumococcal infection in splenectomised children.

As with all haemolytic anaemia, the red cell precursors have a higher percentage in S phase compared with normal individuals. This predisposes these cells to infection with parvovirus B19, the normal aetiological agent for Fifth's disease, resulting in a transient red cell aplasia. The aplasia is self limiting and does not recur because of the development of anti-parvovirus antibodies. Transfusion is only indicated to prevent cardiac failure.

Red cell enzyma defects

Red cells do not have mitochondria and ATP production occurs only as a result of the glycolytic pathway. The pentose phosphate shunt produces reduced glutathione (GSH) involved in the removal of free oxygen radicals, preventing oxidation of the red cell membrane and cellular proteins. Deficiencies in both enzyme systems, i.e. the glycolytic pathway and the pentose phosphate shunt, therefore lead to haemolytic anaemias.

Glucose-6-phosphate dehydrogenase (G6PD) deficiency. The first enzyme of the pentose phosphate shunt is the commonest in which enzyme abnormalities occur. These are particularly common in the Mediterranean areas, Africa and South East Asia, leading to haemolysis, particularly in the presence of other oxidating agents (Table 28.4) when massive intravascular haemolysis can lead to a sudden fall in haemoglobin, haemoglobinuria and even death.

The enzyme is coded for by a gene on the X chromosome and hence the defect is commonest in hemizygous boys. Affected females can occur as the offspring of heterozygous females and affected males. Because of the gene frequency of the abnormal genes of G6PD this situation is commoner than in other X-linked diseases, e.g. haemophilia.

Table 23.5 Common oxidative agents causing haemolysis in G6PD-deficient individuals*

Naphthalene moth balls

Water-soluble vitamin K_1 (in high doses)

Vitamin C

Fava bean (broad beans or pollen)

Drugs:

Antimalarials	— primaquine, quinine
Sulphonamides	+ sulphones
Nitrofurans	
Analgesics	— phenacetin, acetylsalicylic acid (large doses

* more detailed texts should be consulted before prescribing any drugs for G6PD-deficient individuals

The clinical picture varies according to the genetic abnormality of the enzyme. In blacks, the defect results in an enzyme which has a shorter half-life and young red cells have virtually normal enzyme activity. This results in a disease which is less severe than that generally seen in other groups.

The diagnosis is confirmed by analysis of the activity of the enzyme. The disease is managed by advising the patient or parents how to avoid the agents which can precipitate attacks of haemolysis.

If other red cell enzyme defects are suspected of causing haemolytic anaemia, the patient or samples of their blood must be sent to specialist centres where the enzyme activities can be fully investigated.

Extrinsic

Immune haemolytic anaemias

Haemolytic disease of the newborn (HDN). This is due to blood group antigen incompatibility between the mother and the fetus and the presence in the mother of IgG antibodies to this fetal antigen. Clinically the disease varies in its presentation:

1. Intrauterine death.
2. Hydropic infant.
3. Anaemia and jaundice at birth.
4. Early neonatal jaundice.

Antibodies in the maternal circulation are natural or acquired. Of the former, antibodies to antigens of the ABO system are the commonest but rarely cause clinically significant disease because:

a. They are usually IgM and therefore do not cross the placenta.

b. A and B antigens are expressed only weakly on fetal and neonatal blood cells.

Acquired antibodies develop following exposure to antigens either by blood transfusion or following feto-maternal bleeds in previous pregnancies. In the natural course of events, anti-D is the commonest cause of haemolytic disease of the newborn in Caucasians and the one most associated with severe disease. The incidence of haemolytic disease of the newborn due to anti-D is decreasing due to:

a. Transfusion of only rhesus-D-negative blood

to the rhesus-D-negative women of childbearing age. (Where D-positive blood has been inadvertently given large doses of anti-D immunoglobulin may reduce the risk of sensitisation.)

b. Administration of anti-D to all rhesus-D-negative women delivering rhesus-D-positive infants within 72 hours of birth in sufficient doses to prevent sensitisation. The size of the feto-maternal bleed therefore needs to be assessed by the Kleihauer test (95% of foto-maternal bleeds will be covered by 1500 μg of anti-D.)

c. Administration of anti-D to any rhesus-D-negative women having an abortion or obstetric manoeuvre. (A loop-hole exists when women abort early prior to the diagnosis of pregnancy.)

d. And more recently, to prevent the slight risk of sensitisation due to spontaneous bleed during the first pregnancy, primiparous rhesus-D-negative women without anti-D antibodies can be given anti-D during the last trimester of pregnancy. These doses are too low to affect the infant but will protect from sensitisation from spontaneous bleeds occurring during this time.

Because of the reduced incidence of anti-D antibodies other red cell antibodies are becoming relatively commoner causes of haemolytic disease of the newborn. These include within the rhesus system C, E c, e, and outside the rhesus system Duffy, Kell and Kidd antigens.

Recognition of mothers at risk. All mothers regardless of rhesus D status should have their sera investigated for atypical antibodies at booking and during the third trimester. Any abnormal results should be followed up regularly to assess any increase in antibodies and the progress of the fetus monitored.

Diagnosis and management of HDN. Diagnosis of HDN depends on the demonstrating evidence of increased haemolysis in association with positive direct antibody tests on the fetal red cells and antibody in the maternal serum.

Exchange transfusion in HDN. Affected infants may need exchange transfusion with blood negative for the appropriate antigen and cross matched against the maternal serum. Such blood should be arranged to be on standby from the time the mother goes into labour, and should be as fresh as possibly (usually 72 hours) to reduce the metabolic load on the neonate. In cases where compatible blood will not be easily available, appropriate blood or donors may have to be on standby from the 36th week onward.

The indications for exchange transfusion are:

1. At birth Hb 12.0 g/dl and a cord bilirubin of greater than 100 μmol/l.
2. To prevent the bilirubin rising to levels associated with kernicterus (in a full-term, otherwise healthy infant 400–450 μmol/l).

Exchange transfusion replaces antigen-positive blood with antigen-negative cells and also removes some of the antibodies and bilirubin.

It must be remembered that O Rhesus-D-negative blood may not be appropriate in an emergency *unless* the antibody causing haemolytic disease is known to be anti-D, as the blood may not be negative for any of the other red cell antigens likely to be associated with HDN.

Autoimmune haemolytic anaemia (AIHA). In children AIHA is usually a self-limiting disorder associated with a recent viral infection. The diagnosis is based on falling haemoglobin levels, a reticulocytosis and positive DAGT. It usually responds to a short course of steroid therapy (starting prednisolone 60 mg/m^2/day) and rarely relapses on cessation of therapy, thus splenectomy is rarely indicated in paediatric AIHA. However, it may be the presenting symptom of SLE in children and appropriate investigation should always be undertaken.

Non-immune haemolytic anaemia

Microangiopathic haemolytic anaemias. Red cell destruction with typical pathological features including burr cells and microspherocytes are secondary to abnormal flow and often associated with abnormal blood vessel walls secondary to fibrin deposition. Important underlying causes include thrombotic thrombocytopenic purpura, haemolytic uraemic syndrome, giant haemangioma, abnormal cardiac valves (including prostheses) and disseminated intravascular coagulation.

Vitamin E deficiency. Vitamin E protects lipids from peroxidation by free oxygen radicals. In preterm infants low vitamin E levels, low red cell enzyme levels, and possible concomitant oxidant drug therapy, e.g. vitamin K or iron therapy, combine to predispose the infant to a haemolytic anaemia due to membrane oxidation. This can be prevented by vitamin E supplements.

RED CELL HYPOPLASIA/APLASIA

In the adult, pure red cell aplasia (PRCA) is frequently associated with immune disturbance, e.g. secondary to autoimmune disease, lymphoid tumours especially thymoma or caused by autoantibodies to red cell precursors or erythropoietin. In children the spectrum of causes of red cell aplasia is different.

Blackfan–Diamond syndrome

This congenital disorder of erythropoiesis usually presents in the first year of life and may be associated with physical abnormalities, but in contrast to Fanconi's anaemia (see pp. 291) the chromosomes are normal. It has been considered that the disease lay primarily in the lymphoid system but now an abnormality in the erythroid progenitor cells is considered more likely.

Two-thirds of cases will respond to steroids. Patients can usually be maintained at the haemoglobin of 10 g/dl on acceptable doses of prednisolone which it may be possible to reduce as the child matures. The steroid-resistant cases can be treated with anabolic steroids, antithymocyte globulin, blood transfusion or bone marrow transplantation.

Transient erythroblastopenia of childhood

This occurs classically in healthy toddlers (1–4 years) who develop increasing pallor over several weeks. The anaemia is normochromic normocytic; other peripheral blood findings depend on the stage of the disease at diagnosis. Prior to recovery there will be no reticulocytosis and the bone marrow, if examined, will be devoid of erythroid precursors. However, spontaneous recovery occurs with the appearance of erythroid precursors in the marrow and reticulocytes in the peripheral blood. Some patients will be first seen at this stage. The

disease may be associated with a recent viral infection (*not* parvovirus). Diagnosis is made on clinical history and the peripheral blood findings. Bone marrow examination and blood transfusion are rarely necessary.

Aplasia, in patients with haemolytic anaemia, due to parvovirus B19

Erythroid precursors in patients with haemolytic anaemia (e.g. hereditary spherocytosis, sickle cell disease, thalassaemia, pyruvate kinase deficiency) are susceptible to infection with parvovirus which results in a transient pure red cell aplasia (see pp. 285). Transfusion may be necessary if the low haemoglobin levels results in cardiac failure. The virus is the aetiological agent of Fifth's disease. In immunocompromised patients, persistent parvovirus infection may cause chronic red cell aplasia.

ERYTHROCYTOSIS

Polycythaemia rubra vera is rare in infants. The causes of high haemoglobin differ from adults:

1. In the neonate — delayed clamping of the cord.
2. Congenital hypothyroidism.
3. High-affinity haemoglobins.
4. Rare familial inherited disorders of erythropoiesis.

PLATELET DISORDERS

THROMBOCYTOPENIA

Neonatal thrombocytopenia

Neonatal thrombocytopenia due to increased platelet destruction

This may be due to disseminated intravascular coagulation (DIC) or immune destruction. In the latter case the IgG platelet antibodies are maternally derived. They may be secondary to maternal disease, idiopathic thrombocytopenic purpura (ITP) or systemic lupus erythematosus (SLE) and severe thrombocytopenia may develop in the infant even if the mother maintains a normal platelet count. However, a second cause of immune destruction is analogous to that seen in haemolytic disease of the newborn but, because platelet antigen mismatches are uncommon, the disease is rare. It occurs when the infant expresses a common platelet antigen (usually Pl^{A1}) which the mother does not express, and to which she has been sensitised.

In immune thrombocytopenia the infant platelet count will rise as the maternal antibody concentration falls, but for some weeks the infant may be at risk of bleeding. If the antibody is anti Pl^{A1}, then Pl^{A1} negative platelet will survive normally in the circulation and transfusion of these can be used to protect the infant until an adequate platelet count is attained. Transfused platelet will survive poorly in the neonate with thrombocytopenia secondary to ITP, but intravenous IgG (which can be administered to the mother prior to delivery), or steroid therapy may increase the platelet count. In severe bleeding episodes, platelet transfusions may be helpful for the short term.

Congenital thrombocytopenia due to failure of platelet production

This may occur as the result of:

1. Intrauterine infection:
   a. Toxoplasma
   b. Rubella
   c. Cytomegalovirus
   d. Herpes
   e. Syphilis
2. Fanconi's anaemia
3. TAR (thrombocytopenia with absent radii)
4. Other congenital megakaryocytic abnormalities

Idiopathic thrombocytopenic purpura

Autoimmune thrombocytopenia in children is usually secondary to a viral infection and will completely recover in 80% of cases. In the remainder, it will progress to chronic disease similar to that seen in adults.

If the thrombocytopenia is mild no treatment is needed; however, if there are clinical problems such as large haematomas or conjunctival haemor-

rhages treatment may be necessary. Classically, the disease is managed with oral steroids which usually results in an increased platelet count after about 5 days. More rapid rises are achieved with intravenous IgG or high-dose steroids intravenously. Because the incidence of intracranial haemorrhage is less than 0.1% of all patients presenting with ITP, it would be necessary to conduct a trial with more than 6000 patients to show any advantage for intravenous IgG in the prevention of this complication.

Before starting therapy, a bone marrow examination should be performed to confirm the diagnosis (increased megakaryocytes in an otherwise normal marrow). Platelet antibody studies may be helpful but are not always diagnostic and results may not be available soon enough to influence decisions on therapy.

Patients who do not remit or who relapse when steroid therapy is stopped may progress to chronic ITP. If the thrombocytopenia is asymptomatic, therapy is not indicated. Relapsed patients may have satisfactory response to low doses of steroids. Steroid refractory patients may respond to intravenous gamma globulin or splenectomy. Cytotoxic therapy (cyclophosphamide or azathoprine) is used only as a last resort in children.

THROMBOCYTOSIS

Elevated platelet counts in children are rarely due to primary bone marrow disorder; they are usually secondary to blood loss or infection. High levels of platelet count are particularly obvious in the second or third week of Kawasaki's disease.

DISORDERS OF NEUTROPHILS

Disorders of neutrophils can be divided into quantitative and qualitative defects. Both are fortunately rare.

Quantitative defects

Symptoms of neutropenia rarely develop when the neutrophil count is over $1 \times 10^9/l$ and risk of severe bacterial infection, including septicaemia, occurs only if the count is less than $0.5 \times 10^9/l$.

Causes of neutropenia in infancy and childhood

1. Congenital familial.
2. Immune:
   a. Isoimmune neonatal
   b. Autoimmune
3. Drug induced.
4. Secondary to infection.
5. Cyclical neutropenia.

Children with neutropenia should be evaluated for its aetiology and clinical severity. Patients may have identical peripheral blood count and dramatically different clinical features, possibly because the peripheral blood count does not totally reflect the total neutrophil pool.

Neutropenias associated with infections and some drug-induced neutropenias will remit when the initiating agent is removed.

Qualitative defects of neutrophil function

Normal neutrophil function involves many steps:

1 Adherence to vascular endothelial cells and diapedesis through vessel walls.
2. Migration to sites of inflammation along gradients of numerous chemotactic molecules.
3. Phagocytosis of agents — bacteria, fungi which have been rendered more sensitive to phagocytosis by opsonising agents — into phagosomes.
4. Killing of bacteria by fusion of neutrophil granules and lysosomes and generation of killing molecules, e.g. superoxide.

These functions may be abnormal in congenital defects of neutrophils, e.g.:

1. Failure of neutrophils to adhere to tissue and hence inability to migrate to sites of inflammation. These are due to abnormalities of the adhesion molecule receptors on neutrophil surfaces (LFA-1).
2. Failure to respond to chemotactic stimuli, e.g. lazy leucocyte syndrome.
3. Failure of phagocytosis of micro-organisms, e.g. neutrophil actin dysfunction.
4. Abnormal granules, e.g. Chediak–Higashi syndrome, may impede cell motility and phagocytosis.
5. Disorders of oxidative metabolism, e.g. chronic granulomatous disease.

Abnormalities of neutrophil function may occur secondary to diseases which are associated with reduced chemotactic and/or opsonising activity.

These disorders predispose to a variety of bacterial and fungal infections. The precise diagnosis is difficult and is made on the basis of specific tests of neutrophil function. The easiest to diagnose in the general haematology laboratory is chronic granulomatous disease in which the affected neutrophils have the inability to produce superoxides and fail to reduce nitroblue tetrazolium (NBT) to a dark blue colour.

Recombinant DNA technology has made available for therapeutic purposes cytokines which influence neutrophil function and these have been shown to be useful in some congenital disorders of neutrophil function, e.g. γ interferon has been shown to enhance neutrophil function in chronic granulomatous disease and granulocyte-colony stimulating factor (G-CSF) has been shown to increase neutrophil counts in cyclical neutropenia and some cases of congenital neutropenia and is now considered the treatment of choice.

FAILURE OF ALL CELLULAR MARROW ELEMENTS

Aplastic anaemia

Failure of all the cellular bone marrow elements may be idiopathic or secondary to known aetiological agents. In children, exposure to toxins, some drugs (e.g. chloramphenicol, phenylbutazone, anticonvulsants), organic solvents, or viral infections, e.g. hepatitis A, are among the commoner associations. The clinical outcome of aplastic anaemia depends on the degree of pancytopenia. The following are bad prognostic features:

1. Platelet counts of less than $10 \times 10^9/l$.
2. Reticulocytes of less than $10 \times 10^{10}/l$.
3. Neutrophils of less than $0.5 \times 10^9/l$.

In such severely affected patients, death is likely to occur from infection or bleeding, usually the former, within months of diagnosis. Bone marrow transplantation from an HLA-identical sibling donor offers the best chance of survival. Anti-thymocytic globulin in combination with steroids is the best treatment in the absence of suitable donors. More mildly affected individuals have a spectrum of problems varying from transfusion dependence, bleeding diathesis and infection, to minimal clinical problems. They may improve on androgen or steroid therapy.

Fanconi's anaemia

This is a constitutional disorder usually inherited as an autosomal recessive which is characterised by increased chromosome fragility, especially demonstrated by mitomycin C, nitrogen mustard or isonicotinic acid in vitro. The classical patient is of small stature, with congenital abnormalities particularly affecting the skeleton, heart, kidneys, and has abnormal pigmentation (café-au-lait spots). The patient does not always present with classical clinical features; often only partially expressed phenotypes occur. Evidence of bone marrow failure is not usually present at birth but gradually develops during childhood leading to bleeding diatheses, anaemia, and sensitivity to infection.

The peripheral blood count may respond to androgens or steroids and bone marrow transplantation has been used, although because of the inherited nature of this disorder, screening of donors is particularly important.

Malignant transformation to acute myelomonocytic leukaemia is a well-recognised complication of Fanconi's anaemia.

COAGULATION DISORDERS

The normal range of coagulation tests in paediatric patients is different from adults (Table 23.6), but individual clotting factors attain normal adult levels at different rates — a fact which must be taken into consideration when diagnosing coagulation factor deficiencies in children. Factor VIII is present in normal levels at birth. Factor IX is within the normal adult range at 6 months, but the mean values continue to be low for several years.

Haemorrhagic disease of the newborn (HDN)

Vitamin K is necessary for the post-translational modification of the proteins of Factors II, VII, IX and X. In the absence of vitamin K, abnormal proteins — protein(s) induced by vitamin K absence or antagonism (PIVKAS) — are produced. Because of immaturity of the bowel flora, the neonate depends entirely on dietary vitamin K to satisfy its daily needs. Both cows' milk and formula feeds have higher vitamin K content than maternal milk. Classical HDN due to vitamin K deficiency occurs during the second to fourth week of life and can be prevented by oral (2 mg) or intramuscular (1 mg) vitamin K1 administered at birth.

Non-classical forms of the HDN have recently been recognised. The early form (up to 1 week of age) is associated with maternal drug ingestion including warfarin, anticonvulsants and antituberculous chemotherapy. Late HDN occurring at 1–3 months of age is now recognised and associated with failure of vitamin K prophylaxis at birth and breast feeding. It may present with intracranial haemorrhage which is often precipitated by diarrhoea. The American Academy of Pediatrics has recommended that breast-fed infants with sustained diarrhoea for 4 days should be given prophylactic intramuscular vitamin K. Late vitamin K deficiency may also be a presenting symptom of underlying bowel disease or warfarin ingestion.

Disseminated intravascular coagulation (DIC)

DIC is the result of a generalised trigger to the

Table 23.6 Coagulation screening test results in infants

Age	Kaolin-cephalin coagulation time	Prothrombin time	Thrombin time	Fibrinogen
Preterm	Prolonged	Prolonged	N	N
Full term	Prolonged	N	N	N
3/12	N	N	N	N

N = normal

Table 23.7 Laboratory findings in DIC

Blood film	Red cell fragmentation
Platelet count	↓
Kaolin-cephalin coagulation time	Prolonged
Prothrombin time	Prolonged
Thrombin time	Prolonged
Fibrinogen	N or ↓
Fibrin degradation products	↑

N = normal

coagulation system which results in the consumption of coagulation factors and intravascular fibrin deposition. The dual results of this are the loss of haemostatic competence and small vessel occlusion. Abnormal coagulation tests (Table 23.7) reflect these processes. In children, DIC is nearly always secondary to infection. Management involves treating the underlying cause and replacing the consumed coagulation factors and platelets. This should be combined with adequate heparinisation if there is a significant risk of thrombosis, which is particularly important in meningococcal-associated DIC.

The preterm infant is particularly predisposed to DIC, because of low levels of coagulation factors and inhibitors e.g. antithrombin III as well as immaturity of both the reticulo-endothelial system (leading to impaired clearance of activated clotting factors) and the bone marrow which fails to compensate for increased platelet consumption.

Congenital coagulation factor deficiencies

Isolated inherited disorders of all coagulation factors have been recognised. The three commonest are (1) Factor VIII: C deficiency (haemophilia), (2)

Factor IX deficiency (Christmas disease) and (3) von Willebrand's disease (due to an abnormal von Willebrand factor which is the carrier for VIII: C and binds platelets to endothelium). The first two are inherited as X-linked recessive disorders and the latter autosomally (usually dominant).

Presentation

1. Neonatally:
   a. Intracranial haemorrhage (usually associated with difficult labour)
   b. Bleeding from the umbilical stump
2. Later:
   a. Haemarthroses
   b. Deep muscle haematomas
   c. Haematuria
   d. Intracranial bleeding

Diagnosis of coagulation factor disorders

The pattern of screening coagulation factor results is shown in Table 23.8. A suspicion of the disease is confirmed by assaying individual coagulation factors.

Management of acute bleeds

This involves

1. Pain relief — opiates may be necessary.
2. Replacing intravenously the absent factor in sufficient quantities to maintain a haemostatic level over an adequate period of time to allow healing of the bleeding points. Both Factor VIII and Factor IX are available as freeze-dried concentrates which means the bleeds can be treated promptly at home. Hospital admission of such patients is only necessary for major bleeds.
3. Resting the affected part.

Table 23.8 Coagulation tests in inherited coagulation defects

Disease	BT	Kaolin-cephalin coagulation time	Prothrombin time	Thrombin time	Factor VIII: C	Factor IX	VWF*
Haemophilia	N	↑	N	N	↓	N	N or ↑
Christmas disease	N	↑	N	N	N	↓	N
von Willebrand's disease	↑	↑	N	N	↓	N	↓

* VWF (von Willebrand factor) can be measured by VIII Rag, or Ristocetin, induced platelet aggregation

Both patients and families therefore need education into the management of the disease and regular multidisciplinary (dentist, physiotherapist, othopaedic surgeon, haematologist) follow-up to assess:

1. Any long-term damage as a consequence of repeated bleeding.

2. Adequate dental care.

3. To look for the development of antibodies to coagulation factors especially severe haemophiliacs (Factor VIII: C <1%) who may develop antibodies to administered Factor VIII.

4. To monitor the effects of repeated administration of coagulation factor concentrates. Liver damage resulting from non-A, non-B hepatitis and HIV infection (prior to production of HIV-free concentrates) are the most important of these. Recombinant protein or monoclonal antibody-purified preparations are being studied.

Severe congenital bleeding disorders cause chronic problems to the affected individual and to the family. Support therefore is necessary not only for the patient but also for his immediate family, together with adequate education of the people he is likely to come into contact with at school and socially. The patients should be educated in adopting a reasonable lifestyle, taught to give intravenous injections safely, to seek advice when necessary and given HIV counselling when appropriate.

CIRCULATING ANTICOAGULANTS

The coagulation system is balanced by a series of circulating anticoagulants, a congenital deficiency of which predisposes to thrombosis. In the newborn, low levels of these factors are found physiologically and balance the low levels of coagulation factors seen at this time. The best recognised disorders are deficiencies of anti-thrombin III, protein C and protein S. These deficiencies generally predispose to venous thrombosis in affected heterozygous adults. However, protein C deficiency may be inherited as an autosomal recessive disorder; the homozygous state presents early in infancy with purpura fulminans which is usually fatal.

ANTENATAL DIAGNOSIS

Because of the relative ease of sampling fetal blood compared to other fetal tissue, antenatal diagnosis of haematological disease during the second trimester of pregnancy has been established for many years. Identification of haematological inherited disorders by DNA analysis of chorionic villae has made first trimester diagnosis possible in a great many cases. The list of haematological diseases which can be diagnosed antenatally is growing rapidly and includes: sickle cell disease, haemophilia, chronic granulomatous disease, and thalassaemia. Thus diagnosis of heterozygous carrier states in individuals must be accompanied by adequate genetic counselling and the offering of antenatal diagnosis if this is required.

REFERENCES

Dollman P R, Sumer M A 1979 Percentile curves for haemoglobin and red cell volume in infancy and childhood. Journal of Pediatrics 94: 26
Matoth et al 1971 Postnatal changes in some red cell parameters. Acta Paediatrica Scandinavica 60: 317

FURTHER READING

Baehner R L (ed) 1980 Pediatric hematology (Pediatric Clinics of North America), vol 27, no 2. Saunders, Philadelphia
Oski F A (ed) 1987 Pediatric hematology (Oncology Clinics of North America), vol 1, no 3. Saunders, Philadelphia
Willoughby M L N (ed) 1977 Paediatric haematology. Churchill Livingstone, Edinburgh

24. Oncology

P. Morris-Jones

EPIDEMIOLOGY AND AETIOLOGY

Malignant diseases are rare in childhood. They occur in 1 in 10 000 children per year; from birth to 15 years a child has a 1 in 600 chance of developing a malignancy, compared with a 1 in 5 chance in adult life. The types of malignant disease in childhood are very different from those in adults. Embryonic tumours of mesenchymal origin, central nervous system tumours and reticuloendothelial malignancy predominate in childhood in contrast to the carcinomas of adult life. The incidence of the different types of childhood cancers seen in the UK is shown in Table 24.1.

There are significant differences in the tumours seen in Africa and the Far East. Some of these differences are probably environmental while others are more likely to be of genetic or racial origin. There are, for example, very few cases of Ewing's tumour in African children or in American blacks, but the high incidence of Burkitt's lymphoma in certain areas of Africa is not seen in the American black population. Despite these differences the majority of childhood tumours remain sporadic in origin.

There are, however, certain factors which carry an increased risk of malignancy in childhood; hemihypertrophy carries an increased risk of Wilms' tumour, adrenocortical carcinoma and liver tumours. The actual risk factor is unknown as the true incidence of hemihypertrophy is difficult to ascertain. Congenital aniridia usually occurs as an autosomal dominant trait, but when it occurs sporadically the risk of Wilms' tumour in the child is increased to 1000 times above normal. Chromosomal banding techniques have

Table 24.1 Incidence of malignant disease 1954–83: Manchester Children's Tumour Registry

Malignancy	Incidence per 10^6 persons
Acute lymphoblastic leukaemia	26.3
Acute non-lymphoblastic leukaemia	5.8
Other leukaemia	1.0
Hodgkin's disease	3.7
Non-Hodgkin's lymphoma	4.7
Other lymphoreticular system	2.8
Ependymoma	3.0
Adult astrocytoma	3.6
Juvenile astrocytoma	5.6
Medulloblastoma	5.1
Other central nervous system	6.2
Neuroblastoma	6.4
Retinoblastoma	2.7
Wilms' tumour	5.4
Hepatoblastoma	0.5
Osteosarcoma	2.5
Ewing's tumour	1.9
Rhabdomyosarcoma	4.0
Other soft tissue sarcoma	1.4
Germ cell tumours	2.7
Epithelial tumours	2.3
Other and unspecified neoplasms	2.5

shown that these children, who are usually mentally retarded, have a small deletion of chromosome 11. Certain constitutional chromosome disorders carry a known excess risk of cancer and these are shown in Table 24.2. The

Table 24.2 Constitutional chromosomal abnormalities associated with increased tumour susceptibility

Chromosomal anomaly	Cancer type
Trisomy 21 (Down's syndrome)	Acute lymphoblastic leukaemia
Trisomy 18	Wilms' tumour
Turner's syndrome	Neurogenic tumours
XY gonadal dysgenesis	Gonadoblastoma
Klinefelter's syndrome (XXY)	Acute leukaemia, teratoma, breast carcinoma
D deletion (13q-)	Retinoblastoma

banding techniques have also shown acquired chromosome changes in malignant cell; these include the Philadelphia chromosome in chronic myeloid leukaemia, trisomy 8 in acute myelogenous leukaemia and translocations of chromosomes 8, 11 and 14 in lymphomas. Approximately 10% of known single gene traits have malignancy as a complication. The better known of these include familial polyposis of the colon, von Recklinhausen's syndrome, tuberous sclerosis and several of the immunodeficiency syndromes.

The only malignant disease which is certainly inherited is retinoblastoma. This tumour occurs in two forms: unilateral when it is rarely inherited, and bilateral when it is inherited as an autosomal dominant trait, in these cases, the tumour is frequently multifocal in origin. Bilateral and multifocal forms of Wilms' tumour and neuroblastoma may also be inherited.

Very few environmental factors have been identified as a cause of childhood cancer. Prenatal exposure to diagnostic radiation does increase the risk but this is really only important when exposure is in the first trimester. Stillboestrol given during pregnancy has been shown to increase vaginal and cervical adenocarcinoma in the daughters and hypotrophic testes and low sperm counts in the sons. Other possible transplacental carcinogens include diphenylhydantoin and barbiturates.

ACUTE LEUKAEMIAS

Diagnosis

Approximately 85% of all children who develop leukaemia have the acute lymphoblastic type; the majority of the remainder have acute myeloid, myelomonocytic or monocytic disease. The peak incidence of acute lymphoblastic leukaemia (ALL) in childhood is between 2 and 6 years, but it can occur at birth and is seen throughout childhood. The non-lymphoid leukaemias show no peak. Children with Down's syndrome (trisomy 21) have a 15 times greater risk of developing leukaemia and develop the disease at an earlier age.

Most children with leukaemia present with vague non-specific symptoms; pallor, lassitude, irritability and bone pain are common. Lymphadenopathy, hepatosplenomegaly and a petechial rash are frequently found on examination. Hypertrophy of the gums is common in acute myelomonocytic and monocytic leukaemias. The association of these findings with anaemia, thrombocytopenia and circulating blast cells usually makes the diagnosis simple. Some children with leukaemia do not have organomegaly or abnormal cells in the peripheral blood and a bone marrow examination is necessary to differentiate the disease from aplastic anaemia. Infectious mononucleosis has many features commonly seen in leukaemia, but the atypical lymphocytes characteristic of the disease are heterogeneous in appearance, and significant anaemia or thrombocytopenia are rare. Idiopathic thrombocytopenic purpura is usually seen following a viral infection in an otherwise healthy child and a low platelet count is the only abnormality of the peripheral blood.

Once the diagnosis of leukaemia is made, the child should be referred to a major paediatric oncology unit. This is to allow optimum therapy by using a more detailed and complex classification of the disease; the majority of children with acute lymphoblastic leukaemia have small cells known as L_1. In the L_2 subgroup the blast cells are large, they account for about 10% of childhood cases. The L_3 group have very primitive cells which carry surface markers characteristic of B-lymphocytes and account for about 1–2% of childhood cases. T-cell surface markers can be demonstrated in about 10–15% of children with lymphoblastic leukaemia. Most of these children are boys and in older age groups; they have high white cell counts and anterior mediastinal masses. The majority of cases of childhood leukaemia

(70%) have receptors for a specific ALL antigen and are classified as having common ALL; they usually have L_1 cells and the best prognosis. Another group without cell markers (null cells) have an intermediate outlook. Further phenotypes continue to be identified by immunological techniques.

Treatment of acute lymphoblastic leukaemia

Treatment can be divided into three phases:

1. Induction of remission. This is usually achieved by use of steroids, in conjunction with vincristine sulphate and asparaginase and an anthracycline such as doxorubicin (Adriamycin). The term remission means that the child's symptoms and clinical signs have regressed and that the bone marrow contains less than 5% of blast cells and other normal marrow elements are present in normal proportions. This phase is usually complete by the end of 4 weeks of treatment.

2. Consolidation and central nervous system prophylaxis. This involves further cytoreduction and may use other drugs or further courses of those used in the induction phase. Treatment of the central nervous system is essential to prevent the later overt development of leukaemic disease there. Some authorities advocate the use of intrathecal drugs alone, usually methotrexate, but more frequently it is combined with cranial irradiation. New studies may show that this is unnecessary.

3. Maintenance. This consists of repeated cycles of treatment using several drugs. The mainstays are 6-mercaptopurine and methotrexate often combined with pulses of cytosine arabinoside, vincristine and steroids. Treatment with these drugs is usually continued for 2 years; the optimum length of maintenance therapy has not yet been established.

Many protocols have been devised which have been shown to be very successful in the management of ALL and 5-year disease-free survival rates in excess of 60% are common. A proportion of children relapse while still on therapy; the majority of these will respond to further therapy but usually relapse again and median survival time after relapse is approximately 9 months. Of the remainder who come off therapy, about 10% will

relapse in the first year and decreasing numbers relapse in the next few years. Few relapses have been described after 4 years off therapy. With more detailed subclassification, it has been possible to delineate prognostic factors, the majority of failures occur in children:

1. Under the age of 2 and over the age of 10 years.
2. Presenting with high white cell counts at diagnosis.
3. With anterior mediastinal masses — who usually also have T-cell markers.
4. With CNS disease at diagnosis.
5. Who are black.
6. Who are boys and develop isolated testicular disease.

Patients falling into the first three of these categories probably benefit from the use of treatment programmes involving even more intensive therapy and the use of more drugs. Whether or not it is possible to eradicate central nervous system leukaemia without inflicting late damage on the central nervous system is not yet known, certainly the repeated use of intrathecal drugs and irradiation produce a deterioration in mental function. Only a very small proportion of children with bone marrow relapse will ultimately survive, but bone marrow transplant may benefit approximately 20% of these cases.

Treatment of acute non-lymphocytic leukaemias (ANLL)

The general principles of management are similar to those of ALL. The most widely used and useful drugs are, the anthracyclines (daunorubicin and doxorubicin, cytosine arabinoside and thioguanine). Remission induction can be obtained in about 70% of patients. Consolidation is given with the same agents, including central nervous system prophylaxis. Remission is not achieved without a period of severe hypoplasia and these children need special supportive care if they are not to succumb to uncontrolled bleeding, coagulation problems and severe infections. They should not be treated outside special units.

Whether or not maintenance therapy has any part to play in patients with ANLL is questionable and, indeed, in patients with a suitable donor bone marrow transplant is the treatment of choice once remission is obtained. Those without donors may well benefit from autologous transplant following induction of remission and cytoreductive consolidation.

DIAGNOSIS AND TREATMENT OF THE CHRONIC LEUKAEMIAS

Adult-type chronic granulocytic leukaemia

This type of leukaemia shows the Philadelphia (Ph[1]) chromosome; it accounts for approximately 1.5% of childhood leukaemias. The clinical presentation in childhood is varied; signs and symptoms may be insidious in onset. The symptoms are related to anaemia, marrow hyperplasia and splenomegaly and give rise to malaise, pallor, bone pain and a feeling of upper abdominal fullness. There is usually a mild anaemia, an associated marked leucocytosis usually greater than $100 \times 10^9/1$ and a normal platelet count. The majority are mature cells.

There is a group of children with Ph[1] chromosome leukaemia who present as acute lymphoblastic leukaemia and, if cytogenetic studies are not available, may be suspected on the basis of failure to respond to usual therapy. Another group may present in blast cell crisis with morphology suggestive of acute myeloid leukaemia.

The most appropriate method of treatment depends on the findings at presentation. Busulphan is the drug of choice in the chronic phase, while the other forms show better response to similar therapy for acute disease. None of these patients have a good long-term prognosis and should be considered for transplantation in remission.

Juvenile chronic myeloid leukaemia

There is a skin rash, hepatosplenomegaly, lymphadenopathy, thrombocytopenia and a significantly raised fetal haemoglobin. The disease runs an acute course and is unresponsive to chemotherapy.

TUMOURS OF THE CENTRAL NERVOUS SYSTEM

These tumours make up the largest group of solid tumours in childhood, approximately 20%. They differ from those of adult life in that 70% of them occur in structures below the tentorium. The histological subtypes also differ; almost half the malignant tumours in adults are glioblastomas while they only account for about 10% of childhood tumours; high grade astrocytomas considered by many to be a variant of glioblastomas account for another 5%. There is also a group of astrocytic tumours arising in the brain stem in which, because of the site, histological verification is difficult; most of these are probably malignant and they account for 10% of the total. Medulloblastomas and primitive neuroectodermal tumours are a common group in childhood, about 20% of the total, while they are very rare in adult life. Ependymomas, most of which occur infratentorially, are also more common in children than adults. Teratomas, pineal tumours, cranio-pharyngiomas and pituitary tumours are rare but, nevertheless, important diagnostically as they may present initially with precocious puberty, diabetes insipidus, growth failure or the diencephalic syndrome.

Diagnosis and treatment

Most children with brain tumours present with symptoms and signs directly related to raised intracranial pressure and to the focal effects of the mass. The rise in intracranial pressure is usually due to cerebral oedema or to a block in the cerebrospinal fluid pathways and only rarely to the volume of the lesion itself. Symptoms include headache, vomiting and impaired vision.

A common false localising signs is a sixth nerve palsy. Enlargement of the cranium may occur in young children, but convulsions are rare. As so many childhood brain tumours arise in the cerebellum and brain stem, a disturbance of gait and balance is common. Children may be noticed to become clumsy, to walk into furniture or to have deteriorating handwriting. Many of these tumours are benign astrocytomas amenable to surgical removal, but delay in diagnosis may lead to permanent impairment of vision from raised intracranial pressure. Pontine tumours produce similar symptoms and, in addition, defects in the lower cranial nerves with palatal weakness and swallowing difficulties. Spinal tumours, if intramedullary, produce symmetrical weakness and wasting, while extramedullary tumours produce nerve root effects.

CT scanning has made the diagnosis of brain tumours much simpler as it has removed the need for invasive techniques and, in those children with suggestive symptoms and sign, this investigative procedure should be carried out. Stereotactic biopsy techniques have also increased the frequency of histological diagnosis in previously inaccessible sites.

At the present time surgery is the treatment of choice for all central nervous system tumours. Total removal is rarely possible except in the case of cerebellar astrocytomas and the occasional supratentorial low grade glioma. With improved surgical techniques, the use of the dissecting microscope and better supportive care, the surgery is improving and more aggressive surgery holds out the best chance of cure.

Radiation therapy is effective is dealing with small residual portions of the more benign gliomas, but there is no significant evidence of its effect in malignant gliomas. It plays a very important role in the management of medulloblastomas in which whole central nervous system irradiation is essential to obtain a cure as the tumour tends to seed the meninges. The dose is critical and unfortunately the level of radiation necessary is associated with subsequent growth hormone deficiency and learning problems. X-ray therapy is also essential for the treatment of ependymomas which, because of their site, can rarely be removed surgically. The brain stem tumours diagnosed only radiologically show an approximate 25% long-term response to radiation.

Chemotherapy has, as yet, not been fully evaluated in the treatment of brain tumours. There is no doubt that the majority of the tumours do show a response; this has been demonstrated most frequently in recurrent disease. Some patients have had long-term second remissions with clinical and radiological evidence of regression of disease.

There are problems inherent in the use of chemotherapy but the often quoted one of the need for the drug to cross the blood–brain barrier is probably not significant with brain tumours, as the barrier is usually non-functional. It is hoped that with a more optimistic approach by neurosurgeons adjuvant chemotherapy will be used more frequently.

THE LYMPHOMAS

Hodgkin's disease

Most children with this disease present with painless enlargement of one or more lymph node groups, with giant binucleate cells, known as Reed–Sternberg cells, and distorted lymphoid architecture. There are four histological subtypes:

1. Lymphocyte predominance.
2. Nodular sclerosis.
3. Mixed cellularity.
4. Lymphocyte depletion.

The degree of malignancy increases from type 1–4 and there is a decreasingly good prognosis. It is essential, once the diagnosis has been made, to establish the histological subtype and the extent of disease, as these determine appropriate treatment. Four stages (I–IV) of disease have been delineated and subdivided into A and B dependent on the absence or presence of constitutional disturbance, 10% weight loss in 6 weeks, fever, or night sweats.

Stage I disease is limited to one lymphatic region or extranodal site other than liver, bone marrow, skin or lungs. Stage II is involvement of two or more lymph node regions on the same side of the diaphragm. Stage III disease includes involvement of nodes or extranodal sites on both sides of the diaphragm, and stage IV disease means diffuse involvement of liver, spleen, lungs, skin, bone marrow or central nervous system with or without nodal involvement.

Investigations used to establish the stage of disease include lymphangiography, staging laparotomy and splenectomy. Lymphangiography may be technically very difficult in young children and is not without complications. Staging laparotomy and splenectomy also have serious implications and there is a high rate of infectious complications. CT scans do not provide very accurate indication of splenic disease; in view of these problems it is considered justifiable to defer or omit splenectomy in young children.

Chemotherapy is probably the preferable treatment in children under the age of 8 years irrespective of stage, as there is less interference with growth of bone and soft tissue. The commonly used combinations of drugs do, however, have the disadvantage of possibly inducing sterility. In older children with unequivocal stage

I disease the treatment of choice at present is involved field radiation. Radiation and chemotherapy or chemotherapy alone are best in stages II and III and chemotherapy with consideration of radiation to areas of bulky disease for stage IV. Various combinations of drugs have been shown to be effective, the majority include nitrogen mustard, procarbazine and a vinca alkaloid; other drugs which have been used are Adriamycin, cyclophosphamide and bleomycin.

Five-year survival rates of more than 90% have been achieved for stage I disease, 70–90% survival rates are possible for stages II, III and IV.

Non-Hodgkin's lymphomas

This term includes all the malignant solid tumours of the lymphoid system other than Hodgkin's disease. They are a difficult group of disorders to categorise satisfactorily; there are nodular and diffuse forms. The diffuse form is the commoner non-Hodgkin's lymphoma in childhood and also has the worse prognosis.

Children with these tumours present in a wide variety of ways. Cervical lymph node enlargement is common but is rarely the only site of disease. Mediastinal involvement is often seen, the child presenting with cough, superior vena caval syndrome or airways obstruction; tumours arising in this site usually carry T-cell markers and tend to progress to marrow involvement at an early stage. Primary gastrointestinal disease accounts for about 30% of patients, the tumour is usually in the ileum, caecum or ascending colon and the child frequently presents with intussusception. Other sites include retroperitoneal and mesenteric nodes, tonsil, adenoid, bone and gonad.

Burkitt's lymphoma is characterised by a particular histological picture and, when it occurs in Africa, presents with clinical symptoms of primary jaw lesions, abdominal disease or a paraspinal mass causing paraplegia. The same histological picture is found in non-African children but is not associated with jaw lesions, an abdominal tumour is then the commonest.

No truly effective staging system has been evolved for non-Hodgkin's lymphoma in childhood as the different histological types have different patterns of spread. There is some doubt as to whether stage I disease ever really occurs and, for this reason, systemic chemotherapy is the primary form of therapy; radiation has been used for treatment of bulk disease but this is losing favour. Spread to the central nervous system is so frequent that prophylactic therapy is probably indicated in all cases except localised abdominal disease. The most effective chemotherapy programmes are now achieving 2-year disease-free rates of 50–70%. They involve intensive cyclical treatment with several drugs to minimise the development of resistance.

HISTIOCYTOSIS

Controversy continues about the exact aetiology of this group of disorders. A new classification has recently been proposed in which Langerhans cell histiocytosis is differentiated from all other types. There is infiltration of normal tissues by histiocytes and the disorder includes: histiocytic medullary reticulosis; familial haemophagocytic reticulosis; and the spectrum of histiocytosis X which includes Letterer–Siwe disease, Hand–Schüller–Christian disease and unifocal eosinophilic granuloma. Most of these disorders carry a poor prognosis and it is only the localised disease without evidence of organ disfunction occurring in the older child in which the outlook is good. Various treatment regimens have been tried; children with Letterer–Siwe disease may respond to combinations of vincristine, steroids and alkylating agents, but the disease often recurs. Single eosinophilic granulomas may regress spontaneously or respond to currettage or low-dose irradiation. Chemotherapy is the treatment of choice for multiple lesions and careful evaluation of pituitary function is necessary as these patients often have growth hormone failure and diabetes insipidus from involvement of the pituitary.

NEPHROBLASTOMA

Nephroblastoma accounts for around 4% of childhood malignancy; the tumours are bilateral in about 10% of cases. The peak incidence is between the ages of 2 and 6 years. Most children present with an increase in abdominal size, but haematuria is also common and children with this complaint who do not have a urinary tract infection should always be further investigated. Once the diagnosis is suspected the treatment of choice is surgery and there are very few children in whom total nephrectomy with removal of tumour is not possible. The histology of the tumour should be carefully assessed as it is now established that there are some pathological types of tumour which carry a bad prognosis. It is also important to stage the extent of spread of the tumour. Without this knowledge it is not possible to continue with optimum therapy. Tumours of good histology which are confined to the kidney do not require radiation therapy and probably need only short courses of chemotherapy, while those with rupture of the capsule, regional node involvement or poor histology need radiation therapy and at least two-drug chemotherapy. With these methods of treatment between 85% and 90% of these children should survive.

Patients with metastatic disease to lungs are still curable and, using three or four drugs, usually vincristine, actinomycin and Adriamycin, and radiotherapy, about 50% can be expected to survive. Liver metastases have a less favourable outcome. Bilateral tumours are often very responsive to chemotherapy and surgery is either used primarily to remove the worst affected kidney or after drug treatment to resect residual disease.

NEUROBLASTOMA

These tumours of the sympathetic nervous system have so far defied response to the advances in treatment seen in other childhood tumours. They are primarily tumours of young children and arise most often in the adrenal gland, mediastinum or coeliac axis, with smaller numbers in the cervical ganglia or the pelvis. A high proportion present with evidence of widespread metastases to bone; there may be periorbital haemorrhage making non-accidental injury one of the differential diagnoses. There is a group (stage IVS) which presents at birth or in the first few months of life with a small primary tumour, and spreads to liver, bone marrow or skin, but there are no frank bone lesions. These babies usually have spontaneous regression of their disease and require no treatment.

Patients who present with localised disease have best chance of cure if their tumour can be completely excised. Chemotherapy will achieve considerable regression of tumour but surgical removal is necessary to achieve cure. Newer methods of therapy using drugs to achieve regression, removal of bone marrow prior to further intensive therapy and replacement of marrow after treatment, are now used. The results are encouraging and improved survival rates are being achieved.

SOFT TISSUE SARCOMAS

Soft tissue sarcomas originate in embryonic mesenchymal tissue and arise in many different sites. The commonest type in childhood are the rhabdomyosarcomas which arise in muscle and although not all tumours exhibit rhabdomyoblasts they tend to behave in the same clinical way. Treatment of this group of tumours is one of the success stories of paediatric oncology. They have a tendency to metastasise early and to spread locally by infiltration so, at diagnosis, they are rarely confined to the tissue or organ of origin. Metastases are present at diagnosis in about 25% of patients and bone marrow involvement is found in about 20%. Four pathological subgroups are recognised: embryonal; pleomorphic; alveolar; mixed. The alveolar histology is primarily seen in extremity lesions and carries a particularly bad prognosis. The wide variety of sites of origin of rhabdomyosarcomas makes it difficult to generalise about therapy; 30% arise in the head and neck and many of these are in structures adjacent to the meninges where there is a tendency to spread to the central nervous system. Other common sites are the orbit (15%), genitourinary system (30%), and the extremities and trunk (15%). Initial investigations should include a very thorough search for both local spread and metastatic disease. CT scans are very helpful and frequently demonstrate more extensive disease than is clinically apparent.

The major advance in therapy has occurred since adjuvant chemotherapy has been introduced. It has been particularly effective in the presurgical reduction of tumour mass, and has enabled surgeons to carry out conservative resections with retention of normal function, as opposed to massive mutilative surgery. This makes it particularly important that children with these tumours should be referred to specialist centres for full evaluation before treatment rather than after surgery. Radiation therapy has an important role, particularly in the treatment of residual disease after chemotherapy in sites not amenable to surgery. The combination of vincristine, actinomycin D and cyclophosphamide has been shown to be the most effective. Adriamycin also has an effect in these tumours but is probably not essential to the optimum management of stage I and II cases. Ifosfamide has more recently been demonstrated as a very effective agent.

Other soft tissue sarcomas in childhood, such as fibrosarcomas, liposarcomas, leiomyosarcomas, synovial sarcomas and haemangiopericytomas are very rare and no standardised treatment programmes have been evolved. They should undoubtedly be referred to specialised centres and therapy similar to that for rhabdomyosarcomas is probably the best.

BONE TUMOURS

Osteogenic sarcomas and Ewing's tumours account for about 5% of childhood malignancy. The former is a tumour of bone-forming mesenchymal cells while the latter is a non-osseous small cell sarcoma. Both tumours have a maximum incidence in the second decade but while 70% of all Ewing's tumours are seen before the age of 20 years, 50% of osteogenic sarcomas occur in adults. Both tumours are commoner in males. The commonest site for both is in the long bones, but osteogenic sarcomas tend to occur in the metaphyseal region, while Ewing's tumour is more often found in the shaft and is also relatively more common in the pelvic bones. The two tumours present with pain and swelling, pain usually preceding other symptoms and signs by several weeks. The radiological appearances of osteogenic sarcoma include loss of normal trabecular pattern, lytic lesions and new bone formation, and soft tissue extensions often show calcification. Ewing's tumours produce localised rarefaction and periosteal reaction resembling onion skin layers from layers of new bone formation. Both tumours require biopsy to confirm the diagnosis.

The treatment of osteogenic sarcoma has undergone several changes in the last 15 years. There are increasing data indicating that several cytotoxic agents are effective in preventing or diminishing the number and frequency of metastases. Very high dose methotrexate, Adriamycin, cisplatin and bleomycin have all been shown to cause regression of lung metastases and are now used. A small number of orthopaedic units are now undertaking wide excision of the tumour and prosthetic replacement of the involved bone. This treatment is preferable to amputation as the early functional results are very encouraging and do not in any way undermine cure, providing full chemotherapy is also given. Single centre studies have produced 40–70% 5-year survival rates.

The most effective treatment of Ewing's tumours (with vincristine, cyclophosphamide or ifosfamide, actinomycin D and Adriamycin) now consists of primary chemotherapy and resection of tumour whenever possible, otherwise with radiation to residual disease. The tumour is radiosensitive providing sufficient dose can be delivered, but Ewing's tumour, like osteogenic sarcoma, has a great tendency to develop metastases. In about 20% of cases metastases are present at diagnosis and many others become overt within a year but some can be delayed for periods of up to 10 years.

GERM CELL TUMOURS AND MALIGNANT TERATOMAS

Germ cell tumours originate in those cells which eventually differentiate into the ovum and sperm. Tumours of these cells can therefore arise within the gonads or anywhere along the migration path during fetal life. The histology of the tumour depends on the point in maturation at which the abnormal growth occurs, pure yolk sac tumours (endodermal sinus tumours) can occur both in the gonads and in extragonadal sites. These tumours are always associated with an elevation of α-feto protein concentrations; the measurement of this marker is an excellent guide to the complete removal of the tumour and to the development of metastases. When the germ cells have already differentiated and matured along somatic pathways then the resulting tumour is a teratoma; the tumour comprises a variety of different tissues foreign to the part and may be benign or malignant. All these tumours are best treated by surgery when complete removal is possible and then by chemotherapy. The vinca alkaloids, cyclophosphamide, actinomycin D, bleomycin and cisplatin have all been shown to be effective in various combinations.

Non-germ cell gonadal tumours of childhood include Leydig and Sertoli cell tumours, granulosa cell and theca cell tumours and adenocarcinomas.

RETINOBLASTOMA

Retinoblastoma is the commonest ocular malignancy of childhood. Significant cure rates for this tumour have been possible since the beginning of the century. Bilateral cases have the inherited autosomal dominant form of the disease and their offspring have a 50% chance of developing retinoblastomas. The majority of children present in the first 2 years of life. The abnormal white pupil so often described as the common presentation is really an indication of a large tumour unless it arises in the macula. A squint is often present at an early stage. Treatment varies according to the extent of disease; enucleation is usually the treatment of choice in unilateral cases unless the disease is diagnosed at an early stage when radiotherapy may be curative without loss of vision. In bilateral disease, careful evaluation of each eye is necessary and the therapeutic decision is based on the size and location of the tumours.

One should note the chance of second malignancies in these children; there is a well-documented association between retinoblastoma and osteogenic sarcoma. This second tumour may arise in the site of previous irradiation or in bone remote from the orbit.

CURRENT SURVIVAL RATES

Cancer survival rates for children with all forms of malignant disease have improved considerably over the last few years and Table 24.3 indicates the 5-year survival for the cohort of children diagnosed between 1974 and 1983 in the North West of England (Manchester Children's Tumour

Table 24.3 Survival figures 1974–83: Manchester Children's Tumour Registry

Malignancy	% surviving 5 years
Acute lymphoblastic leukaemia	47
Acute non-lymphoblastic leukaemia	21
Hodgkin's disease	91
Non-Hodgkin's lymphoma	46
Ependymoma	29
Adult astrocytoma	24
Juvenile astrocytoma	83
Medulloblastoma	41
Neuroblastoma	28
Retinoblastoma	67
Wilms' tumour	85
Osteosarcoma	39
Ewing's tumour	41
Rhabdomyosarcoma	54
Germ cell tumours	64

Registry). These figures account for all children diagnosed whether or not they received any treatment and give a more accurate figure than the selected results of children treated in specialised centres on specific protocols. They also emphasise the importance of referral of children to such special centres where improved results can be obtained.

TOXICITY OF THERAPY

Immediate effects

There are many immediate complications of the modern treatment of childhood malignancy. Severe and rapidly spreading infections are a major problem, so unexplained fever in these patients requires immediate investigation and treatment with intravenous broad-spectrum antibiotics. Viral infections such as measles, chickenpox and herpes simplex can be fatal; fungal infections and *Pneumocystis carinii* are also quite common.

The children run a considerable risk of nutritional deficiency which may be due to: anorexia associated with the disease or the drugs; vomiting again due to disease or therapy; or malabsorption.

Every effort should be made to induce the patients to take normal foods by mouth but it may be necessary to supplement with high-calorie liquid foods and total parenteral nutrition may sometimes be required.

Long-term effects

As more children have survived childhood malignancy, it is clear that a considerable price has to be paid. In order to achieve a cure, certain side-effects are inevitable, most of these are due to interference with normal growth by surgery and radiation, endocrine deficiencies produced by radiation and chemotherapeutic effects on the gonads, pituitary, and thyroid glands, and developmental and learning problems produced by cranial irradiation. Many of these problems can be minimised or treated by appropriate replacement therapy, but vigilance is necessary in detecting further problems generated by the newer aggressive treatment programmes. Primary neoplasms have been shown to occur with 10% greater frequency in patients cured of one malignancy in childhood. These have been reported within a few months of the first to as long as 30 years later. Approximately 50% of the reported cases have arisen in sites of previous irradiation, 30% in patients with known tendencies such as retinoblastoma and basal cell carcinoma syndrome, and the remainder where no single underlying cause can be determined.

PSYCHOSOCIAL PROBLEMS

A family with a child with cancer is under great stress, the chronic nature of the diseases, the disruptive pattern of prolonged chemotherapy and the long-term insecurity associated with the uncertain future take a very significant toll. Those families in which psychosocial problems pre-exist are particularly vulnerable and require constant support. Community services are not geared to provide this and new methods of help need exploration. Considerable progress has been made in the cure of cancer in childhood and at the present rate of cure, 1 in 1000 20 year olds will soon be survivors of childhood cancer. If they are to be considered truly cured, all services concerned with their care must be aware of their needs. At the moment their general care lags behind the advances in cure. Too many survivors of malignancy are sentenced to be classified as handicapped, because the community will not accept them as normal adults.

FURTHER READING

Altman A J, Schwartz A D 1978 Malignant diseases of infancy, childhood and adolescence. Vol XVIII Major problems in clinical paediatrics. W B Saunders, Philadelphia
Fraumeni J F (ed) 1975 Persons at high risk of cancer: an approach to cancer aetiology and control. Academic, New York
Marsden H B, Steward J K (eds) 1976 Recent results in cancer research: tumours in children, 2nd edn. Springer, Berlin
Morris Jones P H (ed) 1979 Topics in paediatrics I, haematology and oncology. Pitman Medical, Tunbridge Wells
Mulvihill J J, Miller R W, Fraumeni J F (eds) 1977

Genetics of human cancer, vol III. Raven, New York
Nesbit M E 1985 Clinics in oncology — July, 1985. Late effects in successfully treated children with cancer. W B Saunders, Philadelphia
Sutow W W, Vietti T J, Fernback D J (eds) 1977 Clinical paediatric oncology, 2nd edn. C.V. Mosby, St Louis
Voute P A, Barrett A, Blood H J G, Lemerle J, Neidhardt M K 1986 Cancer in children, clinical management, 2nd edn. Springer, Berlin
Waterhouse J, Muir C, Correa P, Powell J (eds) 1976 Cancer incidence in five continents, vol III (IARC scientific publication no 15) International Agency for Research on Cancer, Lyon

25. Neurology

S. Lingam

Neurological disorders needing referral include central nervous system infections, epilepsy, headaches, blackouts, developmental delay, neurological handicap and learning problems; disorders such as myasthenia gravis and degenerative disease are rare. The GP needs to recognise deviations from normal rather than know neurological diseases in detail.

CENTRAL NERVOUS SYSTEM INFECTIONS

Infections of the central nervous system include meningitis and encephalitis and, rarely, brain abscess; the clinical and pathological features depend on extent of involvement and type and virulence of the infecting organism.

Meningitis

Meningitis is inflammation of the meninges; it may be due to many organisms, including bacteria and viruses. Spread to the meninges is either haematogenous through the choroid plexus, or from localised infection, such as otitis media or sinusitis.

Recurrent bacterial meningitis is often due to anatomical continuity between the meninges and the external environment, such as a midline dermal sinus. Only rarely is recurrent meningitis due to an immunodeficiency disorder.

Bacterial meningitis

The predominant infecting organisms causing meningitis vary with age in childhood, as detailed below:

1. Under 28 days (neonate)

   a. Group B streptococcus
   b. *Escherichia coli* (K strains)
   c. *Listeria monocytogenes*
   d. *Pseudomonas aeruginosa*
2. 1 month–2 years
   a. *Haemophilus influenzae*
   b. *Neisseria meningitidis* (meningococcus)
   c. *Streptococcus pneumoniae*
3. 2 years–5 years
   a. *Neisseria meningitidis*
   b. *Haemophilus influenzae*
   c. *Streptococcus pneumoniae*
4. Over 5 years
   a. *Streptococcus pneumoniae*
   b. *Neisseria meningitidis*

Bacterial invasion causes inflammation and hyperaemia of the meninges, followed by neutrophil migration into the subarachnoid space and pus formation. The pus may block the outflow of CSF causing hydrocephalus.

Clinically, there is sudden onset of fever, headache, photophobia, nausea and vomiting, and nuchal or spinal rigidity. Infants usually are irritable with a high-pitched cry and have a bulging fontanelle.

Convulsions and coma are bad prognostic signs. On examination the child is irritable, drowsy, and has neck stiffness (inability to passively flex the neck forward or touch the chest with the chin) and tripod sign (when asked to sit up the child adopts a tripod position with both hands stretched aside and head in extension to avoid a leptomeningeal traction). Kernig's and Brudzinski's signs may be present. These are tested as follows: Kernig's sign — lay the child on the back. Flex one of the legs at hip and knee, then straighten the knee. There will be resistance and pain. Brudzinski's sign — lay the child supine. With one of your hands behind the head flex the neck forward. While doing this there will be flexion of the hips and knees. These are the signs of meningeal irritation which are often present in meningitis; these signs may also be present due to other causes — meningism following subarachnoid haemorrhage, or neck stiffness from painful cervical adenitis. Sixth, third and fourth cranial nerve palsies may also be present. Papilloedema is rare but if it is present it is a poor prognostic sign indicating brain oedema. The major problem is that meningitis often produces no neck stiffness under 18 months of age.

The diagnosis is confirmed by laboratory examination of the cerebrospinal fluid (CSF). Raised intracranial pressure should be excluded before lumbar puncture; it is contraindicated if the child has papilloedema, is very drowsy, or in coma. The CSF findings in several infective conditions are shown in Table 25.1. In bacterial meningitis, neutrophils and organisms may be identified on microscopic examination of the CSF; the protein is raised and the sugar low. Culture of lumbar fluid confirms the infection and will help to reach a decision about antibiotic therapy.

Peripheral blood count, blood urea and electrolytes, and blood sugar should be determined at the time of lumbar puncture.

Non-culture methods of diagnosis, such as latex agglutination of specific antibody, are now becoming reliable. Soluble polysaccharide of the bacteria pneumococcus, meningococcus (groups A, C and D), *Haemophilus influenzae*, streptococcus and *Esch. coli* can be identified by counter current immunoelectrophoresis. Such tests are useful if bacterial cultures are negative because of antibiotic treatment or for rapid diagnosis.

Antibacterial chemotherapy should be given *as soon as the diagnosis is suspected* — if the CSF appears cloudy or there is a purpuric rash. It should be started without lumbar puncture in those for whom it is contraindicated. The drug chosen depends on the likely organisms or those found on culture or seen on microscopy. If the organism is not known, the antibiotics given empirically could be a third-generation cephalosporin or a combination of ampicillin and chloramphenicol. The drug of choice for meningococcal or pneumococcal meningitis is benzylpenicillin. All antibiotics are given intravenously for 10–14 days.

In the newborn period the place of chloramphenicol is now controversial; penicillin and an aminoglycoside, or cephalosporin are often used.

Meningitis is contagious and it is important to provide antibiotic prophylaxis to close contacts in infection due to *Haemophilus influenzae* or meningococcus. Preschool and nursery children, and household contacts should be considered for chemoprophylaxis with rifampicin; this has been shown to prevent secondary cases. Vaccination against some strains of meningococcus (groups A and C) is possible; but in the UK most infections are due to serotype B. Vaccination against *Haemophilus influenzae* is given to children between 2 and 5 years in some countries such as the USA; a new vaccine has been used in Finland in the first year of life.

Table 25.1 CSF findings in infective conditions

Diagnosis	Cell type/ml	Protein (g/l)	Glucose (mmol/l)	Smear (Gram stain)	Other test
Normal	0–5 (lymphocytes)	0.1–0.45	2.8–4.8	Negative	—
Bacterial	200–2000 (mostly polymorphs)	Increased	Very low	Positive	Latex tests
Viral	100–1000 or more (mostly lymphocytes)	Normal or slightly raised 0.45–0.85	Normal (low in mumps)	Negative	Viral isolation. Paired sera for antibodies
Tuberculosis	100–1000 or more (mostly lymphocytes)	Increased 0.6–5	Low 0.5–2	Ziehl–Neelsen stain Immunofluorescence	
Lesions outside subarachnoid space	Often increased 50–1000 (both lymphocytes and polymorphs)	Normal or increased	Normal	Negative	Cultures usually negative

Pneumococcal polysaccharide vaccines against B and C serogroups are available to children at risk — those with sickle cell disease or who have had a splenectomy. Long-term treatment with penicillin is another method of prophylaxis.

Complications of bacterial meningitis

Ventriculitis is the commonest problem encountered in young infants, and is difficult to treat. Ventriculitis should be suspected in any young child who responds poorly to therapy and in whom CSF pleocytosis persists despite adequate therapy. The mortality is high, and if untreated, severe mental impairment and physical disability is common.

A block in the circulation of CSF causes enlarged ventricles which can be demonstrated by CT scan, or ultrasound in the newborn.

Intraventricular antibiotics and surgical drainage are required; this is achieved by the insertion of a reservoir through which CSF may be obtained and antibiotics instilled. Intrathecal antibiotic therapy is not useful as antibiotics will not flow against the direction of CSF to reach the meninges or the ventricles.

Subdural effusion is seen in young children with meningitis due to *Haemophilus influenzae* and pneumococcus but is less common with meningococcus. The diagnosis should be suspected if the temperature persists, if CSF cultures continue to be positive despite adequate therapy, or if there is a focal or persistent convulsion with positive neurological signs such as weakness or hemiplegia. Diagnosis is established by CT scan, and surgical drainage is required.

Electrolyte disturbances are a common complication of meningitis. They are often only transient and may be due to vomiting alone or development of inappropriate antidiuretic hormone secretion.

Meningococcal infection

This is a serious disease which affects any age, but preschool children are most susceptible. If the organism, which resides in the upper respiratory tract, invades the blood, it causes a septicaemia. The child characteristically develops a purpuric or petechial rash; there may also be signs of meningitis.

Meningococcaemia without meningitis has a worse prognosis than with meningitis, and children may die very quickly. Haemorrhage into the adrenal glands (Waterhouse–Friderichsen syndrome) is a well-known complication of meningococcaemia with a high mortality despite the use of steroids. Disseminated intravascular coagulation occurs, and septicaemic shock due to bacterial endotoxin.

The organism can be seen or isolated from CSF, blood culture or material obtained by puncturing a purpuric spot. Intracellular Gram-negative diplococci are seen on the smear. Treatment is 10–14 days of intravenous benzylpenicillin (penicillin G).

Meningococcal disease is a medical emergency. In general practice, if the disease is suspected, parenteral penicillin must be given at once before transfer to hospital.

Chronic meningococcaemia without meningitis is a different disease; this is an immune complex disorder in which there is an intermittent fever, purpuric rash, chronic arthritis, and pneumonitis, with or without serous effusion. Penicillin is the treatment of choice.

Recurrent meningitis should alert the doctor to the possibility of an abnormal connection between the upper airway or ear and the meninges, or an immune deficiency.

Neonatal meningitis

The signs and symptoms of meningitis in neonates and young infants are not clear cut; they include unstable temperature, hypotonia and apnoea. The diagnosis should be considered in any baby with septicaemia or urinary tract infection. The infants at risk are those born preterm and those born after a complicated delivery, prolonged rupture of membranes or maternal infection; long lines for intravenous feeding, umbilical catheters and endotracheal tubes also increase the risk. A common cause of meningitis used to be spina bifida (Fig. 25.1).

Hyponatraemia and hypoglycaemia are common; fluids should be restricted and intravenous glucose given as necessary. The progress of the illness should be followed with repeated ultrasound scans. The mortality of neonatal bacterial meningitis is about 25%. The morbidity is high —

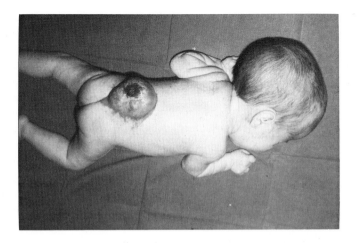

Fig. 25.1 Spina bifida.

including hydrocephalus, mental handicap and cerebral palsy.

Cerebral abscess

An abscess in the brain may occur as a complication of bacterial meningitis, especially following a septic focus such as otitis media, sinusitis with osteomyelitis of the skull, face lesion, or a skull fracture through a sinus or mastoid. It may also occur as a complication of cyanotic congenital heart disease. Clinical features depend on the site of the abscess; there may be fever, malaise, headache, vomiting and focal fits. Localising signs such as hemiplegia, visual defects or evidence of raised intracranial pressure may be present. A high index of suspicion is required to make the diagnosis, confirmation is by CT scan. An EEG may locate an abscess by showing slow wave activity. Lumbar puncture is dangerous if there is raised intracranial pressure.

Tuberculous meningitis

Children are at risk of developing TB meningitis from contact with open tuberculosis (usually from a relative). The onset is usually gradual, during the initial primary tuberculous complex stage TB may not be suspected; miliary TB develops later with generalised clinical features (weight loss, sweating, intermittent fever) and eventual meningitis. The child may initially have personality change, irritability and headache; vomiting, marked constipation and prolonged anorexia then develop followed over a week or so by increasing drowsiness, photophobia and worsening headache. There may be neck stiffness, opisthotonus, sixth nerve palsy, squint, papilloedema, choroidal tubercles or nystagmus. If the diagnosis is missed the child goes on to coma and convulsions with decerebrate rigidity, markedly raised intracranial pressure and often death.

A high index of suspicion is required to make a diagnosis. A tuberculin tests is performed in all children in whom the disease is suspected, although it is important to remember that in 25% of established cases there is anergy and a negative test. Examination of the CSF confirms the diagnosis; acid-fast bacilli may be seen on Ziehl-Neelsen staining, or by immuno-fluoresence. Confirmation by culture will take several weeks.

The prognosis has improved with medical and neurosurgical management; long-term morbidity is considerable with visual and hearing deficits, hydrocephalus, mental retardation, spasticity and post-meningitic epilepsy occurring.

Viral meningitis

Clinical onset is often gradual with fever, headache, vomiting, anorexia and neuralgia leading to clinical signs of meningitis; some children have associated features of encephalitis with marked drowsiness and convulsions. The clinical examination may reveal parotid swelling in mumps meningitis, or diarrhoea and rash in enteroviral meningitis.

The diagnosis depends on CSF findings; CSF is usually clear, the pressure is normal, protein is only mildly elevated, the sugar is normal, except in mumps meningitis where it is low; lymphocytes predominate and no organisms are seen on staining. Electron microscopy of a spun CSF specimen may show viral particles; the diagnosis is often only established later with culture or in retrospect by serology.

No specific treatment is usually required; there is often confusion between viral meningitis and partially treated bacterial meningitis and, if in doubt, assume bacterial meningitis and treat appropriately. Antiviral therapy (acyclovir) should be considered in severe cases and if herpes simplex is suspected, particularly if signs of focal encephalitis also supervene. Analgesia is needed for headache paracetamol is often sufficient.

Mortality and morbidity is low, but some children have residual problems in the form of easy tiredness, behaviour changes, headache and weakness.

Encephalitis

Encephalitis is an infection of the brain substance, encephalopathy refers to inflammation of the brain due to non-infective causes (metabolic or toxic). In encephalitis, there may be direct invasion by the virus or an immunological perivascular response. Acute encephalitis is usually due to a virus and is more serious than viral meningitis as it often results in permanent brain damage.

The herpes virus is an important cause in children as it can cause serious brain damage.

Severe headaches and vomiting are common. Clinically there is altered consciousness, disorientation, confusion, delirium. In severe cases convulsions and coma occur.

In herpes encephalitis the initial symptomatology may be non-specific and includes fever, vomiting, a refusal to feed, mild coryza, lethargy and behaviour disturbance. Herpetic skin lesions or cold sores may be present several weeks before the onset of symptoms or at the same time. It is important to ask if any other family members have had herpes infection. Focal convulsions occur between the second and fourth day of the illness, together with focal neurological signs such as flaccid or spastic hemiplegia, unilateral cranial nerve involvement and unilateral choreiform or dystonic movements. The typical EEG in herpes encephalitis (periodic slow waves) may help to make the diagnosis. Management includes treatment of cerebral oedema and antiviral drug (acyclovir). The prognosis is poor with late treatment, many children die or are left with permanent disabilities; early treatment with an antiviral drug may improve the diagnosis.

HEADACHE

Headache is a common symptom in children. In infants it produces irritability and screaming; an older child can describe the pain. The pain is due to irritation, pressure or traction on pain-sensitive structures in the head or neck; the brain itself is relatively insensitive to pain. The main causes of headache are shown in Table 25.2.

Acute headache

Acute headache may be severe. In many cases, the child has a fever with a virus infection, but a neurological cause needs to be considered, especially if there is associated vomiting or alteration in consciousness. If there is a suggestion of meningitis (see p. 305) admission to hospital and a lumbar puncture are necessary.

Children with concussion following head injury may have severe headaches. Analgesics may be given, but sedation should be avoided. If there is progressive deterioration in the level of consciousness, then immediate neurosurgical referral is indicated.

Chronic headache

Chronic headaches are distressing to both child and parents and are a common cause of missing school. Doctors are often unable to give a clear-cut explanation. The headaches may be progressive, with gradual increase in frequency and duration, or persistent, remaining unchanged in frequency and duration over a period of time.

Table 25.2   Causes of headaches

Acute		Chronic			
With vomiting	Without vomiting	Progressive with vomiting and fits	Without vomiting (no fits)	Persistent with vomiting	Without vomiting
Simple febrile illness	Simple febrile illness	Raised intracranial pressure	Trigeminal neuralgia	Migraine	Tension headache
Meningitis	Poisoning and intoxication, e.g. glue sniffing	Space-occupying lesions, tumours abscess, cyst, chronic subdural haemorrhage	Glosso-pharyngeal neuralgia vasculitis		Malocclusion
Encephalitis					Poor head or neck posture
Subarachnoid, intracranial or acute subdural haemorrhage		Pseudotumour cerebri (benign intracranial hypertension)			Referred pain
					Sinusitis
Concussion of the brain		Hypertensive encephalopathy			Rhinitis
					Toothache
		Lead poisoning			Cervical spondylosis

Progressive headache

Increased intracranial pressure may present as progressive headache with vomiting; there may be focal neurological signs or papilloedema. A space-occupying lesion such as tumour or abscess should then be suspected. Early morning headaches or those which wake the child are usually serious, but migraine can also cause this.

A skull X-ray may show calcification in the lesion or evidence of raised intracranial pressure (copper-beaten appearance, suture seperation), while a CT scan may show the lesion.

Hypertension and lead poisoning must also be excluded. Progressive headache without vomiting is generally due to local irritation or pressure; trigeminal or glossopharyngeal neuralgia are good examples. The problem should be recognised as the pain may respond to analgesic agents or to carbamazepine.

Persistent headache

Headaches which are recurrent are unlikely to be due to raised intracranial pressure; migraine and its variants are relatively common. The incidence of migraine is 50 per 1000 which is eight times more frequent than epilepsy. There is often a positive family history (in 80%). Migrainous attacks are rare under the age of 2 years but do occur in early childhood; they are more common in the prepubertal period and boys are affected twice as often as girls. In adolescents and adults migraine is commoner in females. Where there is a strong family history, attacks may begin early in life. Infants may present with crying and vomiting and they are often labelled as windy or colicky babies.

The vomiting and abdominal pain persist in childhood and become more pronounced; the child is often then diagnosed as periodic syndrome. Migraine is only diagnosed when the headache becomes the main feature.

Young infants are not able to complain of headache but are usually irritable or pale during an attack. Older children often have a history of travel sickness or sleep disturbance and nightmares.

Various factors may act as a trigger; food (milk products, egg, chocolate, tea, coffee, nuts), food colouring (tartrazine) and additives. Emotional upset, tension, psychosocial deprivation, learning problems, intercurrent mild illness, severe exercise, mild head injury, exercise and bright sunshine are also known to precipitate an attack in a susceptible individual.

There are four types of migraine: classical migraine and common migraine, which have a preceding aura; cluster headache and complicated migraine, which may not have an aura. The type of aura depends on which arteries are involved and on the degree of vasoconstriction. The commonest is a visual hallucination due to ophthalmic artery involvement, this includes flashing lights, field defects (blind spot), and microscopia (objects looking smaller than they are).

Mesenteric artery constriction causes gastro-intestinal aura (nausea, vomiting, sensation of fullness), while hemianaesthesia and aphasia occur if the cranial arteries are involved.

Classical migraine

The headache in classical migraine is unilateral (hemicrania), often frontal or temporal but bi-frontal or occipital headache may also occur. It is described as throbbing and severe. Photophobia or vertigo may be present; the child tends to lie down in a dark room and go to sleep. The duration of the attack is variable; most children improve after sleep but some attacks may last for as long as 2–3 days.

Common migraine

Here the aura is less well defined than in classical migraine; the headaches are diffuse and the child often has nausea or vomiting. He looks ill and is pale. Headache intensity may be decreased by pressure over the vessels.

Cluster headache

Here the headaches may recur daily for several days at a time with prolonged trouble-free periods between attacks. There is neither aura nor photophobia. The pain is severe and throbbing but often of short duration (30–90 minutes) and usually occurs in the orbital or temporal regions. Conjunctival redness, oedema, lacrimation, pulsation of the eye, and urinary frequency may be present. Cluster headaches are commoner in males. The headache usually responds to simple analgesics and the child does not seem to prefer a dark room.

Complicated migraine

This form has a varied presentation which may include periodic syndrome, abdominal migraine or rare forms such as ophthalmoplegic, hemiplegic, alternating hemiplegic, basilar artery, convulsive or psychomotor migraine. Complicated migraine may lead to mental retardation especially if it is the alternating hemiplegic type. There is presumably neuronal death secondary to prolonged and frequent arterial vasoconstriction. There may be brain infarction resulting in permanent visual defects, ophthalmoplegia, aphasia or hemiplegia.

Treatment

If there is clear evidence of food intolerance then the offending substances should be avoided; remember that many food products may contain substances such as milk, and advice from a dietician should be obtained.

In classical migraine the child should lie down in a quiet dark room; analgesia may help. Ergotamine is only helpful in common migraine where vasodilatation is the main feature; in children with the complicated form it is contraindicated as it may increase symptoms due to excessive vasoconstriction. Anti-emetic and anti-vertigo agents are useful as symptomatic adjuncts. Frequent (more than two attacks a month) or severe attacks may respond to continuous migraine prophylaxis. Pizotifen may be helpful; parents and children should be warned that it may take 3–4 weeks before any benefit is seen and the importance of regular therapy should be emphasised. Beta-blockers (such as propranolol) help only in acute attacks but are not useful in prophylaxis. Assurance should be given that migraine tends to improve with age, but may recur in adolescence, and that there is no serious disease present. The child should be regarded as normal and otherwise healthy.

Functional or tension headache

Functional or tension headache is usually vague but persistent; it is non-throbbing and may be diffuse or occur bilaterally in the vertex or occiput. Inquiries should be made about family or school stress, insomnia or depression. Drug medication is not usually of help, apart from mild analgesics. Often advice from a child guidance clinic or child psychiatrist may be indicated.

Referred headache

These are due to excessive muscle contraction as occurs in poor head or neck posture, or dental malocclusion. Non-paralytic squint, myopia and astigmatism are usually not causes of headaches in children, but may interfere with visual function and therefore must be corrected. Detailed examination of the sinuses, eyes, teeth, and cervical region may suggest the site of origin. Management involves analgesia and treatment of the cause.

Headaches, regardless of cause, are a significant symptom to the child and a sympathetic approach is required from the physician, family and school for satisfactory management.

CONVULSIONS

The terminology can be confusing. The terms convulsions, seizures, fits and epileptic attacks are by no means synonymous although sometimes considered to be so in the lay mind. It is important to clarify what has been observed by the parent, what preceded it and what the child's condition was like following the episode; their use of the word 'fit' may refer to a genuine seizure or to a temper tantrum, night terror or rigor.

A convulsion is characterised by alteration in motor, sensory or automatic function, with or without loss of consciousness and associated with abnormal neuronal electrical discharges; this is a symptom of an underlying disorder and is not in itself a diagnosis.

Most individuals can be induced into having a convulsion depending on the stimulus and their 'seizure threshold', which is thought to be reduced in young individuals, and by (1) structural abnormalities of the brain such as hydrocephalus, cysts, tumour or abscess; (2) chemical abnormalities, including hypoglycaemia and hypocalcaemia; (3) stimuli such as fever (causing febrile convulsions), flashing lights (causing photogenic or television seizures), and psychogenic factors such as stress.

A suitable history, or direct observation, is required to diagnose the occurrence of convulsions and an electroencephalogram (EEG) is helpful in confirming it. It is important to remember that in some children who have definitely had convulsions, the EEG may be normal between fits.

Telemetric and 24-hour recordings of EEG during normal activity may be useful investigations in some children.

There are four components to a seizure:

1. Prodrome. This may last a few hours or even days. There may be a change in behaviour, mood, appetite or sleep pattern which may be recognisable by parents or the child himself.

2. Aura. Fifty per cent of children give a history of an aura or warning which may be visual, auditory or olfactory;

3. Convulsion. (See Table 25.3) The pattern depends on the site of the abnormal electrical discharges.

4. Post-ictal. The child may be confused, drowsy or have automatisms.

Epilepsy

Epilepsy is a condition in which there is a tendency to recurrent seizures. The incidence is roughly 5–7 per 1000. A single convulsion for which there is a correctable cause such as hypoglycaemia is not strictly epilepsy.

In 80% of childhood epilepsy no cause is apparent (idiopathic epilepsy); secondary causes include central nervous system malformation or infection, metabolic abnormalities, trauma, cerebrovascular disease, tumours, drugs and drug withdrawals, degenerative disease and the neurocutaneous syndromes, such as tuberous sclerosis. Idiopathic epilepsy is frequently familial but with no specific inheritance pattern; several secondary epilepsies may be inherited such as those associated with tuberous sclerosis, phenylketonuria and degenerative diseases.

Classification

Epilepsy is classified into:

1. Generalised.
2. Partial or focal epilepsy.

In generalised epilepsy the seizures are generalised from onset and originate from both hemispheres, whereas in focal epilepsy there is a single focus within the brain. Generalised epilepsy is further subdivided into primary and secondary depending on whether the seizures originate from

Table 25.3 International classification of seizures

Type	Clinical feature	Origin of focus	EEG	Aetiology	Most effective anticonvulsant
1. Partial seizures (those beginning focally)					
a. Partial seizures with elementary (motor or sensory) symptoms	No loss of consciousness	Cortical, single focus	Focal	Focal anatomical lesion — tumour, cyst, abscess, scar (head injury), vascular malformation	Carbamazepine Phenytoin (Phenobarbitone)
b. Partial seizures with complex symptoms (temporal lobe epilepsy)	Loss of consciousness	Cortical, temporal lobe focus	Temporal lobe spikes	Temporal lobe sclerosis, cyst, tumour	Carbamazepine Phenytoin (Phenobarbitone)
c. Partial seizures with secondary generalisation	Initial focal then grand mal with aura	Cortical focus with spread to other cortical parts	Asymmetrical		Valproate Phenytoin Carbamazepine Combination of carbamazepine and valproate Phenobarbitone
2. Generalised seizures (those without focal onset)					
a. Petit mal	Absences	Cortical	Bilateral, symmetrical 3 per second spike and wave pattern	Idiopathic (genetic)	Valproate Ethosuximide
b. Grand mal	Tonic-clonic	Cortical, central	Bilateral, symmetrical discharges	Idiopathic (genetic)	Valproate Phenobarbitone Phenytoin Carbamazepine
c. Myoclonic	Often on wakening or drifting off to sleep. May be very frequent	Cortical, central	Typical 2 per second spike and wave; polyspike complexes	Idiopathic, degenerative disorders; a few may be benign (benign myoclonic epilepsy)	Valproate, clonazepam, clobazam Carbamazepine Steroid, ACTH Ketogenic diet
d. infantile spasms	Salaam fits, lightening spasms	Cortical, multifocal	High voltage disorganised — hypsarrhythmia	Idiopathic or symptomatic (tuberous sclerosis, triple immunisation, birth asphyxia)	ACTH, Nitrazepam Valproate
e. Akinetic	Drop attack	Cortical, multifocal	Atypical spike and wave complexes, mixed often polyspikes		Valproate Nitrazepam Clobazam
3. Unilateral seizures	Unilateral, grand mal	Cortical, unilateral	Unilateral discharges	Focal anatomical lesion — tumour, vascular malformation, cyst	Carbamazepine Phenytoin
4. Unclassified seizures					

normal cortex (primary) or from cortex which is damaged (secondary).

Primary generalised epilepsy is often familial and there is normal intelligence and neurological examination. Children with the secondary form are often mentally retarded and invariably have some neurological abnormality such as spastic quadriplegia, optic atrophy, microcephaly or ataxia. With focal epilepsy intelligence is usually normal and there may be a focal neurological abnormality. The seizure type should be included in describing the type of epilepsy. The international classification of seizures is shown in Table 25.3. If there are several seizure types then the patient should be classified by the predominant type.

Partial seizures

These originate from a single focus within the brain and may be elementary (focal) or complex. Focal convulsions may be motor or sensory depending on which part of the cortex is involved; motor and sensory components may, however, coexist.

Typically, there is no loss of consciousness although if the electrical discharge spreads to involve other areas of the brain then the seizure may become generalised (partial seizures with secondary generalisation).

Partial seizure with elementary motor symptoms (partial motor seizure)

The motor symptoms depend on which part of the motor cortex is involved and are evident in the contralateral limb or body; the thumb is most often affected. In Jacksonian seizures, jerking usually starts in one part, such as the thumb, and spreads to the fingers, then to the hand and eventually involves one-half of the body.

Partial seizure with elementary sensory symptoms (partial sensory seizure)

The focus of origin of the seizure is in the sensory cortex and, depending on the area, results in either a somatic or special sensory seizure. The somatic form presents with tingling, numbness or warmth of a part of the body and, because of the proximity with motor cortex, a degree of motor involvement in the form of short tonic spasms or posturing also occurs. Special sensory seizures originate in the occipital or temporal lobe and involve the auditory, visual, olfactory or taste area; there may be vertigo, flashing lights or hallucination of smell, sound (hearing voices, noise, music) or vision (objects looking larger than normal).

Partial seizures with complex symptoms (complex partial seizures)

These were previously known as temporal lobe epilepsy or psychomotor epilepsy and form about one-quarter of all, and 50% of focal seizures. The convulsion starts in the temporal lobe but can spread to involve other parts of the cortex. Temporal lobe damage may be due to:

1. Chronic neurological disease or an insult which has damaged the brain, such as birth asphyxia, meningitis, tuberous sclerosis, or head injury.
2. Prolonged or recurrent seizures, including febrile convulsions, lasting more than 30 minutes in young children may cause neuronal damage of the hypocampal areas of the temporal lobe.
3. Space-occupying lesions in the temporal lobe, such as cysts, tumours, or tuberous sclerosis.

These convulsions present in various ways:

1. With an aura which may include visceral or special sense experiences such as nausea, vertigo, olfactory (unpleasant smell) or auditory (hearing voices, music) hallucinations, or the well-known *déjà vu* (a sense of familiarity in an unfamiliar setting) or *jamais vu* (a sense of unfamiliarity in a familiar setting) phenomena. Mood upsets in the form of fear or anxiety are common. If the dominant hemisphere is involved then speech may be affected (dysphasia or aphasia).
2. Staring attacks which may resemble petit mal epilepsy where the child stops what he is doing; there may be impairment of consciousness, the attack usually lasts 2–5 minutes and the child often experiences post-ictal confusion.
3. Automatisms which may be simple or complex and may last a few minutes or hours. Simple automatisms include grimacing, lip smacking,

chewing, sucking, picking at clothes, toys or hair. Complex automatisms include violent running, undressing, walking about aimlessly, screaming and scratching.

The diagnosis may be difficult if only an aura in the form of sensory phenomenon or automatisms occur; usually there is a combination. These seizures are of short duration and begin and end abruptly. An EEG may show spikes at the temporal region. Children who do not respond readily to anticonvulsant therapy (carbamazepine or phenytoin) should be further investigated with CT scan to exclude a space-occupying lesion or scar.

Partial seizures with secondary generalisation

These are focal seizures which become generalised, and the child loses consciousness. The EEG often shows asymmetrical discharge involving one hemisphere more than the other, the hemisphere with the initial focus shows more spikes.

Therapy of partial seizures

Both elementary and complex forms often respond well to carbamazepine or phenytoin. Intractable temporal lobe epilepsy may require surgical removal of the temporal lobe.

Partial seizures with a secondary generalisation respond well to sodium valproate alone, or in combination with carbamazepine.

Children with partial complex seizures may have psychological disturbances, personality disorders, memory loss and reduced learning ability. The parents and the school should be appropriately counselled; in severe cases a child psychiatrist or child guidance clinic will be helpful.

Generalised seizures

Epileptic discharges originate in both hemispheres or in a deep-seated focus and result in a generalised convulsion (Table 25.3).

Petit mal or absence attacks

These are frequent, abrupt in onset and brief (5–20 seconds) episodes of unconsciousness associated with cessation of activity; they are more common in girls aged 5–12 years. During the attack the child may show motor or other automatisms such as staring, blinking, chewing or lip smacking. There is no post-ictal phase and the child is usually unaware of the seizure but may be embarrassed by an associated incontinence. Petit mal status (absence attacks continuing for more than 30 minutes) is uncommon.

The seizures are associated with characteristic EEG changes, bilateral symmetrical spike and wave complexes occurring at a rate of 3 per second and which can be provoked by hyperventilation. The prognosis of petit mal is good, except if it develops before 5 years or after 12 years of age, or if there is a pre-existing neurological abnormality or mental retardation; these children later develop other seizures such as grand mal or myoclonic attacks.

Drugs of choice in petit mal are sodium valproate or ethosuximide. Sodium valproate is given orally at 20–30 mg/kg daily in divided doses; some children may require up to 50–60 mg/kg daily. Treatment should be continued for two symptom-free years; withdrawal after prolonged therapy should be slow (3–4 months).

Grand mal (generalised motor tonic-clonic seizures)

Approximately 80% of children with epilepsy have grand mal seizures. The seizures begin abruptly and usually without warning; there is a loss of consciousness and the child falls to the ground; a generalised tonic (rigid) phase then occurs, during which time there is apnoea, cyanosis and deviation of the eyes, followed by a clonic phase. There is rapid generalised jerking movements of all four limbs, the child may bite his tongue, respirations are irregular and pharyngeal secretions are increased with frothing of saliva. Urinary and faecal incontinence and a short period of tachycardia and hyperventilation may occur.

A phase of relaxation occurs; the child is limp, respirations and heart rate become normal and then post-ictal sleep of variable duration follows. After this the child may be irritable, confused, may complain of headache or tiredness and there may be paralysis, ataxia and slurred speech. In some children there is not a full seizure and there may be only a tonic or clonic phase.

The long-term pharmacological management of grand mal involves anticonvulsant drugs. Carbamazepine is the drug of choice; phenobarbitone, sodium valproate and phenytoin are also used. The major side-effects of the common anticoagulant drugs are shown in Table 25.4. Sodium valproate side-effects include transient hair loss, obesity, enuresis, thrombocytopenia and, rarely, disturbance of liver metabolism with raised blood ammonia concentration and encephalopathy. Carbamazepine may cause drowsiness, and very rarely produces haematological disorders; it may improve behavioural disorders, unlike phenobarbitone which makes them worse. Carbamazepine and sodium valproate are often useful in combination in difficult of cases.

The duration of drug therapy is arbitrary; usually a 1–2 year seizure-free period is felt to be necessary before slowly discontinuing drugs. This should be done one drug at a time and over several months. The EEG does not provide an adequate guide to discontinuation.

Myoclonic epilepsy

This is a brief, involuntary, single or multiple jerk of an extremity. Sleep myoclonus is a normal phenomenon and occurs when drifting off to sleep or when awakening. Myoclonic epilepsy may be idiopathic (primary) or complex (secondary); secondary causes include metabolic abnormalities (such as uraemia), neuroallergic reactions (such as post-infectious or post-immunisation encephalopathy) and hypoxic brain damage. Infantile spasms, benign myoclonus of early infancy, myoclonic astatic epilepsy of adolescence and eyelid myoclonia with absences are sometimes put into this group; the international classification of seizures puts infantile spasms and akinetic attacks under a separate heading:

1. Lennox–Gastaut syndrome. A form of myoclonic jerks which occur in older children. There may be associated grand mal and petit mal seizures. The EEG shows slow spike and wave discharges. This is one of the most severe forms of epilepsy and the attacks are often intractable to

Table 25.4 Main adverse effects of anticonvulsants

Anticonvulsant	Adverse effects on the nervous system	Other adverse effects
Carbamazepine	Drowsiness Ataxia Transient diplopia	Hyponatraemia Bone marrow depression Thrombocytopenia Erythema multiforme
Clonazepam	Drowsiness Aggressiveness Muscular hypotonia	Salivary or bronchial hypersecretion in infants
Ethosuximide	Lethargy Unsteadiness	Nausea Vomiting Rashes Bone marrow depression
Phenobarbitone Primidone	Drowsiness Hyperactivity in children Mental slowing Irritability Ataxia	Rashes (bullous, erythema) Folate deficiency
Phenytoin	Drowsiness Mental slowing, confusion Ataxia Increased seizures Diplopia, nystagmus Hallucination Dyskinesis Neuropathy	Nausea, vomiting, constipation Rashes (bullous, purpuric Acne Coarsening of facial features Hirsutism Gum hypertrophy Folate deficiency — anaemia Osteomalacia/rickets Bone marrow suppression T-cell suppression
Sodium valproate	Sedation Ataxia Tremor	Nausea, vomiting, diarrhoea Transient alopecia Weight gain Hepatotoxicity with raised ammonia Pancreatitis Enuresis

conventional therapy; sodium valproate alone or in combination with carbamazepine, nitrazepam, clobazam or acetazolamide may be helpful. If the attacks are resistant then a ketogenic diet or steroids (prednisolone) should be tried. The prognosis is poor and good control is achieved in only

20%; the remainder become progressively mentally retarded, and continue to have fits.

2. Benign myoclonic epilepsy of childhood. Children between 3 and 8 years are usually affected; myoclonus occurs in the upper limb and frequent violent falls are common. The EEG in this condition shows 3 per second spike and wave, or polyspike wave complexes. This form of epilepsy responds well to sodium valproate with a good prognosis. Therapy should be continued until adult life.

3. Myoclonic epilepsy of adolescence. This is similar to the benign myoclonic form in childhood but appears in puberty and is more common in females, particularly at period times. There may be sleep myoclonus and grand mal seizures may coexist. The prognosis is good. Sodium valproate is the drug of choice.

4. Myoclonic absences. These are rare and consist of a brief interruption of consciousness as in petit mal absences together with myoclonus and automatisms. A combination of sodium valproate and ethosuximide is used.

5. Eyelid myoclonia with absences. This is a rare form of myoclonic epilepsy with typical absences, jerking of the eyelids and upward deviation of the eyes. The attacks are photosensitive and are induced by a bright light or repetitive blinking. They can be confirmed by EEG with photic stimulation and respond to a combination of sodium valproate and ethosuximide.

Minor status epilepticus

This is sometimes considered to be a variant of myoclonic epilepsy. It may be suspected in children with predominantly grand mal epilepsy who despite adequate control continue to show a fluctuating deterioration in intellectual or motor function. There is often head nodding, eye flickering, dribbling, slurred speech and confusion. A pseudodementia or pseudoataxia may be present and disappear when the attacks are relieved. The EEG shows a marked abnormality with prolonged electrical storms of 1.5–4 cycles per second spikes and waves, mixed sharp elements or spikes, together with ill-defined complexes.

Treatment is difficult; steroids (prednisolone or ACTH) and ketogenic diet have been used. Intravenous cholormethiazole or continuous clonazepam may need to be tried in resistant cases.

Akinetic epilepsy

In this form of epilepsy the child has sudden loss of muscle tone and falls but recovers quickly. These attacks are socially embarrassing and may cause physical trauma, bruises and haematomas. Loss of consciousness is absent or minimal and there is no post-ictal phase. The attacks occur alone or in combination with other forms of seizures. Treatment is difficult; clonazepam, clobazam, sodium valproate, ketogenic diet and steroids can be tried alone or in various combinations.

Infantile spasms (salaam attacks or West's syndrome)

This affects young children, aged 3 months to 1 year. The parents first notice brief, but frequent, flexor spasms. The child gives a short cry, shoots out his arms and flexes his body and legs giving a salaam or greeting posture. The attacks last a few seconds but recur in succession with about 15–30 attacks a minute. The parents often describe the episode as colic. There may be fit-free periods of several minutes or hours.

The child shows failure in developmental progression and even regression. Infantile spasms may be secondary to pre-existing neurological abnormality such as severe birth asphyxia, metabolic disease, infection or tuberous sclerosis. In the majority, however, no pre-existing neurological abnormality is obvious. The EEG shows a typical chaotic pattern with a total disorganisation of cortical activity with high voltage slow waves and spikes which are termed hypsarrhythmia (*hyps* means mountain-like).

Treatment should be started at diagnosis; untreated attacks may burn out leaving the child severely retarded and with other types of seizures. The treatment of hypsarrhythmia is ACTH with or without nitrazepam in combination. The prognosis is generally poor — epilepsy, mental retardation, cerebral palsy, and other developmental disabilities are seen in 90% of the children. Children with normal development before the infantile spasms and those in whom the attacks started after 6 months of age do better, provided they are treated early (within 1 month from the time when attacks were first noticed).

Epilepsia partialis continua

This is a rare type of epilepsy in which the discharges originate in an isolated area of the motor cortex so that prolonged focal seizures without loss of consciousness occur. The attacks may be prolonged and difficult to treat; in addition to anticonvulsants, ACTH or prednisolone, or lobectomy may have to be considered.

Unclassified seizures

Reflex epilepsy

Attacks begin in childhood or early puberty (age 6–15 years) and are more common in females. Grand mal or petit mal seizures are precipitated by certain sensory stimuli (especially visual or auditory); an example is television or photosensitive epilepsy which is induced by flickering light. The attacks are induced by sitting close to a poorly adjusted television set, or by flashing lights in discothèques. The EEG with photic stimulation may induce attacks; spike discharges may be seen. The photosensitive child should be advised to watch television from a distance of at least 3 metres, and the room should not be darkened. They should be advised to cover one eye when approaching the television set to adjust the channel, when suddenly facing a bright light or entering a discothèque. Tinted sunglasses may be helpful in bright sunlight. If drug treatment is required sodium valproate is used.

Benign focal epilepsy of childhood (benign Rolandic epilepsy)

This form of partial epilepsy starts at 7–10 years of age, disappears by 15 years and is commoner in males. A family history is present in 15% of cases. Attacks occur during sleep or often on awakening;

during the attacks the child wakes up, salivates and may have mild jerks of limbs, lips or tongue. He may be unable to speak but is conscious. Some children have tonic-clonic seizures. The EEG is characteristic with unilateral or, rarely, bilateral spikes over the Rolandic or Sylvian region. The attacks often respond to carbamazepine.

Status epilepticus

A series of seizures without recovery of consciousness between attacks, or any seizure lasting more than 30 minutes should be considered as status epilepticus.

This is a medical emergency, because continuous seizures cause brain hypoxia, cerebral oedema, hyperpyrexia and dehydration; the cause needs to be determined. Status epilepticus may be seen if there is a sudden withdrawal of anticonvulsants in children who have had long-term treatment with these drugs; the drugs should then be recommenced.

The treatment of choice for status epilepticus is a diazepam preparation given intravenously, or by the rectal route (Fig. 25.2). Drug absorption from the rectum is good, and control of convulsions is achieved quickly. Each dose is 0.3 mg/kg up to 10 mg maximum (or 1 mg per year of age plus 1 mg). Continuous diazepam at a dose of 0.3 mg/kg/hour may be given as continuous rectal or continuous intravenous infusion. There is no place for intramuscular diazepam as it is slowly absorbed.

Other drugs which may be helpful include phenobarbitone, phenytoin, and rectal or intramuscular paraldehyde. Rectal paraldehyde is given preferably mixed with equal volumes of an oil. The modern plastic syringes are resistant to paraldehyde, but the drug should be administered soon after drawing up.

If the convulsion lasts more than 6–8 hours the child should be treated for cerebral oedema with intravenous mannitol, and phenobarbitone. Intravenous chlormethiazole may be effective in resistant cases. Supportive care includes an adequate calorie and fluid intake by the nasogastric or intravenous route, control of body temperature, and chest physiotherapy if prolonged sedation is

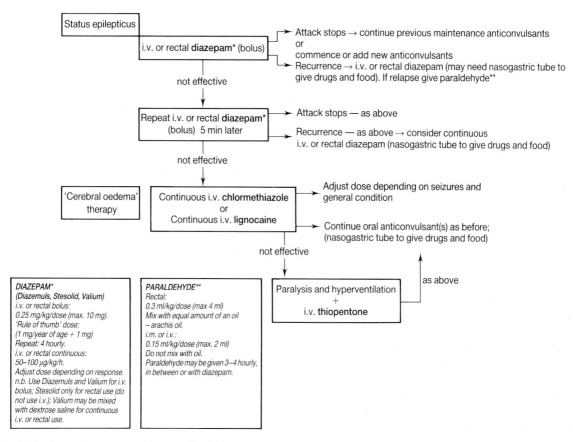

Fig. 25.2 Drug management of status epilepticus.

required. Resistant cases become comatose due to brain cell death or coning.

General management of epilepsy

The parents should be taught the principles of maintaining an airway and an appropriate posture to prevent aspiration of vomit. At home the parents can be taught to administer rectal diazepam in selected cases. Medical advice should be sought with any prolonged convulsions.

Long-term anticonvulsant medication depends on the seizure type rather than the cause of the seizures (see p. 313). The aim is to use a single drug, but occasionally combinations are necessary.

Compliance should be monitored by occasional blood or salivary levels, especially if a child on anticonvulsants is admitted to hospital with seiz-ures, or to check for toxicity (e.g. phenytoin excess may precipitate seizures). Parents should be advised of known drug side-effects. Drug levels are needed to check compliance and only occasionally to adjust medication.

School medical officers and teachers also need to be kept informed about progress and drug therapy. Both drug treatment and the disorder may affect school performance. A child on anticonvulsants can be encouraged to participate in all school activities, including sports; swimming is allowed if epilepsy control is good and there is adequate supervision.

Parents should be counselled and reassured that most epileptics are able to lead normal lives. Over-protection should be discouraged. Convulsions are common in children with mental retardation and in those with behaviour problems. Advice from a child psychiatrist and child guidance clinic may be helpful, particularly with temporal lobe epilepsy. Maladjusted children can even induce seizures; some children may improve with conditioning techniques such as denial or rewards, or with hypnosis. There is some evidence that in a few children dietary manipulation results in improvement of seizure control (in those with seizures triggered by food intolerance).

Febrile convulsions

A febrile convulsion is a seizure occurring in a child between 6 months and 6 years in association with fever and in the absence of intracranial infection, without previous evidence of cerebral pathology or history of convulsion in the absence of fever. Between 3% and 5% of children have at least one febrile convulsion. A typical attack is a brief, single and generalised grand mal seizure. In some children the convulsion may be prolonged (more than 30 minutes) and present as status epilepticus. It may be recurrent during the same febrile illness and post-ictal sleep is common.

Any infection may provoke a febrile convulsion; middle ear, viral upper respiratory tract, gastrointestinal and urinary infections are the most common. In the young child (under 18 months) many authorities advocate routine lumbar puncture after the first febrile convulsion if no definite source of fever is obvious as it is difficult to exclude meningitis. Lumbar puncture should be performed in any child if the fever does not respond to antipyretics and if there is suspicion of meningitis.

Febrile convulsions are thought to occur because of a genetically (autosomal dominant) determined low seizure threshold; if either parent or a sibling has had febrile convulsions the risk is up to 50%. In monozygotic twins the concordance of febrile convulsions is 80%. Males are affected twice as frequently as females.

The trigger in the susceptible child is the rate of rise and height of fever; a child with low threshold may convulse with a minimal rise in temperature whereas those with a higher threshold may only have seizures after a marked rise. Children with a history of cerebral problems (damage or malformation) have low seizure threshold and

the incidence of convulsions associated with temperature in these children is 20%.

Febrile convulsions are often recurrent and 50% of affected children may have more than one, while approximately 20% may have as many as four; recurrence is more common in girls. The recurrence risk is as high as 50% if the first fit occurred under 18 months of age, while it is only 10% after 3 years. Five to 10 per cent of children with febrile convulsions develop epilepsy later.

The aim of management is to stop the acute convulsion and prevent recurrence. Temperature control is important and is achieved by antipyretic drugs and simple measures, such as undressing the child and tepid sponging. In children (under 12 years) aspirin should be avoided as it can trigger Reye's syndrome.

The parents should be instructed about first aid, temperature control and the use of rectal diazepam. Parents should contact their doctor after every convulsion because admission to hospital is indicated for some children.

The long-term management is still controversial but the following plan is reasonable:

1. A child whose first fit is short and uncomplicated (simple febrile convulsions), and for whom there is no family history requires no investigation or prophylaxis — if parents prefer they should be given a supply of rectal diazepam;
2. A child with simple febrile convulsions with strong family history (first-degree relative) of febrile convulsions or epilepsy should be considered for prophylaxis and investigations. A child under 18 months of age and females are more at risk of recurrence and perhaps this group of children should be considered for prophylaxis;
3. A child who has a fit which is prolonged (15 minutes or more) or in whom there is an association with a Todd's paralysis should be investigated and prophylactic anticonvulsants considered;
4. A child who had two or more febrile convulsions (and certainly after the third convulsion) with or without family history should also be considered for investigations and prophylaxis.

Preliminary investigations included:

1. Search for an infection site, particularly meningitis and urinary tract infection (a lumbar

puncture is essential in children under 18 months and on those who have any suspicion of meningitis. It is contraindicated in presence of coma;

2. Metabolic screen (urine amino acids particularly if the child shows slow development), including plasma calcium and fasting blood sugar; and

3. An EEG. The EEG should be performed at least 3 weeks following the seizure in order to obtain a baseline: this will usually be normal but mild abnormalities may be seen. EEG abnormalities may suggest a poor prognosis and the need for careful follow-up.

The anticonvulsant chosen for prophylaxis may vary; generally rectal diazepam is all that is needed. Parents should be instructed to use 5 mg diazepam rectally for children under 15 kg; and 10 mg for over 15 kg as soon as convulsion begins. If the child has had three or four convulsions in one year, and parents have difficulty in using rectal diazepam or if parents prefer another preventive measure, prophylaxis by regular phenobarbitone (5 mg/kg daily as single or two divided doses) is effective and cheap, but it may cause severe and unacceptable hyperactivity (30%); sodium valproate (20 mg/kg dose, in two divided doses) has been also shown to reduce recurrent convulsions, but it should not be given as the first choice because of liver toxicity; liver function test should be performed before and 6 weeks after commencement of sodium valproate.

The duration of regular prophylactic therapy is also controversial; it should probably be given until the child has had at least one seizure-free year. Compliance is important; if a dose is omitted for a day or two, a double dose can be given and then regular prophylaxis continued. Drugs should be discontinued slowly. The prognosis for febrile convulsions is good and most children grow out of the problem.

Neonatal convulsions

Convulsions in the newborn period occur in 1% of all live births. In the majority, the cause is perinatal hypoxia or birth trauma as these cause brain ischaemia, cerebral oedema and haemorrhage. Other causes include metabolic conditions (hypoglycaemia, hypocalcaemia, inborn error of metabolism) and infection (meningitis, septicaemia). The convulsion may present as generalised or focal tonic-clonic seizures or apnoea and cyanosis due to tonic phase.

Management is symptomatic with anticonvulsant drugs and specific drugs depending on the cause. Prognosis in both the short and long term depends on the cause.

MIMICS OF EPILEPSY

Several conditions may be misdiagnosed as epilepsy. These include breath-holding attacks, forms of migraine, vertigo and syncope.

Breath-holding attacks

These are a form of anoxic syncopal attacks which occur in 1- to 5-year-old children; the peak incidence is at 1–2 years. These episodes may involve brief loss of consciousness. The episodes are precipitated by pain, mild trauma or follow temper tantrums. In a typical attack, the child begins to cry aloud and then suddenly stops breathing in expiration and becomes cyanosed, until unconsciousness supervenes.

During an attack muscle tone is increased, and opisthotonic arching may occur. The episode may last for 30 minutes; if it is prolonged a few convulsive twichings or clonic spasms may occur.

The EEG and other neurological investigations are normal, but are not usually indicated. For most children, no treatment is required and the child will grow out of the attacks.

Syncope

A prolonged syncopal attack may rarely be followed by convulsion. Syncope is more common in adolescent girls and should be distinguished from vertigo. Prolonged standing, fasting, emotional upset, the prospect of an unfavourable procedure (such as dental treatment) or seeing a distressing event (such as blood in life or on a screen) can induce syncope.

Observations of pallor, sweating and a slow pulse reinforce the diagnosis. Such children should receive dental treatment in a supine position and can be taught to move their leg muscles if they feel an attack coming on (feeling faint, distortion of sound or vision). An attack of unconsciousness can be precipitated by hyperventilation when distressed or excited.

There may also be awareness of a distorted sound or vision and the child may experience tingling of the extremities and around the mouth. In the infant or toddler, regurgitation or vomiting of food, an unexpected noise or bump, or a painful state, can precipitate a syncopal episode, often with eye rolling and stiffening but little twitching.

This has a reflex cardiovascular cause, and is usually benign, self-limiting and of no serious significance. Anticonvulsants are unnecessary.

INVOLUNTARY MOVEMENTS

Tics are the commonest involuntary movements in childhood, although they are not common in the preschool years. They are habit spasms which are brief, repetitive, involuntary and usually involve movements of the eyes, face and limbs, such as repetitive blinking or shaking of the head. They tend to be stereotyped, increased by anxiety and often have a genetic basis. They are best ignored as far as possible, although some parents find this difficult, especially if there are other tensions in the household or the child has other problems, (such as learning difficulties).

Psychological techniques such as relaxation exercises, or operant conditioning have been used with varying degrees of success, but they are at least harmless.

Drug treatment is often unsatisfactory but moderate doses of diazepam, haloperidol with benzhexol to prevent dystonic reactions, or tetrabenazine can be used. Placebo treatment is worth considering.

A severe form is Gilles de la Tourette's syndrome where the tics are uncontrollable and multifocal; during these tics the child makes a grunting, coughing or barking noise. Self-mutilation and aggressive behaviour may be troublesome. The syndrome is most commonly seen in boys aged 5–10 years. No cause for the disorder has been identified. Haloperidol can be tried.

Athetosis is slow, writhing movements of the limbs, usually associated with grimaces. Hypotonia, speech and swallowing difficulties are very common. These are common in children with cerebral palsy due to severe birth asphyxia or kernicterus. Drug therapy is not helpful.

Chorea, refers to characteristic involuntary, purposeless, sudden jerky irregular movements of the face, trunk or extremities, waxing and waning grip; speech difficulties are often present. Chorea and athetosis often coexist (choreoathetosis) in children with cerebral palsy.

Sydenham's chorea — a manifestation of rheumatic fever — is now rare. The associated hypotonia is usually marked. Serial samples of handwriting will show deterioration and the child may show emotional lability. Slight choreiform movement (chorea minima) is commonly seen in otherwise normal primary school children. Drug treatment of chorea is usually unnecessary. Tetrabenazine is the most effective agent but can cause depression or parkinsonian features.

Central tremor is a fine oscillating movement of the hands present throughout the full range of movement. A slight tremor may be seen in children when anxious or fatigued; some, however, show a marked exaggeration of this to an extent which may impair manipulative activities and handwriting. The condition may be familial. Treatment is often unnecessary but propranolol is the most effective drug. Weighted bracelets can also be helpful.

MOTOR DISORDERS

The normal variation in motor development can be misleading; many preterm babies and some term babies show an extended posture and may appear stiff in early infancy, but few have serious motor disorder later; 7% of normal children do not crawl, but move about by rolling, creeping or bottom shuffling and tend to be more hypotonic than children who crawl, however, they generally walk normally 6–8 months later. The mean walking age for non-crawlers is about 2 years. There are a number of pathological causes of hypotonia and delayed walking; these include the hypotonic phase of ataxic or choreoathetoid cerebral palsy or disorders such as muscular dystrophy. At least one-quarter of boys with Duchenne dystrophy are

Should you pay prescription charges? Read all the statements in **Part 1** opposite. You don't have to pay a prescription charge if any of the statements apply to you (the patient) on the day you are asked to pay. (A valid War Pension exemption certificate only entitles you to free prescriptions for your accepted disablement.) Put a cross in the first box in **Part 1** that applies to you, read the declaration and complete and sign **Part 3**.

Benefits which DO NOT provide exemption. You are NOT entitled to exemption from prescription charges because you receive Pension Credit Savings Credit, Incapacity Benefit, Disability Living Allowance, Contributions based Jobseeker's Allowance or Contributions based Employment and Support Allowance. Only those benefits listed in **Part 1** provide exemption. An HC3 certificate does not entitle you to free prescriptions.

Evidence. You may be asked to provide evidence to show that you do not have to pay. You could show the relevant benefit award notice, or an exemption or pre-payment certificate. If you cannot show evidence at that time you can still get your prescription items free but your Primary Care Trust will check your entitlement later if you do not show proof (see paragraph about Penalty Charges).

If you have to pay a prescription charge. You (or your representative) should put in **Part 2** the amount you have paid and then sign and complete **Part 3**.

Need help with the cost of prescription charges? You can get information by ringing 0845 850 1166 or by reading leaflets HC11 or HC12. You may be able to get these leaflets from your GP surgery or pharmacy. Or ring 0845 610 1112 to get one, or go to www.dh.gov.uk/helpwithhealthcosts

Not entitled to free prescriptions? Pre-pay to reduce the cost. If you think you will have to get more than 4 items in 3 months or 14 items in 12 months it will be cheaper to buy a pre-payment certificate (PPC). Phone 0845 850 0030 to find out the cost, or order a PPC and pay by credit or debit card. You can pay for a 12 month PPC by direct debit instalment payments. Buy on-line at www.ppa.org.uk To pay by cheque get an application form (FP95) from your pharmacy or go to www.dh.gov.uk/helpwithhealthcosts The FP95 tells you what to do.

Do you need a refund? If you are unsure if you are entitled to free prescriptions you should pay for the prescription item(s) and ask for a receipt form FP57. **You must get the FP57 form when you pay for the item(s), you cannot get the form later.** If you find you didn't have to pay, you can claim your money back up to 3 months after paying. The FP57 form tells you what to do.

Patient Representative. If you are unable to collect your prescription yourself, someone can take your completed form for you. You must complete **Part 1**. Your representative must complete **Parts 2 and 3**. Anyone who collects a **Schedule 2 or 3 controlled drug must sign the box in Part 1 when they collect the item(s)** and provide proof of identity if requested.

Data collection. Information about the prescription items on this form will be processed centrally to pay monies due to the pharmacist, doctor or appliance contractor for the items they have supplied to you. The NHS will also use the information to analyse what has been prescribed and the cost. The Counter Fraud and Security Management Service, a division of the NHS Business Services Authority, may use information from this form to prevent and detect fraud and incorrectness in the NHS.

Penalty Charges. If it is found that you should have paid for your prescription items, you will face penalty charges and may be prosecuted under the powers introduced by the Health Act 1999. Routine checks are carried out on exemption claims including some where proof may have been shown. You may be contacted in the course of such checks.

PATIENTS – please read the notes overleaf

late to walk (after 18 months); this should allow the identification of some cases so that genetic counselling can be given.

The commonest motor disorders in childhood are the perceptual motor, balancing and apraxic disorders of so-called clumsy children. These are children whose motor abilities lag behind their general abilities by 2 years or more. Their problems and the cause of their dysfunction are multiple, in only a minority is there a perinatal or genetic cause. The subject has not received the attention of impairment of language, vision or hearing, yet motor skill is important for children in everyday activities, play and writing.

The interested clinician will observe impaired motor performance amongst many children with speech or learning difficulties, behavioural problems or functional symptoms as well as more specific diagnoses such as epilepsy and hydrocephalus. The subject is controversial and many approaches and names are given to the various aspects of the problem (minimal brain damage, minimal cerebral dysfunction, hyperactivity, maladjustment). There is no clear cut-off point between normal and clumsy children. Different children, families and teachers react differently to similar degrees of motor incompetence.

It is also true that the prognosis is good for most young, clumsy children who have merely a maturational lag. Even they are better managed if their movement difficulties are appreciated. The outcome, however, for more severely clumsy children, especially older ones, is less clear. Some retain the difficulties in adult life and some run into significant conduct disorders or other psychiatric disorders. There can be misperception of some clumsy children if the poor motor competence is not recognised. They can become more difficult, frustrated or depressed, and parents or teachers may be wrongly blamed. Remedial techniques require further evaluation and will never be sufficiently available to meet the needs of all such children. Widely discrepant abilities present great problems to class teachers and parents. Acceptance of each child's strengths and weaknesses is important for the child, who should be encouraged to find activities (e.g. swimming or chess) which may be enjoyable, successful and relaxing. Children

with greatest difficulties on testing may need a specialist opinion to exclude specific neurological disorders.

Thereafter, a plan of management using existing resources has to be worked out between the school or family doctor, the teacher, the educational psychologist, the parents and the child. There are no medical solutions.

HEAD INJURIES

Head trauma is a common cause of death in childhood, while the sequelae of head injuries such as post-traumatic epilepsy, abnormal behaviour or impairment of intellectual performance may be permanent. Injuries occur at home, in the playground, as a result of traffic accidents, or may be non-accidental. The majority are due to falls from a height (trees, windows), or against an object. The skull in infants is relatively thin and elastic and thereby protects the brain and reduces the concussive effects of trauma; over 5 years of age the effects are similar to those of adults as the skull is now a rigid structure with little capacity to expand if there is haemorrhage or oedema. *Contre-coup* injury is common in children. This is when an injury, usually a blow or blunt injury on one side of the head, causes the brain to hit against the opposite skull vault.

Several types of head injury exist:

1. Contusion (of the head). There is only a bruise on the head with the brain unaffected. There is no loss of consciousness, the child may have dizziness, nausea or vomiting. Skull X-rays are not necessary. The parents however should be given a head injury observation chart.

2. Concussion (of the brain). Here there is loss of consciousness, often brief, but may be prolonged for hours or days. Irritability, dizziness, nausea and vomiting are associated. Headaches may be severe and persist for several days or even weeks. Retrograde and post-traumatic amnesia are often present; prolonged retrograde amnesia suggests a poor prognosis. A child with concussion should have a skull X-ray and requires admission to hospital for observation. If there is progressive deterioration, particularly in consciousness, severe concussion with brain oedema or intracranial haemorrhage should be suspected. Progressive bradycardia with increasing hypertension suggests raised intracranial pressure whereas a falling blood pressure or unequal pupils may indicate intracranial bleeding. Urgent neurosurgical referral is required. Every patient with deterioration should be assumed to have bleeding until proven otherwise (by CT scan) as it is not possible to separate the two clinically.

3. Brain contusion. Bruising of the brain is often a result of *contre-coup* or *coup* injury. Microscopic haemorrhages are seen in the brain substances; with severe contusion marked damage occurs. Contusion of the brain is difficult to diagnose clinically; in *contre-coup* injuries the signs and symptoms are on the opposite side of the head to that which was injured. There may be a hemiplegia or convulsion.

4. Cephalhaematomas and laceration of the scalp. These are common and clinically visible. Profuse bleeding from small lacerations is often frightening to the parents and to the child; simple cleaning and suturing is required.

Skull fractures

These may be simple and linear, depressed or compound. Simple fracture is common and usually of no major clinical significance, although skull X-ray is indicated to confirm the fracture and admission to hospital for observation is advisable. The haematoma subsides spontaneously; routine antibiotic cover is not necessary. Depressed fractures need surgical correction; the cause is often a blow or fall on a sharp object. The depression may be clinically apparent but is confirmed on X-ray.

Compound fractures are serious. A compound basal skull fracture is accompanied by CSF leak through the nose or ears which can be confirmed by finding glucose in secretions (by Clinistix), and by evidence of haemorrhage around the eyes. There is a risk of central nervous system infection.

Penetrating head injuries and open head injuries are easy to diagnose, the point of penetration may be obvious and the brain may occasionally be exposed through the wound. There is a risk of infection and damage to the brain substance; the prognosis in most cases is surprisingly good. Neurosurgical referral is important.

Indications for skull X-ray in children include head trauma with unconsciousness, penetrating injury, less than 1 year of age, cephalohaematoma, a depression palpable in the scalp, haemorrhage around the eyes, CSF otorrhoea or rhinorrhoea, blood in the middle ear, focal neurological signs and fits, coma or marked lethargy.

Subdural collection

This may occur as a result of trauma or as an effusion associated with meningitis. The child may present with focal convulsions, raised intracranial pressure, or in infants with enlarging head circumference. The history gives a clue, and the diagnosis is confirmed by skull X-ray, CT scan, angiography, or diagnostic subdural taps. Management is symptomatic; but surgical drainage may be necessary, if there is raised intracranial pressure or if there are chronic subdural effusions — seen in young children following non-accidental injury. The prognosis is variable and depends on the cause and the result of the pressure effects of the subdural collection.

PROGRESSIVE DEMENTIA IN INFANCY AND CHILDHOOD

Here there is a progressive deterioration in either mental or physical function, or both, as a result of progressive central nervous system pathology.

The cause may be an inborn error of metabolism, neurodegenerative disease, persistent encephalitis, infiltrative tumour, or chronic drug or metal intoxication (e.g. toluene or lead poisoning). Minor motor status, hypothyroidism, and low pressure hydrocephalus may present as pseudodementia which disappears with therapy.

Most children with this group of disorders are normal at birth; a history of arrest or regression of development and loss of skills or progressive dementia is present. It is important to establish the diagnosis so that appropriate genetic counselling can be given. Treatment such as bone marrow transplantation are being developed for some metabolic disorders (mucopolysaccharidoses).

INBORN ERRORS OF METABOLISM

These are recessive inherited disorders where enzyme deficiencies cause either the deficiency of an essential metabolite or the accumulation of a toxic one.

Eight major subgroups exist; disorders of amino acid metabolism (phenylketonuria); disorders of carbohydrate metabolism (galactosaemia, glycogen storage disease); mucopolysaccharidosis, neurolipidosis and disorders of glycoprotein metabolism (fucosidosis, mannosidosis); organic acidurias (proprionic aciduria, methylmalonic aciduria, lactic acidaemia); disorders of lipid metabolism (gangliosidosis); disorders of metal metabolism (Wilson's disease); and disorders of purine metabolism (Lesch–Nyhan syndrome, porphyrias).

MUSCLE DISORDERS IN CHILDREN

Neuromuscular disorders may be broadly classified as myopathy or neuropathy. Myopathy refers to conditions in which there is an abnormality of muscle function, attributed to pathological clinical abnormality or abnormal electrical discharges in the muscle fibres or interstitial tissues of voluntary muscles; the cause of which is *not* a disorder of the central or peripheral nervous system. Neuropathy is a result of denervation; the muscle undergoes degeneration.

There are a large number of rare neuromuscular disorders and their precise diagnosis requires a specialist opinion; usually serum creatine kinase (creatine phosphokinase, electromyelography, nerve conduction studies and biopsy of muscle (sometimes also sural nerve) may be necessary to allow a diagnosis and permit genetic counselling for such conditions as muscular dystrophy, spinal muscular atrophy, congenital neuropathy or myopathy.

Children affected by neuromuscular disease such as chronic spinal muscular atrophy are weak, hypotonic and hyporeflexic. In Duchenne muscular dystrophy the mean IQ is 85 and affected boys may present with delayed language development.

Myopathy may be due to inflammatory, metabolic or endocrine causes; they may be congenital (congenital structural myopathy — a term usually reserved for myopathies which show characteristic histological features with light and electron microscopic findings). Muscular dystrophy is a term used for progressive genetic myopathies which present with distinct clinical and histological features. In some, particularly in Duchenne or Becker muscular dystrophy, there is enlargement of muscles (true muscular hypertrophy) and later pseudohypertrophy (due to replacement of the muscle fat). Some muscular dystrophies are associated with myotonia and they are classified as dystrophia myotonica. Congenital myopathic disorders are rare.

Muscular dystrophy

Duchenne muscular dystrophy is the most common and most severe of the muscular dystrophies. It is inherited as an X-linked recessive trait, occurs in 1 in 4000 male live births. It characteristically has an early onset (before 3 years), symmetrical proximal muscle involvement (pelvic and pectoral girdle), pseudohypertrophy of calves and deltoid, progressive weakness leading to inability to walk within 10 years of the onset of symptoms, and death by respiratory or cardiac failure in the first or second decade.

The boy's gait is typically waddling; he shows lumbar lordosis, and because of contractures may walk tip-toe. The child shows Gowers' manoeuvre (he climbs up his legs, when asked to rise from sitting or lying on the floor). There is a high level of creatine kinase in the plasma. Boys with Duchenne muscular dystrophy are mentally slow (the cause of this is not clear) and cardiac involvement occurs in most (tachycardia, tall R waves in the right precordial leads, deep Q waves in the limb leads) and myocardial failure is a common cause of death.

The gene locus and gene product (dystrophin) which are defective in Duchenne muscular dystrophy have been identified, dystrophin in muscle is absent (in Becker muscular dystrophy dystrophin is abnormal). The pathogenesis of the disease is still poorly understood. Carrier detection and prenatal diagnosis (by chorionic villi biopsy or amniocentesis) is much more reliable because of gene mapping studies. Carrier mothers have raised creatine kinase, and slightly increased calf muscle bulk.

Becker muscular dystrophy, which is also inherited in an X-linked recessive manner, is characterised by later onset (5–25 years) and a more benign progression, so that total crippling and death occur much later. The mean age when Becker patients become chairbound is 27 years (compared to 8.5 years for Duchenne); the age of death is 42 years and 16 years respectively. Becker muscular dystrophy has several similarities with Duchenne; weakness first occurs in the pelvic girdle and thighs, then the pectoral girdle and upper limb, proximal muscles are affected more than distal, deep tendon reflexes are generally diminished and finally become non-existent, marked pseudohypertrophy of calf and deltoid muscle occurs, and there is cardiac involvement. In both conditions the creatine kinase is raised in the initial stages and becomes less as the condition worsens; electromyography (EMG) shows myopathic changes and muscle biopsy are similar; therefore the diagnosis is made on clinical grounds.

Spinal muscular atrophy

Spinal muscular atrophy is a neuropathic disorder caused by degeneration of the anterior horn cells. There is bulbar muscle involvement in some form thus it is not confined only to spinal cord, brain stem nuclei may also be involved.

The early-onset form is congenital in origin (Werdnig–Hoffmann disease); and the childhood onset form can occur at any age. These disorders are all due to different gene mutations, but resemble each other in phenotypic expression.

Certain common features are seen. They are familial disorders. They are progressive (although the tempo may be fast or slow). Painless muscle weakness and wasting affecting chiefly the limbs and trunk occurs, with no sensory or sphincter disturbances nor intellectual impairment. Muscle tone is reduced or normal, and the deep tendon reflexes are diminished. Muscle fasciculation is often present in affected muscles. In Werdnig–Hoffman disease, tongue fasciculation is seen in the newborn period. The EMG reveals evidence of denervation and muscle biopsy shows group atrophy. Muscle enzymes, EEG and CSF are normal. The final diagnosis may be confirmed at autopsy, which shows selective loss of anterior horn cells in cord and brain stem.

There is no specific treatment; death occurs from chest infection. Although it is true that the earlier the onset, the worse the prognosis, this is not invariable. The Werdnig–Hoffmann type with onset at birth may survive beyond infancy (or even into the teens). Generally, it can be said that those with congenital onset have the following fates: 60% are dead by 1 year, 50% are dead by 4 years. In survivors, scoliosis and contractures further limit activity.

In those with onset in childhood, the prognosis in terms of survival and quality of life can be surprisingly good. Of those with an onset from 3 to 18 years of age, more than a quarter will still be alive after 20 years of illness.

Diseases which are incurable are not untreatable, and muscular dystrophy and spinal muscular atrophy are good examples. Treatment is multidisciplinary, including genetic counselling, orthopaedic surgery to release contractures, and physiotherapy to prevent contractures. Such children are managed by the multidisciplinary team.

26. Surgical disorders

J.A.S. Dickson

THE NEWBORN

Congenital abnormalities of all systems are the major cause of surgical problems in the newborn period.

The gastrointestinal tract

Oesophageal atresia

Oesophageal atresia has an incidence of 1 in 3000–5000 live births. In the commonest form (85%) the upper oesophagus ends blindly in the upper mediastinum while the lower oesophagus arises by a fistula from the trachea. The other variants include atresia without fistula and fistula without atresia. Fifty per cent of these babies have anomalies in other systems.

Diagnosis. Polyhydramnios is present in up to one-third of mothers with babies with oesophageal atresia. After birth, the baby is unable to swallow saliva, drools from the mouth and may choke on a feed. Spill-over of saliva into the trachea may cause choking and cyanosis. Air forced into the distal oesophagus through the fistula produces abdominal distension and may lead to acid reflux into the trachea. The diagnosis is confirmed by an inability to pass a 10–12 gauge catheter into the stomach; if the tube is held up at 10–12 cm the diagnosis is established. Plain X-rays show the site of arrest of the tube while the presence of gas in the abdomen suggests a fistula.

Treatment. In the majority, primary surgical correction is possible. The rest will require a delayed repair or an oesophageal replacement around 1 year of age. About 85% of babies with oesophageal atresia now survive and deaths are due to abnormalities in other systems.

Intestinal obstruction

The signs and symptoms in the newborn are: bile-stained or persistent vomiting; abdominal distension; and delayed passage of meconium.

Green vomit in the newborn must be assumed to be due to intestinal obstruction until proved otherwise. The level of the obstruction may be indicated by the degree and type of abdominal distension; in high small bowel obstruction it is upper abdominal, in low small bowel obstruction it is central, and in large bowel obstruction in the flanks and across the epigastrium. Over 90% of term babies pass meconium within 24 hours of birth. Delay is associated with prematurity and birth asphyxia but if longer than 48 hours an obstruction should be suspected. In proximal obstructions the distribution of the gas in the gut on plain abdominal X-rays is usually diagnostic.

Duodenal obstruction

Duodenal obstruction, which is seen in 1 in 5000–6000 live births, may be due to atresia, stenosis, diaphragm or associated with an annular pancreas. The obstruction is commonest in the second part of the duodenum distal to the ampulla of Vater. Other congenital abnormalities are common and 30% have Down's syndrome.

Diagnosis. Maternal polyhydramnios is present in about 30%; an ultrasound examination of the mother can identify the dilated fetal stomach and duodenum. After birth vomiting, usually but not always bile stained, frequently precedes feeding. All feeds are vomited. Abdominal distension varies with the fullness of the stomach. The passage of meconium is delayed. Plain abdominal X-rays show the classical double-bubble sign of gas in the stomach and the dilated proximal duodenum.

Treatment. If the diagnosis is delayed, loss of acid gastric contents leads to a metabolic alkalosis which will require correction. The dilated duodenum is anastomosed to the duodenum immediately distal to the obstruction. Delayed transit across the anastomosis is common. This can be overcome by total parenteral nutrition, of by passing a tube across the anastomosis at the time of the operation. Around 70% of babies should survive.

Jejunal, ileal and colonic atresias

These are probably due to some intrauterine accident occuring in previously normal bowel. All the signs of obstruction are present. The incidence is about 1 per 6000 live births with colonic atresias accounting for 10%. Plain X-rays show multiple fluid levels in increasingly distended gut ending in one very large loop.

Treatment. The operation involves resection and anastomosis. Survival rates are round 80%.

Cystic fibrosis should be excluded by a sweat test in all babies with small bowel atresia or evidence of meconium peritonitis.

Meconium ileus

Meconium ileus is the earliest and the most acute intestinal complication of cystic fibrosis. The obstruction, seen in 15% of such babies, is due to impaction of a bolus of abnormally viscid meconium in the distal small bowel. Volvulus, meconium peritonitis or a small bowel atresia may complicate the disorder.

Diagnosis. Abdominal distension, present at birth, is a major feature; bile-stained vomiting occurs early and no meconium is passed. Plain abdominal X-rays show evidence of obstruction with stippling in the right iliac fossa or dilated loops with relative absence of fluid levels. A gastrografin enema will outline a microcolon containing small plugs of mucus, a narrow terminal ileum and a proximal dilated segment. The obstruction is relieved by the enema in up to one-half of the uncomplicated cases; complicated cases, and those not relieved by the enema, require surgery. Full treatment for cystic fibrosis should be started at once and the diagnosis confirmed by raised serum immunoreactive trypsin (IRT) levels and a sweat test.

Malrotation and volvulus neonatorum

The anatomical features of malrotation of the gut are failure of rotation of the duodenum with the duodeno-jejunal junction lying to the right of the midline, and non-rotation of the colon with the caecum lying in the epigastrium. This leaves a narrow unstable mesenteric isthmus around which the bowel can twist, causing an obstruction in the second part of the duodenum which may rapidly progress to strangulation of the midgut loop.

Diagnosis. Volvulus should be suspected in those babies who, after initial normal progress, suddenly develop a duodenal obstruction. In doubtful cases, a barium meal will show the level of the obstruction or the abnormal position of the duodenum.

Treatment. Urgent surgical untwisting of the volvulus is required, followed by a derotation of the gut and widening of the mesenteric root.

Hirschsprung's disease (congenital intestinal aganglionosis)

This can present at any stage in childhood. The incidence is 1 in 5000–6000 live births.

In over 90%, symptoms start in the first week of life. The underlying abnormality is the absence of parasympathetic ganglion cells from the wall of the gut. The distal rectum is always involved, but the proximal extent varies. The condition is conventionally divided into short-segment disease, where the aganglionosis does not extend proximal to the junction of sigmoid and descending colon (65–75% of all cases), and long-segment disease where more proximal colon is affected. The picture may be complicated at any stage by necrotising enterocolitis.

Diagnosis. The commonest early symptom is delayed passage of meconium. Abdominal distension follows and there is a reluctance to feed and reflex vomiting. Bilious vomiting usually occurs later. Rectal examination may lead to an explosive decompression or merely disclose an empty distal rectum. The differential diagnosis includes functional obstruction, seen in prematurity or after a traumatic labour, and asphyxia and the meconium plug syndrome. Where there is total colonic aganglionosis it must be distinguished from other small bowel obstructions.

Plain abdominal X-rays and a barium enema will confirm the diagnosis in 70% of cases but must be confirmed by a suction rectal biopsy. It is essential that at least 12 hours should elapse between a rectal washout or rectal examination and the barium studies. The barium enema will show essentially normal distal bowel (the narrow segment) expanding rapidly at the point of transition (the cone) into the dilated proximal ganglionic gut. This gives both the diagnosis and length of the aganglionic segment.

Treatment. The initial treatment is a colostomy in an area of ganglionic gut. At the age of 6 months to 1 year a pull-through operation is performed, resecting the aganglionic segment and bringing ganglionic bowel down to the anal canal by one of the techniques described by Swenson, Duhamel or Soave. Following surgery most children will gain adequate bowel control but at a later date than their peers. A few have problems with failure of relaxation of the internal sphincter and require later dilatation or sphincterotomy.

The meconium plug syndrome

A few neonates have an apparent obstruction which is relieved by a contrast or saline enema. It is important to exclude Hirschsprung's disease by biopsy and cystic fibrosis by a sweat test.

Anorectal anomalies

Anorectal anomalies are generally obvious at the initial newborn examination. Lesions can be divided into low or high, depending on the level at which the rectum ends; if the rectum ends above the pelvic floor the lesion is supralevator or high, if below it is translevator or low. In most of these babies the rectum ends as a fistula joining the posterior urethra (high lesions) or the perineal skin (low lesions) in the male, and the upper vagina (high lesions) or the vaginal introitus or perineal skin (low lesions) in the female. Two further variants occur in the female. In the most severe form, the persistent cloaca, the urethra, vagina and rectum all reach the perineum through a common channel. Intermediate lesions also occur. Associated anomalies, particularly oesophageal and duodenal atresia, are common and abnormalities of the renal tract are seen in 40%.

Diagnosis. The initial assessment should be made by examination of the perineum and gentle probing for the fistula. Plain abdominal X-rays exclude other gut anomalies and obstructions and a lateral view of the sacrum gives some indication of the state of the pelvic floor and innervation of the rectum which is usually normal if more than three sacral segments are present. In high and most intermediate lesions, a preliminary colostomy relieves the obstruction and allows time for full investigation. The distal gut is outlined with a water-soluble contrast introduced through the colostomy, renal ultrasound and micturating cystourethrogram outline the renal tract. Low anomalies can be corrected by an immediate perineal operation. High anomalies are repaired by a pull-through operation when the baby is around 6–9 months of age.

Necrotising enterocolitis

Necrotising enterocolitis is seen in pre-term babies, after birth asphyxia or shock, in cyanotic heart disease, particularly after surgery, after umbilical vein catheterisation and exchange transfusion, in Hirschsprung's disease, and sometimes for no obvious reason. The underlying pathology is an area of necrosis of the gut wall which varies in its extent in length and depth of the wall. The aetiology, apart from general agreement that ischaemia and secondary bacterial infection are involved, is obscure.

Diagnosis. The condition should be suspected in any at-risk neonate who becomes less active, has temperature instability, gastric retention or abdominal distension. Blood in the stools increases the probability and plain abdominal X-rays are usually diagnostic. The early X-ray signs are those of bowel wall oedema and increased fluid between dilated loops. Intramural gas (pneumatosis intestinalis), which may progress to free gas from a perforation or gas in the portal veins in the liver, confirms the diagnosis.

Treatment. The treatment is initially medical and includes: stop oral intake and start nasogastric suction; intravenous fluids and i.v. feeding; i.v. antibiotics such as gentamicin, penicillin and metronidazole; close monitoring of vital signs, haemoglobin, platelets, because of the risk of disseminated intravascular coagulation, acid-base balance, and daily abdominal X-rays.

Surgery is reserved for patients who fail to respond or develop a perforation or obstruction. On recovery, late stricture formation is seen in at least 20% of cases.

Exomphalos

Exomphalos is a useful term to cover all congenital abnormalities with herniation of gut at the umbilicus. These should be subdivided into:

1. Hernia into the cord. Here there is only a small defect at the base of the umbilical cord. Reduction of the hernia and surgical repair usually present no problem.

2. Omphalocele. This is a defect of the muscle of the abdominal wall where the sac has a wide base and contains liver. Associated anomalies such as cardiac defects or extroversion of the bladder are common. Minor defects can be repaired but large defects present a major surgical problem.

3. Gastroschisis. Here there is a short transverse defect alongside the umbilicus through which the gut prolapses. The cause is probably an early antenatal rupture of hernia into the cord. Treatment is complicated by the difficulty of returning the gut to the contracted abdomen and delay in return of function of the gut. Antenatal diagnosis of these lesions is now common.

Diaphragmatic hernia

Congenital diaphragmatic hernias occur at three sites, oesophageal hiatus, which is discussed under gastro-oesophageal reflux, posterolateral or Bochdalek's hernia, and retrosternal or Morgagni's hernia.

The posterolateral hernia, most frequently (80%) on the left side, allows gut into the chest during intrauterine development. The lung on the affected side fails to develop and, in the most severe forms, displacement of the mediastinum causes underdevelopment of the opposite lung. This is an urgent neonatal emergency. As air is swallowed the gut in the chest expands and progressively compresses the lungs. The diagnosis should be suspected in any newborn with respiratory distress, cyanosis and apparent dextrocardia, particularly if the abdomen is scaphoid.

A plain chest X-ray will usually give the diagnosis. Bowel loops are seen on the affected side, the mediastinum is displaced, the opposite lung collapsed and the abdomen is empty.

Treatment. Emergency treatment is directed at deflating the gut with a nasogastric tube and positive pressure ventilation through an endotracheal tube. Ventilation through a face-mask will only force more air into the gut and increase the pressure on the lungs. Surgery, which can be delayed until the infant's condition in stable, involves return of the gut to the abdomen and repair of the diaphragm. Currently extracorporeal membrane oxygenation is being tried to improve the survival rate in special centres. Survival depends on the amount of lung present and complications such as persistent fetal circulatory pattern; around 60% of babies survive. Long-term lung function in survivors is usually normal.

Neural tube defects

These comprise spina bifida, anenecephaly, encephalocele and hydrocephalus and have an incidence of between 5 and 6 per 1000 live births. The term spina bifida covers all defects of the vertebral neural arch.

Spina bifida occulta, where the defect is a split in the bony arch without meningeal or skin protrusion, is most often discovered as an incidental finding during X-ray examination of the lumbosacral spine. The presence of a hairy patch, capillary haemangioma, or dermal sinus may point to the underlying defect which is then not strictly occult, and may rarely be associated with spinal cord involvement, a tethered filum terminale or diastematomyelia — splitting of the cord. A true dermal sinus, which is situated in the midline, has a lining of modified pink skin which leads down to the theca, and must be distinguished from the common postanal dimple or sinus. This is skin lined, lies over the tip of the coccyx, and apart from the uncommon complication of local sepsis from retained stool, is of no significance. A dermal sinus requires full investigation and excision.

A meningocele, the least common form of spina bifida, is a skin-covered lesion with cystic protrusion of the meninges, but without underlying neurological involvement. With lipoma of the cauda equina, a similar bulge over the spine occurs and is filled with fatty tissue intimately involved with the cord, nerve roots and often meningeal distension. There is often both a primary neurological defect and a risk of deterioration secondary to differential growth of the spine stretching a fixed cord.

In meningomyelocele, an abnormal cord is adherent to the surface of the sac often at a raw plaque; in the most severe form, myeloschisis or rachischisis, the whole cord lies open on the surface for several segments. The neurological deficit varies with the level and nature of the lesion from pure sacral lesions with only bladder and anal involvement to total paralysis caudal to a thoracic defect. Mixed upper and lower motor neurone lesions are common. Most (70–80%) of the severe defects develop progressive hydrocephalus secondary to an associated Arnold–Chiari malformation, where there is displacement of the hind brain and fourth ventricle through the foramen magnum into the vertebral canal and prolapse of the cerebellar tonsils. Defects in the midline of the skull (cranium bifidum), most commonly frontal or occipital, may similarly be meningoceles without underlying brain damage or contain abnormal brain tissue and are then known as encephaloceles. These lesions are also often associated with hydrocephalus.

Hydrocephalus is also caused by other blockages of the cerebrospinal fluid pathway; in the cerebral aqueduct, at the exit foramina of the fourth ventricle, or secondary to intracranial bleeding or meningitis with blockage of the basal cysterns, and most rarely by posterior fossa tumours.

Management

There is now general agreement that the treatment should be planned in the light of the probable immediate and late outcome. In spina bifida there is a policy of selection of those children most likely to benefit from immediate surgery, i.e. within 24 hours of birth. Adverse factors against surgery, include: severe paralysis of the lower limbs, total paraplegia or hip flexors only acting; severe hydrocephalus, a head circumference 2 cm above the 90th centile corrected for weight and gestational age; gross kyphosis; or other associated major abnormalities or severe cerebral birth trauma.

These criteria will exclude about 60% of cases from early surgery. After early closure, even of the less severe defects, 70% develop hydrocephalus, requiring control by one of the valve systems (Holter, Pudenz, Hakim, etc.) with ventriculoatrial or ventriculoperitoneal shunting.

The management of severely affected babies without operation is more controversial. If fed normally, but given no other treatment apart from dressing of the back, up to 50% survive. The spinal lesion epithelialises in 1 to 3 months but most develop hydrocephalus. These survivors can be later transferred to the full treatment regimen without disadvantage.

The immediate orthopaedic assessment is confined to determining the degree of fixed deformity and the extent of voluntary and reflex muscle activity. Passive manipulation of fixed deformities, e.g. talipes, should start at once. Splints must be used with care to avoid damage to anaesthetic skin.

Early urological investigation, similarly, is limited to assessing bladder function from the pattern of micturition and the extent of bladder filling. Outflow obstruction is recognised by a persistently full bladder and constant dribbling. Total bladder and bladder neck paralysis, in which the bladder is either easily expressible or never full, is the safer lesion. Regular expression is only of value for babies with flaccid bladders without outflow obstruction.

Long-term management

Even the less severely affected children, who now

form most of the survivors, have life-long medical problems.

Valve complications.

1. Blockage. All valves block eventually. Some children will no longer be valve dependent when this happens, but many of these lead a precarious existence with permanently increased intracranial pressure and are liable to acute problems following minor head injuries or intercurrent infection. The blockage is equally common at upper and lower ends; in the ventricle, choroid plexus or brain may plug the catheter while at the lower end, as growth proceeds, the catheter becomes too short and is pulled out of the atrium with blockage in the venous system. In the peritoneum the catheter may simply retract from the cavity or a CSF pocket may become walled off from the general peritoneal cavity. The signs and symptoms of blockage are headache, altered state of consciousness, convulsions, vomiting, squint and down-turning of the eyes, increased tension in the anterior fontanelle and over the spinal defect, dilated scalp veins and papilloedema. Acute blockage must be treated urgently by the appropriate operative revision. Around puberty children, both those who have not previously required a shunt and those with shunts which have been non-functional for long periods, are at risk of developing acute hydrocephalus.

2. Valve colonisation. Between 5% and 15% of valves become colonised by organisms of low pathogenicity, most frequently *Staphylococcus epidermidis*. The signs of this are a general malaise, low-grade pyrexia, anaemia and, when a vascular shunt has been used, splenomegaly, proteinuria and haematuria. Colonisation may cause blockage of the shunt system especially in the peritoneum. Treatment involves control of systemic infection by appropriate antibacterial agents and replacement of the infected valve by a new clean system.

Urological management.

The renal tract is at risk from disordered bladder and sphincter contraction, which lead to incomplete bladder emptying with infected residual urine, ureteric reflux and back pressure on the kidney. Regular urine culture is essential and ultrasound examination should be performed annually unless the system is stable. Isotope renograms are the investigation of choice if there is evidence of deterioration. Micturition cystourethrography is useful to demonstrate reflux and bladder-outflow obstruction. Around 30% of these children can achieve acceptable levels of urinary continence. Cystomanometry is probably the most valuable means of assessing the prospects and deciding the method of treatment. Overactive detrusor contractions can be damped by imipramine, oxybutynin or terodiline and sphincter obstruction may respond to prazosin. Bladder expression by an adult, or for older children by themselves, with or without drugs, helps to get complete emptying.

Sphincter obstruction not responding to drugs should be relieved by external sphincterotomy. Contrary to expectations, by permitting complete emptying of the bladder, this may improve continence. For the remainder, diversion by conduits of ileum or colon to the anterior abdominal wall is much less favoured than in the past. Alternatives include penile appliances for males, and intermittent non-sterile self catheterisation for both sexes and indwelling catheters for girls. In children with full mobility and adequate bowel control implantable artificial sphincters are under trial.

INGUINO-SCROTAL PROBLEMS

Hernia and hydrocele

Inguinal hernias in childhood are almost always of the indirect type and due to the persistence of the processus vaginalis. Direct hernias are rare, but may be seen in association with lower abdomen muscular deficiencies. Femoral hernias are rarer still. Indirect hernias occur in 1–2% of boys and in about 1 in 500 girls; approximately 60% are right sided, 25% left sided and 15% bilateral. They are much commoner in preterm babies.

Primary hydroceles similarly are secondary to patency of the processus vaginalis. In some cases, this is obvious as the hydrocele is reducible, that is a communicating hydrocele or fluid hernia, while in others it is valvular and although there are fluctuations in size during the day, fluid cannot be returned to the abdomen. Hydroceles of the spermatic cord are also collections of fluid in persistent loculi of the processus, and communicate with the peritoneal cavity.

Diagnosis

The commonest presenting symptom is a swelling which may be confined to the inguinal region or extend down the spermatic cord into the scrotum. In the first year of life the swelling usually appears after a bout of crying or coughing and may become irreducible, even at first presentation; irreducibility or strangulation becomes less common as the child gets older. If the swelling is present at the time of examination and reduces, the diagnosis is easy; if the swelling is irreducible the differential diagnosis is between an obstructed hernia, a hydrocele, an incompletely descended testis, and inguinal adenitis or abscess. An obstructed hernia is tender, may surround the testis, and always extends up to the external inguinal ring. Inguinal lymph nodes lie lateral to the external inguinal ring and are often multiple; there may be an obvious primary septic lesion in the drainage area. A hydrocele of the spermatic cord presents as a swelling in the cord above and separate from the testis. If in doubt, it is usually safest to presume that an irreducible lump is either a strangulated hernia or a torted, undescended testis. When no swelling is present at the time of examination, careful palpation of the cord, rolling it over the pubic bone, will reveal the thickening due to the sac and the walls of the sac slipping on each other may be felt. For an experienced examiner this, together with the history is adequate for surgical intervention. Children over 4 years are able to co-operate by coughing, lying down and standing up, making the diagnosis easier.

Management

Non-communicating hydroceles are common in the first few months of life. Their fine valvular communications close spontaneously and do not require treatment. Those still present by the first birthday require exploration. Inguinal hernias do not recover spontaneously and, provided an experienced paediatric surgeon and anaesthetist are available, the only reason to delay operation in an otherwise fit baby is extreme prematurity. It is best to wait until a weight of 2000 g, or for very preterm babies gestational age of 44 weeks, is reached before surgery. The operation for inguinal hernias and hydroceles is essentially the same, involving simple division of the processus vaginalis at the internal inguinal ring; no repair is required. In the UK, bilateral explorations are usually restricted to children who have definite signs on both sides. The operation on an irreducible hernia in a baby is one of the most difficult in surgery; fortunately full strangulation of the gut with the risk of perforation is rare. The greatest risk is to the blood supply of the testis. It is usually best to sedate the child, nurse him in the head-down position and as soon as he is relaxed, either spontaneous reduction will occur or gentle to firm pressure will achieve reduction. After a successful reduction, operation should be delayed by 2–3 days to allow the oedema to subside. When reduction fails an urgent operation is required.

Undescended testis

The testis normally descends into the scrotum before the end of the eighth month of pregnancy; incomplete descent is seen at birth in only 2.7% of full-term boys, but in 21% of preterm boys. Most of these testes descend in the course of the subsequent 9 months. Spontaneous descent after the age of 1 year, when the prevalence of incomplete descent is only 0.5–0.7%, probably occurs only rarely.

The incompletely descended testis must be differentiated from the ectopic, the retractile and the absent testis. The ectopic testis lies in a position outside the normal line of descent, most commonly lateral to the external ring, the inguinal ectopic testis, and only rarely in the femoral, perineal or penile positions. A retractile testis has descended normally, but is pulled out of the scrotum by the action of the cremaster muscle. It has now been recognised that a few apparently adequately descended testes ascend in later childhood. Testes may be congenitally absent or disappear following torsion.

Diagnosis

The testis is most easily felt in the neonatal period, and most difficult to feel around the ages of 3–5 years, with palpation becoming easier again towards puberty as the organ enlarges and the cremaster relaxes. Palpation requires a warm and relaxed patient who is lying down, and a gentle examiner with warm hands. The testis should be milked down towards the scrotum by one hand, stroking along the line of the inguinal canal from the internal to the external ring, where it can be caught by the fingers of the other hand and pulled as far into the scrotum as it will come. If there is any doubt, pulling the thighs into the fully flexed, slightly abducted position, like squatting, will usually make a retractile testis descend into the scrotum.

Indications and timing for operation

Spermatogenesis will not occur normally in a testis left undescended until puberty. Changes in ultra-structure can be recognised after the first birthday, and more obvious changes on light microscopy after the fifth birthday. While early placement of the testis in the scrotum has not been definitely shown to improve fertility, it is the only hope. Most undescended testes are associated with an inguinal hernia, and have an increased risk of un-dergoing torsion, and a slight, but definitely increased risk of the later development of malig-nancy. The teasing and emotional problems of having only one testis in the scrotum provide a further powerful reason for orchidopexy.

The operation should, therefore, be performed certainly before the fifth birthday and where there are skilled paediatric services, probably shortly after the first birthday. At operation, absence will be confirmed, any hernias can be corrected and torsion prevented, but there is probably no long-term effect on the development of malignancy.

Torsion of the testis

Testicular torsion may be major or minor. In tor-sion major, the whole testis and epididymis twists on the spermatic cord, usually within the tunica vaginalis (intravaginal). This is generally secon-dary to an abnormal anatomical position of the testis, horizontal, clapperbell testis, or undes-cended. The underlying abnormality must be assumed to be bilateral. If a torsion is not cor-rected within 6 hours, some testicular damage is inevitable and this damage increases with time.

Torsion minor, which is commoner in the boy under 10 years of age than torsion major, is a torsion of the hydatid of Morgagni, a small embryological remnant on the upper pole of the testis or epididymis.

Torsion is a sudden and painful event. The pain is abdominal as well as local, and in the descended testis the swollen and tender scrotum makes the diagnosis obvious. Epididymitis, except in associa-tion with other problems, such as a chronically infected bladder associated with spina bifida, is rare in childhood and should be considered only when torsion has been excluded by operation. In torsion minor, the symptoms are less acute and the tenderness may be clearly localised over a tender dark nodule at the upper pole of the testis. Rarely, an acute hydrocele develops in children with a fine patent processus vaginalis in response to an inter-current infection and mimics an acute scrotal emergency.

Management

External reduction has been suggested but few surgeons have had real success with this and, be-sides, early fixation is required. Urgent exploration and reduction of the torsion is therefore recom-mended. An avascular testis should be excised. Both the affected and the normal testis should be fixed in the scrotum to prevent recurrence. In tor-sion minor the hydatid is excised. If the diagnosis has been delayed, it is important to remember that the symptoms will subside in about a week even without treatment.

Idiopathic scrotal oedema

This is an acute swelling of the soft tissues of the scrotum. The area is red and oedematous, the swelling extends up into the groin and may be tender, but a normal cord and non-tender testis can generally be palpated through the swelling. The whole condition usually subsides spon-taneously within 2–3 days. The cause is obscure and antibiotics and antihistamines have been used in treatment but it is doubtful whether they make much difference. An association with perianal lesions has been described.

Testicular tumours

These are rare. Teratoma, orchioblastoma or yolk sac tumour and rhabdomyosarcoma present as painless, testicular swellings. They may be confused with hydroceles. They should be excised urgently.

Circumcision

Phimosis

The foreskin is normally adherent to the glans penis at birth. Separation occurs over the first years of life and, in the majority, the skin can be pushed back freely by the age of 5 years. Provided there is an adequate external meatus no attempt to retract the foreskin should be made before then. The meatus is best assessed by observing the urinary stream or by pulling the skin forwards away from the pubis. A thin or spraying stream suggests obstruction, ballooning of the prepuce during micturition is usually normal and does not of itself indicate obstruction. Fewer than 5% of normal boys require circumcision for these reasons. Where the prepuce is still non-retractile at 5 years, freeing any residual adhesions and retraction using Emla cream for anaesthetic is simple and satisfactory.

Cicatrical phimosis is seen in older children. The prepuce is obviously scarred, the urinary stream is poor and often painful, bleeding is common and ballooning unusual. It has been assumed that this is caused by forceful retraction or an infected balanitis, but there is little evidence to support this. Histologically the lesion is balanitis xerotica obliterans.

Posthitis and balanitis

Posthitis (or inflammation of skin of the prepuce) is part of a nappy rash and is a contraindication to circumcision. Balanitis which is infection under the prepuce, occurs with a widely open prepuce as well as with stenosis and obstructed drainage. Immediate treatment includes warm bathing, local antibiotics and rarely a surgical dorsal slit of the prepuce. Circumcision is indicated after healing.

Smegma collections develop during separation of the prepuce. They appear as white swellings over the glans. Left alone they discharge spontaneously. The rare true preputial cysts are treated by circumcision.

Other indications

Circumcision is also demanded for religious, cultural, or simply social reasons. It is impossible to prevent its performance for religious and cultural reasons but it should not be recommended on a purely social basis. It is probably best delayed, if possible, until after the child is out of napkins. It should also be avoided in children with hypospadias until it is clear that the skin will not be required for repair. In Jewish children it is necessary to discuss the problems with the Mohel.

Complications of circumcision include infection, haemorrhage (haemophilia may present in this way), damage to the penis, meatal ulceration and stenosis, and recurrence. Meatal ulceration is rarely seen in a glans protected by the prepuce but commonly follows circumcision. The symptoms are pain and bleeding on micturition and sometimes acute retention of urine. The diagnosis is obvious on examination of the penis; retention is usually relieved by sitting the child in a warm bath. The ulceration should be treated by a local ointment such as a topical steroid. If healing is associated with meatal stenosis a formal meatotomy is required.

Hypospadias, epispadias, ectopia vesicae

In hypospadias the external urethral opening is on the ventral surface of the penis. It may be glandular, coronal, penile, peno-scrotal, scrotal, or perineal. In epispadias the urethral opening is on the dorsal surface of the penis. There is again a gradation of severity from splitting of the glans, a long dorsal defect of the penile shaft to total extraversion of the bladder (ectopia vesicae).

The aim of treatment is to produce a straight penis with a normal urinary stream and preferably the urethral opening at the apex of the glans. Hypospadias is the commonest of these anomalies. In the most minor degree, glandular hypospadias, there is only a cleft glans associated with a hooded prepuce not united at the fraenum. Provided the urinary stream is straight no treatment is required.

There may be a chordee, or ventral bowing of the penis, which must be corrected. The chordee correction is performed at around 18 months of age and the repair of the hypospadias at around 3–4 years of age is preferable, so that the young boy is micturating normally when he goes to school. In this group there is a slight increase in the incidence of upper urinary tract anomalies, but ultrasound of the kidneys is only indicated in the more severe forms of hypospadias. In the more severe degrees of hypospadias, particularly if the testes are undescended, it is essential to establish the sex of the infant before starting treatment as errors can be made. The hooded appearance of the prepuce in glandular hypospadias may be a cosmetic indication for circumcision.

Epispadias is a much more complex anomaly, often involving deficiencies in the bladder neck, and can occur in both sexes. Female epispadias can be recognised by the bifid clitoris and widely open urethra; it is a rare cause of urinary incontinence. In the male, the penis is short and there is reverse chordee. It is essential to check on the upper urinary tract and bladder neck by renal ultrasound and voiding cystourethrogram. Repair is best delayed until it is possible to say whether the child is continent, which is usually by 4–5 years of age. Penile lengthening may be required before the repair. If the bladder neck is deficient it will also require repair, but this is a less satisfactory procedure and continence is not always achieved.

Extraversion of the bladder (ectopia vesicae) also occurs in both sexes. The bladder is open on the anterior abdominal wall, there is a generalised deficiency of the abdominal wall often with an associated omphalocele, the symphysis pubis is widely separated, the anus is anteriorly placed and, in the male, there is epispadias. The upper urinary tract is usually normal at birth but the ureters may become obstructed as their orifices prolapse through the abdominal wall defect. When the bladder is of reasonable size an early repair of the bladder and epispadias can be attempted. Results, even in specialised units, are still disappointing. For those children where repair fails and those with bladders too small for the attempt, a urinary diversion with bladder excision is required; currently for children with good bowel control, there is renewed interest in variants of the ureterosigmoid anastomosis.

BREAST LESIONS

Breast lesions are seen in childhood and include: neonatal hypertrophy with or without secondary infection, prepubertal mastitis, precocious development, absence of one or both breasts, gynaecomastia in boys, and adolescent hypertrophy in girls.

Breast enlargement with secretion is common in the neonatal period. Left alone most cases resolve within a few weeks. Expression of milk predisposes to abscess formation. Abscesses are nearly always caused by a penicillin-resistant staphylococcus and should be treated by a systemic β-lactamase-resistant penicillin such as flucloxacillin, and by early incision if pus has formed. Extension of the abscess due to delayed treatment may destroy breast tissue and cause large skin defects.

Prepubertal mastitis is seen at around 8–12 years of age in both sexes; one or both breast discs become enlarged and painful, simultaneously or sequentially. The condition is usually self-limiting and the breast returns to its normal prepubertal size within a few weeks. Biopsy should be avoided as it is almost certain to cause permanent damage to the breast.

Precocious breast development under 8 years of age should be investigated to exclude the various causes of precocious puberty.

Male gynaecomastia is seen at puberty. It nearly always regresses spontaneously but embarrassment makes many boys request treatment. Simple bilateral mastectomy is sometimes justified.

Absent breasts require plastic surgery early in puberty as the skin must be stretched to accommodate a prosthesis.

Overgrowth of the female breast at puberty develops usually after 15 years of age but is seen earlier and can be sufficiently severe to require reduction mammoplasty.

Breast tumours are almost unknown before puberty.

DEFECTS AT THE UMBILICUS

The umbilical cord contains the umbilical vein,

two umbilical arteries and possibly vestigial remnants of the vitello-intestinal duct and the urachus. A discharge may therefore be due to infection in one of the vessels, particularly after therapeutic cannulation, or less frequently bowel content from the vitello-intestinal duct, or urine from a urachal fistula. A persistent vitello-intestinal duct must be excised at a formal laparotomy. With a urachal fistula full studies of the urinary tract, particularly to exclude outflow obstruction, are essential before surgical closure.

An umbilical polyp is most often a pyogenic granuloma; this responds to treatment with silver nitrate, simple ligation, or surgical diathermy. The rarer protrusion of a vitello-intestinal remanant of bowel mucosa (often gastric) can be recognised by its velvety appearance, surrounding excoriation, and failure to respond to simple measures. It should be excised.

Hernias at the umbilicus are very common, especially in children of African ancestry. In the true umbilical hernia there is a circular defect under the cicatrix, which varies from the just palpable to the large defects admitting several fingers. The bulge tends to alarm the child's parents but strangulation of gut is unusual and spontaneous rupture very uncommon. As the natural tendency is for the ring to close spontaneously, considerable patience in advised, even for large defects, as reduction in the size makes the operation easier. Operative repair should not usually be considered before 5 years and only very seldom under 2 years of age. The surgical technique should retain the umbilical cicatrix. A few small defects, particularly in older children, may trap omentum or peritoneal fat and cause intermittent acute central abdominal pain.

A supraumbilical hernia is really a form of epigastric hernia. The defect is immediately above the umbilical scar and is transverse. This and epigastric hernias further up the linea alba, do not have a hernial sac, may be painful from trapping of extraperitoneal fat and do not close spontaneously. Operation is therefore recommended.

THE ABDOMEN

Appendicitis

Appendicitis can occur at all ages, but is uncommon before the second birthday. While the cause remains obscure, it is obstruction of the lumen, for example secondary to a faecolith, lymphoid swelling, or previous scarring, which leads to progressive diseases, which can be dangerous because of the risk of perforation, local abscess formation, and general peritonitis. In the classical presentation, the diagnosis is easy. Abdominal pain, initially central, moves to the right side of the abdomen, the tongue is coated and the breath fetid, and there is vomiting following the onset of the pain. Pyrexia is usual, but in early cases the temperature does not often exceed 38°C except in young children in whom, early in the disease, it can be much higher. Tenderness and guarding in the right iliac fossa are the essential clinical signs in confirming the diagnosis. In children over the age of 5 years, with pelvic appendicitis without definite abdominal signs, a rectal examination will reveal the anterior tenderness. In those with definite abdominal signs, the rectal examination usually adds little to the diagnosis and, in children under the age of 5 years in whom an abscess is not suspected, often very little information is obtained. In cases of doubt, a polymorphonuclear leucocytosis is sometimes helpful confirmation of the presence of acute pyogenic infection. A plain supine abdominal X-ray may also be helpful in difficult cases, showing the evidence of oedematous bowel in the right iliac fossa, localised fluid levels, or even the presence of a calcified faecalith.

When the child is not acutely ill and the diagnosis in doubt, a period of observation of 6–12 hours is safe and helpful. Two-thirds of the children admitted to hospital for acute abdominal pain recover spontaneously without a definite diagnosis being made. For these the term acute Non-Specific Abdominal Pain (NSAP) is useful.

Helpful markers to exclude some of the differential diagnoses include:

1. Simple colic — the pain is central and of short duration and abdominal tenderness and pyrexia are absent

2. Mesenteric adenitis — this is usually associated with an upper respiratory infection or tonsillitis. The temperature is often high and the abdominal tenderness central and diffuse.

3. In viral or bacterial bowel infection there is

diarrhoea, and any tenderness is over the whole colon

4. In urinary tract infection the pain is either over the bladder or in the loins, there is dysuria, and pus cells are found in the urine on microscopy

5. In pneumonia, there should be chest signs, but if these are obscured there is still flaring of the alae nasi, often tachypnoea, the pain is usually upper abdominal and guarding is absent

6. The predominant symptom in infectious hepatitis is severe anorexia, which precedes jaundice and pain

7. Intussusception is commoner under the age of 2 years and colic is particularly severe

8. Most children who have been starving for over 12 hours have acetone in their breath. In diabetes mellitus, there should be a longer history and blood and urine sugar levels are raised.

The possibility of appendicitis coinciding with an upper respiratory tract infection or measles must always be remembered.

Management

The treatment of acute uncomplicated appendicitis is appendicectomy. Where the diagnosis is delayed and an abscess has formed, simple drainage or conservative treatment followed by appendicectomy 6–8 weeks later may be preferable.

In generalised peritonitis, rehydration with intravenous fluids and control of infection by antibiotics such as metronidazole and gentamicin, augmentin, or a second- or third-generation cephalosporin must precede surgery. Complications include local wound sepsis, intraperitoneal abscesses, and late adhesion obstruction.

Meckel's diverticulum

Meckel's diverticulum, which is a persistence of the intestinal end of the vitello-intestinal duct, arises from the antimesenteric border of the distal ileum. It is present in 2% of the population and most cause no problems. The complications, in order of frequency, are bleeding secondary to ectopic gastric mucosa, intestinal obstruction from intussusception, volvulus around, or an internal hernia behind, a persisting band, and acute inflammation.

Bleeding from a Meckel's diverticulum usually starts in the first year of life, is painless and can be severe. Confirmation of the diagnosis between episodes is difficult, but a technetium-99 pertechnetate scan will often show a hot spot over the ectopic gastric mucosa on the gamma camera image. The treatment includes blood replacement, followed by laparotomy with excision of the diverticulum including its base.

Intussusception

Intussusception is an invagination of one segment of bowel into the adjoining, usually distal, segment. In older children the process is often initiated by abnormalities such as polyps, cysts, or a Meckel's diverticulum. The more common form, which occurs in children between the ages of 3 months and 2 years, often has no obvious cause. The apex in the terminal ileum or at the ileo-caecal valve is carried round the gut by peristalsis; with very delayed diagnosis it may appear at the anus.

Clinically, the children are typically previously fit and have recently had an upper respiratory tract infection. The first symptom is violent crying caused by severe colic. This comes in waves and is followed by vomiting of stomach contents and emptying of normal stool from the bowel. In between the spasms of pain, the infant looks pale and anxious. Many babies go on to pass a stool of mixed blood and mucus, 'redcurrant jelly', or blood may be seen on the examining finger after rectal examination. This is not essential for the diagnosis. Gentle palpation of the abdomen during a quiet interval will usually reveal the mobile sausage-shaped mass lying in the line of the colon. Failure to feel this may be due to its position, as under the liver, or muscle guarding as the intussusception is tender, or abdominal distension. Delay in diagnosis leads to rapidly progressive signs of small intestinal obstruction with copious bile-stained or faecal vomiting, pyrexia and dehydration. Plain abdominal radiographs, supine and erect, are helpful; the caecal gas shadow is absent, there are dilated loops of small bowel with fluid levels, the intussusception itself may be seen, and there is evidence of peritoneal oedema in the right iliac fossa. Ultrasound examination of the abdomen has largely replaced the contrast enema for diagnosis.

An intussusception is an acute surgical emergency and the rare deaths are nearly always due to delays in diagnosis and treatment. Intravenous fluid replacement and the administration of antibiotics are often needed. Where the child is fit and the history short, generally under 24 hours, a contrast enema can also be used to achieve reduction. Surgical reduction is still frequently required. An irreducible intussusception requires resection and a primary anastomosis. Recurrence is seen in 5% of cases. The typical cry permits the diagnosis to be made early; some of these reduce spontaneously, the others should be managed as described with possibly a freer use of operation to exclude an anatomical lead point.

Chronic inflammatory bowel disease

Ulcerative colitis and Crohn's disease are rare in children. In the majority of cases the conditions are easily distinguished but in about one-fifth the signs and symptoms overlap. Crohn's disease is being seen with increasing frequency.

Ulcerative colitis

This affects the large bowel. There is mucosal inflammation and ulceration; the muscle layers are only affected when there is toxic megacolon. The disease has a long and intermittent course of remission and relapses; as in adults it is premalignant, but the time before the development of malignant change is longer than the 10 years quoted as critical in adults. The symptoms are chronic diarrhoea with blood and slime in the stools. Anaemia and failure to thrive are usual, anal fissures are common, and systemic complications, such as arthritis, iritis and liver disease are sometimes seen. The diagnosis is made from the history and confirmed by sigmoidoscopy and biopsy. Barium enema and colonoscopy show the severity and extent of the disease and are necessary in the long-term follow up to look for malignant change. The drugs of proved efficacy in treatment

are steroids to induce remission and sulphasalazine as maintenance.

The indications for surgery include: toxic megacolon as an emergency; chronic disease leading to growth failure, delayed puberty or loss of schooling; and severe local or systemic complications. The usual operation in children was a total colectomy with a terminal ileostomy and preservation of the rectum. In some cases bowel continuity can be restored later by ileo-rectal anastomosis or a mucosal core-out and endorectal pull through. A variety of small bowel pouches are being tried to reduce stool frequency.

Crohn's disease

Crohn's disease is a chronic granulomatous disease of the gut of unknown aetiology. It affects the full thickness of the intestinal wall with the ileocaecal region the commonest site, but any part of the gut can be affected, and multiple lesions are common. Perianal lesions and mouth ulcers are also common; systemic lesions do occur but with less frequency that in ulcerative colitis. Finger clubbing is seen in one-quarter of patients.

The disease runs a long and intermittent course. The initial symptoms are often those of vague ill health with failure to thrive or grow, anorexia, diarrhoea, and abdominal pain. As a result the diagnosis is usually not made until a year or more after the start of symptoms. Once it has been suspected, the diagnosis can be confirmed by barium studies and sigmoidoscopy or colonoscopy with biopsy of an accessible lesion. The typical string sign of a narrowed segment of terminal ileum can be shown by both barium meal and barium enema examinations. Earlier radiological signs are loss of the mucosal pattern and evidence of fissuring and oedema of the bowel wall. Endoscopically the lesions vary from small aphthous-like ulcers to areas of cobblestone mucosa, fissuring, and segments of narrowing. The histological features are those of granuloma formation with giant and epithelioid cells.

Neither surgery nor medical management is satisfactory as the disease recurs in 80% of patients. Drug of proven effect are steroids and sulphasalazine or mesalazine; azathioprine and metronidazole have also been used. The indications for surgical excision of the affected segment are similar to those for ulcerative colitis, but the lesions are frequently multiple and the tendency to recurrence and faecal fistulae and sinuses is high.

The use of elemental and exclusion diets have also produced remission.

A carefully timed excision of isolated ileocaecal disease can permit a normal pubertal growth spurt.

Oesophageal varices

Oesophageal varices are rare in childhood. The obstruction to portal blood flow is seen after portal vein thrombosis in the neonatal period and usually following dehydration or septicaemia, liver disease in cystic fibrosis, α-1-anti-trypsin deficiency, after operation for biliary atresia, after hepatic necrosis and in congenital hepatic fibrosis.

Haematemesis, often very severe, is the normal presenting symptom; splenomegaly is usual, the liver is often normal, but is enlarged if diseased. The diagnosis is confirmed on oesophagoscopy or by a barium swallow. The first acute bleeds usually stop spontaneously. Treatment includes passing a nasogastric tube and the use of iced-water stomach wash-outs, oral neomycin and lactulose, blood replacement, pitressin intravenously and if this fails propranolol and balloon compression with a Sengstaken tube. When these measures fail oesophageal transection is usually successful. Control of the varices should probably be attempted by injection sclerotherapy, leaving any shunt as late as possible to allow normal liver growth and avoid porto-systemic encephalopathy.

Chronic abdominal pain

Only around 5% of children with recurrent abdominal pain (Apley's little belly achers) have a detectable organic lesion. Management demands a detailed history and careful clinical examination to exclude organic disease. Parental and GP concern is usually centred around the possibility of appendicitis, which in fact is one of the least likely causes. Over investigation must be avoided as it is unproductive and promotes anxiety as it proceeds. Reasonable routine screening tests include items such as a full blood count, ESR, routine urine testing with microscopy and culture, and a plain abdominal X-ray. After organic disease has been excluded, the child and his family must be reassured and, where appropriate, acceptable alterations in diet and family organisation advised.

Hiatus hernia and gastro-oesophageal reflux

The oesophagogastric junction, the lower oesophageal sphincter and oesophageal vestibule- should all lie in the abdomen, with the lower oesophagus held to the right crus of the diaphragm by the phreno-oesophageal ligaments. Two types of hernia occur at the hiatus. With the paraoesophageal or rolling hernia, which is rare in children, the fundus of the stomach rolls into the peritoneal sac protruding through an enlarged hiatus. The common hernia is the sliding hernia in which the oesophagogastric junction is displaced into the chest. Gastro-oesophageal reflux is usually associated with a sliding hernia but can occur without any demonstrable evidence of herniation, particularly in infants. Reflux and herniation are not synonymous, but most frequently occur together.

In the infant reflux occurs easily but, presumably because of the lower acidity of the stomach contents in the first 3 months of life, it is less damaging to the oesophageal mucosa. Reflux rarely occurs during sleep. This explains the ease with which small babies can be 'burped', the frequency of posseting (regurgitation of small amounts of curdled feed), and the more persistent vomiting which usually stops spontaneously towards the end of the first year of life. Reflux is least likely to occur when the baby lies prone.

Clinical features, diagnosis and prognosis

The outstanding symptom is regurgitation and/or vomiting starting in the first week of life, occurring after and between feeds. The vomit does not contain bile but may be stained with blood. Minor degrees of reflux recover spontaneously, and in the majority of infants the vomiting resolves by 12 months of age. More severe reflux can be associated with failure to thrive, aspiration of gastric contents with chronic recurrent pulmonary infection, ulceration of the lower oesophagus leading to acute or chronic bleeding, dysphagia from spasm and finally stricture formation. It is also likely that reflux is one of the causes of excessive crying, irritability and sleep disturbance.

There is a clear association between hiatus hernia and congenital hypertrophic pyloric stenosis. Reflux is common in severely mentally retarded children in whom it must be distinguished from rumination. Occasionally reflux presents in older children with symptoms similar to those seen in adults — heartburn and dysphagia, particularly on stooping or bending.

Investigation

A barium swallow is essential to study the mechanism of swallowing, look for the presence of spasm or stricture in the lower oesophagus, and study the stomach, pylorus and duodenum. The most important features are the positions of the oesophageal vestibule and lower sphincter. Ultrasound examination, which is non-invasive, can demonstrate fluid reflux in children even when a barium study has failed to show it. Oesophagoscopy — preferably with a flexible fibre optic instrument — also allows examination of the stomach, pylorus and first part of the duodenum, differentiates stricture from spasm and demonstrates oesophagitis better than barium. A 24 hour pH study produces the most physiological assessment of what is happening in the lower oesophagus.

Management

A baby who is thriving and has no evidence of oesophagitis or recurrent chest infection needs no investigation or treatment. Investigations are reserved for those babies with severe vomiting, failure to thrive, recurrent chest infection, haematemesis, possibly severe sleep disturbance, and certainly dysphagia, suggesting early stricture formation. For those with minor symptoms, thickening the feeds and mild antacids are helpful. In babies under the age of 6 months alginate antacid (Gaviscon) should not be used, because of its high sodium content.

Posture. It has been traditional to maintain babies with symptomatic reflux in an infant hernia seat with the back angled at 60° to the horizontal. It seems reasonable for the less severe cases to recommend this sitting position at 60° from 1–1.5 hours after feeds and that the child should sleep prone at night. In the more severe cases, nursing on a special frame prone at 60° may be helpful. H_2 antagonists (cimetidine and ranitidine) reduce the gastric acid output and may speed the healing of the oesophagitis.

Surgery. This is only indicated for those infants in whom medical measures fail to control the reflux and who fail to thrive, become anaemic, or develop a stricture. The Nissen fundoplication, or Belsey Mark IV operation, are the most frequently performed procedures, In these, after mobilization to ensure an adequate length of oesophagus within the abdomen, the body of the stomach is wrapped around and sutured in front of the oesophagus. 'Dumping' has been reported following the Nissen operation, even without any procedure on the pylorus.

Peptic ulceration

Peptic ulceration, gastric and duodenal, is seen only rarely in childhood. There are usually diagnostic pointers in the history: a positive family history, loss of appetite, epigastric pain, relief of pain with vomiting and alkali, waking at night, and association with school or family stress. A barium swallow and meal is probably still indicated as the first investigation, but the diagnosis must be confirmed by endoscopy.

If an ulcer is found, the treatment is similar to that for adults, including drugs such as cimetidine or ranitidine.

Gastrointestinal bleeding

Bleeding from the upper gastrointestinal tract can present as the vomiting of fresh or altered blood (coffee grounds). More rarely the blood is only recognised in the stool, usually as melaena, but in babies and younger children it can appear as fresh blood; the type of the bleeding, varying from fresh red to melaena, usually indicates the proximity of the source to the anus, but the speed of intestinal transit may make this misleading. It is frequently impossible to determine the cause of minor bleeding from the anus. Minor rectal bleeding is of minimal significance and the first need is to identify those cases requiring fuller investigation. Severe bleeding, as shown by finding a sizeable quantity of blood or clot in the stool or a fall in the haemoglobin level, recurrent bleeding, and bleeding associated with colic or vomiting should be investigated.

The bleeding and clotting times must, of course, be checked to exclude a haemorrhagic tendency. In the newborn, swallowed maternal blood is a common cause of melaena. Swallowed blood from lesions of the nose or throat should be considered at all ages and the presence of blood in the stool confirmed by routine chemical testing (Tables 26.1, 26.2).

Constipation

In children, constipation is a source of complaint for the parents rather than the child. Investigation is required when there is a general upset with loss of appetite, severe straining at stool with bleeding, and faecal soiling. The problem, often starting around the time of toilet training, is variously described as holding back, idiopathic megarectum, obstipation, and it responds well to encouragement and an adequate aperient regimen. A rectal examination is essential to exclude anal stenosis and other obstructive lesions and to confirm that the anal canal is dilated and loaded down to the anal verge. The anal reflex should also be tested to exclude a neuropathic rectum, although this in isolation from bladder problems is improbable. Wash-outs and enemas should be required only rarely. Those children with a history starting in the neonatal period, who fail to thrive, or do not respond to the aperient regimen require investigation to exclude Hirschsprung's disease and anal achalasia. A barium enema is helpful in Hirschsprung's disease, but when the aganglionic segment and is shorter than about 3–4 cm it is not diagnostic. Suction rectal biopsies taken at 3, 4 and 5 cm from the anal verge will establish or exclude the diagnosis of Hirschsprung's disease.

Anorectal manometry is essential for the diagnosis of anal achalasia in which there is a failure of relaxation of the internal sphincter which is also seen in Hirschsprung's disease, but no histological abnormality. This and many of the other less clearly established abnormalities respond well initially to an anal sphincter stretch under anaesthesia, combined with encouragement and aperients. Relapse is probably best treated by a formal internal sphincterotomy.

Hirschsprung's disease in the older child

While most children with Hirschsprung's disease are diagnosed in the neonatal period, a few with less severe symptoms present later and even in adult life. Constipation starting from birth is very suggestive, but attacks of enterocolitis may cause confusion with intermittent diarrhoea. Failure to thrive is usual but not invariable. With short and

Table 26.1 Gastrointestinal bleeding: haematemesis

Age	Bleed	Cause	Vomit	Investigation
Infant	Minor	Pyloric stenosis	Coffee grounds	Test feed
				Barium meal, ultrasound
		Reflux oesophagitis		Barium swallow, pH study
	Severe	'Stress' peptic ulcer	Fresh blood	Barium meal
Older	Minor	Hiatus hernia with	Coffee grounds	Barium swallow and endoscopy
		Reflux oesophagitis		
	Severe	Acute gastric erosions		Barium meal and endoscopy
		Peptic ulcer		Barium meal and endoscopy
		Mallory–Weiss syndrome*		Endoscopy
		Oesophageal varices		Barium swallow and endoscopy

*The Mallory–Weiss ulcer is a longitudinal split in the oesophageal mucosa caused by severe vomiting

Table 26.2 Gastrointestinal bleeding: rectal bleeding

Age	Bleed	General condition	Cause	Stool	Investigation
Neonate	Minor	Well	Anal fissure	Blood steaked	Local examination
		Well	Haemorrhagic disease of the newborn	Fresh blood	Prothrombin time
			Mucosal erosions	Blood streaked	None
	Major	Ill	Necrotising enterocolitis	Blood and stool mixed	Plain X-ray
		Ill	Volvulus	Fresh blood	Plain X-ray Barium meal Laparotomy
Toddler	Minor	Well	Fissure-in-ano	Blood streaked	Local examination
	Mixed	Ill	Intussusception	Fresh blood and mucus	Clinical examination Barium enema, ultrasound
	Major	Usually well	Meckel's diverticulum	Fresh blood or melaena	Technetium scan
Older	Minor	Well	Fissure-in-ano Polyps Infective diarrhoea	Blood streaked Fresh blood Blood and pus Blood and mucus	Local examination Sigmoidoscopy Stool culture
	Mixed		Ulcerative colitis	Blood and mucus	Barium enema Colonoscopy
			Peptic ulcer	Melaena	Barium meal Endoscopy
	Major		Oesophageal varices	Mixed blood and melaena	Barium meal Oesophagoscopy

long-segment colonic disease the clinical signs are chronic large bowel distension with an empty lower rectum. With short-segment disease the faecal mass is forced distally into the aganglionic segment and may reach the anal verge with consequent soiling and present a picture very similar to simple rectal inertia.

A rectal biopsy is required for diagnosis. Where the aganglionic segment is less than 5 cm long, an extended internal sphincterotomy may be adequate. For most a formal pull-through operation is required.

Minor anorectal problems

Anal fissure

Anal fissures are a common cause of rectal bleeding and pain on defaecation. The blood streaks the stool and the toilet paper. Pain on defaecation is usual but not always present. In the infant, fissures may be multiple and part of a napkin rash.

In the older child, the fissure follows tearing of the anal canal from passage of a hard stool.

The diagnosis is made by examination of the anal canal with gentle eversion of the anal verge. Rectal examination should not be attempted while the pain is acute. Very often there is a skin tag or sental pile, making the outer end of the fissure. Treatment involves keeping the bowel motions soft by aperients. Local anaesthetic ointments are helpful only for older children who can apply them personally before a bowel action. Those few fissures which do not respond to simple measures will heal after a sphincter stretch under anaesthesia. If this is necessary, it is wise to perform a biopsy to exclude chronic inflammatory bowel disease.

Child abuse

Fissure-in-ano, dilated perianal veins and constipation may be due to child abuse. Reflex anal dilatation, the spontaneous opening of the anal canal in response to parting of the buttocks in the absence of severe constipation, is a suspicious but not pathognonomic sign.

Perianal abscess and fistula-in-ano. Perianal abscesses follow infection of a perianal haematoma or an anal gland and present as painful fluctuant swellings at the anal verge. The treatment is to incise and lay open the abscess under general anaesthesia. Abscesses arising in anal glands tend to recur as the gland opens into the anal canal and a fistula forms. This will only heal after laying the whole track open.

A chronic fistula must always be biopsied as it may also be secondary to chronic inflammatory bowel disease.

Ischio-rectal abscesses. These arise from infection deep in the space lateral to the rectum but are rare in children. They present with pyrexia and a painful, tender mass lateral to the anus, and require antibiotic treatment and early incision to prevent formation of a high anorectal fistula.

Rectal prolapse

Rectal prolapse is common in children. It occurs after straining at stool or with acute or chronic diarrhoea. The causes of chronic diarrhoea, especially cystic fibrosis, must be excluded. Most prolapses are of mucosa only and will recover spontaneously. Prolapse of the full thickness of the rectal wall is rarer but occurs particularly in patients with paralysis of the pelvic floor muscles. Simple management includes a mild aperient to keep the stool soft, abandoning potty training, and strapping the buttocks together. Where this is ineffective a submucous injection of phenol in almond oil will usually suffice, reserving circumferential perianal suture for those few resistant to all other measures.

THE HEAD AND NECK

Congenital defects arise from failures of fusion, inclusion of dermal elements at fusion lines, and persistence of remnants of structures from embryological development.

Pierre Robin syndrome

A small lower jaw (micrognathia), often associated with a median cleft palate, allows the tongue to prolapse into the nasopharynx obstructing the airway.

If the child is tube-fed nursed fully prone, an adequate airway can be maintained. The growth of the lower jaw usually compensates and after a few months it is found that the airway can be maintained.

Choanal atresia

Babies are obligate nose breathers and obstruction at the back of the nasal airway causes severe distress. Unilateral obstructions are often discovered accidentally or later, but bilateral obstructions cause severe cyanosis, and respiratory distress relieved on crying. An oropharyngeal airway strapped into position will maintain the airway for the few hours necessary for transfer for surgery. The obstruction is excised and the nasal airway kept open by leaving plastic tubes in situ.

Cleft lip (hare lip)

Cleft lip and palate result from failure of fusion of fusion of the embryological facial processes. The incidence is about 1 per 600 live births. Embryologically and functionally clefts are now divided into defects anterior and posterior to the incisive foramen behind the incisor teeth in the hard palate. Anterior clefts are inherited separately from isolated clefts of the hard and soft palate.

In anterior defects the problem is essentially cosmetic, while in posterior defects failure of closure of the oropharynx from the nasopharynx prevents normal sucking and swallowing, and speech. Babies with combined defects have both problems. The aims of treatment are that the child should look well, feed well, and speak well. All plans for treatment are compromises in an attempt to achieve these.

Appearance

Repair of the lip is usually delayed until around 3 months of age as it is technically easier at this age and size, but it can be done in the neonatal period. Until the lip has been repaired reassurance for the parents (photographs of previous repairs are very helpful here) is important. It is relatively easy to get a good cosmetic repair of a unilateral lip defect but in bilateral clefts secondary operations are often required. Correction of the nose is more difficult and this may also require secondary operation.

Feeding

Feeding should not be a problem with lip and alveolar defects as the gums can achieve a seal on the nipple or teat adequate for sucking. With palatal defects sucking is not possible. A few babies will require tube feeding initially, but most can be taught to feed from a spoon tipping the milk well back over the tongue. Various modified teats for bottles and palatal obturators have also been recommended and for those determined to breast feed the milk can be expressed either onto a spoon or directly into the baby's mouth.

Speech

Palatal repair, which is essential for normal speech, is usually undertaken around 12–15 months of age. The earlier the successful repair the sooner feeding and speech problems can be overcome, extensive early dissection increases the risk, however, of intereference with the growth of the maxilla.

Throughout management it is essential to control the upper alveolar (gum) arch by orthodontic appliances to improve its position before, and prevent collapse after operation. Speech is not often a problem after a satisfactory palatal closure and minor defects can be improved by speech therapy, but continued failure of closure of the oropharyngeal isthmus or persistent fistulae in the hard palate require later correction by closure of the fistulae and a pharyngoplasty when growth is nearer completion. Abnormalities at the inner end of the Eustachian tube, often aggravated by surgery, increase the risks of middle ear infection and any subsequent deafness will lead to further speech problems. Careful otological supervision and hearing tests are therefore essential.

Other facial clefts

Midline clefts of the upper lip are rare, technically easy to repair and important chiefly for their as-
sociation with other midline defects such as single nostril, absence of posterior pituitary gland, absent corpus callosum and cerebral cortical defects. Lateral clefts of the face are also rare.

Inclusion dermoids

Inclusion dermoids are epithelial-lined cysts occurring at fusion lines. The commonest, the external angular dermoid, lies deep to the lateral end of the eyebrow and above the outer canthus of the eye. It is oval and set in a depression in the bone and rarely may communicate through a defect in the skull with an intracranial extension. Skin and muscle are freely mobile over the cyst which is also mobile over the bone. The common sites for inclusion dermoids are given below:

Orbit — external and internal angular.
Ear — posterior to pinna.
Nasal — extends deep into the nasal cavity.
Scalp — over anterior and posterior fontanelles.

All should be excised at a convenient time, say between 3 months and a year of age, as they may increase in size and become infected.

Pre-auricular sinuses

These are common. The opening is a small pit on the front of the helix of the ear. The deep part ramifies unpredictably in front of the ear. Uninfected sinuses are of no significance. Infection often presents as an abscess over the parotid and will not heal until the sinus has been excised completely.

Thyroglossal cysts and ectopic thyroid

The thyroid gland develops from a downgrowth arising at the site of the foramen caecum on the tongue. Normally, no remnants are left in the line of descent, but any which do persist may develop into cysts at any point along the track. These cysts are tethered to the hyoid bone and therefore move up on protrusion of the tongue as well as on swallowing. A thyroglossal sinus develops from spontaneous rupture or surgical incision of an infected cyst, or after incomplete surgical removal.

Ectopic thyroid tissue can be seen at the base of

the tongue or mimicking a cyst in the neck. This is solid, will take up radio-iodine on isotope scanning, and will usually regress on thyroxine therapy. The mass at the back of the tongue should only be excised if the swelling persists after treatment. Ectopic thyroid in the neck should not be excised as it may be the only thyroid tissue present. Many of these children with only ectopic thyroid tissue are bordering on hypothyroidism.

Branchial fistula and cyst

The site of the second branchial cleft is represented in the tonsillar fossa. This cleft may persist throughout its length leaving a fistula from the lower anterior border of the sternomastoid muscle to the tonsil.

These fistulae leak saliva, frequently become infected and should be excised. Partial persistence of the track produces a cyst in the anterior triangle of the neck, which can usually only be distinguished from an enlarged lymph node at operation.

Enlarged cervical lymph nodes

Enlargement of the cervical lymph nodes is seen in acute infection, chronic infection and in the rare conditions of leukaemia and Hodgkin's disease. Transient swelling of the nodes is seen with oropharyngeal infections. Pyogenic infection, most commonly staphylococcal, is very common, particularly in the upper deep cervical group including the tonsillar node. The progression to abscess formation is common and very often no obvious focus is found. The infection presents as a red tender swelling below the angle of the mandible in the upper neck. In the most severe cases, there is general malaise with fever and trismus which makes swallowing difficult. An antistaphylococcal antibiotic, such flucloxacillin, is indicated. In less severe situations the value of antibiotic therapy is doubtful and very often it aborts the infection, only for it to flare up again on stopping treatment. When pus is present, surgical drainage is essential. The differentiation of chronic infection such as mycobacterial or fungal infection from neoplasia is best achieved by biopsy. In general, a lymph node which has been persistently enlarged and is not definitely showing signs of regression over a period of 3 months should be excised for biopsy.

Swellings of the salivary glands

Parotid

The commonest cause of parotid swelling is epidemic parotitis (mumps). This should only cause confusion when the swelling is unilateral. Acute pyogenic parotitis is very rare outside infancy. Recurrent subacute parotitis may be associated with stenosis of the duct orifice or dilatation of the duct radicles (sialectasis). Management is difficult as frequently no pathogenic organism can be cultured from the saliva. Despite this, ampicillin is usually given and most cases repond rapidly. Recurrence is common, but the condition eventually burns itself out over a period of years.

Submandibular glands

These are similarly affected by recurrent infection but stone formation in the duct is also seen. This is most easily diagnosed by palpation along the duct in the floor of the mouth. Stones should be removed. Unlike the parotid, the submandibular gland can easily be excised if recurrent infection and swelling become troublesome.

27. Miscellaneous problems

J. Mackinnon

JOINT DISORDERS

Children with joint symptoms can sometimes present a difficult diagnostic problem. A careful history and thorough physical examination are, as usual, the cornerstone of diagnosis. The history should reveal the type and pattern of onset of symptoms and the examination should determine exactly which structures are involved (joints, tendons, bursae, pericardium, blood vessels, heart valves, eyes, skin). The age and sex of the patient and the pattern of joint and extra-articular involvement will help to classify the various juvenile chronic arthritides. Symptoms which must be taken seriously include limp, pain on movement or 'loss of function' of any limb or joint and unilateral symptoms. A joint which is hot, swollen or tender might be infected. It is also important to recognise simple postviral arthropathy and not to label it as a chronic arthritis.

Laboratory investigations, such as the erythrocyte sedimentation rate (ESR), should identify those conditions which are inflammatory and simple radiology can usually separate those conditions due to abnormalities of articular cartilage or the bony epiphyses.

The commoner causes of arthritis in childhood are listed in Table 27.1.

Growing pains

A common symptom in children is a diffuse, vague, recurrent, poorly localised ache in the legs, usually worse at night. There is loss of function and in some instances the symptoms suggest attention seeking. In children with very mobile joints, strenuous exercise may produce these vague symptoms. There are no abnormal physical signs and laboratory tests are normal. Simple reassurance is all that is required.

Table 27.1 Causes of arthritis in childhood

Trauma	
Infection	Haemophilus, staphylococcus, tuberculosis, viruses
Post-infective	Dysentery, rheumatic fever
Allergic	Henoch–Schönlein purpura, food and drug allergy
Connective tissue	Juvenile chronic arthritis (see Table 27.2)
Blood disorders	Leukaemia, haemophilia, sickle cell anaemia
Malignancy	Neuroblastoma

Traumatic and orthopaedic conditions

Hip pain due to Perthes disease or slipped epiphysis can be diagnosed radiologically. Inflammation of the tibial tubercle (Osgood–Schlatter's disease) causes local tenderness, sometimes with a knee effusion. Overuse of a joint which has an underlying abnormality (e.g. chondromalacia patellae or osteochondritis dissecans) may provoke pain or effusion which is recurrent or slow to resolve. Laboratory tests to exclude active inflammation are normal.

Septic arthritis

Infection of the joint tissues may occur from either haematogenous spread or from a direct penetrating wound. The joint is hot, swollen and tender and the child toxic and febrile. A similar picture may occur with osteomyelitis in which a sterile sympathetic effusion into a nearby joint can occur. Maximal clinical tenderness over bone outside the joint margins will differentiate this from a septic arthritis. If bone or joint infection is suspected, aspiration of joint fluid for Gram staining and culture is essential. Blood cultures should also be taken. X-ray changes of bone infection are usually absent in the early stages of the disease; bone scanning is more reliable. Delay in diagnosis of joint or bone infection may lead to irreparable tissue damage.

The usual causal organisms are *Staphylococcus aureus*, *Haemophilus influenzae*, streptococci or pseudomonas. The possibility of gonococcal arthritis in adolescents and the predilection of salmonella, *Streptococcus pneumoniae* and haemophilus for the bones and joints of children with sickle cell anaemia should be remembered. Antibiotic therapy should be given intravenously for a minimum of 2 weeks and then continued orally until all evidence of joint infection has disappeared and the ESR is normal. Open drainage or repeated aspiration of pus from the infected joint may be necessary. Splinting of joints in the position of neutral function may make the patient more comfortable.

Viral diseases

Joint symptoms occur late in viral diseases such as mumps, rubella or glandular fever. An appropriate history of contact, characteristic physical signs and a rising antibody titre or positive Monospot test will help make the diagnosis. Arthritis may occur after rubella immunisation. Swollen joints may precede the onset of anorexia, liver tenderness and jaundice in infectious hepatitis. Simple analgesia is all that is required as treatment for these self-limiting arthropathies.

Post-infective arthritis

Rheumatic fever (arthritis, carditis, erythema marginatum, chorea and rheumatic nodules) may occur 10–14 days after an infection with a β-haemolytic streptococcus. Joint symptoms which accompany a sore throat are, however, unlikely to be due to rheumatic fever. Enteritis due to salmonella or shigella may be followed by a reactive arthritis (sterile synovitis) which is self limiting.

Allergic arthritis

The purpuric rash of Henoch–Schönlein purpura with its characteristic extensor distribution is the commonest vasculitis of childhood. The associated migratory arthropathy affecting large joints lasts a few days, although in a few cases may be more prolonged. There is usually associated abdominal pain with or without blood in the stools, haematuria, and patches of urticaria affecting the hands, feet and forehead. Food or drug allergy or urticaria from any cause may also produce a transient synovitis.

Connective tissue disease

There are several subgroups of juvenile chronic arthritis, distinguished by age of onset, sex, the pattern of joint involvement and extra-articular manifestations, and certain laboratory tests as shown in Table 27.2.

Management of chronic arthritis

1. Suppression of disease activity. Non-steroidal anti-inflammatory drugs have largely superceded the use of aspirin, particularly since the association between aspirin and Reye's syndrome has been apparent. It is still, however, appropriate to use aspirin in orthopaedics in children, 80–90 mg/kg/day. Naproxen 10 mg/kg/day is a useful non-steroidal anti-inflammatory drug. With severe systemic involvement steroids may be necessary.

2. Physiotherapy aimed at maintenance of joint mobility, strengthening weakened muscles and prevention of contractures is an important part of management. The use of a tricycle encourages exercise and mobility without full weight bearing. Hydrotherapy will ease muscle spasm and make movement of stiff joints easier. Night splinting of joints in the neutral position may help prevent deformity.

3. Slit lamp examination to detect early iridocyclitis is vital, particularly in antinuclear an-

Table 27.2 Juvenile chronic arthritis

	Girls: boys	Age of onset	Joints affected	Other manifestations	Antinuclear antibodies	Rheumatoid factor	Differential diagnosis	Complications	
								Severe arthritis	Iridocyclitis
Chronic arthritis of childhood									
Systemic onset (Still's disease)	4:5	Any	Any	High remitting fever, pink maculopapular rash, splenomegaly, lymphadenopathy, pericarditis	Negative	Negative	Glandular fever, leukaemia, neuroblastoma, rheumatic fever	25%	None
Polyarticular	8:1	Any	Any	Low grade fever, mild anaemia, growth retardation	25%	Negative	Gut arthropathy, psoriasis	15%	Rare
Pauciarticular (Type 1)	4:1	Early childhood	1–4 large (hips and sacroiliacs spared)	Few	50%	Negative	Single joint infection, TB	Rare	50%
Juvenile rheumatoid arthritis (IgM rheumatoid factor positive)	6:1	Late childhood	Any but particularly small joints of hands and feet	Low grade fever, anaemia, subcutaneous nodules, vasculitis, erosions on X-ray	75%	100%	Resembles adult rheumatoid	50%	Scleritis
Juvenile ankylosing spondylitis (Pauciarticular type 2)	1:10	Late childhood	Few large (hips and sacroiliac involvement common)	HLA B27 positive (75%)	Negative	Negative		Some have ankylosing spondylitis on follow up	5–10%

tibody-positive patients. This should be done every 6 months. Treatment with local steroid drops is usually adequate, but alternate day systemic steroids may be required to suppress a more active uveitis.

4. Education of the child can usually continue in his normal school, although in some of the more severe cases a sympathetic flexible attitude is required to make life easier for a child who may not be as mobile as his peers. Education of the family about the nature and prognosis of the disease and proper support in more severe cases is another important part of treatment of the child and his family. With early diagnosis and appropriate treatment approximately 80% of children with chronic arthritis may enter adult life with little or no disability.

ORTHOPAEDICS

Borderline orthopaedic abnormalities

There are several variations of normal lower limb postures which cause anxiety to parents. These are usually related to the position into which the baby was folded in utero. Treatment for these conditions used to be prescribed before it was recognised that a very high spontaneous rate of resolution towards more normal or acceptable posture took place.

Intoeing

Three common causes of intoeing occur:

1. In the foot itself, metatarsus varus.
2. In the lower leg, medial tibial torsion associated with lateral bowing of the tibia.
3. In the femur, persistent femoral anteversion.

1. Metatarsus varus. Metatarsus varus is an adduction deformity of the forefoot. The heel is always in the normal neutral position and the forefoot, which is frequently highly mobile, can be passively abducted. No treatment is needed.

This condition is sometimes mistaken for a true club foot or talipes equinovarus. In true talipes the heel is high, the Achilles tendon short and the heel in varus deformity. It is usually difficult or frankly impossible to passively correct the abnormal pos-

ition of the foot and all cases of obvious or suspected talipes should be referred to an orthopaedic specialist for appropriate treatment.

2. Tibial torsion. The foot is normal but rotated medially in relation to the knee, so that when the patellae are pointing directly forwards, the feet are turned in and when the feet are parallel and pointing forwards the patallae point outwards, like a divergent patellar squint! This condition is commonly associated with lateral bowing of the tibiae and normally corrects by the age of 4 or 5. Forward bowing of the tibia is pathological.

3. Persistent femoral anteversion. In this condition the femoral neck remains markedly anteverted in relation to the shaft, with the result that the range of internal rotation of the hip is much greater than the more restricted external rotation. The feet and knees are normally aligned, but the child is most comfortable with the hips internally rotated which makes the patellae converge and the feet take up an intoeing position. This position usually corrects by the age of 8. If a particularly ugly posture is still present as a result of failure of spontaneous correction, then a femoral derotation osteotomy may improve the situation, but in very few cases is this justified.

Out-toe gait

This is the opposite of intoeing and is due to persistent femoral retroversion. External rotation at the hip is easy and there is little internal rotation.

Knock knees

Provided they are not associated with any other abnormality such as rickets, they will correct spontaneously.

Flat feet

Most children when they first walk have flat feet, but as the medial arch develops this gradually disappears. Providing the feet are pain free, mobile, and the medial arch can be restored by dorsiflexion of the big toe or standing on tiptoe, the condition is benign.

Painful stiff feet are pathological. They may be

due to juvenile arthritis or infection of the subtalar joint. Feet of unequal size may suggest an occult spinal dysraphism.

Hip disorders

Each age group has its own likely hip disorder (Table 27.3).

Congenital dislocation of the hip (CDH)

This is due to an abnormal development of the acetabulum, femoral head, capsule or other soft tissue; the head of the femur may become partially or completely dislocated. Failure to diagnose and treat this condition early may lead to permanent abnormalities of the hip joint. Every newborn should be examined carefully for signs of unstable hips which include the limitation of abduction of flexed hip, and the ability to dislocate the femoral head over the posterior rim of the acetabulum by pressing downwards and backwards with the thumb, or relocate the femoral head back into the acetabulum by applying pressure forwards with fingers on the greater trochanter (see Fig. 10.1).

Asymmetry of the creases on the thigh or unequal leg lengths may also lead one to suspect the diagnosis. A single examination at birth is not sufficient, the hips should be flexed and abducted at screening examinations as limitation of abduction may appear after 4 or 5 months of age.

If a child has one or more of the following features which are known to be associated with an increased incidence of CDH, or if he presents signs or symptoms referable to the hip or leg, he should be carefully examined:

1. Family history of CDH.
2. Female sex.
3. First born child.
4. History of oligohydramnios in pregnancy.
5 Breech delivery.
6 Presence of talipes.

Table 27.3 Hip disorders of various age groups

Age (years)	Disorder
0–5	Congenital dislocation
5–10	Perthes disease
10–15	Slipped epiphysis

Hips which are dislocatable clunk rather than click. A hip which is completely stable in a dislocated position may not clunk at all and may only be detected clinically by asymmetry of the legs or a high index of suspicion, thus leading to appropriate radiological investigation. The use of ultrasound examination of the hips is particularly helpful if there is clinical uncertainty about their normality. Despite careful screening some children with CDH present late. They may present because they walk late with a limp, or asymmetry of the legs, sometimes the CDH is detected on an X-ray taken for other reasons.

Treatment consists of some form of abduction splintage which will usually stabilise the hip. Persistent instability may need an open reduction and the likelihood of this being necessary increases with delayed diagnosis.

Other hip disorders

As mentioned above, Perthes disease and slipped epiphysis usually occur in late childhood or early adolescence; trauma and infection may occur at any age. These conditions may present with symptoms of synovitis: limp, pain in the hip and pain referred to the knee (Fig. 27.1).

Constitutional symptoms and signs of infection, together with pain, muscle spasm and swelling of the hip joint require aspiration of the joint for a proper bacteriological diagnosis. This is most important as failure to diagnose an infective arthritis early can lead to irremedial damage.

Perthes disease. Perthes disease is due to aseptic necrosis of the femoral head epiphysis which presents with signs of synovitis. There are three stages of the condition, each of which lasts for about 9 months.

1. Aseptic necrosis. Initially there are no radiological changes but after a few weeks the epiphysis becomes more dense.

2. Revascularisation. The radiological changes becomes more mottled.

3. Reossification. The femoral head is gradually reformed. Avoidance of weight bearing prevents flattening of the femoral head (like a mushroom). If this flattening is masked the incongruity between the femoral head and the acetabulum may

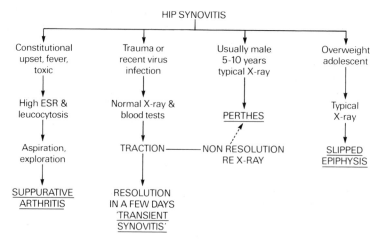

Fig. 27.1 Investigation of a painful hip.

lead to osteoarthritic changes in the joint in later life.

Slipped epiphysis. This condition affects the adolescent and radiographical appearances of the hip usually shows a postero-inferior slip of the femoral epiphysis which is best seen in the lateral projection. Immobilisation may be sufficient to arrest the process, but some form of internal fixation is usually required.

DENTAL EDUCATION AND THE PAEDIATRICIAN

Eruption

The first tooth normally erupts into the mouth at around 6 months of age and the full complement of 20 deciduous teeth is acquired by 5 years. Natal teeth, present at birth, need to be removed if they are loose and in danger of being dislodged and inhaled, if they ulcerate the tongue or if they cause discomfort to the mother during breast feeding.

Teething is the facile excuse given for many symptoms occurring between 6 months and 3 years. Increased salivation and some discomfort in the mouth are understandable; fits, unexplained fever or diarrhoea and vomiting ascribed to teething are not. It is an easy and dangerous excuse for the unwary.

The permanent dentition begins to erupt between 5 and 6 years. The full number of 28 permanent teeth have normally appeared by 13–15 years but the four wisdom teeth erupt later, usually by 25 years, making a full total of 32 teeth.

Caries

Dental caries involves the progressive destruction of the calcified dental tissues. Complete destruction of teeth affected by caries can occur if left untreated. By 2 years of age the average child has two carious lesions. In England and Wales, approximately one-third of adults over the age of 16 have no natural teeth at all, largely because of carious destruction. The deposition of salivary polysaccharides matted together with bacteria produces a layer of dental plaque on the teeth. A diet rich in sugary foods and sweets provides the substrate on which the bacteria feed and produce acids in the mouth, which decalcify the enamel and gradually destroy the organic matrix of the tooth.

Prevention

Studies done in the 1940s have shown that if drinking water contains one part per million of fluoride, the prevalence of dental caries is more than halved. This was initially shown by epidemiological surveys in areas with and without natural fluoridation and was confirmed when deficient areas had fluoride added to the water supply. In those areas of the country where the water is not fluoridated, the daily consumption of half a fluoride tablet (each tablet contains 2.2 mg sodium fluoride) between the ages of 6 months and 2 years and one tablet daily until 12 years, will have a significant effect in preventing dental caries. Compliance with this is not usually very good. Fluoridation of the water supply would be preferable; at present, only 10% of the population of the UK drink water containing one part per million of fluoride. Excess fluoride intake can cause mottling of the teeth. The area dental officer will have information about fluoride levels in the local water supply.

Dental care

Fluoride tablets should be allowed to dissolve in the mouth for their topical effect on the teeth. Proper tooth brushing to remove dental plaque should be taught from an early age and a parent should assist in cleaning the teeth until the child is competent to do it by himself. The use of a fluoride-containing toothpaste after the age of 4 years is recommended. Children younger than this tend to swallow the toothpaste which contains appreciable amounts of fluoride.

The consumption of highly refined carbohydrate between meals is cariogenic and should be discouraged, but since these snacks are almost part of the daily pattern of eating in children, substitution of low-sucrose foods such as fresh fruit, cheese, nuts or vegetables should be attempted. It is better, if sweets are allowed, to concentrate their consumption to one particular part of the week when the craving can be satisfied ad libitum.

The practice of giving bottles or dummies containing sweetened liquids as a pacifier is to be deplored. This may produce rampant decay of the upper teeth. (The lower ones are usually protected by the tongue.)

Regular visits by children to the dentist should be encouraged, if only to watch other members of the family having treatment. The establishment of a good relationship with a sympathetic dentist may be very useful for dental education and save a lot of time and discomfort later in life.

COMMON SKIN PROBLEMS

Napkin rash

This may be caused by:

1. Seborrhoeic dermatitis.
2. Chemical irritation (napkin dermatitis).
3. Candidiasis.
4. Eczema (atopic dermatitis).
5. Napkin psoriasis.
6. Intertrigo.

1. Seborrhoeic dermatitis. A transient non-itchy condition seen in babies under 3 months old. It is characterised by greasy scaling affecting the scalp (cradle cap), axillae, flexures, eyebrows, backs of ears, trunk and shoulders as well as the napkin area. It will usually disappear spontaneously, but troublesome cases do respond to 1% hydrocortisone cream or ointment.

2. Napkin dermatitis (ammoniacal dermatitis). This occurs when wet soiled napkins are left unchanged for long periods; it may imply some degree of neglect. Ammonia produced by interaction of stool bacteria and urine irritates the skin. The rash affects only skin in the napkin area; it does not affect the skin flexures such as the groin, and it may lead to severe umbilicate pustules or ulcers. Treatment consists of changing napkins frequently, or if possible not using napkins at all for a day or two and exposing the affected area. Napkins should be rinsed carefully in water containing a small amount of vinegar. Zinc and castor oil cream will usually clear up the dermatitis. If there is associated fungal infection this should also be treated.

3. Candidiasis, superimposed on napkin dermatitis is common, particularly if the baby has oral thrush. Initially the perianal skin becomes macerated, then an erythematous sharply defined area involving the genitalia develops. Satellite lesions around the main eruption are typical of candidiasis. Topical application of nystatin, clotrimazole or miconazole, together with oral administration of nystatin suspension to clear up the gastrointestinal candidiasis, is usually effective. Proprietary formulations containing nystatin, hydrocortisone and clioquinol are useful when treating infected napkin or seborrhoeic dermatitis.

4. Eczema is uncommon in babies younger than 3 months. It is usually associated with a family history of atopic conditions. The rash is invariably itchy and there are usually widespread lesions involving the face and flexures in the elbows and behind the knees. Topical corticosteroids, antihistamines for the itching, emulsifying ointment used in the bath instead of soap and avoidance of conditions which will tend to make the child sweat should all be prescribed (see Ch. 15).

5. Napkin psoriasis resembles true psoriasis with well-defined, slightly raised erythematous scaly plaques in the napkin area, which may spread up the trunk. The flexures are usually involved. The condition usually responds to a weak topical steroid, only some of the affected babies will have psoriasis later in childhood.

6. Intertrigo results from constant rubbing together of opposed skin surfaces. This is particularly common in fat babies and easily treated by frequent washing and a sprinkling of dusting powder onto the affected areas to reduce friction. Plastic pants, which encourage sweating, should be avoided.

In all these conditions, if topical steroids are used, 1% hydrocortisone is always sufficient. Fluorinated steroids should *never* be used.

Impetigo

Impetigo is a skin infection caused by a β-haemolytic group A streptococcus or *Staphylococcus aureus*. The portal of entry is usually a crack in the skin and lesions are common around the nostrils and angles of the mouth, or on eczematous skin. Picking and scratching results in further spread of the lesions. The infection starts as small vesicles which rapidly burst, exude and then become covered with characteristic golden 'stuck-on' crusts. Treatment of a small area of localised impetigo can be satisfactorily accomplished with 3% chlortetracycline ointment.

The crusts should be removed twice daily by gentle soaking and friction with a mild antiseptic and cotton wool, followed by application of the antibiotic ointment. In more extensive infection local treatment is not usually sufficient and systemic antibiotics are necessary; erythromycin will normally be adequate. If the patient is a nasal staphylococcus carrier, chlorhexidine and neomycin cream (Naseptin) can be applied nightly. The patient should use his own towel, keep his nails short and refrain from picking or scratching the lesions.

Predisposing factors such as lice and scabies should be sought and treated. Cross-infection in schools is particularly common. Nephritis can occasionally occur following impetigo caused by a nephritogenic strain of streptococcus.

Scabies

Scabies is due to infestation with a burrowing mite, *Sarcoptes scabiei*. The female digs into the superficial layers of the skin making a small burrow in which she lays her eggs, one or two per day.

The clinical presentation is with a widespread erythematous papular rash which is intensely itchy, particularly at night when the skin is warm. The diagnostic lesion is the burrow, but these are not always found in the same distribution as the rash. Using an auriscope torch and magnifying lens (but no speculum) burrows can most easily be found in the finger webs and the inner surfaces of the wrists. Fewer burrows will be found in the vest and pants area, the feet and ankles. The face is not normally involved except occasionally in babies. Adult female mites can be lifted from the end of a burrow with a bevelled needle and examined under the microscope.

Treatment is with an emulsion of benzyl benzoate. A single application to all the skin surfaces below the neck will cure 99% of cases. The whole family must be treated simultaneously if re-infestation from an untreated person is to be prevented. Until all the dead mites are shed from the skin, their continued presence may cause itching, but this does not mean that treatment has been unsuccessful.

Fungal infections

Fungal infections account for 3–5% of new referrals to a dermatology clinic. Recognition is important because inappropriate treatment with steroids results in a reduction of the inflammation and irritation, but a more widespread invasion of the skin by fungus makes proper treatment much more difficult.

The three commonest fungus infections are those due to dermatophytes (ringworm), tinea versicolor and candidiasis.

Dermatophytes

Dermatophytes cause scalp, groin and body ringworm and athlete's foot. Body ringworm is most commonly acquired from animals (cats, cattle) and is more inflammatory and itchy than the others mentioned. The usual lesion is a circular scaling itchy patch with a raised edge. This is most easily seen on the trunk. Maceration of the skin between the toes with papules and vesicles on the soles of the feet occurs in athlete's foot. In the groin a scaling patch spreading onto the scrotum and inner thigh is seen. In the scalp a typical circular patch occurs in which the hair has broken off close to the scalp. Nail infection causes thickening and separation of the nail from its bed (onycholysis). The nail is discoloured and crumbly.

Diagnosis is confirmed by showing that skin scrapings examined under the microscope contain hyphae. Fluorescence under Wood's light is a useful way of screening large numbers of school children.

Differential diagnosis is from eczema, seborrhoeic dermatitis or psoriasis (which is not usually as itchy as ringworm and does not cause hair loss on the scalp), and compulsive hair pulling (trichotillomania).

Treatment using Whitfield's ointment or specific antifungal agents such as tolnaftate, clotrimazole or miconazole is usually sufficient for localised eruptions provided it is continued for at least 2 weeks. Generalised relapsing or obstinate infections, particularly of the nails and scalp, are best treated with oral griseofulvin.

Tinea versicolor

Tinea versicolor is a mild yeast infection causing a series of hyperpigmented scaling patches usually affecting the trunk, neck and face. There may be more widespread pale fluorescent patches seen under Wood's light. Topical treatment with antifungal agents (clotrimazole) is effective but should continue for several weeks or the condition may relapse.

Warts and verrucae

Warts and verrucae are caused by viruses. Most lesions will disappear if left alone due to the reduction of immunity in the host. A verruca in a weight-bearing area can be painful and may need to be frozen with liquid nitrogen and curetted by a chiropodist. Providing they are covered with a waterproof plaster, verrucae need not exclude a child from swimming. A number of simple proprietry applications for warts and verrucae are available at the chemist, salicylic acid in collodion or podophyllin paint is as effective as any other method of treating warts.

28. Tropical child health in the non-industrialised world

M. C. K. Chan

Three in four children today live in tropical developing countries where poverty and malnutrition associated with diarrhoeal diseases interacting with infections and parasitic disease contribute to an appalling mortality rate amongst preschool children, 20–50 times more than in Western Europe. Infants who survive the perils of parturition are likely to die from neonatal tetanus or septicaemia.

MALNUTRITION

Infants and children have greater nutritional requirements than adults because they are growing. Poverty and disasters, either natural or man made, lead to starvation which inevitably affects children most severely. The replacement of breast feeding by bottle feeding in developing countries, has led to rampant infantile diarrhoea and malnutrition in the form of marasmus. Malnutrition is responsible for millions of childhood deaths annually, either directly or in combination with infections. These factors are reflected in the causes of death of young children in non-industrialised countries compared with those in the developed world (Table 28.1).

The major forms of malnutrition are marasmus and kwashiorkor with a spectrum of features between the two, in addition to deficiencies of vitamins, iron, folates and trace elements (see Ch. 11).

Marasmus

Marasmus is associated with an absolute deficiency of calories, proteins and other essential nutrients. This stage affects infants and young children who

Table 28.1 The main causes of death in children aged 1–4 years in non-industrialised and developed countries (WHO 1976)

Cause of death	% of deaths
Non-industrialised countries	
Diarrhoeal diseases	10–40
Respiratory infections	20–30
Accidents	1–10
Congenital defects	1–5
Developed countries	
Accidents	18–37
Congenital defects	8–18
Malignant neoplasms	10–15
Respiratory infections	5–12

have a marked deficit in both weight and height. Gross wasting of subcutaneous fat and muscles makes these suffering children look wizened but with abdominal distension due to wasting of the abdominal wall through which peristalsis is visible (Fig. 28.1). Marasmic children, in common with others who are malnourished, have impaired immune function of both cellular and humoral systems and succumb to infections. Yet, in spite of these severe changes there is no hepatomegaly, oedema or hair changes, and the child is alert and hungry (Fig. 28.2). Marasmus is the result of chronic diarrhoea and malabsorption or chronic inadequate food intake.

Kwashiorkor

Kwashiorkor (first described in 1933 by Cecily Williams in West Africa) is a syndrome seen in underdeveloped tropical countries in children taken off breast milk and given a diet low in nutrients. Its pathogenesis is incompletely understood, although recent research indicates an association

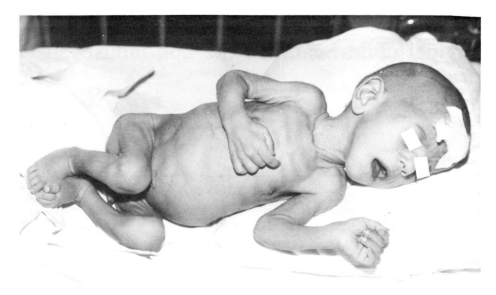

Fig. 28.1 A 3-month-old Asian infant weighing 3 kg with marasmus after recurrent episodes of diarrhoea. He had been bottle fed since birth.

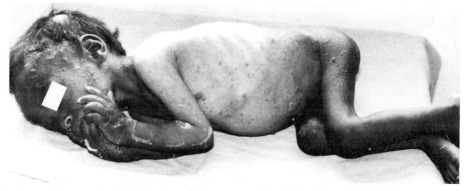

Fig. 28.2 This 2-year-old marasmic child looks alert and hungry, and is suffering from chickenpox.

with mycotoxin from contaminated food. Aflatoxin produced by the mould *Aspergillus flavus* is not destroyed by cooking. When ingested aflatoxin accumulates in the liver where it is thought to be toxic and its effects probably produce kwashiorkor. Clinical features are related to gross disturbance of protein, water and electrolyte metabolism manifested by oedema associated with hypoalbuminaemia, retarded growth and dermatoses in a miserable apathetic child. Skin changes include hypopigmentation, patches of hyperpigmentation described as 'black paint' that tend to desquamate leaving raw areas similar to second-degree burns, and 'crazy paving' usually on the legs. Hair loses its lustre, falls off easily, becomes red and sparse and may show the *flag* sign (variation in colour reflecting periods of normal and abnormal nutrition). Visceral organs undergo pathological changes including fatty infiltration of the liver, atrophy of intestinal mucosa and the reticulo-endothelial system, and pancreatic fibrosis. Severe cerebral atrophy or brain shrinkage has been found on computed tomography of young children with kwashiorkor.

These severe forms of malnutrition have recently been reported in British children fed on macrobiotic food by their vegetarian parents.

Nutritional anaemias due to iron and folate deficiency, avitaminosis A and rickets are the other manifestations of malnutrition. Vitamin A deficiency affects epithelial tissues of the eyes, respiratory tract and intestines. Eye problems associated with xerophthalmia range from night blindness to frank, ulcerating keratomalacia. The immune system is depressed in vitamin A deficiency and causes frequent respiratory infections and diarrhoea that may be fatal. Vitamin A deficiency may be due to dietary deficiency alone, but it is often precipitated by measles, diarrhoea and intestinal parasites.

Prevention of malnutrition

Children in the underprivileged world are in urgent need of better nutrition, clean water, improved sanitation, and protection against specific infections and parasites to cope with life in a hostile environment, but the most important health need of children in the tropics is breast feeding. This is the best safeguard against malnutrition and gastrointestinal infection in infants. Unfortunately, breast feeding is being abandoned for artificial feeding and indications are that this trend will continue. Contributory factors to the decline in breast feeding are complex and involve the employment of women outside the home, separation of mothers and babies in hospitals, parental ignorance of infant nutrition, the aggressive sales techniques of milk marketing firms, and changing social values associated with urbanisation. The World Health Organisation (WHO) code of practice for the marketing of breast milk substitutes was introduced in 1981 to curb unethical promotion of artificial milk, particularly in developing countries. Most member countries of the WHO have accepted this code which has raised public awareness of the benefits of breast milk and the problems of bottle feeding. However, it has not persuaded many middle class women in non-industrialised countries to give up bottle feeding and breast feed their babies. Infant feeding practices in affluent countries also have a sig-

nificant influence on women in urban areas of the developing world where the trend against breast feeding has been most obvious. It is hoped, therefore, that the present increase in breast feeding being practised in Western Europe and North America, together with the worldwide concern for childhood nutrition, will encourage more women in developing countries to breast feed their babies.

Asian rickets

Rickets affects all age groups of Asians from the Indian subcontinent living in the UK with those in northern cities most at risk. Neonatal rickets occurs in babies born of mothers with osteomalacia, infantile rickets affects toddlers, and adolescents (mostly girls) have late rickets. The child with rickets complains of progressively severe pain in the legs which, if untreated, leads to deformity of the knees (genu valgum) and pelvis.

Risk factors for rickets in Asian children include maternal deficiency of vitamin D during pregnancy and lactation, strict vegetarian diets, and limited exposure to sunlight. In 1981 the 'Stop Rickets' campaign was launched by the Minister of Health in Britain. Daily doses of 10 μg vitamin D were offered to Asian and other immigrant children at risk from rickets. In Glasgow where there was a high prevalence of rickets in Asian children, this suboptimal vitamin D supplementation greatly reduced severe rickets. However, vitamin D deficiency persists in Asian adolescent girls who need annual supplements in the autumn.

DISEASES IMPORTED INTO THE UK

It is estimated that 1 in 15 persons in the UK is exposed to diseases from the tropics. In 1986, 1.25 million British residents visited malarious areas. There are more than 2 million people from the New Commonwealth now living in Britain. Therefore, all doctors in primary health care must be aware of the common childhood diseases which have been imported into this country. These diseases fall broadly into three groups: tropical diseases, communicable diseases of public health significance and inherited disorders.

1. **Tropical diseases**:
   a. Malaria — chiefly *Plasmodium falciparum* and *Plasmodium vivax*
   b. Intestinal helminths — ascaris, trichuris and hookworm
   c. Nutritional rickets in Asians
   d. Schistosomiasis
   e. Leishmaniasis
   f. Skin infections — fungal and parasitic
2. **Communicable diseases**:
   a. Tuberculosis — pulmonary and disseminated
   b. Diarrhoeal diseases — salmonella, shigella, giardia and *Entamoeba histolytica*
   c. Viral hepatitis
   d. Viral haemorrhagic fevers — Lassa, Ebola and dengue
3. **Inherited disorders**
   a. Thalassaemias — α-thalassaemia and β-thalassaemia
   b. Haemoglobinopathies — sickle cell disease (HbS) and haemoglobin E disease
   c. Glucose-6-phosphate dehydrogenase (G6PD) deficiency presenting as neonatal jaundice, favism, and drug-induced haemolytic anaemia

Malaria

A worldwide resurgence of malaria occurred during the 1970s, killing about a million African children every year. This resurgence was reflected in Britain by a sharp annual increase of imported malaria in that period. The upward trend has continued during the decade 1977 to 1986 with a 51% increase from 1529 to 2309 cases being reported to the Malaria Reference Laboratory. Infection with *P. falciparum*, mainly acquired in Africa, has risen from one-fifth to one-third of all cases, with about 1200 cases of *P. vivax* mostly from Asia reported annually, constituting 65% of all infections. Resident ethnic minority groups, temporary residents from West Africa and tourists who visit Kenya are at high risk. Infection rates are highest in immigrants settled in Britain who visit relatives: 316 and 331 per 100 000 for Africa and Asia respectively, 120 and 39 in tourists, and 228 and 38 in business travellers to those regions. Children

under 15 years had the highest attack rate for malaria of 176 per 100 000 travellers in 1986, more than double the rate in the age group 35–54 years. This may be associated with poor compliance with prophylaxis.

Deaths from malaria were only associated with *P. falciparum* infections, the majority being in persons of British origin who had either not taken prophylactic drugs or had been on inappropriate medicines.

Clinical presentation

Congenital malaria occurs through transplacental infection in babies born to non-immune women. However, because of the parasite's lifecycle, symptoms may not develop for up to a month after birth. Congenital infection may occur with *P. falciparum*, *P. vivax* and *P. malariae*. Infected infants develop fever, jaundice, pallor, and abdominal distension with splenomegaly from the age of 1–4 weeks.

Childhood malaria does not usually manifest the periodic fever and rigors so characteristic of malaria in adults. *Plasmodium vivax* infection is the usual form of malaria contracted by Asian children born in this country while on holiday in the Indian subcontinent. The incubation period is long, averaging 2 weeks to 9 months because *P. vivax* has an exoerythrocytic phase in the host's liver from which merozoites can escape, weeks or months after the initial infection, to complete the lifecycle. Fever (39–40°C) is sometimes accompanied by rigors and vomiting. The child is flushed and hepatosplenomegaly is present. Anaemia is not a feature of vivax malaria. Although distressing, this disease is rarely fatal.

Plasmodium falciparum infection, on the other hand, is frequently a fatal disease in young African children living in highly endemic areas. Death usually results from cerebral malaria or acute overwhelming infection. Some children achieve a relative tolerance to the parasite after several attacks of falciparum infection and are asymptomatic in spite of hepatosplenomegaly, parasites in their blood and anaemia. Children suffering an acute attack of falciparum malaria develop a high, continuous fever (38–40°C), anaemia (haemoglobin less than 9 g/dl), an enlarged tender liver and splenomegaly. Febrile convulsions often occur and can be distinguished from cerebral malaria because the loss of consciousness lasts only for a few minutes.

The clinical diagnosis of *P. falciparum* malaria can be difficult to make in white children in this country. Besides the non-specific clinical picture and the low index of suspicion on the part of the doctor, these children have usually taken anti-malarial prophylaxis. However, the dosage was either inadequate or the drugs were stopped soon after returning to the UK. In areas of chloroquine-resistant *P. falciparum* malaria, inappropriate prophylactic drugs may have been taken. These problems are illustrated in the following case.

Case history.

A 12-year-old white girl born in Zambia moved to England after her second birthday. Her next visit to the tropics had been a month's holiday in Nairobi and Mombassa. She had taken pyrimethamine 25 mg weekly while abroad but stopped when she arrived home. Two days after the holiday she developed a fever and cough which was diagnosed as pleurisy. She did not improve on penicillin for 10 days, after which she attended her doctor presenting with anorexia, vomiting, abdominal pain and fever (38°C). A tentative diagnosis of hepatitis was made and she was nursed at home. Four weeks after her return from Africa she had jaundice (serum bilirubin 90 μmol/l). One week later she was admitted to hospital with drowsiness and vomiting. She was ill with marked pallor and a temperature of 38°C on admission but without jaundice. She had an enlarged spleen, 1 cm, a haemic heart murmur, but no abnormal neurological signs and a normal cerebrospinal fluid. Blood investigations showed heavy parasitaemia with *P. falciparum*, and haemolytic anaemia (haemoglobin 3 g/dl, reticulocytes 25%). She was given a transfusion of packed red cells and chloroquine treatment with dramatic improvement: she was discharged from hospital 4 days later.

This case emphasises the need for antimalarial prophylaxis to be continued for 4–6 weeks after leaving a malarious area to ensure the eradication of all forms of *P. falciparum*.

Cerebral malaria is a serious complication of *P. falciparum* infection that can be rapidly fatal and calls for immediate treatment. Capillaries supplying the brain are blocked with parasitised erythrocytes and produce foci of cerebral necrosis. The child with cerebral malaria presents with fever for a few days followed by repeated convulsions with alteration of the level of consciousness and coma. There are hardly any focal CNS signs; some children show minimal signs of meningeal irritation, but retinal haemorrhages are often present. The cerebrospinal fluid is usually normal and this distinguishes cerebral malaria from septic meningitis and viral encephalitides. In young children, the mortality rate from cerebral malaria even with the best available treatment is 25% and there is a significant morbidity from neurological sequelae in survivors.

Chloroquine-resistant strains of *P. falciparum* have been proliferating and spreading in South America (in the late 1950s), South-east Asia (1960s) and East Africa (1980s). These resistant strains have recently been found also in India, particularly on the East coast, and in parts of Central and West Africa. Their existence has created problems in the prevention and treatment of malaria.

Diagnosis

Malaria can only be diagnosed by microscopic blood examination, preferably of a thick film stained with Field's stain. A thin blood film should also be examined to determine the intensity of infection and the type of malarial parasite, factors which determine the method of treatment and the drug to be prescribed. Parasitaemia above 2% requires immediate treatment, while the patient with high parasitaemia (5% or more) has severe malaria and should be given parenteral therapy and intensive care. If the pathologist is not experienced in identifying the type of plasmodium, blood films should be sent for confirmation to laboratories such as the Liverpool School of Tropical Medicine or the Hospital for Tropical Diseases, London.

Treatment

The aim of treatment is the eradication of parasites with appropriate drugs. In *acute attacks*, chloroquine will effectively eliminate sensitive strains of *P. falciparum*, *P. vivax*, *P. malariae* and *P. ovale*, but will not prevent relapses of *P. vivax* and *P. ovale*. The widespread development of chloroquine-resistant *P. falciparum* has led to the increasing use of quinine, which binds plasmodial DNA, as the drug of choice. *Quinine* may be given by mouth in a dose of 10 mg per kg body weight every 8 hours for 7 days followed by a single dose of Fansidar (Table 28.2). Side-effects of quinine include abdominal pain, blurred vision, cardiac arrythmias (prolonged QT interval and flattening of the T-wave), central nervous system depression, dysphonia, giddiness, hypotension, rashes, tinnitus, tremors and urticaria. Unusual complications are hypersensitivy reactions, haemolysis, leucopenia, thrombocytopenia, granulomatous hepatitis and ochronosis. Hypoglycaemia and hypotension may occasionally follow rapid intravenous infusion.

Chloroquine is still effective, and possibly superior to quinine when the parasite (*P. vivax, P. malariae, P. ovale, P. falciparum*) is sensitive to it. The schedule and dosages of chloroquine are given in Table 28.2. Resistance of *P. falciparum* to chloroquine is classified according to clinical response and blood parasitaemia as follows:

RI   Clinical cure with no parasites after chloroquine therapy is followed within 3 weeks with reappearance of parasites in the blood.

RII   Clinical improvement with reduction in blood parasites is followed by increase in parasitaemia soon after chloroquine is stopped.

RIII   No improvement in clinical state nor effect on parasitaemia after a therapeutic course of chloroquine.

Oral, intramuscular and subcutaneous administration of chloroquine seldom causes side-effects. Intravenous chloroquine has caused hypotension and cardiac arrhythmias, particularly in African children. Minor side-effects include abdominal discomfort, nausea, vomiting, dizziness, blurred vision and generalised pruritus.

Severe malaria occurs with *P. falciparum* infection only and manifests with high blood parasitaemia (more than 5%) with or without clinical features of *cerebral malaria* such as frequent convulsions followed by coma, or profound anaemia (Hb<5 g/dl), pulmonary oedema, bleeding associated with coagulopathy, renal failure and hypoglycaemia. Management of severe malaria requires prompt control of convulsions with paraldehyde (per rectum or i.m.) or diazepam (i.v.) and tepid sponging, assessment of hydration and detection of pulmonary oedema. Fluid intake and output should be recorded hourly with monitoring of vital signs. Rectal or other means of measuring core temperature should be recorded continuously with an electronic thermometer if possible. Antimalarial drugs should be given by intravenous infusion but oral medication instituted as soon as possible. *Quinine* dihydrochloride 10 mg/kg well diluted in 30 ml 5% dextrose is infused intravenously over 4 hours followed by the same dose infused over 8 hours. This regimen of slow infusion prevents transient high concentrations of

Table 28.2   Treatment regimens for acute malaria in non-immune children

Drug	Starting dose	Subsequent dose	Course duration
Quinine	10 mg/kg	10 mg/kg 8-hourly	7 days
Chloroquine or amodiaquine			
15 kg or less	10 mg/kg	10 mg/kg after 6 hours 5 mg/kg daily for 2 days	3 days
More than 15 kg	10 mg/kg	5 mg/kg after 6 hours 5 mg/kg daily for 2 days	3 days
Fansidar			
15 kg or less	½ tablet	—	—
15+–20 kg	1 tablet	—	—
20+–30 kg	1½ tablets	—	—
30+–50 kg	2 tablet	—	—
50+ kg	3 tablet	—	—

quinine which would be toxic to the cardiovascular system. Oral treatment should replace the parenteral route as soon as possible. The total course of treatment for severe malaria is 7 days. This is followed by Fansidar. In chloroquine-sensitive areas, *chloroquine* 5 mg/kg diluted in 30 ml 5% dextrose may be given by slow intravenous infusion over 4 hours. A second intravenous dose may be repeated 12 hours after the first dose. The total dose infused should not exceed 25 mg/kg. The rate of chloroquine infusion must be carefully monitored and the infusion rate reduced if blood pressure falls. Rapid bolus infusions or injections of intravenous chloroquine may cause lethal hypotension and should never be given. Parenteral chloroquine seems to produce more severe side-effects in children than in adults. This is so with intramuscular chloroquine and, therefore, the dose by this route must not exceed 2.5 mg/kg.

Patients with *P. vivax* and *P. ovale* infections are treated with a course of oral chloroquine followed by primaquine to eradicate the exoerythrocytic form of the parasite to prevent relapses. Although primaquine is effective, it has a narrow margin of safety between therapeutic and toxic dosages, and is not usually given to young children. *Primaquine* is used for 14 days after a course of chloroquine in the following dosages:

Body weight: Daily dose:
10–30 kg   3.75 mg
31–40 kg   5–7.5 mg
41–60 kg   7.5–15 mg

Children with glucose-6-phosphate dehydrogenase (G6PD) deficiency may develop haemolytic anaemia or methaemoglobinaemia with primaquine. Afro-Caribbean children with G6PD A– enzyme deficiency may still use primaquine but

the daily dose is given once a week for 8 weeks. This modified regimen gives a cure without significant haemolysis and has also been used in Thailand. However, this modification does not prevent haemolysis in children with Mediterranean and Chinese variants of G6PD deficiency.

Prevention

Travellers to endemic regions may be protected from malaria by taking measures such as chemoprophylaxis, protection against mosquito bites, and seeking immediate medical attention in case of fever.

Chemoprophylaxis with appropriate drugs should be given to all non-immune children and adults entering a malaria endemic area. It should be started preferably 1 week before entry and not later than the first day of exposure; it must be taken regularly and continued for 4–6 weeks after the last exposure. Antimalarial drugs in common use such as chloroquine and proguanil are bitter, and therefore may be difficult to administer to young children. However, every effort must be made to ensure regular chemoprophylaxis. A guide to drug dosages for chemoprophylaxis is given in Table 28.3.

Children indigenous to an endemic area are at greatest risk of severe malarial infection and mortality in the first 5 years of life. Ideally, the young child should be protected from malaria by all means including chemoprophylaxis, and prompt treatment be given when there is an acute attack. Older children would not require continuous prophylaxis as this would interfere with development of immunity. Chemoprophylaxis given during seasonal peaks of malaria transmission will reduce the severity of parasitaemia without interfering with development of immunity, and will

Table 28.3 A guide to malaria chemoprophylaxis in non-immune children 1988

Drug	Interval	Dosage: age of child and fraction of adult dose					
		By weight	<6 weeks	6 weeks–1 year	1+–5 years	5+–12 years	>12 years
Proquanil	Daily	5 mg/kg	$\frac{1}{8}$	$\frac{1}{4}$	$\frac{1}{2}$	$\frac{3}{4}$	Adult 200 mg
Chloroquine	Weekly	10 mg/kg	$\frac{1}{8}$	$\frac{1}{4}$	$\frac{1}{2}$	$\frac{3}{4}$	Adult 300 mg
Maloprim*	Weekly	—	Not recommended	$\frac{1}{8}-\frac{1}{4}$	$\frac{1}{2}$	$\frac{3}{4}$	Adult 1 tablet

* Contains dapsone 100 mg and pyrimethamine 12.5 mg in 1 tablet.

assist in promoting normal growth. However, continuous chemoprophylaxis is justified in children with homozygous sickle cell disease (sickle cell anaemia) in whom severe haemolytic crises are often precipitated by malaria. Community-wide chemoprophylaxis for indigenous children is no longer recommended because of poor compliance and irregular drug supplies. Instead, all children should receive treatment for malaria if they are febrile.

In regions where there is no evidence of chloroquine resistance, proguanil (5 mg/kg) daily or chloroquine (10 mg/kg) weekly gives adequate protection. Where chloroquine resistance is commonplace (India, East and Central Africa; Fig. 28.3) proguanil daily and chloroquine weekly are recommended. In some regions such as the Pacific islands and Thailand where chloroquine resistance is commonplace and the combination of proguanil and chloroquine is apparently ineffective, the current recommendation is chloroquine and Maloprim (dapsone and pyrimethamine) weekly for chemoprophylaxis.

The widespread use of chemoprophylactic agents against *P. falciparum* infection has uncovered side-effects. Proguanil may cause mild gastric irritation. Prolonged use of chloroquine in large doses may lead to neuroretinitis and visual impairment, but this complication is very rare even after 5 years of regular use in adults. Ophthalmic examination is advised after 6 years of chloroquine administration. Blood concentrations of chloroquine are higher than normal in the presence of renal and hepatic damage. Maloprim produces methaemoglobinaemia and haemolysis in some susceptible subjects such as those with G6PD deficiency; a major side-effect is life-threatening agranulocytosis usually associated with high dosage (twice the recommended dose) in adults. Fansidar and amodiaquine are no longer recommended for chemoprophylactic use because of fatalities reported in the mid-1980s from hepatitis, agranulocytosis and Stevens–Johnson syndrome.

The most important point to remember about chemoprophylaxis is that protection is not absolute and that breakthrough infection can occur with any of the drugs recommended anywhere in the world.

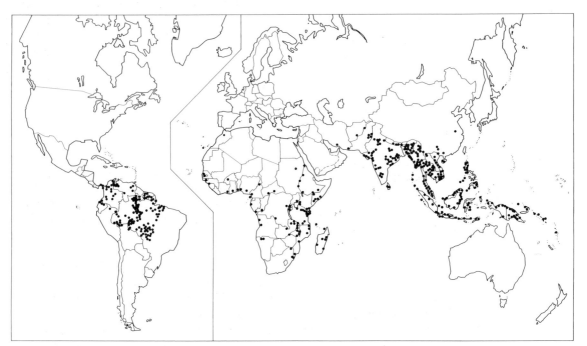

Fig. 28.3 Areas where chloroquine-resistant *Plasmodium falciparum* has been reported. Reproduced by permission, from 'World Malaria Situation 1986–87'. Weekly Epidemiological Record 64 (33): 251 (1989).

Therefore, personal *protection against mosquito bites* is important and may be achieved by using nets around the bed at night especially for babies and young children, taking care to tuck in the net under the mattress, after checking that there are no mosquitoes inside. Increased protection may be obtained by impregnating the net with permethrin or deltamethrin because mosquitoes are repelled even if the bed net is torn. Arms and legs should be covered after sunset, and insect repellant, such as dimethyl phthalate or *N, N*-diethyl-3-toluamide (DEET), applied on exposed skin.

Newer drugs for malaria

Mefloquine, a drug structurally related to quinine, is a very active schizonticide but is slow in action, and it has been used in combination with Fansidar or quinine against chloroquine-resistant *P. falciparum*. However, resistance to both Fansidar and Mefloquine has been reported in Thailand. Qinghaosu (artemisinin) isolated from the leaves and flowers of the plant, *Artemisia annua* L. by Chinese scientists in 1972 is a fast-acting blood schizontocide. Its antimalarial activity is increased by the formation of esters and ethers. Clinical trials of qinghaosu and its derivatives given orally or intravenously have shown potency against drug-resistant parasites. Antibiotics such as erythromycin, tetracycline and cotrimoxazole also have antimalarial activity against resistant *P. falciparum*. Clinical trials using oral Halofantrine has shown high concentration and rapid absorption when taken with a fatty meal. If this is confirmed, it would be a good drug for young children taking milk feeds.

Vaccines against *P. falciparum* are being developed but it will be some years before a suitable product for clinical trial is produced.

Intestinal helminths

The absence of proper sanitation for disposal of excreta and the use of untreated human faeces for manure contribute to the high incidence of ascariasis, trichuris and hookworm in tropical rural communities.

Ascariasis

Ascaris lumbricoides is found in many children, some of whom have multiple infestations with other helminths. Larvae in the lungs may cause pneumonitis with symptoms of asthma, transient migratory pulmonary infiltration seen on radiograph, and eosinophilia — features that constitute Loeffler's syndrome. Adult ascaris worms produce abdominal colic, nausea and vomiting, but heavy infestation may lead to intestinal obstruction, intussusception, peritonitis, cholecystitis, cholangitis and obstructive jaundice.

Levamisole is considered to be the drug of choice because it is very effective against ascaris and is well tolerated; mild nausea and vomiting has been reported in 1% of treated patients. A single oral dose of 3 mg/kg with a maximum of 150 mg for adults is adequate treatment for ascariasis. Levamisole should be avoided in patients with advanced liver or kidney disease; it should not be given with tetrachloroethylene in multiple infestations. Mebendazole is active against ascaris but is not recommended for children under 2 years of age. Pyrantel is an effective broad-spectrum antihelminthic drug which in a single oral dose of 10 mg/kg (maximum 1 g) is sufficient to eradicate roundworms. Piperazine citrate in a single dose of 2 g/m^2 body surface area or 3–4 g is effective treatment for ascaris, but multiple doses may cause neurotoxicity with ataxia, hypotonia, incoordination and drowsiness.

Whipworm

Trichuris trichiura (whipworm) infection is common in young children and symptoms are related to the number of worms present in the bowel. Heavy infection presents with abdominal pain, diarrhoea, malnutrition with pica, blood in the stools, tenesmus and rectal prolapse. The worms attach to the mucosa of the rectum and sigmoid colon and cause bleeding ulcers that result in iron deficiency anaemia. Malnutrition may be severe enough to cause bone age retardation. Finger clubbing is a feature of heavy infestation secondary to increased vagal stimulation caused by chronic diarrhoea. Many infected children have concomitant amoebiasis and shigellosis. Complete eradication of trichuris infection is difficult and only two drugs are effective for treatment: pyrantel and mebendazole. Pyrantel may be used in children over 6 months in a single dose of 10 mg/kg (maximum 1 g for adults); and mebendazole for those over 2 years of age in a dose of 100 mg daily for 3 days.

Hookworms

Ancylostoma duodenale and *Necator americanus* exclusively parasitise man. Larvae penetrate the skin of bare-footed children producing a dermatitis *ground itch*, at the site of entry and migrate to the lungs where they may cause cough and fever. Adult worms are attached to the jejunal mucosa and live by sucking blood from the host. Iron deficiency anaemia results when the worm load is large. Treatment requires correction of the anaemia and expulsion of the worms. Pyrantel is very effective against hookworms in a single dose 10 mg/kg given daily for 3 days. Bephenium is used in a single dose of 2.5 g for children weighing more than 10 kg, and repeated after 1 or 2 days. Tetrachloroethylene is widely used in the tropics as it is cheap and effective. A suspension in a single oral dose of 0.1 ml/kg up to a dose of 5 ml for an adult is given in the morning before food. If a mixed infection with ascaris is suspected, this should be treated first because tetrachloroethylene activates migration of round worms and may lead to intestinal obstruction. Thiabendazole 50 mg/kg body weight up to a maximum of 3 g in a single dose is also effective treatment for hookworms and other helminths.

Schistosomiasis

Schistosomiasis is second only to malaria as a major tropical disease affecting 200 million people in the world. The disease is acquired in childhood through exposure to infected streams, rivers and irrigation canals where certain snails, the intermediate host, survive. Man-made lakes and irrigation schemes have become sources of infection and spread of schistosomiasis in the tropics. There are three major species of schistosomes (helminthic flukes), *Schistosoma haematobium* (in Africa and the Middle East), *S. mansoni* (Africa,

Central and South America) and *S. japonicum* (Far East). *Schistosoma mansoni* and *S. japonicum* affect the large bowel and liver while *S. haematobium* affects the urinary tract.

The development of symptoms depends upon the worm load, the number of ova laid and the immune response of the host. White children are likely to present with anorexia, malaise, prolonged fever, dry irritating cough, urticaria and loss of weight. Investigations show marked eosinophilia and patchy pulmonary infiltration on X-ray in some cases. Children in endemic areas do not present with constitutional symptoms; those infected with *S. mansoni* and *S. japonicum* have diarrhoea with blood and mucus while haematuria and dysuria are symptomatic of *S. haematobium* infection. Chronic infections with *S. haemotobium* can cause hydronephrosis which is reversible with early treatment and, later, irreversible fibrosis and calcification of the bladder. Portal hypertension from liver fibrosis is a complication of *S. mansoni* and *S. japonicum* infections. Recurrent salmonella infections are likely to develop in subjects with schistosomiasis, the micro-organisms living in the integumen of schistosomes. Praziquantel is highly effective against *S. mansoni* and *S. haematobium* in a single dose of 40 mg/kg taken after a meal. Against *S. japonicum* better results are obtained with two 30 mg/kg doses taken 4 hours apart. No serious toxic effects have been reported.

Leishmaniasis

Leishmaniasis is a parasitic disease due to protozoa spread by sandflies. Two major syndromes are recognised:

1. Visceral leishmaniasis (kala azar) affecting the reticuloendothelial system is a systemic illness.
2. Cutaneous leishmaniasis in which parasites are restricted to the macrophages of the skin and sometimes adjacent mucous membranes.

Endemic areas exist in China, India, the Middle East, Mediterranean countries, Africa and Central and South America. Visceral leishmaniasis attacks children under 8 years, who present with prolonged fever seldom over 39°C, loss of weight, hepatosplenomegaly, and lymphadenopathy. Infants are toxaemic. Anaemia is usually severe (haemoglobin less than 7 g/dl), normochromic, normocytic, associated with leucopenia and thrombocytopenia. Secondary bacterial infection and bleeding are complications. The disease is sometimes mistaken for acute leukaemia when the bone marrow is examined. Visceral leishmaniasis is a diagnosis to be considered in a child with prolonged fever who has been on holiday in the Mediterranean. Pentamidine 4 mg/kg body weight or sodium stibogluconate (Pentostam) 10 mg/kg (maximum 600 mg) given by injection daily for 10 days is the treatment. Allopurinol 20 mg/kg daily in patients with visceral leishmaniasis has shown promising results when antimicrobials have failed.

Tuberculosis

Tuberculosis is a common and dangerous disease in young children in many developing countries. Haematogenous spread of tubercle bacilli is frequent in poorly nourished children and affects lymph nodes, meninges, peritoneum, bone and joints and rarely, kidneys. The notification rates of tuberculosis in previously untreated children per 100 000 population of England for 1983 were 2.4 for whites; 27 for Indians born in Britain, 48 for Pakistanis and Bangladeshis born in Britain, and 62 and 63 respectively for those born in the Indian subcontinent. The majority (76%) of children in 1983 had respiratory diseases. Tuberculin testing of all immigrant children on arrival is recommended and BCG given to all who have a weak or no reaction. A weak or minimal tuberculin reaction in the presence of active tuberculosis may occur in: very malnourished children; severe disseminated infection; following measles; patients on immunosuppressive drugs; the first weeks of an infection; or faulty technique or inactive tuberculin. BCG vaccination is currently offered in the UK to: newborn infants of non-Caucasian families, tuberculin-negative children of new immigrants, and tuberculin-negative children aged 12 or 13 years when routinely tested in schools.

DIARRHOEAL DISEASES

Acute diarrhoea with its serious consequences of dehydration, electrolyte imbalance and nutritional impairment is a major cause of morbidity and mortality in developing countries (Table 28.1). About 5 million deaths from diarrhoea occur worldwide each year in preschool children. Viruses, bacteria and parasites have been identified as causal agents of acute diarrhoea in infants and children.

Rotavirus infection is an important cause of acute diarrhoea in some developing countries, e.g. Bangladesh, but its precise role in other countries has still to be established. Rotavirus vaccines have been studied in field trials but none has been recommended for routine use.

Shigellae and salmonellae are the most frequently identified bacterial pathogens. Although enterotoxogenic *Escherichia coli* has been identified in nurseries in industrialised countries and in adults with travellers' diarrhoea, its role in acute infantile diarrhoea awaits clarification. Campylobacter has been cultured from stools of children with acute diarrhoea in tropical Africa. Untreated, the infection tends to persist for 7–14 days with apparent recovery followed by relapse of symptoms mistaken for acute appendicitis.

Giardiasis and amoebiasis are the two major diarrhoeal diseases caused by parasites. In the highlands of Papua New Guinea, a syndrome of severe abdominal distension, vomiting and diarrhoea in breast-fed infants under 6 months of age has been described in association with heavy infestation of *Strongyloides fuelleborni*. Other features of this infection are ascites and oedema with hypoproteinaemia, and eosinophilia. The disease is rapidly fatal unless treated with mebendazole 25 mg/kg body weight.

Management of diarrhoea in developing countries

In 1978, the World Health Organisation launched a global diarrhoeal diseases control programme with the support of UNICEF. The immediate objective of this programme was to reduce diarrhoea-related mortality and malnutrition in children by widespread implementation of oral rehydration therapy and improved feeding practices. Nearly 100 countries have incorporated the control of diarrhoeal diseases as an integral part of primary health care after a decade of the diarrhoea diseases control programme.

Clinical management of diarrhoea is based on the principle of replacement of lost fluid and electrolytes. The first step in management is the identification of dehydration and the assessment of its severity in the child with diarrhoea. The severely dehydrated child requires parenteral fluid therapy to correct shock by rapid restoration of circulatory volume. Lesser degrees of dehydration can be managed successfully with oral fluids, which if given early in the course of diarrhoea, prevent the development of circulatory failure and the use of expensive equipment and fluids for parenteral therapy. The solution recommended by the World Health Organisation for oral therapy is oral rehydration salts (ORS) solution containing:

Glucose	110 mmol/l
Na^+	90 mmol/l
CL^-	80 mmol/l
K^+	20 mmol/l
HCO^-_3	30 mmol/l

The solution is made from glucose 20 g, sodium chloride 3.5 g, sodium bicarbonate 2.5 g and potassium chloride 1.5 g dissolved in one litre of clean drinking water. This ORS solution is satisfactory for the management of hypo-osmolar dehydration found in most developing countries, but its content of sodium is too high for use in young infants or children suspected of hyperosmolar dehydration.

Initial oral rehydration should be complete within 4–6 hours when skin turgor and pulse will return to normal and urine flow will have begun. Mild to moderate cases, passing stool every 2 hours, will require 100–200 ml of ORS solution per kg bodyweight daily. After 4–6 hours the same amount of oral fluids is given if signs of dehydration persist. As stool frequency decreases, less ORS solution is offered until the patient returns to normal. Infants with diarrhoea are encouraged to breast feed during oral rehydration. Vomiting is not a contraindication to oral therapy.

Oral rehydration with ORS solution is effective, simple and safe in the management of acute diarrhoea worldwide. When provided early in the disease, it substantially reduces death rates and hospitalisation. Oral rehydration therapy could prevent 20–25% of the 14 million deaths a year among the world's preschool children.

Investigators at the International Centre for Diarrhoeal Diseases Research, Bangladesh have found that using cooked rice powder instead of glucose produces a version of ORS which reduces the duration of the disease by 30%, reduces stool volume by 40%, and reduces vomiting by 60%. This rice-based ORS could help to maintain the child's nutrition by reducing the diarrhoea and restoring normal appetite, therefore breaking the cycle of malnutrition and diarrhoea.

Amoebiasis

This disease, caused by the protozoon *Entamoeba histolytica*, produces a severe illness in malnourished young children in the tropics. Infection occurs by swallowing cysts usually in contaminated water. Water may be made safe by boiling or by treatment with 3 parts per million of iodine or hypochlorite. The parasite invades the large intestine producing mucosal ulcers from the terminal ileum to the perineum. Haematogenous spread to the liver with abscess formation occurs even in mild infections. Most children present with mild diarrhoea which may become chronic or relapsing; the stools are loose, containing excess mucus and some blood. Fever and constitutional disturbance may not be evident, but abdominal discomfort, tenesmus and tenderness over the colon are present. The severest form of amoebiasis may be acute, simulating bacillary dysentery, and be complicated by colonic perforation and peritonitis with a high mortality. Cutaneous ulceration in the perineum is another complication.

Women with untreated amoebic dysentery can infect their newborn infants during parturition.

Diagnosis of amoebiasis is made by examination of a fresh warm stool for haematophagenous trophozoites of *E. histolytica*.

Metronidazole 40 mg/kg bodyweight given orally in three divided doses daily (maximum 2400 mg) for 5 days is safe and effective treatment for acute invasive amoebic dysentery. The parasites disappear from the stools within 24 hours.

Diloxanide furoate (Furamide) is the drug of choice in chronic infections in which only cysts and not vegetative forms of *E. histolytica* are present in the faeces.

Giardiasis

Giardia lamblia is a flagellate protozoon which lives in the duodenum and jejunum of the host. Surveys of primary school children in Rangoon and Mexico City showed prevalence rates of 21% and 13.7% respectively. Breast milk is protective and giardia is rarely found in infants under 4 months of age. A first infection with giardia in developing countries occurs in late infancy and early childhood. If left untreated, symptoms improve spontaneously but many become asymptomatic cyst excreters. Symptoms vary from mild to severe diarrhoea which may become prolonged and result in failure to thrive. Giardia infection is associated with malabsorption and the passage of pale, frothy, offensive stools. Diagnosis is made by finding oval cysts or, sometimes, trophozoites in freshly voided stools. When stool examination is negative, duodenal juice aspirates should be examined for trophozoites. An ELISA test has been developed for detection of giardia antigens in faeces.

Transmission of the parasite is by the ingestion of contaminated food and water.

Metronidazole 20 mg/kg body weight daily (maximum 800 mg) in four divided doses for 5 days or tinidazole 50 mg/kg/day as a single dose for 3 days are effective for treatment but repeated courses may be necessary.

Cryptosporidia

These parasites have been found in 4–10% of diarrhoeal episodes in children in many parts of the world, usually without other pathogens being present. It seems to cause more diarrhoea than other parasites. Cryptosporidial diarrhoea can be fatal in patients with acquired immune deficiency syndrome (AIDS). In children, it causes self-limiting watery diarrhoea with weight loss, and if ORS and feeding are not given promptly, dehydration and malnutrition will result. Laboratory diagnosis is made by microscopic examination of stool stained by the modified Ziehl–Neelson 'in cold' or

Kinyoun methods for ovoid cysts that appear bright red.

Management consists of correcting dehydration and children should be fed as soon as possible. No drugs have been found to be effective against cryptosporidia.

Shigellosis

Shigellae are Gram-negative bacilli that can invade the mucosa of the colon and cause dysentery, acute severe diarrhoea with mucus, pus and blood in the stools. There are four subgroups: *Shigella dysenteriae*, *Sh. flexneri*, *Sh. boydii* and *Sh. sonnei*, listed in order of severity of illness produced in man. *Shigella flexneri* tends to be the dominant species in the tropics, although *Sh. dysenteriae* has been responsible for epidemics in Central America; *Sh. sonnei* is the dominant species in the UK. After a short incubation (2–3 days) there is an abrupt onset of fever, abdominal cramps and pain, vomiting and diarrhoea. Initially the stools are loose and yellow-green but later, mucus, pus and blood are passed. Young children may present with febrile convulsions and signs of meningeal irritation.

A very severe form of infection with *Sh. shigae*, (subtype of *Sh. dysenteriae*) may produce gangrene of the colon and prove rapidly fatal.

When diarrhoea is the main symptom, the illness can be distinguished from salmonellosis, *E. coli* enteritis and staphylococcal food poisoning by culturing the stools.

The most important aspects of treatment are the early recognition and correction of dehydration and shock and restoration of fluid and electrolyte balance. In severe systemic infection with *Sh. dysenteriae* and *Sh. flexneri* subtypes, co-trimoxazole should be administered for 5–7 days. Control of cross-infection is necessary.

Salmonellosis

Salmonellae are motile, non-lactose fermenting Gram-negative bacilli; there are more than 1000 species. *Salmonella typhi*, *S. paratyphi A* and *S. paratyphi B* cause typhoid or enteric fever while the other species are associated with food poisoning. These pathogens are heat sensitive.

Food poisoning results when frozen poultry and meat are not completely thawed before cooking.

Typhoid fever

Typhoid fever reported in the UK is an imported disease, 80–85% of cases having acquired the infection in the Indian subcontinent and the Mediterranean. Around one-half of cases occur in children, mainly from immigrant households who have visited the Indian subcontinent.

The infection is usually acquired from food and drink contaminated by a human carrier. *Salmonella typhi* invades the mucous membranes and Peyer's patches of the upper small intestine to enter the reticuloendothelial system and blood, producing bacteraemia. Fever is high and persistent associated with delirium, the temperature seldom returning to normal. The child has anorexia, vomiting and diarrhoea. Headache is a frequent complaint and signs of meningeal irritation are present in some cases. A palpable spleen is almost always found in typhoid fever. Complications are rare if treatment is instituted early, but may include toxic myocarditis, detectable by electrocardiography, and perforation and haemorrhage in the small intestine. Leucopenia is present in 25% and thrombocytopenia in 15% of patients. Although typhoid fever is a major illness, some untreated cases may resolve spontaneously.

Laboratory diagnosis of typhoid fever depends upon culture of *S. typhi*, *S. paratyphi* A or B from blood and stools. Serology is of limited value because the Widal reaction is useful in patients not normally resident in typhoid endemic areas who have not been given TAB vaccine. A rise in O antigen titre suggests an active infection but a rise in H antigen titre suggests previous infection or immunisation.

Management consists of symptomatic treatment of fever and the use of antimicrobial agents, namely, chloramphenicol (50 mg/kg daily), co-trimoxazole, or amoxycillin (100 mg/kg daily) for up to 3 weeks. In a large series from Durban, amoxycillin was found to be superior to chloramphenicol because there was no recurrence of fever, no persistent carriers and only 2% failure of response in African children.

It is important to realise the association between schistosomiasis and persistent salmonella infection in children from the tropics. Salmonellae reside in the integumen of schistosomes but will be eradicated with treatment for schistosomiasis. There is also a high frequency of salmonella osteomyelitis in West African children with sickle cell disease, probably due to tissue hypoxia from thrombotic crises.

Viral haemorrhagic fevers

The media have drawn attention to the hazards of Lassa fever, Marburg and Ebola virus diseases being imported from Africa. The high mortality and infectivity of these diseases have prompted the establishment of high security isolation units in England which have very rarely been used. In fact, these exotic diseases are exceedingly rarely encountered in the UK when compared with cases of imported malaria, tuberculosis and typhoid. Fever and rash, often haemorrhagic, are features of these diseases and dengue haemorrhagic fever which is a major public health problem affecting children in South-east Asia. These diseases should be suspected in children with fever who have recently arrived from endemic areas. However, it is important that malaria and typhoid be excluded by blood examination.

INHERITED DISORDERS

There are three major genetic disorders involving the red cell prevalent in the tropics and subtropics: thalassaemias, haemoglobinopathies and glucose-6-phosphate-dehydrogenase (G6PD) deficiency (see p. 360). These inherited disorders are found in Africa, South-east Asia, the Mediterranean and Middle East, and wherever there are migrants from these areas, e.g. the Caribbean, the Americas, Australia and Europe. The world distribution of these genetic conditions is similar to that of endemic malaria, past or present. It is postulated that the prevalence of these genes is related to the advantage endowed to heterozygous carriers to cope successfully with *P. falciparum* malaria. Evidence from epidemiological and clinical research favour this postulate in heterozygous carriers of sickle cell haemoglobin (HbS). However, homozygous subjects appear to have a distinct disadvantage when exposed to infections, drugs and other environmental factors.

Thalassaemia

Thalassaemia is a genetically determined anaemia found in Cypriots, Indians, Arabs, Vietnamese and Chinese. It is an inherited disorder of haemoglobin synthesis in which there is a reduction in the rate of synthesis of one globin chain and an excess of the partner chain produced at the normal rate. The chain produced in excess precipitates in the bone marrow and erythrocytes causing ineffective erythropoiesis, decreased red-cell survival and chronic anaemia. There are two main types of thalassaemia: α-thalassaemia and β-thalassaemia, both inherited in an autosomal recessive manner.

Homozygous β-thalassaemia

This is a severe anaemia in children who die unless frequent blood transfusions are given. Although affected infants are normal at birth, anaemia of insidious onset is obvious after the third month together with poor feeding, pallor and splenomegaly. There is stunting of growth and hyperplasia of the maxillae resulting in a characteristic appearance, the thalassaemia facies (Fig. 28.4). Regular blood transfusions are needed but these and the increased intestinal iron absorption lead to haemosiderosis and death from cardiac failure in the second and third decades. This dismal outlook has been modified by early diagnosis and the regular use of iron chelating agents. The blood pictures resembles iron deficiency anaemia but with many target cells, tear-drop cells and red cell fragments. Fetal haemoglobin (HbF) concentrations are increased (10–90%). The basis of treatment is the correction of anaemia without inducing iron overload. The haemoglobin concentration should be raised to the normal range and maintained by blood transfusions. Excess iron is removed by desferrioxamine 25–50 mg/kg administered by overnight subcutaneous infusion with a syringe pump. Ascorbic acid is given to enhance the action of desferrioxamine. Young children have been maintained in negative iron balance by this method. Most of the 30 000

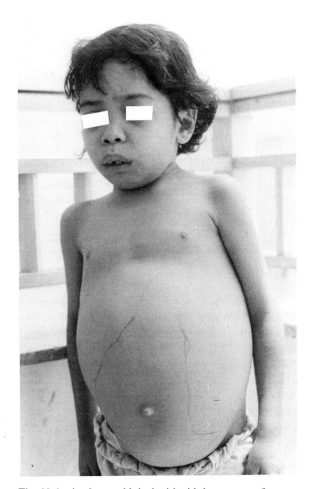

Fig. 28.4 An 8-year-old Arab girl with homozygous β thalassaemia. She has gross hepatosplenomegaly and hypertrophy of the maxillae (producing the thalassaemia facies) as a result of chronic anaemia.

children with thalassaemia born each year live in Asia and the Middle East where subcutaneous treatment is neither practical nor affordable. For them less expensive oral iron chelating drugs would be most helpful. Three groups of oral agents are currently being assessed: pyridoxal isonicotinoyl hydrazone, the hydroxypyridones, and a polyanionic amine N,N'-bis (2 hydroxybenzoyl) ethylenediamine N,N'-diacetic acid. Only one has been used in humans, 1,2-dimethyl-3-hydroxypyrid-4-one, and its efficacy is similar to parenteral desferrioxamine at daily dosages of 40–100 mg/kg.

Haemoglobin H

This disease is a form of α-thalassaemia prevalent in some Mediterranean countries and South-east Asia. Most subjects have moderate anaemia (haemoglobin 8–9 g/dl), splenomegaly and a normal life expectancy. Anaemia may be severe during infection, pregnancy or from haemolysis induced by oxidant drugs e.g. sulphonamides. The red cells are hypochromic and microcytic with fragmentation, basophilic stippling and target cells. The mean cell volume (MCV) and mean cell haemoglobin (MCH) are low. On incubation of the red cells with brilliant cresyl blue for 30 minutes, numerous HbH inclusion bodies are visible.

Haemoglobinopathies

A haemoglobinopathy is a structural haemoglobin variant resulting from substitution of an amino acid in one of the globin chains, e.g. HbS (sickle cell haemoglobin), in which glutamic acid is replaced by valine in position 6 of the β chain. Haemoglobinopathies are transmitted by autosomal recessive inheritance; the parents are heterozygous (HbAS) and the affected child is homozygous (HbSS).

Sickle cell disease

Sickle cell disease occurs in the homozygous individual (HbSS) who does not possess any normal adult haemoglobin (HbA). Sickling or polymerisation of HbS molecules into filaments occurs when the erythrocyte is deoxygenated. Anaemia is obvious in the 6-month-old infant in whom fetal haemoglobin concentration is declining and insufficient to protect red cells from sickling. Other clinical features in infancy include dactylitis, pneumococcal infections and anaemic crisis from acute splenic sequestration (sudden splenic enlargement and circulatory collapse). The latter two complications contribute to a mortality rate of 10% in Jamaican infants with sickle cell anaemia. Older children suffer vaso-occlusive crises consisting of sudden onset of bone pain in the limbs, joints, spine and chest, or abdominal pain accompanied by nausea and vomiting. The child will resent examination of the affected part because of pain. Symptoms are due to ischaemia and may last from hours to days. Infection (particularly malaria) is often a precipitating factor, with accompanying fever, dehydration and tachycardia. Aplastic crises are serious, occurring when marrow erythropoiesis suddenly ceases, and are related to parvoviral infections or folate deficiency. Severe anaemia develops rapidly to precipitate life-threatening cardiac failure.

Diagnosis of sickle cell disease depends on identifying sickle cells on blood film and electrophoresis of haemoglobin which shows the presence of HbS and absence of HbA.

Prompt treatment of any infection or fever is most important in the prevention of vaso-occlusive crises. The child with pain should be given bed rest, hydration, analgesics and antimicrobial agents. Blood transfusion is required in the presence of severe anaemia. Folic acid supplements and prophylactic penicillin should be provided.

Prognosis is good in the UK. Symptoms tend to decrease as the child grows older. The disease is mild in Saudi Arabs and those who have high concentrations of fetal haemoglobin in adulthood.

Haemoglobin E

Haemoglobin E found mainly in South-east Asians is the next most frequent abnormal haemoglobin. The homozygous individual has mild anaemia (haemoglobin 9–10 g/dl), decreased red-cell lifespan and microcytosis. Anaemia may be marked in the presence of infection, pregnancy and nutritional deficiency.

Glucose-6-phosphate-dehydrogenase (G6PD) deficiency

More than 400 million people with glucose-6-phosphate-dehydrogenase deficiency are to be found in South-east Asia, the Mediterranean and Middle Eastern countries, Africa, the Caribbean, and wherever these peoples have emigrated. Deficiency of this red-cell enzyme is associated with neonatal hyperbilirubinaemia, acute haemolytic anaemia and chronic haemolytic disease.

The enzyme G6PD catalyses the conversion of glucose-6-phosphate to 6-phosphogluconate and the reduction of nicotinamide adenine dinucleotide (NADP) to NADPH. The latter participates in the production of reduced glutathione which protects the red-cell membrane from damage by oxidative free radicals (e.g. hydrogen peroxide). There are about 300 variants of the G6PD enzyme, with activity ranging from less than 10% to twice the normal level. Variants with moderate and severe enzyme deficiency are liable to haemolysis when exposed to drugs and chemicals (Table 28.4).

Neonatal hyperbilirubinaemia

Neonatal hyperbilirubinaemia due to G6PD deficiency has been observed in Chinese, Greek and African infants. Jaundice appears on the second day, usually in male infants (G6PD deficiency is an X-linked recessive inherited condition), and hyperbilirubinaemia is frequent on the third to fifth days but sometimes occurs in the second week in Chinese infants. Kernicterus develops rapidly, particularly in preterm infants and those with severe infections. Anaemia is variable and splenomegaly uncommon. Serum bilirubin concentration is usually high (350 μmol/l) and unconjugated. In the tropics serum bilirubin concentrations of 700 μmol/l have been recorded in infants on admission to hospital. There is a simple test for detecting G6PD enzyme using a few drops of blood and based on a colour change when NADP is converted to NADPH. Management of these severely jaundiced babies is with blood exchange transfusions and phototherapy. It is important to identify the agent which induced the haemolysis. In South-east Asia and West Africa, naphthalene in mothballs is usually responsible as it can be absorbed through the skin and lungs. Infants in contact with linen stored in naphthalene develop hyperbilirubinaemia rapidly leading to kernicterus and permanent neurological sequelae.

Acute haemolytic anaemia

This condition is precipitated when G6PD-deficient children are prescribed drugs or exposed to certain chemicals, listed in Table 28.4. Symptoms are similar to those of favism but the outcome is seldom fatal.

Table 28.4 Drugs and chemicals to be avoided in G6PD deficiency

Antimalarials:	primaquine, pamaquine, pentaquine
Sulphonamides:	sulphanilamide, sulphapyridine, sulphadimidine, sulphacetamide, salicylazosulphapyridine (Salazopyrin)
Sulphones:	diaphenylsulphone (dapsone)*, sulphoxone*, glucosulphone sodium (Promin), sulphamethoxazole (in cotrimoxazole)
Antibacterial agents:	nitrofurans — nitrofurantoin, furazolidone, nitrofurazone nalidixic acid
Antihelminthics:	niridazole, stibophan
Analgesics:	acetophenetidin (phenacetin), acetylsalicylic acid (asprin) in large doses.
Miscellaneous:	dimercaprol (BAL), phenylhydrazine*, arsine*, acetylphenylhydrazine*, probenecid, vitamin K water-soluble analogues
Chemicals:	naphthalene (mothballs)*, methylene blue, toluidine blue
Fava bean (*Vicia fava*)	

Note: G6PD deficiency is genetically heterogeneous; different genetic variants have different susceptibility to haemolytic risk from drugs. A drug found to be safe in some G6PD-deficient subjects may not be equally safe in others.
* These drugs and chemicals may cause haemolysis in normal individuals if given in large doses.

Favism is a disorder of young children, usually male, who suffer acute haemolysis following inhalation of the pollen or ingestion of the beans of *Vicia fava*. It has been recognised since antiquity in Greece and China, and is a serious complication of G6PD deficiency. There appears to be a familial predisposition as only some G6PD-deficient children develop favism while others are unaffected. Symptoms consist of headache, dizziness, nausea, vomiting, chills, fever, pallor and lumbar pain. Haemoglobinuria appears within a few hours followed by jaundice. A typical attack lasts for 2–6 days and deaths occur within the first 48 hours.

Anaemia is usually severe in acute haemolysis and renal failure is a potential complication.

Prevention of haemolysis

There is a case for screening newborn infants of susceptible genetic origin for G6PD enzyme and to give advice about the avoidance of potentially harmful drugs, chemicals and food to those who have G6PD deficiency.

MEDICAL ADVICE AND IMMUNISATIONS FOR TRAVEL TO THE TROPICS

Protection should be given against the major diseases of childhood prevalent in the tropics and subtropics, such as malaria, tuberculosis, poliomyelitis, tetanus, diphtheria, pertussis, measles and yellow fever.

Immunisations should be given as detailed in Table 28.5.

Table 28.5 Age of immunisation for some major childhood diseases

Vaccine	Age
BCG	Neonatal period onwards
Diphtheria/ pertussis tetanus (DPT)	First dose can be given at 2 months. Two further doses given at monthly intervals in the tropics.
Poliomyelitis	Both killed and live vaccines can be given simultaneously with DPT
Measles	9 months onwards
Yellow fever	After 9 months

Smallpox vaccination is no longer mandatory for travel abroad now that the disease has been eradicated worldwide. The vaccine causes complications in children with eczema and skin eruptions. Cholera and typhoid vaccinations are not recommended for infants.

Malaria chemoprophylaxis is essential when travelling to endemic areas (see p. 363).

Personal hygiene and health can be maintained by giving infants extra fluids in the tropics, boiling suspect water for drinking, avoiding bathing in infected rivers and pools and wearing shoes outside the house. A supply of disposable needles is recommended because of HIV and AIDS.

FURTHER READING

Black J 1985 The new paediatrics: child health in ethnic minorities. BMJ, London
Hendrickse R G (ed) 1981 Paediatrics in the tropics: current review. Oxford University Press. Oxford
Stanfield J P, Brueton M, Chan M C K, Parkin J M, Waterston A (eds) 1991 Diseases of children in the sub-tropics and tropics, 5th edn. Edward Arnold, London
WHO 1976 New trends and approaches in the delivery of maternal and child care in health services. 6th Report of the WHO Expert Committee on MCH. Technical Report Services 600. WHO, Geneva
WHO 1988 Vaccination certificate requirements and health advice for international travel. WHO, Geneva, p 50

29. Emergency procedures

M. Cummins

Acute medical emergencies are common in young children and may be caused by illness or accident. In 1987 accidents and injuries caused 20% of deaths in children aged 0–4 years, 31% in the 5–14-year-old age group and approximately 120 000 hospital admissions. Ill children should be transfered to hospital but medical assistance in the home, the clinic or at the site of an accident may be life-saving.

CARDIORESPIRATORY ARREST

The child appears blue or very pale; there are no respiratory movements, the carotid and femoral pulses are not palpable and the heart sounds are inaudible. Events preceding the cardiorespiratory arrest should be determined; a history of illness, drug intake, respiratory difficulty, blood loss or accident may be helpful in management.

Management

Prompt resuscitation is vital in order to maintain cerebral circulation (Table 29.1). This is ideally carried out by a team in a hospital setting but may need to be attempted anywhere. Equipment for paediatric resuscitation is listed in Table 29.2; the basic items should be kept in all family doctors' surgeries and childrens' clinics.

Establish ventilation

Lie the child on a hard flat surface. Suck out the mouth and pharynx. Pull the chin forwards by lifting the angle of the mandible and perform endotracheal intubation and positive pressure ventilation. Bag and mask ventilation using oxygen or

Table 29.1 Management of cardiorespiratory arrest

Cardiorespiratory arrest	— Lie flat — Clear airway

Ventilation	— Bag + mask + O_2
	  Endotracheal intubation +
	  IPPV + O_2
	  Mouth-to-mouth

Circulation	— External cardiac massage (4 compressions: 1 breath)
i.v. infusion	— Sodium bicarbonate (8.4% 2–3 ml/kg)
ECG monitor	— Drugs i.v. or intracardiac

Table 29.2 Equipment for management of cardiac arrest

Suction apparatus

Airway

Bag and mask, e.g. Ambubag, Penlon bag

Paediatric laryngoscope

Endotracheal tube with connections (sizes 3.0–7.5 mm)

Oxygen

ECG machine

Defibrillator

Intravenous cannulae sizes 18, 20, 22, FG

Paediatric infusion set

Cutdown pack

Infusion pump

air should however be sufficient. Chest wall movements will be visible if adequate ventilation is taking place. Tracheostomy is rarely needed, but may be necessary, for example, after foreign body inhalation or severe upper airways obstruction. Mouth-to-mouth ventilation must be used if no equipment is available. There is concern about the transmission of HIV infection with mouth-to-mouth, but the risk are thought to be slight and at present there are no recorded cases of infection transmitted in this way.

Restore circulation

External cardiac massage (ECM) should begin at once with rhythmic compression of the sternum at a rate of 60–100 per minute; the faster rate is used in infants. The pressure of two fingers on the lower sternum is sufficient in young infants. A palpable femoral pulse is a sign of adequate cardiac output. The rate of ECM to artificial ventilation is 4 to 1. An intravenous infusion of dextrose/saline or plasma should be started immediately. The antecubital fossa is often the easiest site for insertion of a cannula; the jugular and scalp vein sites may interfere with the giving of artificial respiration; if a cut-down is needed the long saphenous vein at the ankle, anterior to the medial malleolus, is the best site. Sodium bicarbonate (2–3 mmol/kg) is given to correct any metabolic acidaemia caused by inadequate peripheral circulation (Table 29.3); further alkali administration should be determined by blood gas status. In young children care must be taken not to give excessive volumes of fluid as this may cause circulatory overload.

If there is evidence of serious blood loss or severe dehydration then plasma (10–20 ml/kg) or blood should be given to restore blood volume.

Drugs

Drugs (Table 29.3) should be given intravenously or if necessary intracardiac, there is no place for

Table 29.3 Drugs which may be used during resuscitation at cardiac arrest

Sodium bicarbonate 8.4%	— 2–3 ml/kg (2–3 mmol/kg)
Adrenaline 1:10 000	— 0.1–0.2 ml/kg (1 ml/year up to 10/ml)
Calcium gluconate 10%	— 0.1–0.2 ml/kg (1 ml/year up to 10 ml)
Lignocaine	— 0.5–4 mg/kg dose (then continuous infusion at 0.5–3 mg/kg/hour)
Dopamine	— 5–20 µg/kg/min

intramuscular administration. An ECG machine should have been attached so that any arrhythmia may be identified and treatment monitored. Adrenaline and calcium gluconate are useful for asystole; if there is ventricular fibrillation a DC shock starting at 10 J/s (or 2 J/s/kg) is given; with ventricular tachycardia lignocaine can be tried, while dopamine or isoprenaline infusions are used to maintain circulation and restore blood pressure.

PROLONGED CONVULSIONS

Convulsions, particularly those precipitated by fever, are common in childhood.

The child should be laid semi-prone to maintain a clear airway. It is not necessary to place anything between the teeth. Remember the risk of aspiration if there is vomiting.

Prolonged fits may lead to cerebral oedema and thus be self-perpetuating. Anticonvulsant treatment is therefore urgent, while tepid sponging should be given if there is a high fever.

Drug management outside hospital

Rectal diazepam or intramuscular paraldehyde are the safest and most appropriate anticonvulsant drugs. Rectal diazepam is well absorbed and can be given by a syringe without a needle in a dosage of 0.6–0.8 mg/kg. A repeat dose may be necessary. Paraldehyde (0.2 ml/kg) is given by deep intramuscular injection; although a glass syringe is often used, a plastic syringe can be used if the solution is in the syringe for only a very short while. If the convulsion does not stop the child should immediately be transferred to hospital.

Drug management in hospital

Bolus intravenous diazepam (0.3 mg/kg) can be tried; there is a danger of respiratory depression if large doses are used. Intramuscular diazepam is ineffective. If the convulsion persists a diazepam infusion (0.04 mg/kg/h) may be given. Intravenous phenytoin, phenobarbitone, chlormethiazole or induction of anaesthesia are alternatives in persistent epilepticus.

Advice for parents of children who have recurrent febrile convulsions

If the child develops a high fever but has not yet had a convulsion a tepid sponge with lukewarm water and an appropriate dose of a medicine to reduce the fever (paracetamol elixir or suppository) are used. Administration of rectal diazepam can be taught to parents and should be used if they feel there is an impending convulsion or during a convulsion. Should a fit occur the child should be laid on his side in the semi-prone position and the airway cleared, and medical attention should be sought urgently if the convulsion does not stop within 5 minutes. The GP should be told about the fit whether or not it stops quickly.

UPPER AIRWAYS OBSTRUCTION

The common causes in childhood include laryngotracheobronchitis, croup, epiglottitis, foreign body inhalation, pharyngeal oedema due to allergy, burns or trauma and retropharyngeal abscess. The clinical features are inspiratory stridor, signs of respiratory distress, drooling and sitting forward, cyanosis, drowsiness and respiratory arrest.

In severe cases transfer to hospital is urgent; the doctor should accompany the child and give oxygen if necessary. *The throat must not be examined* unless there is an anaesthetist and resuscitation equipment available as respiratory obstruction may be precipitated.

When obstruction is severe it must be bypassed. This should be carried out by an experienced anaesthetist or surgeon; appropriate endotracheal intubation under general anaesthesia is used but tracheostomy may be necessary. In extreme cases of emergency and when experienced staff are not available a large bore canula (size 14 Medicut) can be inserted safely into the trachea in the midline just below the thyroid cartilage.

SHOCK

This is a clinical syndrome resulting from poor tissue perfusion. Shock may become irreversible and prove fatal even though the underlying cause is corrected. Clinical features include pale, cold skin, poor capillary return, hypotension, tachycardia and tachypnoea. There is initial agitation followed by progressive confusion and coma. Causes of shock include hypovolaemia due to haemorrhage or burns, dehydration from gastroenteritis or diabetic ketoacidosis, septicaemia (from meningococcus, staphylococcus or Gram-negative organisms), meningitis, peritonitis, cardiogenic conditions (e.g. myocarditis, paroxysmal arrhythmia, cardiac tamponade), anaphylaxis, neurogenic agents (e.g. overdose of hypnotics, tranquillisers or anaesthetic agents, or spinal cord injuries), adrenocortical insufficiency (e.g. congenital adrenal hyperplasia), poisoning particularly with salicylates or iron, or respiratory disease causing profound hypoxia (e.g. epiglottitis, staphylococcal pneumonia).

Immediate treatment

1. Lie the child flat.
2. Establish an airway.
3. Endotracheal intubation where appropriate with intermittent positive-pressure ventilation.
4. Oxygen.
5. Elevate the legs except when the cause is respiratory in origin.
6. Start an intravenous infusion; a cut-down may be necessary, administer normal saline or plasma up to 20 ml/kg.
7. Monitor the central venous pressure.
8. Catheterise the bladder.
9. Nurse in intensive care area.
10. Treat underlying cause.
11. Monitor therapy.

Anaphylactic shock

This is an extreme form of allergy causing respiratory distress and circulatory collapse. The offending antigen leads to the release of histamine and related substances resulting in increased capillary permeability and bronchial constriction. Common causes include drugs (e.g. penicillin or anaesthetics), injections (e.g. desensitisation material, radiological contrast media), immunisations, incompatible blood transfusions and insect stings.

Clinical features include erythema, urticaria, itching, angioneurotic oedema, sweating, vomiting, diarrhoea, colicky abdominal pain and cough. Bronchospasm, laryngeal oedema and cardiac arrest may follow.

Management

Remove the suspected agent. Apply a tourniquet above the local site. Adrenaline (0.01 ml/kg of 1:1000 strength to a maximum of 0.5 ml) can be given subcutaneously, together with intravenous or intramuscular antihistamine (0.25 mg/kg of chlorpheniramine or 0.5 mg/kg of promethazine).

In life-threatening situations with circulatory collapse ensure an adequate airway, give oxygen, give adrenaline intravenously (0.01 ml/kg of 1:1000, maximum 0.5 ml or 0.1 ml/kg of 1:10 000, maximum 5 ml) and give plasma expander (20 ml/kg) or saline intravenously. Aminophylline (4 mg/kg) by slow intravenous injection is used for bronchospasm, while intravenous hydrocortisone (50–100 mg) is given if there is a poor response or laryngeal oedema.

HYPOGLYCAEMIA

Hypoglycaemia is most frequently a problem in diabetic children on insulin, but may occur in salicylate, alcohol or oral hypoglycaemic poisoning. Spontaneous hypoglycaemia occurs in glycogen storage disease, ketotic hypoglycaemia, adrenocortical insufficiency, hypopituitarism, prediabetes or if there is excess insulin production such as by an islet cell tumour.

Hypoglycaemia is defined as a blood glucose concentration less than 2.2 mmol/l. Early symptoms include headaches, dizziness, pallor, sweating and associated irritability and mood changes; nightmares may occur. Profound hypoglycaemia causes drowsiness, coma and convulsions.

Mild attacks respond to oral glucose in the form of glucose tablet, sweets, sugar lumps or a sugary drink. All diabetics should have some form of glucose available at all times. If there is impairment of consciousness then the ideal treatment is an intravenous infusion of 10% dextrose (5 ml/kg, 0.5 g/kg) as a bolus, followed by a slow infusion. Stronger glucose solutions are available, but should never exceed 20%. Outside hospital, an in-

tramuscular injection of glucagon (1 mg) should reverse hypoglycaemia.

BURNS

Burns are common in toddlers, usually as a result of domestic accidents. They produce about 40 000 attendances annually in accident and emergency departments. The classification, clinical features and common causes of burns are shown in Tables 29.4 and 29.5. If more than 10% of the body surface area is involved with second or third degree burns then shock may ensue from fluid loss.

Burns are sometimes due to non-accidental injury, but more often are related to overcrowded, disorganised or careless management of the child. Appropriate investigation of the circumstances is necessary and help given to the family.

First aid measures

If there is only involvement of small areas of skin,

Table 29.4   Classification of burns

Type	Skin layers involved	Features	Common causes
First degree	Superficial epidermis	Erythema Pain	Scalds Sunburn
Second degree	Entire epidermis	Erythema Pain Blistered and moist areas	Scalds Contact with hot objects
Third degree	Entire dermis including nerve endings ± underlying tissue	Dry lesion White or charred painless	Open flames Chemicals Electricity Steam

Table 29.5   Percentage surface area of different parts of the body

	Surface area (%)		
	1 year	3 years	10 years
Head	17	15	9
Trunk	36	36	36
Both arms	16	16	18
Both legs	30	32	36
Genitalia	1	1	1

the affected area may be immersed in cold water. It should then be covered with a sterile, but non-adhesive, dressing and bandaged. The dressing should be changed after 48 hours.

Chemical burns, particularly those involving the eye, must be thoroughly irrigated with water; clothes and all traces of the offending agent should be removed.

For all other types and more extensive burns the affected area may be immediately cooled by immersion in cold water, blisters should be left intact and clothes should not be removed. The burns should then be covered with a clean sheet and the child transferred to hospital for assessment.

Burns involving the eye or mouth, genitalia, hands and feet should receive specialist attention even when only a small area is involved.

Emergency hospital management

Maintain the airway; any burn involving the mouth or neck may produce oedema and respiratory obstruction. Emergency intubation or tracheostomy may be needed. If more than 10% of the body surface is involved intravenous fluids will be required to prevent shock from fluid loss. Plasma should be given (10 ml/kg), half in the first 8 hours and the other half during the following 12 hours. Maintenance fluids should also be given.

Packed cell volume, blood urea, electrolytes, blood group and urine specific gravity should be monitored serially. A urinary catheter may be needed to monitor urinary output. Some form of analgesia is usually required for the first 48 hours; intravenous pethidine (0.5 mg/kg) may be needed.

The child is barrier nursed in a warm cubicle lying on sterile towels with the burn exposed until it has dried. Alternatively Flamazine may be applied to the affected areas and covered with dressings. This assists in pain relief. Dressings should be reapplied after a maximum of 48 hours using appropriate analgesia. Antibiotics are not usually necessary unless there is evidence of secondary infection.

The parents will need help and support because of the anxiety and long-term management often required; plastic surgeons must be consulted early.

DEHYDRATION

In the UK and worldwide the commonest cause of dehydration in childhood is gastroenteritis. Dehydration may be classified as hypotonic, isotonic or hypertonic depending on the proportion of water and electrolyte lost and the blood sodium measurement. The physical signs become increasingly obvious as the severity increases (Tables 29.6, 29.7)

Table 29.6 Features of different types of dehydration

	Hypernatraemic dehydration	Isotonic dehydration	Hypotonic dehydration
Plasma Na (mmol/l)	>150	130–150	n130
Losses	Na<H_2O	Na = H_2O	Na>H_2O
Skin texture	Rubbery + thick	Reduced elasticity	Reduced elasticity
Skin colour	Grey	Grey	Grey
Anterior fontanelle	Depressed	Depressed	Very depressed
Pulse	Rapid	Rapid	Rapid
Blood pressure	Normal until late in illness	Low	Very low
Sunken eyes	Not obvious	Present	Present
Convulsions	Yes	No	±
Replace fluid deficit	Slowly + steadily over 48 hours	$\frac{1}{3}$ in 4 hours, $\frac{2}{3}$ in next 16 hours	$\frac{1}{3}$ in 4–6 hours, $\frac{2}{3}$ in next 16 hours
Type of fluid	0.45% saline with 2.5% glucose	0.45% saline or 4% dextrose/physiological saline	0.9% (normal) saline with 5% dextrose

Table 29.7   Fluid replacement in dehydration

	Mild	Moderate	Severe
Degree of dehydration	5%	10%	15%
Loss (ml/kg body weight)	50	100	150
Rehydration	Oral	Intravenous	Intravenous
Replacement volume	Maintenance + 50 ml/kg	Maintenance + 100 ml/kg	Plasma 20 ml/kg then maintenance + 150 ml/kg

Management outside hospital

Mild gastroenteritis can be treated with oral, clear electrolyte-containing (about 50 mmol sodium/l e.g. Dioralyte), solutions of flat Coca-Cola or lemonade. Older children who show evidence of 5% dehydration may be treated at home as long as they are able to take fluid by mouth and are carefully monitored; dehydration, however, may appear rapidly in infancy, and babies with diarrhoea and vomiting may require admission to hospital even if there is no overt evidence of dehydration. Even a single diarrhoea stool can cause dehydration; it must be remembered also that liquid stool in a baby can be mistaken for urine. Hypernatraemia is a problem of the first year of life; many of the signs of dehydration appear late in the illness because of the relative preservation of the intravascular compartment. Fortunately, it is now uncommon, because of the low solute milks which are used for babies and the popularity of breast feeding.

Management in hospital

Clinical assessment; check weight against recent known weights; monitor blood electrolytes, haematocrit and urine specific gravity. Send appropriate bacteriology including blood culture.

With 10% dehydration or persistent vomiting intravenous rehydration is required; plasma (20 ml/kg) or saline should be given initially if there is evidence of shock. Rehydration is based on the extent of dehydration, type of dehydration (as indicated by blood electrolytes), age and weight, maintenance requirements (Table 29.8), and whether fluid losses continue.

Table 29.8   Maintenance fluid requirements at different ages

Age	Volume
1 week–6 months	150
6 months–1 year	120
1–2 years	100
2–4 years	90
4–8 years	80
8–12 years	70
over 12 years	60

POISONING

In England and Wales in 1987 there were 7 child deaths caused by the ingestion of drugs and other poisonous substances (excluding carbon monoxide). About 80 000 children attend accident and emergency departments annually due to poisoning or suspected poisoning. Accidental poisoning is common in young children (less than 4 years old) but is rare among older children of normal intelligence. Intentional drug overdose becomes more common at puberty.

Loss of consciousness or odd behaviour may be presenting symptoms and poison must always be considered in the differential diagnosis of such problems. Young children, fortunately, spill more poison than they swallow. Most deaths, however, occur in the young age group. Poisoning often occurs during periods of domestic upheaval (e.g. moving house, family illness, pregnancy), or in disorganised families where poisons are unwisely left within the reach of toddlers. All parents should be counselled about the risk of poisons when discussing childhood safety and hazards.

Management

Maintain the airway; if there is any sign of respiratory difficulty endotracheal intubation and assisted ventilation may be necessary.

The general condition of the child should be assessed with special attention to the level consciousness, adequacy of respiration, blood pressure and other vital signs. If blood pressure is low or consciousness is impaired an intravenous infusion should be started. Local effects of corrosive poisons may be evident from burns on the mouth or skin or there may be signs of systemic effects of an ingested agent. Examples include pinpoint pupils due to barbiturates, cardiac dysrhythmias due to tricyclic antidepressants, hyperventilation due to salicylate overdosage, and dilated pupils, flushed skin and tachycardia due to atropine-like substances. The nature and time of ingestion are important clinical details. Careful enquiry into circumstances surrounding the poisoning should also be made.

Identification of the poison is important. A MIMS colour identification chart, which should be kept in all casualty departments, may give a clue. The regional poison centre should be consulted regarding contents of mixtures, toxicity of substances and also for information about treatment.

Removal of poison should be induced if the child is fully conscious and the substance is not corrosive or oily. Ipecachuana syrup (15 ml) is given with a drink and usually produces vomiting within 20 minutes. The dose may be repeated if this fails. Gastric lavage is usually reserved for children who have ingested iron-containing medicines, but may also be used when there is a large overdose of drugs. The contraindications to gastric lavage are as with ipecachuana emesis; lavage may be carried out in an intubated child who has a cuffed endotracheal tube in situ. Haemoperfusion and dialysis my be required with certain toxic drugs:

1. Barbiturates.
2. Ethchlorvynol.
3. Glutethimide.
4. Meprobamate.
5. Methaqualone.
6. Salicylates.

7. Chloral hydrate (trichlaethanol derivative).
8. Theophylline.

Forced alkaline diuresis may be of use if phenobarbitone, barbitone or salicylates have been ingested; this should, however, be used with caution in young children because of the risk of metabolic upset. Specific antidotes (Table 29.9) may be available.

Hospital observation is advisable even if there are no apparent ill effects; 6-hourly observation is adequate in most cases. Blood levels of drugs such as paracetamol, salicylate and barbiturates together with blood biochemistry should be estimated. If poisoning is suspected, but is not proven, urine should be sent to the local poisons centre for chromatography testing in order to confirm the diagnosis.

Poisoning with specific agents

Paracetamol

Paracetamol may cause hepatic necrosis; more than 150 mg/kg may cause severe but often reversible liver damage, over 300 mg/kg may cause irreversible liver necrosis and has a high mortality.

Clinical features include on day one, vomiting, on day one to two, abdominal pain, increased serum bilirubin, aspartate transaminase and prothrombin time, progressing to hepatic failure with jaundice, encephalopathy and acute renal failure on days two to seven.

Management. Induce emesis, give methionine, or N-acetyl cystine, give vitamin K if the prothrombin time is prolonged, treat any hepatic failure and provide supportive care. Methionine or N-acetyl cystine will prevent irreversible hepatic

Table 29.9   Specific antidotes for certain poisons

Poison	Antidote
Carbon monoxide	Oxygen
Opiate (morphine, pethidine, dextropropoxyphene (Distalgesic)	Naloxone
Cyanide	Cobalt
Paracetamol	Methionine
Thallium	Prussian Blue

damage by paracetamol if given within 12 hours of ingestion. The likelihood of damage can be predicted from plasma paracetamol levels; if the plasma paracetamol level is above the line joining 200 mg/l at 4 hours and 70 mg/l at 12 hours after ingestion, then the following agents should be given over a 4-hour period: Methionine 2.5 g orally every 4 hours to a total of 10 g, or N-acetyl cystine 150 mg/kg i.v. over 15 minutes, then 50 mg/kg in the next 4 hours, and 100 mg/kg over the following 16 hours. Intravenous glucose should be given (as 5% dextrose initially) in order to prevent hypoglycaemia. Paracetamol overdosage should not be regarded lightly.

Dextropropoxyphene

This substance is usually in a combination with paracetamol (e.g. Distalgesic). The signs are similar to those of opium poisoning, pinpoint pupils, depressed respiration and loss of consciousness. Respiratory failure may occur rapidly, naloxone (0.005–0.01 mg/kg intravenously or intramuscularly) will specifically reverse the effects. The response should be immediate.

Salicylates

Salicylate poisoning in children has become less common. Their availability has been reduced as salicylates are no longer recommended for children under 12 years old because of the risk of Reye's syndrome. Methyl salicylate or oil of wintergreen is highly dangerous; about 4 ml be fatal for infants. The therapeutic administration of salicylate to sick children may cause poisoning because of cumulative effects. Infants are as a rule more susceptible, with the same blood level, to toxic effects than older children. A blood level greater than 30 mg/100 ml (2.2 μmol/l) suggests moderate or severe poisoning.

The clinical features include epigastric pains, nausea and vomiting, pyrexia, sweating, tremor, hyperventilation, oedema and dehydration. The laboratory data includes hyperkalaemia, hypernatraemia or hyponatraemia, respiratory alkalosis, metabolic acidosis (though not in young children), hyperglycaemia, hypoglycaemia and hypoprothrombinaemia.

Management. Up to 12 hours after ingestion induce emesis; an intravenous infusion should be started if the blood salicylate level is greater than 30 mg/dl or there are signs or symptoms as above. Blood salicylate level, electrolytes, glucose, prothrombin time and blood gases should be monitored and any electrolyte, acid-base or blood glucose imbalance treated. Vitamin K should be given. Alkaline diuresis may be used in adolescents while haemoperfusion and dialysis may be required in severe cases (salicylate level greater than 90 mg/dl, 6.6 μmol/l).

Barbiturates

These drugs cause respiratory depression, coma and hypotension. Induce emesis if the child is fully conscious; if drowsy observe in an intensive care area, artificial ventilation may be necessary. The barbiturate blood level confirms the diagnosis. Blood biochemistry should be monitored. Forced alkaline diuresis is useful in barbitone or phenobarbitone poisoning; haemodialysis may be required in severe cases.

Phenothiazines

This group includes chlorpromazine, perphenazine (Fentazin) and prochlorperazine (Stemetil); metoclopramide (Maxolon) is a related compound.

Clinical features include drowsiness, facial grimacing, oculogyric crisis, rigidity, tremor and hypotension.

Management is by symptomatic support; induce emesis, while dyskinesia can be treated with benztropine (Cogentin) 0.03 mg/kg i.v.

Belladonna alkaloids

Atropine, deadly nightshade and lomotil are in this group. A dry mouth and skin, flushing, fever, tachycardia and dilated pupils are seen. Lomotil causes small pupils.

Management is by inducing emesis, symptomatic care and giving naloxone (0.02 mg/kg).

Tricyclic antidepressants

These drugs are now the commonest cause of

death by accidental poisoning in young children; ingestion of more than 10 mg/kg will cause severe symptoms, while more than 20 mg/kg may be fatal.

The major toxic effects are on the cardiovascular (CVS) and central nervous systems (CNS). The drugs are believed to act by blocking re-uptake of noradrenaline and 5-hydroxytryptamine in neurones and by blocking the parasympathetic nervous system (PNS) and peripheral uptake of noradrenaline, plus a quinidine-like action on the heart.

The clinical features include:

1. CVS — all forms of arrhythmia plus hypotension.

2. CNS — hallucinations, convulsions, pyramidal and extrapyramidal signs, coma.

3. PNS — dry mouth, blurred vision, dilated pupils, retention of urine, pyrexia.

4. Respiratory system — respiratory depression, apnoea.

Management. Up to 12 hours after ingestion emesis is induced if the child is fully conscious. The cardiac rhythm, blood gas status and biochemistry should be monitored. Hypoxia and acidosis (these potentiate arrhythmias) and hypovolaemia should be treated. Dopamine is used if hypotension persists without arrhythmia; arrhythmias should be treated after correction of acidosis. Physostigmine (0.5 mg) may be given by slow intravenous infusion in prolonged coma but may cause convulsions or bradycardia.

Iron

Iron tablets are commonly eaten by toddlers when their mothers are pregnant; as few as three ferrous sulphate tablets may be fatal. Serum iron levels greater than 90 μmol/l indicate severe poisoning.

Clinical features include vomiting, gastrointestinal haemorrhage (gastric mucosal necrosis), hypotension if bleeding is severe and grey stools or melaena; after 24 hours encephalopathy (convulsions, coma), metabolic acidosis, renal failure and pulmonary oedema occur, while hepatic necrosis may develop later.

Management. Intramuscular desferrioxamine (1 g) as a chelating agent, gastric lavage with 1%

sodium bicarbonate solution and 5 g of oral desferrioxamine. The serum iron level should be monitored. If there are symptoms or a serum iron level greater than 90 μmol/l then intravenous infusion of desferrioxamine (15 mg/kg every 4 hours, up to 80 mg/kg total) is given. Desferrioxamine may cause hypotension if given too fast.

Button batteries containing mercury

These batteries are easily swallowed by young children and can cause severe caustic injury to the upper gastrointestinal tract. Some makes contain a lethal quantity of mercury for a child. Exhausted batteries are thought to be less toxic than new ones.

Management. Identify brand and type of battery and ask local poisons centre for information. X-ray the chest and abdomen with straight and lateral films: if the battery is lodged in the oesophagus or is leaking it must be removed immediately. If in the stomach or beyond and the edge clear and intact on X-ray, then there is no indication for immediate operation. Give antacids, purgatives and metoclopramide. Check stools for presence of battery. Repeat X-rays after 24 hours. Arrange removal if still in stomach and signs of leakage. If intact in stomach, repeat films after another 24 hours and if the battery has still not passed through the pylorus arrange for removal.

Lead

Lead is a common environmental contaminant; poisoning is usually an insidious process resulting from repeated and often unsuspected exposure. In addition to clinically evident poisoning, it is now suggested that increased blood and tissue lead concentrations may be associated with behaviour disorder, lowered intelligence and minor neurological dysfunction.

Lead may be absorbed from the gut, lungs, and skin; it is bound to erythrocytes, redistributed to liver and kidney and finally excreted or is deposited in bones and teeth. Iron deficiency, common in toddlers, potentiates lead absorption from the gut.

Clinical features of lead excess include lassitude, colicky abdominal pain, constipation, pallor from anaemia and later impaired consciousness, convulsions and raised intracranial pressure. Blue lines in the gums and peripheral nerve palsies are rare. Blood lead levels are, in part, correlated with symptoms:

0–40 μg dl	0–2 μmol l — 'normal'
40–60 μg/dl	2–3 μmol l — asymptomatic
60–100 μg/dl	3–5 μmol/l — symptomatic
>100 μg dl	>5 mol/l — encephalopathy

Investigations may show hypochromic anaemia with normal serum iron, haemolytic anaemia, aminoaciduria and glycosuria, radiodense metaphyseal bands at growing ends of long bones and opaque material may be evident on abdominal X-ray. There may be evidence of raised intracranial pressure on skull X-ray and CT scan.

Management. The management of lead poisoning depends on symptoms: the source of lead intoxication should be identified (pica, old paint), supportive care should be given for convulsions and raised intracranial pressure, and chelating agents to lower the blood lead concentrations. The chelating agents are calcium versenate (calcium — EDTA, 1500 mg/m^2 daily i.v. or i.m.), dimercaprol (BAL, 500 mg/m^2 daily i.m.) and penicillamine (600 mg/m^2 daily orally or i.m.) As a rough guide penicillamine is adequate if the blood lead is 3–4 μmol.l (60–80 mg/dl), calcium versenate is used if there is a higher concentration. Remember the child may be returning home to re-exposure unless the cause is identified and removed.

Poisoning with household products

These substances are generally accidentally ingested by toddlers: most are surprisingly harmless but should nevertheless be kept locked safely out of reach. The National Poisons Information Service will provide details of toxicity and management.

Bleach

Bleach is 3–6% hypochlorite and causes burning sensation, vomiting and abdominal pain; it may produce pharyngeal and laryngeal oedema. Chlorine gas is produced in the stomach and may produce pulmonary oedema. Oral fluids should be encouraged if small amounts are ingested. Gastric lavage should be considered for large quantities.

Abrasive agents

These include oven cleaners (30% caustic soda), kettle descaler (formic acid), dishwashing machine powders (silicates and metasilicates), drain cleaners (caustic soda or sulphuric acid), car battery acid (concentrated sulphuric acid).
All cause ulceration and necrosis of the tissues they contact. Laryngeal oedema and gastric perforation may occur. Formic acid may cause acute renal failure. *Gastric lavage and emesis are contraindicated.* Contrast radiography then endoscopy should be performed if there is evidence of serious damage and laparotomy considered. Antibiotics and steroids should be given for severe cases

Cleaning products containing surfactants

These include carpet shampoo, dishwashing liquid, fabric conditioner, washing powder, general purpose household cleaners, scouring liquids, creams and powders.

Effects include skin irritation, vomiting and diarrhoea. Liberal fluids are given by mouth with demulcent (milk or antacid preparation).

Lavatory cleaners

These contain paradichlorobenzene which causes vomiting and diarrhoea. Purgation is necessary if more than 1 g is ingested.

Disinfectants

Disinfectants may consist of up to 40% isopropyl alcohol (double the potency of ethyl alcohol). They cause local irritation, depression of respiration, drowsiness, stupor and coma; 100 ml of isopropyl alcohol can be fatal in adults. Haemodialysis can be used in severe cases.

Ethyl alcohol poisoning

Ethyl alcohol is contained in many cosmetics as well as beverages. It is rapidly absorbed through the gastric mucosa. It is a nervous system depressant and causes hypoglycaemia by inhibiting gluconeogenesis.

Blood alcohol level and glucose should be measured and emesis induced if the child is fully conscious; if drowsy, an intravenous infusion of 10% dextrose should be started. The blood glucose should be monitored and corrected if required; naloxone may improve the level of consciousness, while haemodialysis and haemoperfusion may be needed in severe cases.

Paraffin poisoning

The danger here is from pulmonary aspiration and severe chemical pneumonitis. Do not induce emesis or perform gastric lavage but rather treat symptomatically.

Solvent abuse

Glue and petrol sniffing are becoming major sociological problems; it usually occurs among male teenagers but even younger children are now involved. It causes drunken behaviour and may be suspected from typical smell on clothes and unexplained mood changes. Glue sniffing has relatively few complications but can cause neurological damage and occasional deaths, while petrol sniffing causes more chronic than acute problems but may cause coma and cardiac arrhythmias.

FURTHER READING

Alpert J J, Reece R (eds) 1979 Paediatric emergencies. Paediatric Clinics of North America 26: 4
Black J A 1979 Paediatric emergencies. Butterworths, London
Grosfield J L (ed) 1975 Childhood trauma. Pediatric Clinics of North America 22: 2
Gutgesell H P, Tacher W A, Geddes L A, Davis J S, Lie J T, McNamara D G 1976 Energy dose for ventricular defibrillation of children. Pediatrics 58: 898
Knusden F U 1979 Rectal administration of diazepam in solution in the acute treatment of convulsions in infants and children — anticonvulsants effect and side effects. Archives of Disease in Childhood 54: 855–857
Lissauer T 1980–81 Paediatric emergencies. Hospital Update (nos 6,7)
McLean W 1980 Child poisoning in England and Wales. Some statistics on admissions to hospital 1964–76. Health Trends 12: 9–12
Vale J A S, Meredith T J (eds) 1981 Poisoning. Update Books, London
Valman H B 1979 Accident and emergency paediatrics, 2nd edn. Blackwell Scientific, Oxford

30. Pharmacology

G. Rylance

Children receive drugs like any other age group but possibly less than the elderly. More than three-quarters of children admitted to hospital are given medicines of some kind, and of those seen outside hospital, more than 50% receive medicine in any 2-week period. Newborn infants receive medication infrequently; antenatally most have been exposed to some sort of clinical agent.

Children handle drugs differently from adults. There are differences between different ages, but also there is a large interindividual variation at the same age. Children are in a continuous state of physical and mental development; the changes are most involved, in the first few weeks and months of life. There is now less need to depend on adult data to supplement available information, as knowledge of paediatric pharmacology has improved. Children will always remain 'therapeutic orphans' to some extent, but this mainly arises from the necessity to test and assess new drugs in adults before using them in children. This time delay before drugs become available for use in children should not be long and all new drugs should be assessed in children at a relatively early stage in patient trials.

This chapter describes the pharmacological basis for a rational approach to paediatric prescribing and therapeutics.

DRUG HANDLING PROCESSES

Absorption, distribution and elimination (pharmacokinetics) are the processes which determine the time-dependent changes in serum concentration of drugs and their metabolites. Pharmacokinetics describe the fate of a drug from its administration to the achievement of a given concentration at recep-tor sites, and how long that concentration will remain there, or rather the rate of its decrease with time at these sites. A knowledge of pharmacokinetic parameters forms a basis for the rational use of drugs by specific dose and frequency regimen calculation.

Absorption

Absorption, or the entry of drug into the circulation, is essential before most drugs can act, although some drugs acting on the skin and those acting following inhalation need not necessarily be absorbed into the blood stream as such. The rate and extent of absorption depends on the route of administration, the physiochemical properties of the drug, such as pK_a, molecular weight and lipid solubility and the site and area of absorbing surfaces. It is necessary for solid drug forms to disintegrate before they can be dissolved and subsequently absorbed. Liquid preparations, which are frequently given to children and perhaps most appropriately for those under 5 years, tend to be absorbed at slightly faster rates than tablets or capsules, but the differences are not usually significant. If faster drug activity is required, the alternative of intravenous administration is now available for most drugs. Liquid preparations can be disadvantageous in that peak concentrations occur earlier and a fluctuation in concentration between doses is seen (see later). There does not seem to be any significant functional difference between older infants, children and adults in the gastrointestinal tract handling of drugs; the newborn baby, however, has an achlorhidric stomach with slow gastric emptying and intestinal transit time. There is a theoretical possibility that the prolonged contact with absorbing surfaces in the intestine may allow an increase in the amount of drug absorbed in newborns, although this does not seem to be clinically significant.

Absorption from intramuscular and subcutaneous sites depends mainly on tissue perfusion. When this is adequate, absorption is similar in children and adults. Differences between individuals depend more on the disease problem and how it affects tissue perfusion, rather than age. There does not seem to be any clinical delay in absorption of drugs as a result of vasomotor instability often seen in newborn infants.

There is evidence that some drugs can be absorbed through the skin; most drugs are, however, not absorbed to any significant extent. The absence of a stratum corneum in the first few weeks of life in preterm babies makes them at particular risk from toxicity arising from drugs intentionally or accidentally applied to the skin, but this fact also occasionally affords therapeutic possibilities for drug administration (see later).

The term 'systemic bioavailability' describes the rate and relative amount of drug that reaches the systemic circulation from a particular dosage form. More usually the term is applied to the amount of drug reaching the systemic circulation following administration at any site, compared to the amount of drug which is available in the circulation following intravenous administration. Bioavailability is usually expressed as a percentage, or as a decimal expression where 1=100%. It would be apparent, therefore, that bioavailability of most drugs administered topically will be low and generally at most in single figures of percentage or below 0.1 as a decimal. By definition, bioavailability of drugs administered intravenously will be 100% or 1. It is important to realise that the rate and extent of absorption is not always greater following administration intramuscularly, than following oral administration. There are many drugs where the rate and extent are similar and some (e.g. chloramphenicol, phenytoin, digoxin) where the rate, but not always the extent, will be greater after oral dosing. Different preparations of the same drug may vary considerably in their bioavailability and although this is not an argument for proprietary drug name prescribing as such, it is important to appreciate that drug effects due to differences in bioavailability may occur when one preparation of a drug is substituted for another.

Distribution

This is a process which regulates the amount of drug reaching specific body compartments or tissues and therefore the concentration of a drug at the receptor site. It is affected by tissue mass, fat content, membrane permeability, blood flow and the degree of protein binding, which all influence the extent and pattern of the distribution process.

Most drugs are bound to proteins in the circulation and are bound intracellularly, but they distribute freely through body water compartments. The relative proportions of these compartments vary with age through childhood. When expressed in relation to body weight, the largest volumes of total and extracellular water are found in the first few months of life and particularly in preterm babies at this time. The greatest change with age occurs in the extracellular water compartment, which is a major determinant of water-soluble drugs (Fig. 30.1).

Most drugs are water soluble and their distribution, which is mainly confined to the extracellular water compartment, is affected by the changes in body compartments. Water-soluble drugs therefore require to be given in larger weight-related doses in early infancy, and especially preterm babies, in order to reach similar concentrations to those in older children. Such doses for which the extent of distribution is the major function relate only to single doses and when drugs are given repeatedly, there are additional drug handling process considerations.

Although some drugs are fat soluble and the relative body fat content changes with age through childhood, it is not possible to be quite as specific in describing the effects of these changes on drug dose requirement.

The passage of drugs across biological membranes is an important part of the distribution process. It appears that the blood–brain barrier is more permeable in the newborn period, although the evidence for this is not specific. There may be an increase of drug passage into cerebral spinal

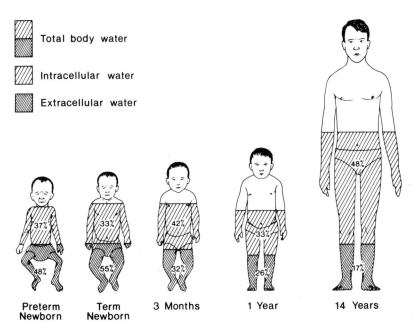

Fig. 30.1 Body fluid compartment proportions.

fluid and some drugs may reach particularly high concentrations in specific tissues, for example, digoxin in cardiac muscle. The degree of extra-cellular binding of drugs to plasma proteins, especially albumin, determines the amount of the pharmacologically active fraction (unbound) of each drug. The reduction in protein binding in the newborn, compared with older children and adults, results mainly from their low and qualitatively different plasma albumin, and is further modified by the displacement of drugs because of higher free fatty acid and bilirubin concentrations. Drug protein binding is lower in the newborn and perhaps infancy, but after 1 year of age, is similar to adults. Lower protein binding has been shown in the newborn for a number of drugs including phenobarbitone, phenytoin, salicylates, sulphonamides, diazoxide, phenylbutazone and ampicillin. It is not easy to predict the net effect of this increase in the pharmacologically active free fraction. There is more free drug available to receptor sites and therefore more activity, but there is also more available for metabolite breakdown and excretion.

Drug distribution is expressed in kinetic terms as an apparent volume of distribution (V_d). This describes, theoretically, the volume of fluid into which the drug appears to be distributed in a concentration equal to that in plasma and therefore indicates the extent to which the drug passes from the vascular space into peripheral tissues. Its usefulness lies in the fact that the dosage requirement (D) to produce a desired plasma concentration (C) can be calculated using the expression: $D = V_d \times C$, provided that the drug is totally absorbed or given intravenously. This equation relates only to a single dose and is relevant at only one point in time. Because elimination processes proceed continuously, that drug concentration will decrease at a rate proportional to the drug's clearance rates unless further drug is administered. The rate at which a drug needs to be given to maintain a desired concentration is the maintenance dose requirement expressed as a dose per unit time.

Apparent volumes of drug distribution in children are greatest in the newborn period and reduce progressively throughout childhood, most rapidly in the first year of life, but remain relatively greater than adult values. This presumably reflects the age-dependent variation in the extracellular fluid compartment (Fig. 30.1) which forms part or whole of the distribution volume.

Elimination

This is the process by which a drug is removed from the body. It is effected either by metabolism (biotransformation) or excretion of the parent drug; the metabolites of some drugs are active and some parent drugs are totally inactive, and so the net pharmacological effect does not necessarily relate solely to these processes individually. The rates of drug elimination vary greatly with age throughout childhood.

Biotransformation

The rate of drug biotransformation probably depends on liver size and the metabolising ability of the appropriate microsomal enzyme system per unit volume of liver. Liver volume per unit body weight is twice as great in the newborn period than in the early teenage years and the relative volume seems to decrease steadily throughout childhood. Little is known about the effects of age on the microsomal enzyme system, but in the newborn period and early infant it is certainly immature. The deficiency in glucuronidation causing physiological jaundice in the newborn is perhaps the best example of this immaturity. It is also responsible for the cardiorespiratory collapse (grey baby syndrome) seen in preterm newborn babies given similar weight-related doses of chloramphenicol to those used in older children. Pharmacokinetic differences between immature, more mature babies and infants explain this toxic effect. A decreased rate of glucuronidation has also been shown for salicylates and nalidixic acid in newborns. There is a similar decrease in the rate of oxidation of paracetamol, phenylbutazone, phenobarbitone, phenytoin and diazepam in the first few weeks of life. These two processes increase in efficiency during the first year of life, reaching and sometimes overtaking adult levels. The rate of maturation of these processes varies quite significantly between individuals and the rate of change can be quite rapid so that over a matter of weeks, a young infant may change from a poorly efficient drug oxidation unit to one which is highly efficient. Some processes, e.g. demethylation and sulphation, proceed at adult rates from birth.

Paracetamol, which is metabolised by both glucuronidation and sulphation, is primarily handled by sulphation in the newborn and young infant who has a decreased ability to conjugate glucuronidation; the sulphated metabolite is therefore the predominant one at this time. In the older child and adult, the ratio of paracetamol glucuronide to sulphate is reversed.

The results and effects of changes in liver size, content and enzyme system maturity changes occurring in early infancy particularly are not predictable. It is known, however, that a number of drug metabolic processes in later infancy and early childhood proceed at greater rates than in older children and adults. The most rapid clearance rates for many drugs at any time in life are therefore found in children in the first few years of life; this involves carbamazepine, diazepam, phenobarbitone, sodium valproate and theophylline. As they get older, children become closer to adults in their rates of metabolism. It is not clear whether the faster rates seen in young children are due solely to the relatively greater liver volumes at this age. Some drugs are affected by first-pass metabolism through the liver and intestine, which reduces their systemic bioavailability; examples include terbutaline, propranolol, methyldopa, morphine and imipramine.

Excretion

Most drugs or their metabolites are ultimately excreted via the kidney, and their elimination is therefore subject to age-dependent developmental changes in glomerular filtration and tubular secretion. Glomerular filtration rates reach adult values, corrected for surface area, between 3 and 5 months of age. Digoxin, gentamicin and tobramycin are excreted by this process and their elimination is therefore slower in the newborn and early infancy periods compared with later infancy and childhood. Tubular secretion reaches adult values (per unit surface area) between 5 and 7 months. The penicillins are excreted in this way and their elimination is therefore slower in the first few months of life.

The rate of drug elimination is best described by the concept of total body clearance, which is a measure of the apparent volume from which drug is removed in a given time; this determines dosage requirements. A more convenient expression of the rate of elimination is the drug half-life, which is the time over which the concentration of drug in plasma is reduced by half. It is dependent on both the clearance and the volume of distribution and has important implications for dose frequency. Compared with adults, the half-lives of most drugs are considerably longer, while their clearance rates are markedly slower in the newborn period and early infancy. In later infancy and throughout childhood, the situation for most drugs is reversed with faster clearance rates and shorter half-lives than in adolescence and adulthood.

PHARMACODYNAMICS

Pharmacodynamics is the measurement of what the drug does to the body; it includes the mechanism of drug action and the relationship between drug effect and the dosage or plasma concentration. Pharmacodynamics of most drugs may be similar in adults and children, but this cannot be always assumed as paradoxical effects do occur; for example, phenobarbitone tends to excite in children and sedate adults, whereas amphetamines tend to produce almost the reverse effect.

ADVERSE REACTIONS

These are the undesirable or unwanted effects of drugs or their metabolites and often represent an extension of the usual pharmacological effects; for example, the anticholinergic effect of atropine which increases the heart rate, may also cause dryness of the mouth and blurred vision. Adverse effects may also arise because of concentration- or dose-related toxicity, idiosyncratic reactions, or allergic effects. Deafness associated with toxic concentrations of gentamicin is an example of dose- or concentration-related toxicity. Malignant hyperpyrexia with suxamethonium is a genetically determined abnormal reaction and is therefore idiosyncratic. Penicillin anaphylaxis and the many skin rashes which directly follow the use of drugs are examples of allergic effects which arise from disturbances of the normal immunological re-

sponse. Most so-called adverse reactions to penicillin are not reactions to the drug but are rather related to coincidental virus infections.

The overall incidence of adverse effects is considerable and approximately 10–15% of all drug-exposed children are reported to suffer adverse effects. The reporting of adverse effects by doctors and parents may not be truly comparable; for example, drowsiness is infrequently recorded by doctors as an adverse effect, whereas it is the commonest one reported by parents. Other likely effects, including nausea, vomiting, diarrhoea, abdominal pain and rashes, are reported equally by parents and doctors. It is likely that the reported incidence of adverse effects is lower than it really is. This is because at any one point in time, long-term problems will not be appreciated, but also perhaps because people charged with the care of children are not always aware of possibilities. Many doctors fail to advise parents of the common, but not particularly serious, adverse effects that might occur; fewer mention the rarer and more serious effects. It is likely that reporting of adverse effects might increase if parents were aware of possible effects of drugs.

The most frequently observed drug reactions seen in children and the system involved are shown in Table 30.1.

DRUG INTERACTIONS

Drug interactions can occur with food and with other drugs. The presence of food generally delays gastric emptying; this usually does not affect the total amount of drug absorbed; in a small number of drugs, for example, erythromycin, rifampicin, isoniazid and penicillins, there is a reduction. The absorption of nitrofurantoin is increased by food, and this and the tendency to produce gastric upset, is why the drug should be administered with or after meals. Drug interactions unrelated to food occur less commonly but are generally more important.

Pharmacodynamic interactions occur between drugs which compete for the same receptor site or which act on the same body system. They may also occur when one drug induces disease or a change in fluid and electrolyte balance which then

Table 30.1 The most frequently observed drug reactions and the likely cause in infants and children outside the newborn period

System	Effect	Drug
Gastrointestinal	Nausea and vomiting	Most drugs
	Diarrhoea	Ampicillin
	Monilial infection	Ampicillin
	Stained teeth	Tetracycline
	Hypersalivation	Clonazepam
Haematological	Bone marrow depression	Chloramphenicol Cytotoxics
	Megaloblastic anaemia	Co-trimoxazole Phenytoin
Cutaneous	Maculopapular rash	Ampicillin Carbamazepine Phenytoin
	Urticaria	Penicillin
	Alopecia	Sodium valproate Cytotoxics
Neurological	Nystagmus	Carbamazepine Phenytoin
	Drowsiness	Antihistamines (decongestants) Carbamazepine Clonazepam Phenobarbitone
	Ataxia	Phenytoin Carbamazepine
	Dyskinesia	Metoclopramide Prochlorperazine
	Hyperkinesis	Phenobarbitone
Metabolic	Hyperkalaemia	Frusemide
	Hyperglycaemia	Prednisolone Thiazides
	Cushingoid syndrome	Corticosteroids
	Short stature	Corticosteroids
Cardiovascular	Bradycardia	Digoxin
	Hypertension	Prednisolone
	Tachycardia	Atropine β_2 agonists

alters the response to another drug, for example, thiazide-induced hypokalaemia increases the possibility of digoxin toxicity.

Pharmacokinetic interactions occur by three main mechanisms:

1. Induction of the hepatic microsomal enzyme system by one drug may increase the rate of elimination of another. This is the basis of most anticonvulsant drug interactions. Carbamazepine, phenobarbitone and rifampicin are examples of potent enzyme-inducing agents. The net effect of induced enzyme activity is to reduce the blood levels of concurrently used drugs. Changes in the doses of the initial drug may be required if these enzyme-inducing drugs are added to existing drug regimens, and conversely when they are withdrawn.

2. Inhibition of liver enzyme microsomal system tends to cause an increase in the drug concentration of a simultaneously administered drug and this therefore causes an increase in that drug's overall effect; for example, chloramphenicol increases the anticonvulsant effect of phenytoin, while erythromycin increases the concentration of simultaneously administered theophylline and this tends to be clinically expressed as theophylline toxicity. Cimetidine is also an enzyme inhibitor, but few of the drugs used concurrently are metabolised by the liver and there is generally therefore no significant clinical effect.

3. Displacement of one drug from its protein binding sites by another drug may cause a greater activity of the displaced drug by an increase in its free fraction. This tends to be a temporary phenomenon as the greater amount of free drug is soon eliminated. Examples of this interaction are the increase in the concentration and effect seen with phenytoin as a result of concurrent use of aspirin, and the displacement of phenytoin by sodium valproate in multiple drug therapy of epilepsy.

The oral hypoglycaemics and warfarin are some of the more common interacting drugs but these are infrequently used in children. The majority of known and clinically significant interactions involve the use of anticonvulsants, rifampicin, erythromycin, cimetidine and chloramphenicol.

PRESCRIBING CONSIDERATIONS

Is a drug really necessary?

This is often the most difficult question in the prescribing process. Although it is easy to be critical of the prescribing habit of other doctors, it is likely that children are exposed to more drugs overall than they need be. The routine use of antibacterial drugs in upper respiratory tract infections is often unnecessary; oral and nasal decongestants are of questionable benefit when one considers the adverse effects involving drowsiness in a quarter of children using them, and the possibility of a stimulant or hypertensive effect. The efficacy of oral antiemetic drugs is also doubtful, although these drugs may be effective when given by intramuscular and rectal routes. The appropriate approach to therapy for diarrhoea is to withdraw food while substituting a suitable fluid and electrolyte mixture, rather than drug therapy. Mild fevers frequently produce no effects in children and routine therapy with paracetamol in all cases may not be appropriate. Aspirin should never be used because of its tendency to cause Reye's syndrome, albeit rarely, but particularly in children with influenzae and chickenpox. The use of a tricyclic antidepressant in children with nocturnal enuresis should be questioned; enuresis is a self-limiting condition and the benefits of these drugs are often only temporary. The dangers of accidental overdose and complications should not be underestimated also in siblings. Children who sleep little and who are frequently, but falsely, labelled hyperactive, are often inappropriately and unsuccessfully given sedatives. Careful explanation of the pros and cons of drug therapy may help parents understand that the child should be managed without medication. However, in some cases parental pressure for treatment is strong and it is important that the doctor is fully aware of the likely benefit and potential disadvantages of drug therapy.

Prophylaxis

Drugs may be used to prevent disease and symptoms of disease. The major indications and most useful drugs for prophylaxis are:

1. Recurrent urinary tract infections; vesicoureteric reflux — trimethoprim, nitrofurantoin.
2. Close family contact of meningococcal disease; close child contacts of *Haemophilus influenzae* disease — rifampicin
3. Further rheumatic fever — phenoxymethylpenicillin.
4. In postsplenectomy children and those with sickle cell disease — phenoxymethylpenicillin and pneumococcal vaccine to proven infection with *Strep. pneumoniae*.
5. Newborn baby exposed to tuberculosis — isoniazid.
6. Bacterial endocarditis in children with known cardiac valve lesions during dental procedures, bladder catheterisation and other procedures likely to result in bacteraemia — amoxycillin, erythromycin, gentamicin.
7. Some abdominal surgery including appendicectomy to reduce complications — metronidazole.

Drug choice

The number of drugs prescribed should be kept to a minimum in order to limit adverse effects and interactions, but also to aid patient compliance. The prescriber should consider clinical benefit of each drug, toxicity, the therapeutic benefit–risk ratio, the administration route and whether a drug effect can be maintained throughout the proposed treatment period. If two drugs have similar profiles, the cheaper drug should be chosen for use. Drugs that can be given once or twice daily are usually of greater advantage than those requiring more frequent administration. It is sometimes helpful to use drugs with established target ranges for optimum use.

The choice of antibacterial therapy is governed by the likely or known causal organism at a given age, the ability of a drug to get into certain tissues, and the tendency for resistance to occur. For example, different organisms are more likely to cause the same disease at different ages; *Haemophilus influenzae* is the most likely bacterial organism to produce acute otitis media in children under 4 years, whereas *Streptococcus pnenumoniae* is the more likely pathogen above this age. Penicillin is used to treat meningococcal meningitis but does not penetrate into the nasopharynx well; rifampicin is the more appropriate prophylaxis of contacts and to clear the organism from this site in an affected case with meningitis. Erythromycin penetrates into nasopharyngeal secretions well and is used to clear the organism in pertussis infection. The use of chloramphenicol in small infants may cause the grey baby syndrome; blood concentrations can be high as a result of unpredictable slow clearance of the drug in some children. The monitoring of blood concentrations should prevent this occurring, but the majority of cases of chloramphenicol poisoning are due to children being given large doses accidentally.

The risks to young siblings when drugs such as tricyclics and opiates are accidentally ingested should also be a consideration. Some drugs should, if possible, never be used in children, for example, tetracycline, which causes staining of teeth. Aspirin is known to be one cause of Reye's syndrome, particularly in children with influenza and chickenpox. There is no indication for the use of this drug in children except in those with juvenile chronic arthritis.

Route of administration/drug formulation

The objective of any therapeutic approach is to achieve an effective drug concentration at the expected site of action as quickly and conveniently as possible. This can usually be achieved in children by the oral route, although the parenteral route is more appropriate when the child is vomiting or is gravely ill, when compliance is uncertain, and when drugs are known to be poorly absorbed from the gastrointestinal tract.

In the younger child, liquid oral preparations are generally preferred, although even young children can be encouraged to swallow tablets or capsules which have some advantages. The longer shelf-life of tablets and capsules lengthens the time necessary between prescription renewal; this may mean better compliance and less danger of sudden withdrawal such as with anticonvulsants, should prescriptions not be replenished on time. Most liquid preparations are absorbed more rapidly than capsules or tablets, although in practice this is not important. The more rapid absorption of liquids may, however, increase the fluctuation in plasma drug concentrations which occurs normally between doses, and may lead to a greater tendency for adverse reactions or even subtherapeutic levels.

It is now accepted that with chronic administration, sucrose-based liquid medicines cause dental caries and gingivitis and their use should be discouraged. Information on the base of each liquid drug should be available from regional drug information centres or pharmacies. Phenytoin suspension is a good example of a preparation requiring vigorous shaking prior to administration as the drug tends to settle towards the bottom of the bottle.

Many parents find rectal drug administration unpleasant. This route cannot be relied upon to produce adequate blood levels of some drugs, for example, theophylline from aminophylline suppositories, without the risk of dangerous toxicity. This route, however, can be useful in some circumstances; for example the child who is convulsing at home can be given rectal diazepam solution from specially designed tubes and the drug will be absorbed at only a slightly slower rate than from intravenous administration. Prochlorperazine suppositories given before cytotoxic therapy can prevent subsequent vomiting. Paracetamol suppositories are effective in reducing temperature in children who are vomiting or in whom oral administration represents a risk arising from a decreased conscious level. Metronidazole suppositories are a relatively cheap and effective means of treating anaerobic infections of the bowel and also reducing complications in certain types of bowel surgery when administered immediately prior to the procedure.

Topical application of drugs is limited to bad skin conditions; there may be a place in the future for transepidermal administration such as theophylline delivery to preterm newborns. If skin is broken or inflamed, however, there is a much reduced barrier to drug absorption and therefore topical agents applied to diseased areas as treatment may cause systemic effects. Extensive nappy rashes, eczema and blistered skin conditions are examples of problems where the risk of toxicity for repeated use of topical agents is increased. Applying topical steroids in young infants with relatively mild napkin rashes can lead to excess steroid absorption. Other problems have been reported following percutaneous absorption of alcohol, iodine, salicic acid, oestrogens, exachloraphine and antibiotics (e.g. neomycin).

Intramuscular injections are frequently painful. Hydrocortisone, aminophylline and paraldehyde are particularly irritant. There is little advantage in the use of this route; where indicated, the quadriceps muscle is the safest site and the upper and outer quarter of the buttock should not be used (the course of the sciatic nerve is more transverse in this area in children than in adults). Babies of low gestational age have little muscle bulk and intramuscular injection is inappropriate in preterm babies.

Inhalation of some drugs is useful and particularly so in the treatment and prevention of asthma. Inhaled salbutamol produces a greater effect than when the drug is given orally and also there is a reduction in the adverse effects. Delivery apparatuses should be geared to the age of the child. In general terms, children below the age of 2 need nebulisers; above this age and up until 4 or $4\frac{1}{2}$ years, drugs can be inhaled from apparatuses based on drug reservoirs which allow aerosol puff systems to be used enhancing and enriching air within certain volumes of plastic reservoirs; children above $4\frac{1}{2}$ can usually be taught to use powdered drug inhalational devices or continue with the spacer systems. Few children below the age of 8 or 9 years can efficiently take drugs directly from aerosol inhalers. These are probably best reserved for children above 10 years. In all cases, technique must be checked as the likeliest cause of poor response to drug therapy relates to deficiencies in the technique of the inhalational administration.

The intravenous route is generally indicated in very sick children and ones in whom peripheral perfusion may be reduced.

Sustained-release preparations, which reduce fluctuation in drug concentration between usual dose intervals, should be particularly useful in children who will metabolise drugs rapidly. Young children, however, under 4 years who might be expected to benefit most in this respect cannot generally swallow large solid preparations. Accommodating the needs of young children by crushing or cutting the tablets usually destroys the sustained-release properties. However, some small granule preparations can be emptied from capsules or sprinkled directly onto food or liquid and so extend the predominantly absorptive phase and reduce wide movements of concentration between doses.

It is rare for children to react to dyes and colouring agents by sensitivity reactions, although occasionally children react to tartrazine in oral liquid preparations.

Dosage

Dose size

Many formulae have been devised to aid the calculation of dosage in children, but most are unsatisfactory as they involve using fractions of adult doses and take no account of the differences in kinetics and dynamics between children and adults. After a single dose, the drug concentration in blood or other body tissue depends on the dose size, route of administration and the apparent volume of distribution. The concentration after what is usually a fairly rapid distribution of most drugs is given by the formula: c (concentration) $= d$ (dose absorbed) $\div aV_d$ (apparent volume of distribution). The background to this may be more readily appreciated by consideration of two containers of different volume each filled completely with water and into which the same amount of dye is sprinkled. The resultant colour will be more dilute in appearance in the larger volume container. Children, and young children particularly preterm infants, have generally larger volumes of distribution than older children and adults. Similar single weight-related doses will therefore produce lower blood concentrations in the newborn, compared to older infants and similarly in older infants compared to older children, because of the relatively larger apparent volumes of distribution. Therefore, the younger the child, the larger will be the weight-related, single dose of a drug. If dose were related to surface area, then the dose required to produce similar drug levels in different ages of children would tend to be the same as volumes of distribution and tissue compartment volumes are similar when related to this parameter. However, the use of surface area for drug dosing is not always practicable as the size tends to be large, increasing any error in the calculation or in measurement of weight and height. In addition, there is generally the need to assess 2 parameters, height and weight, in order to determine the surface area.

In most prescribing circumstances, children need repeated doses and maintenance doses depend on variables other than the apparent volume of distribution which was the only parameter relevant to single dosing. In these circumstances, the steady-state plasma concentration of a drug depends on the systemic clearance (reflecting the sum of all eliminating processes) and the rate of replenishment of the drug. The formula for concentration in maintenance dosing is given by $c = d$ (dose absorbed) $\div$ (elimination rate constant $\times aV_d \times$ dose interval). As the clearance rates of drugs which are metabolised by the liver tend to be greatest after the early neonatal period in infancy and in early childhood, daily weight-related doses of drugs need to be highest in infants and are gradually reduced as the child gets older. In the first few weeks of life, daily weight-related doses are overall lower, since drugs are not cleared as well as at other ages, owing to hepatic immaturity. The weight-related dose per unit time related to age in repeated dosing circumstances is described in Figure 30.2, where the shadow/body ratio represents the relative dose size at different

ages based on a ratio of 1 in the average young adult.

As the clearance of drugs primarily eliminated by the kidney is similar at most ages after about 6 months, weight-related daily doses of these drugs are similar at most ages after about 6 months, e.g. gentamicin. The plasma half-life is often considered to be an index of drug clearance although this is not strictly the case. It does however relate in part to drug elimination. Its importance is in its part in determining the time taken to reach a steady-state concentration after a regular and same dose treatment is started. Unless a loading dose is used a steady-state drug concentration is not reached until after about five or six elimination half-lives have elapsed. If therapy is urgent, it is necessary to give a loading dose, for example, the use of aminophylline in children with acute asthma and anticonvulsants in children presenting with continuing convulsions. It is also appropriate to use loading doses for drugs which have long half-lives, e.g. phenobarbitone. Figure 30.3(a) illustrates the schematic representation of the accumulation of any drug in relation to its half-life. Unless the

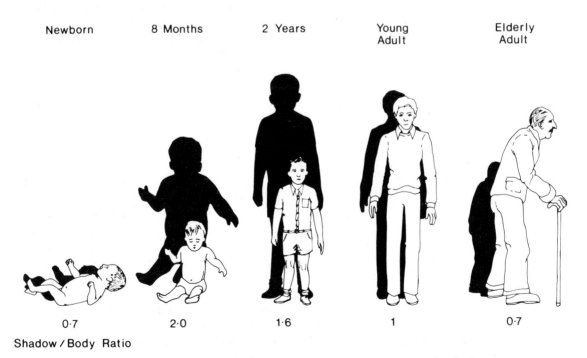

| Newborn | 8 Months | 2 Years | Young Adult | Elderly Adult |

Shadow / Body Ratio

| 0·7 | 2·0 | 1·6 | 1 | 0·7 |

Fig. 30.2 Differences in appropriate weight-related doses of most drugs (shadow indicates relative dose).

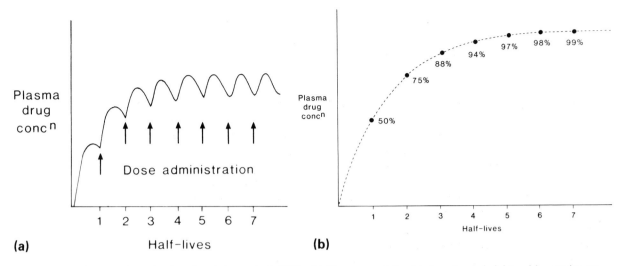

Fig. 30.3 (a) Accumulation of a drug in relation to its half-life. (b) The same relationship in a drug administered by continuous infusion.

drug is given by continuous infusion (a smooth line, Fig. 30.3(b)), drug concentrations tend to rise and fall between dosage times and this is demonstrated in Figure 30.3(a) where dosage times approximate the half-life. The steady-state concentration is one where the amount of drug going into the body is equal to the amount coming out, but fluctuation in drug concentration will occur according to those parts of the dose interval when more drug is entering the systemic circulation (rising phase) and being eliminated (falling phase). Figure 30.4 shows a schematic representation of the accumulation of phenobarbitone in different ages where smooth lines are used to represent a situation as if the drug had been continuously infused. (The time to reach steady state is a function of half-life and is unaffected by the dose frequency.) The difference in time to reach a steady state is shown and also the eventual concentration related to similar weight-related doses and affected by different rates of clearance according to age. The difference in times to reach steady-state concentration has obvious implications for the kind of assessment of drug therapy in relation to dose given and this assessment may be clinical or by measurement of drug plasma level.

If a reliable dose recommendation is not available for a drug, the prescriber should seriously consider whether its use is advisable.

Detailed recommendations are included in most prescribing texts and these relate to clinical use and kinetic studies. It is more important for some drugs to have accurate dosing recommendations and these will be the ones where there is a narrow therapeutic index (small difference between the concentration producing clinical effect and adverse effects). For some drugs such as laxatives, the dose is less important and a range of drug dosage related to age can be given. The same is true for many antibacterial agents which have fairly wide therapeutic indices. The newborn baby is a special case and for most drugs therapeutic indices are lower and more accurate dosing is appropriate.

Dose frequency

For drugs with a clear relationship between blood concentration and clinical effect, an appropriate interval between doses usually approximates the elimination half-life. Half-lives of drugs are important in the determination of fluctuation in concentration between doses and the time taken to reach steady state. For most drugs, longer intervals are required between doses in the newborn and considerably shorter intervals between doses in later infancy and early childhood compared with adults. If these drugs are given at the same frequency to older infants and children as to adults,

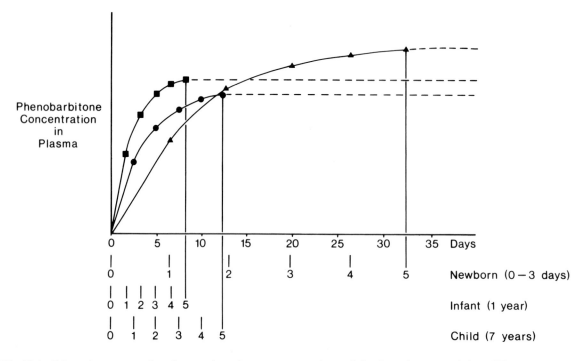

Fig. 30.4 Schematic representation of eventual steady-state concentration and the time taken to reach it at different ages.

large fluctuations in drug concentration between doses occur with the increased risk of adverse effects or decrease in efficacy.

Many commonly used drugs in children have relatively short half-lives, for example theophylline, which is less than 6 hours. If three or more equal dose and time intervals are planned, it is not possible to administer these drugs strictly according to the principles outlined. A relatively long sleep period and the rigidity of the school system mean that children have a shorter day during which drugs may be given, and dose intervals of 4, 8 and 12 (or 8, 4 and 12 hours) would punctuate school and sleep if drugs were to be given strictly three times a day (Fig. 30.5). It is usual to compromise by using a less frequent dose regimen or unequal dose interval pattern; this leads to increased variability of plasma drug concentration. Sustained-release preparations may help in reducing the concentration fluctuation, but relatively few are available. The ideal for many drugs would be a sustained-release liquid preparation.

Where no relationship between drug concentration and effect is known, the frequency of dosing is governed by practical considerations, such as convenience to promote compliance (the fewer doses; the better), and the need to reduce the incidence of adverse effects (mainly gastrointestinal). Generally, one or two doses per day are acceptable; more frequent doses are more likely to be omitted.

Dose modification according to physiological and pathological states

It is always appropriate for the prescriber to consider the usual path of elimination of a drug and any acute or chronic problems in the child which might affect the course and rate of drug elimination.

If there is renal insufficiency, the dose of a drug which is partially or totally eliminated by the kidney should be reduced, either by decreasing the amount given at each dose interval, by lengthening the dose interval, or changing both. An example

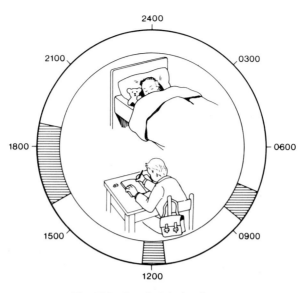

Fig. 30.5 Practical dosing times.

is gentamycin prescribing in newborn babies. In these babies, it is sometimes difficult to avoid exceeding trough levels of 2 mg/ml, which are associated with significant renal toxicity, while at the same time, achieving adequate peak levels without extending the dose interval beyond 12 hours. One can appreciate that by continuing to increase the dose interval in order to get concentration to fall prior to the next dose, one may not have much time spent when drug concentration at peak times is in excess of the minimum inhibitory concentration (MIC) of the organism for which the treatment is given.

The effects of liver disease on drug elimination in children are less easily quantified, but in general, drugs will be cleared less rapidly if there is significant hepatocellular dysfunction. In the newborn, especially preterm babies, there is immaturity of most microsomal enzyme systems and lower or frequent doses of drugs, like theophylline and chloramphenicol, primarily dependent on the liver for their elimination, are necessary. Impaired glucuronidation of paracetamol is compensated for by a relative increase in sulphation in early infancy.

Absorption does not seem to be impaired in most gastrointestinal diseases and although the rate of hepatic metabolism seems to decrease during

fever, there remains little information and doses should be similar as at other times.

Duration of therapy

This should be kept to a miminum. There is increasing evidence that urinary tract infection treatment can be short and in some cases by single dose. Treatment of acute lobar pneumonia when the pneumococcus is the likely causal organism, need continue only for 48 hours after the temperature has returned to normal and clinical improvement is obvious. Treatment of more chronic conditions has also tended to be shorter in recent years; one such example, is the management of tuberculosis where 6 months' therapy, occasionally less, is adequate for the treatment of most pulmonary TB.

Developmental changes in the young influence the duration of therapy for some chronic conditions. The most notable example of this is the developmental change in the brain which allows early cessation of anticonvulsant therapy.

Compliance

This is the ability of individuals to take drugs as

prescribed, to take the right drug in the right dose at the right time and for the right length of time. Only about 50% of children who take medicines for chronic conditions are fully compliant and the same is probably true of those taking medication for acute conditions. Poor compliance may lead to therapeutic failure. The degree of compliance in the young may largely reflect parental attitudes. Most children are dependent on their parents for drug administration or adopt their behaviour and attitude towards therapy. The following steps would be expected to improve compliance:

1. Prescribe the most appropriate medication with full explanation of how it works, how to take it and for how long, how to store it, how it is expected to help and how to recognise problems that might arise. Written as well as verbal information should be given if possible.

2. Plan and discuss the dose regimen at the start of therapy so that an unwritten contract is assumed. This should take account of periods of sleep, mealtimes, school hours and breaks, preferred formulations, easiest unit sizes, and rational and practical dose intervals based on kinetic information. Decide at what times a drug should be taken, the best tablet size or volume of liquid and whether the drug should be taken before, during or after meals. These things should be noted and explained to children and their parents.

3. Choose the most palatable preparation possible. Give information on possible adverse effects, both the most likely and those that are rare.

PRESCRIPTION WRITING

Prescriptions should be clearly written using approved abbreviations. In general, single drugs should be prescribed and the approved name should be used wherever possible. If a particular brand is required, it should be stated thus: diazepam — 'Valium brand' only.

The drug name should be printed in block letters. Metric doses must be used and, wherever possible, decimal points should be avoided. The approved abbreviation of gramme is g, of milligramme is mg and of microgram μg, even so it is advisable for micrograms to be written in full. Except for compound fomulations, substitutes for

dose weights, for example, Caps, Tabs, Vials, should be avoided.

Abbreviations such as 'prn' and 'sos' should not be used. The symptom or sign to be relieved must be written in prescribing instructions of this nature and the maximum frequency of administration should be clearly stated, e.g. 'As required for headache — maximum 4 hourly'. Only the following routes of administration should be abbreviated:

Intravenous   — i.v.
Intramuscular — i.m.
Topical   — top.
Inhalation   — inhal.
Intradermal   — i.d.
Per rectum   — p.r.
Subcutaneous   — s.c.
Intrathecal   — i.t.

Oral and other routes of administration should be written in full. All prescriptions should bear the full signature of the prescriber and, in hospital practice, this should be repeated when the drugs are discontinued.

A choice of route, for example, oral i.m./i.v. should never be offered and no amendment to dose or dose frequency should be made to any existing prescription. In both cases, a change means that the prescription must be rewritten. Although it has been recommended that liquid drug doses should be supplied in 5 ml volumes, it may be necessary, because of stability and palatability, to prescribe the required dose and for the pharmacist to decide on the appropriate volume.

Prescriptions for controlled drugs must state the name and address of the patient, dosage and total number of doses written in both figures and letters, and the frequency of administration.

INFORMATION FOR CHILDREN AND THEIR PARENTS

Children and their parents need to be informed in order to use medicines safely and effectively. The giving of appropriate information is the responsibility of the prescribing doctor. This should be done in full and open discussion with the parents and the child when considering proposed treatment. Non-drug alternatives to usual accepted therapies should be discussed. These may include dietary change, behaviour modification programmes and physiotherapy.

What parents and children need to know

1. The name of the medicine.
2. Reason for using it.
3. When and how to take it.
4. How to know if it is working effectively; and what to do if it is not.
5. What to do if one or more doses are missed.
6. The risks of omitting medication.
7. How long to continue taking it.
8. The most likely side-effects; those that are unlikely but are important and what to do if they occur.
9. Whether other medicines can be taken at the same time.
10. Alternatives to drug therapy.

A specimen information sheet is shown in Table 30.2

Table 30.2 Specimen information sheet

Drug management	Information needed
How drug is to be taken	Dose per formulation and number of units Suggested clock time (to be agreed) Time between doses Time before or after food Duration of treatment
Storage of drug	Container Type of cupboard. Temperature Expiry date Signs of deterioration
How drug is expected to help	Symptoms Consequences of good or bad compliance Time to achieve effect Signs of effect Action to take if no effect
Recognising problems due to the drug	Signs Action to take

MEDICATION IN SCHOOLS

In most cases, medicines do not need to be given during school hours. Even for the commonly used antibiotics, three times daily administration is acceptable for most conditions. However, some drugs need to be used at school and this presents problems for children, their families and teachers. It is understandable why teachers are reluctant to accept third party responsibility for the safe storage and administration of medicine, when one considers the stringent regulations of not dissimilar situations with inpatients (and administration) by nurses. In the latter case, medicines are always locked away, and on a medicine ward round it is necessary for two nurses to be in attendance, each drug given to be signed for and the process checked by another nurse of fairly senior status. Nevertheless, it should be possible to formulate a code of conduct acceptable to all parties by close liaison between parent, child, teacher, school nurse and doctor. There is a clear responsibility on the doctor to consider this specific problem when they advise on and prescribe medication.

DRUGS IN BREAST MILK

Most drugs are excreted in breast milk, but usually in amounts which are too small to harm the baby. Most current recommendations are based on single case data and problems which might occur have been generally overstated and recommendations are overcautious.

The concentration of drug in milk usually, but not always, parallels that in plasma and milk/plasma ratios for most drugs are between 1:3 and 1:1. The total amount available for absorption by the infants is generally small, usually less than 2% of the total maternal dose.

Some infants in the first few weeks of life, such as preterm and jaundiced babies, are at greater than normal potential risk. This risk decreases as kidney and liver function improve with increasing age. In addition, infants with glucose-6-phosphate dehydrogenase (G-6-PD) deficiency and those with an allergic tendency are also at increased risk from some drugs, although these conditions are seldom evident at the time.

Idiosyncratic reactions, unrelated to dose or concentration, can occur despite low milk concentrations, but these are rarely of clinical importance.

APPROACH TO DRUG THERAPY

Although the risk is negligible for most drugs, prescribers should generally be cautious. If drugs are necessary, a suitable preparation can almost always be found and in single dose treatment of almost any drug, there is no risk.

Mothers who require treatment should not be prevented from breast feeding unless there is information to suggest that a drug concerned is unsafe. A few contraindicated drugs include those in cancer chemotherapy (cytotoxics), ergot alkaloids, and radiopharmaceutical agents. Even some of these can be used in specific circumstances when 'time-offs' are built in to the feeding regimen following drug dosing. This may require 48 hours or slightly more off breast feeding. The least potentially toxic drug that is compatible with appropriate therapy of the mother should be used.

Information and advice is usually available from a drug information centre. The likely drug concentration in breast milk and thus the daily dose for a baby on an average milk intake can be calculated. A direct assay of drug concentration in milk may be helpful in checking predicted amounts. The infant's condition can also be closely monitored. Some effects are predictable, like bradycardia and hypoglycaemia with beta-blocking drugs; anticholinergic symptoms with atropine; or sedation with psychotropics. Where appropriate, the baby's blood levels and other related functions, for example, blood film/count and thyroid function, can be checked.

Although this approach is relevant to all drugs that might harm the baby, it is especially important for those drugs for which there is a theoretical risk. These include anticoagulants, antithyroid drugs, atropine, beta-blockers, chloramphenicol, clemastine, diazoxide, diuretics, gold salts, H2-receptor antagonists, isoniazid, lithium, oral hypoglycaemics, naladixic acid, narcotics, non-steroidal anti-inflammatory agents and oral steroids. These drugs are, however, seldom given to breast feeding mothers and there is no evidence that significant poisoning has resulted from their use in practice.

Children can be poisoned accidentally by drugs, poisonous plants and household chemicals. There are a number of background causes:

1. The child's normal exploratory activity, especially in children aged between $1\frac{1}{2}$ and 3 years.
2. The child mistaking medicines for sweets.
3. Inadequate or inappropriate drug storage or supervision.
4. Prescription of excessive doses of drugs by doctors or mistakes by pharmacies.
5. Inappropriate administration by parents as a form of child abuse, or good intentional, but overzealous treatment.
6. Older child or adolescent suicide attempts or 'cries for help'.

Most poisoning could be prevented if child-resistant containers are used and if all other dangerous products were in appropriate containers, correctly used and stored. It is important that drugs can be identified by name of packaging and in household chemicals, that the contents are clearly listed. Legislation has reduced the incidence of poisoning in many countries.

Poisoning as a possible diagnosis should be considered in children presenting with an acute illness, particularly when unusual symptoms are present. As in other cases, the most important feature in diagnosis is to get a thorough medical history. This will then form the basis for further diagnostic approaches and therapeutic interventions.

Diagnostic approach

If a clear history of drug ingestion cannot be obtained, the approach to diagnosis should include the following:

1. Obtaining information about medicines stored in the home or taken by other family/household members.
2. Smelling the breath to detect solvents, looking at the lips and mouth for burns caused by caustic chemicals, and looking for discolouration and parts of tablets retained in the mouth.
3. Examining the contents of the vomit which may afford identification of tablets. A sample of vomitus should be retained where possible for later analysis.
4. Looking for signs and symptoms that may suggest a causative agent, for example, salicy-

lates cause hyperventilation; barbiturates may produce respiratory depression; atropine causes fever, dilated pupils, dry mouth and tachycardia; and phenothiazines and metoclopramide may cause oculogyric crises and dyskinetic posturing.

Immediate management

1. Examine the child. Assess the general condition and particularly the level of consciousness.

2. Secure the airway and resuscitate as necessary.

3. Obtain a history and where possible get information on the name of drug and the amount and time of ingestion.

4. Obtain the container and its label if possible. Always remember that the label is not an absolute guide as to contents which may have been transferred from some other container.

5. Empty the stomach contents unless the patient is convulsing or comatose, more than 4 hours have elapsed since ingestion (or 6 hours in the case of acetylsalicylic acid), or the poisoning is due to corrosive or petroleum products. Ipecachuaha paediatric emetic liquid should be given in a dose of 15 ml with half that for children under 1 year. This should be immediately followed by at least 200 ml of juice or water. The emetic effect is more rapid if the child is asked to run around, or even bounced on someone's knee. Ipecachuaha administration can be repeated after 20 minutes if vomiting has not occurred. Milk retards the emetic effect of ipecachuaha and also increases the gastric absorption of lipid-soluble products and petroleum distillates.

6. Give antidotes or take other specific measures in the few circumstances where these are appropriate (Table 30.3)

7. Activated charcoal (50 g) can help reduce the absorption of a number of drugs, and is particularly useful in tricyclic poisoning. However, rapid ingestion may cause vomiting and its place in the management of acute poisoning compared with emesis induction and gastric lavage remains uncertain.

8. Always contact a Poisons Information Unit or Centre in order to check that all measures have been taken.

Table 30.3 Poison antidotes

Drug	Antidote
Disinfectants	Milk, liberal fluids
Iron	Desferrioxamine (use 2 g/l of water in lavage and leave 10 g in 50 ml in the stomach)
Morphine (and analogues like diphenoxylate)	Naloxone 400 μg (1 ml) intravenously and 400 μg (1 ml) intramuscularly Can be repeated every 2–3 minutes with a maximum of 2.5 mg
Paracetamol	Acetylcystine (in hospital)
Phenothiazines and metoclopramide	Diazepam 0.5 mg/kg up to maximum of 10 mg intravenously or procyclidine hydrochloride or Biperiden

Hospital referral or not

A decision can usually be made on the basis of history and the presence or absence of symptoms. Ingestion of the following substances is always an indication for referral to hospital:

Acetylsalicylic acid
Atropine
Digoxin
Diphenoxylate with atropine
Ergotamine
Iron
Paracetamol
Quinidine
Tricyclic antidepressants
Sustained-release preparations
Toxic chemicals, corrosives
Petroleum products

Children may be kept at home if most other drugs have been taken, if sufficient time for absorption has elapsed and if:

a. They are free of symptoms
b. The general practitioner is informed
c. Delayed problems are not expected
d. The parents can be trusted to contact the doctor or hospital if symptoms occur

THERAPEUTIC DRUG MONITORING

The indications for monitoring drug levels are the same in all ages, but there is a greater clinical importance in children because they vary widely in their handling and response to drugs, and the margin of safety is often narrower. The titration of dose to response is less reliable in children for many commonly used drugs, for example, anticonvulsants.

Therapeutic drug monitoring may be helpful in determining doses most likely to provide safe and effective drug concentrations, in assessing compliance and in the intepretation and understanding of possible drug interactions. Although a number of different body fluids, including saliva, have been used, blood levels are generally the most appropriate unless knowledge of concentration in certain tissues, as in the situation of possible therapeutic failure in the treatment of meningitis, is considered necessary. Effective doses are determined by relating drug concentration in blood to a target range which can be defined as that range of concentration within which maximum pharmacological effect is achieved with the minimum of toxicity. Without appropriate interpretation, a knowledge of drug concentration is clinically useless. For maximum benefit, the prescriber needs to consider the following:

Duration of therapy

Unless a loading dose is given, a steady-state concentration which reflects the dose being given daily will not be reached until about five elimination half-lives have elapsed. Measurement of drug concentration should occur after this time period.

Relationship between elimination half-life and dosing

All drugs fluctuate in concentration between doses unless they are given by continuous infusion. This fluctuation may be acceptable or unacceptable: in the latter, adverse effects may occur or even poor therapeutic control when concentrations are lowest. Blood samples taken immediately before a dose will generally reflect the lowest concentration occurring in the child's body. Although this is often the best time to measure drug levels, it is not always convenient and therefore blood samples taken at other times will produce results which need careful interpretation taking account of the

likely concentration–time profile between doses for that drug and in that age of child.

Combination therapy

Interactions between drugs and changes in concentration as a result of added therapy either by increase or decrease should always be considered.

Active metabolites

Some drugs have active metabolites. Carbamazepine is perhaps the best known one where the activity of the epoxide metabolite is possibly responsible for about a third of the anticonvulsant effect. The relationship between concentration and parent drug may not be close in these situations. For other drugs like primidone, it is usual only to measure the active metabolite — phenobarbitone.

Compliance

If a drug concentration is undetectable, this sug-

Table 30.4 Elimination half-lives, usual dose frequency and target ranges of drugs for which the therapeutic drug monitoring is indicated

Drug	Approximate half-life (h)	Usual dose frequency (times/day)	Target range mg/l (mmol/l where appropriate)
Carbamazepine (note the epoxide metabolite)	6–10	2–3	4–12 (16–50)
Chloramphenicol	2–12	4	Peak 15–25
Digoxin	24–60	1–2	0.5–2.1 ng/ml (0.65–2.6 nmol/l)
Ethosuximide	30–40	1	40–100 (280–700)
Gentamicin	2–4	3	Peak 6–12 Trough <2
Phenobarbitone	30–40	1	10–35 (40–140)
Phenytoin	Varies with dose	2	10–20 (40–80)
Theopylline	3–5	2–3*	10–20 (55–110)

* Wherever possible, sustained release preparations should be used. Prolongation of the phase where absorption predominant reduces fluctuation and allows less frequent dosing than indicated by elimination half-life.

gests that there is poor compliance. When a concentration is lower than expected, it may be that the child has a rapid clearance of the drug, compliance is compromised by reduction in planned dosage, or there may just have been a forgotten recent dose.

It is important that the measurement and interpretation of a child's plasma concentration of drugs is only a small part of information needed in treating children appropriately. Therapeutic drug monitoring complements clinical judgement and in no way replaces it.

Information on drugs for which therapeutic drug monitoring is useful is shown in Table 30.4.

FURTHER READING

British Medical Association and Royal Pharmaceutical Society Britain 1989 British National Formulary. The Pharmaceutical Press, London

Bylance G W (editor-in-chief) 1987 Drugs for children. WHO Regional Office for Europe, Copenhagen

31. The dying child

J. Goodall

A dying child has two main needs: to be relieved of distress and to be understood. In response, members of the caring team must know when to substitute palliative for active treatment and learn the likely level of the child's understanding. Inclusion of the parents is vital. They are likely to be chief comforters and interpreters for their child and yet are already chief mourners. Quality time must be spent in helping them to understand both the philosophy of care and their child's likely grasp of what is going on. A family's ability to cope with bereavement may be governed by the adequacy of terminal care.

PALLIATIVE TREATMENT: SYMPTOM CONTROL

If the threat of death comes suddenly, active intervention is likely to continue almost to the end. Even so, parents must be allowed access and involvement. If the child is dying of an illness known to be fatal, much suffering to both child and family will result from a doctor's inability to give up striving for cure instead of concentrating on comfort. When the course of the illness is clearly downhill, the prescription chart should be reviewed with a checklist of symptoms. Treatment designed for cure, such as cytotoxic therapy, may stop, and drugs for symptomatic relief take over.

Common symptoms in terminal illness are pain or dyspnoea, nausea and vomiting. All these can be reduced or kept away if the principle of *round-the-clock* medication is followed together with the recognition that severe symptoms warrant potent drugs, including opiates. Drug cocktails are to be avoided, as each symptom must be titrated against its own appropriate treatment to achieve control.

The commonest error in terminal care is to prescribe *as required*. This produces a pattern of acute distress followed by oblivion. The aim is rather to keep the child enjoying what remains of life with as clear a mind as possible. Sensitive vigilance is required.

Anxiety will be reduced as distressing symptoms are controlled. Diverting play helps to pre-occupy both patient and parents and may also allow hidden anxieties to be acted out and so perceived and helped. Daily blood tests or the nuisance of a drip are unnecessary worries for a terminally ill child. Thirst is usually satisfied by drinks or ice chips and parents are freer to hold a child who has no intravenous line.

THE CHILD'S LEVEL OF UNDERSTANDING

Proper medical care involves understanding personal needs as well as prescribing drugs. Parents may need anticipatory guidance as to how to inform or answer their dying child and his siblings. Those working with them should be able to explain how a child's mind works. Just as there are normal sequences for locomotor development or physical growth, so there are recognisable stages in conceptual development before adult thinking is achieved. Young children may quietly accept facts whose implications greatly upset older minds, but which are beyond their present ability to comprehend. They are also likely to misinterpret statements with a double meaning.

A child of less than 2 years is egocentric, regarding medical procedures entirely as personal attacks during which close parental support is needed. A normal child of under 6–7 years old still takes things at face value. Thus, a 4-year-old child took fright at the offer to 'show him his bones after the X-ray' and adamantly refused to be X-rayed at all. Fears are of pain and isolation rather than to do with dying. Under-fives frequently regard death as a reversible process, although experience will hasten conceptual understanding regardless of age. The illness and death of another patient may thus heighten a child's insight into his own relapsing illness, so that even a 4-year-old may recognise that 'It might happen to me, too'. Parents should be warned that trust depends on truth. Because in a child's terms time has little meaning, awkward questions may be satisfied by giving an immediate rather than a long-term answer. 'It's not going to happen today and we won't leave you', may well be sufficiently reassuring. Children who confidently expect a personal welcome to Heaven comfort their care-givers as well as themselves. It is better not to talk of God 'taking' a child, rather that He is 'taking care of' her. Even so, if these are not familiar concepts to that family it may be better to use matching ideas, such as death 'being like' going on a journey, or moving house. This can help both dying child and siblings, but to speak of a known and loved companion on the way is the greatest comfort of all.

By early teens the ability to reason in abstract terms has developed and there is a much greater awareness of the implications of death. Reactions of denial, rage or depression may be evident and the dying teenager may deliberately thwart attempts at communication. There may be fears now about the mode of dying which remain unexpressed, sometimes for fear of adding to the parents' grief. To help bring openness between such family members is a painful process, requiring tact and time, but when it can be achieved the tranquillity of having come to terms with what is happening brings real consolation.

FAMILY AND TEAM SUPPORT

When adequate support is available, thought should be given as to whether the child should be allowed to die at home. This may bring advantages to other children in the family whose sorrows are often overlooked in the hospital setting. They should be allowed to see the dead child and invited to attend the funeral, though not forced into either of these actions. Their needs should also be included in bereavement counselling offered to the parents afterwards.

Staff as well as parents find the care of a dying child emotionally taxing and all have their own special needs. Strength may be gained from contact with the hospital chaplain, a psychiatrist or simply others who have passed this way before.

Suffering shared and accepted can be a growing point towards maturity, and many parents and professionals have discovered the paradox that to be with a child facing death has been an experience of enrichment as well as of loss.

FURTHER READING

Bluebond-Langner M 1978 The private worlds of dying children. Princeton University Press, Princeton
Chapman J A, Goodall J 1980 Helping a child to live whilst dying. Lancet 1: 753–745
Cotton 1981 A brother dies at home. Journal of Maternal and Child Health 6: 288–292
Donaldson M 1978 Children's minds. Fontana/Collins, Glasgow
Kubler-Ross E 1969 On death and dying. Macmillan, New York
Piaget J 1926 The language and thought of the child. Routledge and Keegan Paul, London
Rothenburg M B 1967 Reactions of those who treat children with cancer. Pediatrics 40: 507–510
Saunders C M 1984 Management of terminal diseases, 2nd edn. Edward Arnold, London, Ch 14
Zorza R, Zorza V 1980 A way to die: living to the end. Andre Deutsch, London

32. Ethical dilemmas in paediatric care

J. Goodall

Introduction

In today's paediatric practice, all doctors are faced with increasingly difficult ethical questions. Is this an aborted fetus or a very preterm baby needing ventilation? Does this little girl, who so hates venepunctures, really understand anything of what it would mean to her to donate bone marrow, or why nobody else in the family can do it? At the other end of the spectrum, in developing countries, decisions are more likely to be forced by economic rather than ethical considerations, although the distribution of global and local wealth will have already involved moral (or immoral) discrimination. As few doctors have an in-depth training in ethics, how are we to face the multiplication of these and other dilemmas as technology advances but resources lag behind?

What do we mean by ethics?

Whatever our backgrounds, we will have some concept of attitudes and actions being right or wrong. To choose between them is a moral decision, but general agreement within a community as to precepts which determine such decisions constitutes that community's ethical system. Ethics has been defined as the reasoned analysis of duty, but dilemmas arise when we are faced with an uncomfortable mixture of duties. Thus, to remain just, to do good, to do no harm and also to respect individual freedom are all recognisable moral duties. Yet not only may they sometimes clash with each other, even in the mind of the one trying to practise them, but they may be perceived in quite a different light by those at the receiving end. Thus, a child may decry and resist venepunc-

ture, considering this to be a very *bad* thing, whilst the one doing it is full of intention to do *good*.

Ethical systems

Most ethical dilemmas are created by tension existing between conflicting principles and whatever a community's chosen ethical system, this cannot be avoided. In the UK, until recently, both our legal and ethical systems have been based on the Ten Commandments, as moral precepts (given to the early Jews) and the Golden Rule of loving a neighbour as oneself (given to the early Christians). Each human life, individually of unique value, was to be quality controlled primarily by living according to the Maker's instructions, so producing a moral and mutually caring community.

As society has become increasingly pluralistic on the one hand and materialistic on the other, this ethos is less popular and laws have already been adapted to suit the majority view with attempts being made to mould a new ethical system. The old Greek and Roman models of physical perfection and economic prosperity have reappeared and utilitarianism (the greatest happiness for the greatest numbers) an emerging ethic. Alternative systems are humanism, emphasising man's continuing progress through application of intellect, and existentialism with its emphasis on guidance by subjective feeling. All this can be fascinating for armchair debate, but we need realistic and reliable principles to guide us in clinical practice.

Traditionally, the ethical system in medicine has also partly been derived from the views of Hippocrates: our aims have been to preserve life and to prevent suffering. When these two principles clash, how do we strike a balance between them? Reason or feeling may separately arrive at different answers, but each must be used to inform the other. We must also remember that humans are mortal as well as moral entities and that death is a fact of life rather than always being a medical failure.

THE BEST INTERESTS OF THE CHILD

Paediatric dilemmas arise because there are contrary views as to what exactly constitutes an affected child's best interests. We cannot be entirely materialistic, thinking in terms of physical wellbeing alone when knowing as we do the emotional price which a child can pay, as when kept in personal isolation. Like all of us, children have emotional, spiritual and intellectual, as well as physical, components. Unless we remember these, we can abuse them even with protective intent. Dilemmas, therefore, are not merely clinical but also impinge on the child's emotional, social (domestic and legal) and educational status, all against an economic background where what might be most effective is not always what is cost effective. These are not always straightforward choices between right and wrong. Sometimes we have to choose the lesser of two evils, rather than deciding what is unequivocally good. A few true examples will illustrate this:

An asphyxiated neonate was hand ventilated for half an hour when resuscitative attempts were abandoned. Almost at once, gasping began and normal respirations continued but within hours the child started to convulse. What would do most justice to the child?

A bright 14-month-old boy with advanced scoliosis and chest deformity was operated on in what proved to be a fruitless attempt to avoid paraplegia. The anaesthetist had great difficulty with intubation because of associated micrognathia. Whilst still in hospital post operatively, having been put on halo traction, he developed overwhelming pneumonia with carbon dioxide retention. Could further use of technology do more harm than good?

A child of 8 months was brought up with a bruised temple after his father had accidentally dropped him. The story was acceptable until skeletal survey revealed an old, healed rib fracture for which the parents could not account. A place of safety order was imminent until a grandmother mentioned how, in

play, the father often tossed the child up and caught him again, which amused them both. Should their freedom to play this game be curtailed; and if so, how?

A neonate presented with ambiguous genitalia. Testicular tissue was removed from the ovarian site, but a uterus and a vagina were both present and were preserved. After clitoridectomy, the child was brought up as a female, but the surgeon insisted that she should never be told her true condition. The parents questioned this, but how much would the child understand anyway?

An Indian teaching hospital had one ventilator in the paediatric intensive care unit but no one trained in its use. Babies were dying of tetanus, who could have benefited. What would be the best use of resources?

Most paediatric dilemmas are matters either of life and death or of other conflicting interests.

DILEMMAS ABOUT LIFE AND DEATH

In these dilemmas, the question posed is how far to go with intervention when the patient's clinical state has deteriorated beyond reasonable hope of recovery. The principles in tension are first, respect for each fellow human with the continuing desire to preserve another's life and second, compassion for the burden that such a life is carrying and our desire to prevent intolerable suffering. Resuscitation may save a life, but leave a retarded patient. Is it therefore better to stop resuscitation than to take such a risk? Aggressive treatment may prolong survival but may also prolong agony. Has the time now come to relieve symptoms rather than still to hope for cure?

Whose life is it anyway?

Answers to this question may vary and include mention of God, the state, the community or the hospital team as well as making reference to parents and child. The life is clearly the child's, but the parents are normally legally responsible and intimately involved, backed by their own supporters. Amongst these are the professional care givers. In the see-saw of opinion, there are those who say that the right to life must be rigidly upheld and that to withhold aggressive treatment is equivalent to murder. At the other extreme are those who assert that survival can be nothing but a living death and that there is, therefore, a right to die. Passion runs high as these views polarise. The third option, of offering symptomatic relief with the dying child at the heart of the family, is one commonly overlooked by the protagonists (and the press), though not now by practitioners. This approach is not to be confused with active or passive euthanasia, but is the proper care of the incurably ill of whatever age. Table 32.1 should be reviewed in this light.

Resuscitation vs. CNS damage

The dilemma here is that the patient may well die without resuscitation, yet with it may survive to be neurologically disabled. For *neonates* there is little time for discussion. Prompt intervention will govern the severity of residual handicap and is normally embarked upon, respect for life being the overwhelming consideration. If resuscitative efforts fail (half an hour being the usually recommended period of hand ventilation in hypoxia), a decision then has to be taken as to whether further efforts should cease and whether mechanical ventilation is futile therapy, not even to be embarked upon. A preterm or other hypoxic infant may be thought suitable for mechanical ventilation, but then fails to respond. The decision to pull out is

Table 32.1 Dilemmas about life and death: value of life versus burden of life. When treatment may add to disability

1. Resuscitation vs CNS damage:
   Neonatal: extreme prematurity
                      hypoxia, acute or advancing
   Post-neonatal: brain trauma or oedema
                      cardiac or respiratory arrest

2. Aggressive treatment versus palliative care:
   Severe congenital handicap: physical
                                 mental
                                 metabolic
   Severe acquired handicap: brain damage
                                 paraplegia
   Inevitably progressive   degenerative brain disease
      disease: muscular dystrophy
   Excessively burdensome   cytotoxic therapy
      treatment: marrow transplant
                                 very abnormal diet with
                                    poor response
                                 repeated unrewarding
                                    surgery
                                 chronic intensive care
   End-organ failure: kidneys, heart and lungs,
                                    liver

harder to make, but persistently deteriorating oxygenation and repeated discussion with the parents may bring clarity. Where there is no hope of survival, it may be more respectful to the baby and compassionate to the parents to stop intensive care and let parents have a little time in peace with their dying baby, without the intrusion of equipment.

After the neonatal period

In an acute crisis such as a severe head injury, mechanical ventilation is often started in the hope that the patient may rally. If this does not happen it is usual to establish brain death before the ventilator is stopped, although as yet this is only a legal requirement when organs are to be harvested for transplantation. It could be argued that if ventilation is proving to be futile, then it could be discontinued as soon as this is clear. Because many families are comforted to think that organ donation may be possible, this possibility should be discussed with them (together with its practical implications) before life support is stopped.

This kind of dilemma often arises within minutes or hours and has to be resolved within hours or days. Parents and staff may be shocked, and all risk being in a state of denial. Parents may feel dissociated from medical staff and are determined to keep trying, particularly if the child seems outwardly normal. On both sides, anger and depression may interfere with communication, but it is important that this is recognised and that the doctor/family relationship is kept open, with discussion ongoing, every encouragement being given to parents to stay close to their child. In these circumstances feeling needs very much to be informed by reason.

Aggressive and palliative care

Here, decisions are less acute. In a clearly deteriorating clinical state it has to be decided whether prolonged attempts at restoration of life are warranted, or whether it would be better to offer symptomatic relief, knowing now that death is inevitable. Moral philosophers speak of ordinary care replacing extraordinary care, and medical responsibility lies not only in knowing what it is technically possible to do, but also in considering whether it is always appropriate to do it. In a severely handicapped state, the child's life is still of value, whatever the outward appearance may be. In many conditions, the onlookers suffer more than the patient. For years, if ever, such a child may not have the least idea that there is anything wrong, yet there are still the basic needs for personal contact and comfort. When we talk about compassion, we must remember all this (reason informing feeling), yet we may also legitimately question whether it is really respecting life to embark on painful or lengthy therapy which is clearly likely to be futile (feeling thus informing reason). Surgery for some forms of severe congenital handicap may even kill the baby. Likewise, although ventilatory support may save the life of a preterm infant, it cannot indefinitely do so for a teenager with advanced cystic fibrosis or muscular dystrophy. In chronic renal failure, there may be time to dialyse the patient until the right kidney is available for transplant, thus with the hope of normal life again, but in liver failure the only hope is for transplantation of the correctly sized donor organ and time is therefore pressing. Thus, for one child, life can be made tolerable whilst waiting, but the other will soon die unless someone else dies and donates.

Many patients may clearly be dying of their inevitably progressive disease, with no hope of restoration and no point in the prolongation of fruitless therapy (Fig. 32.1). Both the team and the family will have to face the need to change direction, no longer hoping for cure but still aiming at comfort. In these circumstances, both starting and stopping ventilators will be rare events. The normal aim now is to offer palliative care to the end. When in doubt about what to do for the best, senior doctors and nurses should confer and offer parents (and an old enough child) input from a different counsellor if so desired. Optimal therapy is then decided upon mutually and excessively burdensome treatment may be gratefully replaced with symptomatic relief. Pride of place should then be given to quality time for the family together (see Ch. 31).

Balancing options in life and death decisions therefore involves accurate clinical judgement with a clear understanding of the diagnosis, prognosis and options available in management. The final decision about any individual's care may pivot on joint commitment, by parents and professionals, to the preservation of sensitive relationships around and towards the child (Fig. 32.2). Particularly in countries where technology is available, these decisions are likely to get harder as medicine advances and public expectations grow. Yet our focal point should always be the patient who, despite the clinical problems, is not an item of hospital property, but someone with individual personal needs. Such a child's best interests can never be met by snap judgements and it has to be said that life and death decisions are usually extremely difficult.

DILEMMAS OF CONFLICTING INTEREST

Dilemmas of life and death are mainly clinical situations where those taking decisions are, however superficially, known to each other. Except in matters of consent, the final decision in dilemmas over conflicting interests may not involve clinicians at all. Paediatricians expect and are expected to take a clear lead in clinical decision making. Because of their insight into the many aspects of child care, they also have responsibilities as advocates for children. Increasingly, as members of a society paying for health care, they must be cost conscious

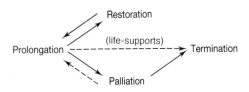

Fig. 32.1   Possible goals in the management of illness.

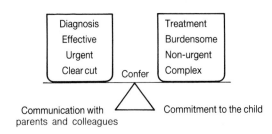

Fig. 32.2   Balancing options in management.

and be ready to advise on the distribution of costly resources. Finally, as ordinary citizens, they have votes and voices to use in seeking to establish the common weal. Thus, professionally, as public servants or as private individuals they can each have a contribution to make. As serious conflicts of interest arise, their special understanding of and relationship with children may be the factors which tip the balance when formulating appropriate recommendations. Paediatric advice may therefore be offered in case conferences, court rooms and resource committees (from local to national level) as well as in clinical settings. Paediatricians have a duty to speak for children in circumstances where they could otherwise be abused, even by those genuinely intending to be their protectors. Table 32.2 is reviewed in this light.

Consent

Young children who cannot possibly understand fully the need for painful treatment, research or the donation of organs, may have consent for such procedures given on their behalf by parents. Those

---

Table 32.2 Dilemmas of conflicting interests: child protection versus child abuse. When caregiver and child may have opposing view points

1. *Consent:*   *informed or enforced:*
   painful treatment
   research on children
   minors as donors

2. *Confidentiality:*   *keeping secrets from the child:*
   adoption
   artificial insemination by donor (AID)
   genetic or chromosomal abnormality
   life-threatening illness

                 telling the child's secrets:
   consultation with other carers
   court proceedings: abuse, divorce

3. *Cost:*   *cost-effective versus most effective:*
   emotional:
   hi-tech, low touch
   seeing through a child's eyes

   economic:
   quality adjusted life years (QALY)
   performance indicators
   prevention better than cure
   global inequalities

---

old enough to understand may not always feel bold enough to refuse, particularly if they are being asked to help another child, or if they want to please the researcher. We must therefore act sensitively and responsibly in these areas, to honour and not exploit a child's trust. A child even as young as 4 years of age may well be spontaneously altruistic and willing even to be hurt on behalf of someone known and loved, but to be hurt on behalf of unknown children requires an ability to weigh up pros and cons which is not usually an easy concept until 10 years of age or more. For a donor who is a minor, being in relationship with the recipient may again be the pivot on which the personal sacrifice is made. Other paediatric research, whether it be therapeutic or non-therapeutic, has ethical as well as medical implications. These should always include the need to see the investigation through the eyes of the child involved, as well as seeing any potential benefit for other children. Ethical committees which have to approve such projects could well benefit from a greater input by clinical psychologists than is at present customary.

Confidentiality; keeping secrets from the child

Here paediatricians may be asked to advise whether and when children should be told private information about themselves. In this computer and case-conference era, it is likely that secrets will at some time leak out and could reach the child by an undesirable and potentially shocking route. An athlete's unexpected chromosomal make-up could be devastatingly newsworthy. It may be wiser to let the child into such a secret casually and by degrees, starting early with factual, basic information before the implications will even be thought about. Thus, 'some people don't have their own babies' would be a simple statement to be built on later by further explanation, both of AID and infertility. The same approach holds for a life-threatening diagnosis.

Telling the child's secrets

A child's own secrets should be regarded as personal and private and his or her permission asked before sharing, for example, in a letter to the headmaster, that the child is being bullied at school. It is easy to overlook that confidences are confidential. Although a wife is not expected to give evidence against her husband, an abused child may be encouraged to give evidence against parents. Cross-questioning in court can be a form of child abuse in itself and even the use of videos as evidence, although done with protective intent, if also done without consent may actually abuse the child's trust. This is an area where those who understand children should share their knowledge, helping when need be to get existing practices changed.

Cost

Here, hospitals and governments have to balance what could be most effective with what would be cost effective. Resources are not limitless, yet neither should they be considered only in cash terms.

Emotional cost

High technology, with the social and personal segregation often involved in its practice, may risk too high a demand on family relationships. Thus, the exclusion of parents from neonatal intensive care units was found to be associated with an increase in child abuse. As old heads do not grow on young shoulders, so children may misconstrue other forms of separation, even those designed for their protection. Thus, being sent into care may be seen to result from the child's own naughtiness rather than due to the parents' unacceptable behaviour. For some children, the emotional cost of feeling rejected is borne for the rest of their lives. Not only may foster homes break down, but their financial cost is high: it could be more effective as well as cost effective to put greater effort into improving understanding within abusing families instead of even temporarily breaking them up.

Economic cost

This is also high for technological mechanisms. Demand usually outstrips supply. As more techniques develop, so their use becomes the norm and the cost of a health service escalates. Clinicians must learn to be responsibly aware of the price of care. The concept of quality-adjusted life years (QALY) evaluates the cost of treatment relative to the consequent survival rates, changes in life expectancy and effect on the quality of life, the aim of such exercises being to give more funding to the most productive procedures. Patients may take the risk to life expectancy implicit in experimental surgery, for the hope of improved life experience. Yet the same money spent on health education or on the herniorrhaphy waiting list could have helped far more people. Can the value of giving hope to one be balanced against the misery of hope delayed for many? Another managerial way of evaluating efficiency is the use of *performance indicators* which compare the turnover of patients and cost of treatment between different centres or departments. These yardsticks, are, of course, largely material and statistics do not give value judgements. However unpalatable clinicians may find resource management, this brings opportunities to help managers understand the human cost implicit in medical care. Facts must be presented with feeling.

Medical and societal ethics may thus overlap, but in the clinical situation the doctor's first concern is to meet the particular patient's need as appropriately as possible with the means available. Due thought must also be given to the emotional cost borne by the patient and the surrounding family, so evident when caring for children. Concentrating only on the material cost of care can be counter productive. Taking the emotional cost into our budgeting may help to show that what could be done is not always what should be done. Even apart from economic considerations, technology should be used with discrimination as a tool rather than being allowed to grow into a devouring tyrant.

Used correctly, the potential and actual benefits of modern advances are clearly enormous. Used indiscriminately, the enormous outlay will bring unsatisfactory return to families, physicians and the public purse alike.

In a personal series of 44 babies with spina bifida, none of whom received surgery, all died within a year, yet in their parents' eyes what discriminated between a child's life having been 'reasonably good' or 'rotten' was whether family interaction had been encouraged. Those who went home lived longer and their parents were happier than those whose care was entirely hospital based, and whose parents remained embittered years later. An entirely cash-centred exercise in the effectiveness of treatment would not expose such unseen and immeasurable facets of care.

Aetiology of cash-consuming disorders

All over the world it is a well-known, but unpopular, fact that much expensive disease is preventable. In the wealthier countries, adult obesity accounts for a significant percentage of morbidity and mortality. In child care worldwide, socioeconomic deprivation is a common cause of prematurity. It may cost about as much as a decent local house to apply the available intensity of care needed to save an extremely preterm baby's life. On the child's going home, poverty remains, as do high risks of further disease and deprivation. It could often be a more effective use of money to improve the social conditions at the root of these costly demands. Prevention is always better than cure and nowhere is this better seen than where global inequalities in the distribution of wealth and health go together. The developed world may present a working medical model but can also export serious mistakes; the purchase of extravagant hospital equipment may threaten village vaccination programmes. Yet we can also learn from developing countries that rich relationships do not depend on material prosperity and that neither quality nor quantity detract from the value perceived in the children themselves.

Those interested in achieving a better balance of care, working at what is best for the world's children, must include such considerations in their own ethical systems. Even so, wherever a child is cared for, the therapy offered must be the best available in that culture which is compatible with the emotional, as well as physical, needs of the patient. Health education and preventive intervention must be practised alongside clinical medicine. Governments will need to be properly informed about economic costs, but it is a political task to allocate resources appropriately. Paediatricians must learn to be better economists and politicians, as well as developing greater skills in evaluating the emotional cost of expensive therapy for their young patients and including this in the reckoning.

CONCLUSION

Ethical dilemmas in paediatric practice should be met in the context of personal relationships. In matters of life and death, family interaction must be guarded right to the end. Where there are other conflicts of interest, the child's viewpoint must be strongly represented as being a crucial, not a minor, factor in their resolution. In life, in death and in the crises between, doctors must always stand firm as advocates for children. This will sometimes involve helping others who may also be trying to speak for a child yet who will need to be enlightened as to how children think before they can truly act in any child's best interests.

FURTHER READING

Autton N 1984 Doctors talking. Mowbray, London

Beauchamp T L, Childress J F 1983 Principles of biomedical ethics, 2nd edn. Oxford University Press, Oxford

Brandon J, Warner J 1977 AID and adoption: some comparisons. British Journal of Social Work 7: 335–41.

Calne R 1987 Prospects for kidney and liver transplantation in children. Hospital Update December: 1030–1036.

Cook D 1983 The moral maze. SPCK, London

Delight E, Goodall J 1990 Love and loss: conversations with parents of babies with spina bifida managed without surgery. Developmental Medicine and Child Neurology Suppl 61 Vol 32, No 8

McCormick R 1974 To save or let die. Journal of American Medical Association 229: 172–176

Pearn J H 1984 The child and clinical research Lancet ii: 510–512

Richardson S A, Goodall J 1984 Trends in the management of spina bifida babies, 1971–1981: home care for the non-surgical group. Journal of Maternal and Child Health 9: 252–257

Scorer G, Wing A 1979 Decision making in medicine. Edward Arnold, London

Smith A S 1987 Qualms about QALYs. Lancet i: 1134–1136 (see also Lancet 1987; i: 1372)

UNICEF 1983 The state of the world's children 1984. Oxford University Press, Oxford

Vipuleadran V, Mason A R, Sunderland R 1988 Cost to the NHS of accidents to children in the West Midlands: notional values for grief, suffering and loss of earnings. British Medical Journal 296: 611

33. Examination technique

D. Harvey   I. Kovar

The hints in this section would apply to most examinations. The DCH is aimed to test knowledge and competence in primary care child health. The examiners' test is to decide whether you would be able to safely advise on and care for a child in primary care. It is not necessary to know the minutiae of rare diseases; it is important to be able to know the effects of these illnesses on children and their families, and to understand in a basic way the principles of management of the disorder. For example, with leukaemia, the examiner will be less concerned with your knowledge of specific drugs than with your understanding of principles of diagnosis (clinical findings, approach to investigations) and management (of pain, anaemia, bleeding, infection, social and family problems). It is important that you should obtain experience in, and feel competent with common problems, such as the clinical diagnosis of acute and chronic disorders of childhood, simple epidemiology, principles of assessment and screening (developmental, hearing, vision, and speech), infant feeding, immunisation, communication with social and educational agencies, common psychological disorders, and genetic counselling.

The examination should not be taken with book knowledge alone. An examining board may not require you to have undertaken a junior post in paediatrics; we would suggest that it is unwise to take this type of exam without a minimum of 6 months' suitable clinical experience. Discussion of clinical problems with friends and teachers, adequate reading around common problems, and confidence in the examination and assessment of well and sick children of different ages ensures the best preparation for this, and indeed any, clinical examination. Remember that the written examination tests theoretical *and* clinical knowledge.

The format of the exam varies slightly from one examining board to another. The common format is a written section with multiple choice questions (around 60), short note questions, and case commentaries or essays, and for successful candidates a clinical examination.

Written questions

Before sitting for a written examination, all candidates should look carefully at their handwriting; it would be even better to ask a colleague to criticise it. Is it legible? If it is not, there is not much hope of impressing the examiner. There is nothing more maddening for an examiner than struggling to understand what a candidate has written. Many candidates seem to make the mistake of writing too fast so that their writing deteriorates. It is better to write less, but clearly, rather than a lot which is illegible. If the view of your friends is that your writing is awful, it would be wise for you to take some professional advice about improving it.

At the top of the examination paper there will be instructions on how to answer it. These must be read very carefully, in order to answer the right number of questions and to know if any of them is compulsory. One should read each question more than once. A plan can then be made for the time available for answering them.

A candidate who does not have English as a first language must make certain of having sufficient command of it to answer the questions easily. If not, it could be sensible to take some instruction on improving it. It is not necessary to worry too much about spelling; it is, of course, useful to be able to spell correctly, but it is more important to write down information clearly and precisely.

Multiple choice questions (MCQ)

Many candidates seem confused by these questions, but they have been shown to test knowledge more satisfactorily than other methods.

Before answering the question, one should be certain of what is being asked. It is usually wise to read the question more than once, perhaps three times would be best. Almost all MCQs have a basic statement which is called the stem, and there are several questions based on it. The stem may be only one word, but is more likely to be a short sentence.

There are several different types of MCQ. One variety asks several, usually five, questions about the stem and only one is correct. The MCQ most commonly used in the UK is known as the 'true, false or don't know' type. There are usually five questions about the stem, but any of the statements can be correct; sometimes all of them are correct, sometimes none, or any other combination. Each item question may be independent of the others. It is important to understand this type of MCQ, as they are the commonest in the DCH. A mark is given for each of the five questions about the stem. If the statement is false and it is answered as false, a mark will be given; similarly if a true statement is answered as true. But a mark will be lost if the answer is wrong. A mark is not lost when a statement is marked as don't know. It is therefore very important *not* to guess. Questions should only be answered as true or false by a candidate who is almost certain of being correct. The answer sheet is usually marked by optical scanner linked to a computer. Care has to be taken to fill in the correct box; nothing is worse than to find out after several questions that you are out of sequence.

MCQs are fairly difficult to set accurately. They are always discussed carefully by the examiners and are evaluated after they have been used to discard any which are ambiguous or do not seem to discriminate well between good and poor candidates. There is no point in having questions which are so difficult that none can answer them or so easy that every candidate gets them right.

It is a good idea to practise MCQs; they should be answered against the clock, in order to mimic the time restraints of a real examination.

Short note questions

It is common to find some questions which start with 'Write short notes on. . . .' or 'Write a brief account of. . . .' Do not be tempted to write too much; it is especially easy to do this when one of the questions is on a subject about which one knows a great deal. It is easy to write too much and to spend so much time that the other questions are skimped; because they are more difficult, they need more thought.

It sometimes helps to make lists or underline some words to draw attention to them. The aim should be to get information over to the examiner in the shortest and clearest fashion.

Essay questions

There seem to be going out of fashion in favour of MCQs and short questions. However, some examinations still expect candidates to write a long account of a subject and to spend about 45 minutes on the answer. It is always possible to find out the type of questions which are asked by writing to the examining board which is organising the exam. They will usually be prepared to send old examination papers, so that candidates can practise.

Whereas a short question can be answered with only short phrases, an essay should be written in normal English prose, with proper sentences. It will be necessary to spend a little time planning what needs to be written. The answer should have a short introduction, then cover the subject in a logical fashion and end with some sort of conclusion. It is quite permissable to include lists or even to draw diagrams to illustrate something which cannot be described easily in words. A judicious amount of underlining may help the examiner.

Clinical examination (long and short cases)

This is usually the most difficult part of the examination. The candidate will be given a time to take the history and examine the child; then the examiner will listen to a presentation of the findings. A statement of the child's problems and a plan for their management will be expected. There is usually not enough time for the history and examination, rarely as much as in an outpatient clinic, so it is important to move fast. This is why a candidate should prepare for the exam by developing a plan of history taking and examination by the constant practice of seeing children. Do not forget important parts of the history, such as the birth, the family's illnesses and living conditions, development and immunisation. If these items are always included in one's daily work, they will not be forgotten in the fluster of the exam. That, after all, is the point of the clinical — to see if the candidate's technique of clinical practice is satisfactory.

Every moment free should be used to do a complete examination of the child, not forgetting important things like taking the blood pressure of older children. If it is impossible to do certain things, this should be explained to the examiner; examples are that one would like to measure a child accurately and to test the hearing.

Ward rounds are good practice. It is necessary to present every small point in the history, but to mention the salient points and demonstrate that a full history and examination have been done. It is permissible, for example to say 'There were no important features in the family history' or 'The rest of the examination was normal'. The examiner can always ask for more details.

If it does not seem possible to make one diagnosis, the examiner should be told so. It is usually more useful to list the child's problems, if any, and to make a plan for management. One should not expect every child to be abnormal; many children in ordinary clinical practice are normal and they appear in an exam. If you think that a child is normal, you should say so. After the long case, another examiner will show a candidate some short cases. The children will usually have some obvious clinical signs, which allow a straightforward diagnosis to be made. Sometimes the examiner may want a demonstration of clinical ability, so the question may be 'Please examine the cardiovascular system'. One must watch out for other related physical signs; thus if a large liver is found, a search should be made for jaundice.

The short cases allow a candidate to demonstrate the ability to approach children properly. It is wise to get down to their level and to remember the dictum 'Never take your child to a paediatrician with a good pair of trousers, because it means that he doesn't kneel on the floor'.

It is difficult to make a recommendation about what to wear for the exam. There are no rules, except to look clean and tidy. Some examiners do not like dress which is too informal, but it is unwise to wear anything too formal and uncomfortable as it might hinder a relaxed attitude to the children. A middle way would seem best.

The viva voce

The oral examination is also less popular with examiners than it was. Certainly some candidates perform less well than they should, because they are so nervous.

The examiners will ask questions or may show X-rays or pictures of patients. They are keen to have practical replies and will pay less attention to esoteric information gleaned from a textbook than knowledge drawn from common clinical work.

As in most parts of the exam, one can only perform well with practice and rehearsal. A good way of preparing oneself is to show X-rays to colleagues who are also taking the exam and to demand quick answers to questions. The questioning can then be reversed. Only by getting used to aggressive questioning can one become used to the nerve-racking pressure of the oral.

Changes in the examinations

New techniques are constantly being introduced. For example, it is possible to show videotapes of children and these can be used to replace parts of the clinical examination. When parts of the exam are shown to be unsatisfactory, they are dropped and replaced by a new type of assessment. One should always check with the examining board to be certain that they have not made any changes.

34. Multiple choice questions

1 **Cot deaths:**
A are more likely to occur in babies of low birth-weight
B are more likely to occur in those whose sibling was previously a cot death
C could have been avoided in 50% of cases
D are usually caused by parental failure
E are associated with negative postmortem findings in over 90% of cases

2 **Vaccines in common use against the following infectious disease contain live organisms:**
A measles
B diphtheria
C rubella
D tuberculosis
E typhoid (monovalent)

3 **Cystic fibrosis is a disease characterised by:**
A changes in exocrine glands
B small bowel mucosal villous atrophy
C fat globules in the stool on microscopy
D a low sweat sodium and chloride concentration
E recessive inheritance

4 **The following statements are true:**
A a steady state concentration will be reached earlier when regular large doses are administered
B drugs eliminated by the kidney should not be given to patients in renal failure
C the grey baby syndrome should not occur if chloramphenicol levels are maintained within the therapeutic range
D the timing of samples for monitoring drugs is unimportant if the drug is in a steady state
E most children require larger weight related doses of most drugs than adults

5 **Pertussis (whooping cough):**
A is only mildly contagious
B is characterised by a spasmodic cough and is often accompanied by vomiting
C is always due to an infection with *Bordatella pertussis*
D may produce subconjunctival haemorrhages
E is hardly ever seen in the first 3 months of life due to passive immunity provided by the mother

6 **In measles:**
A the rash starts peripherally and spreads towards the face
B the rash may desquamate
C Koplik spots appear at the same time as the rash
D blindness is a recognised complication
E viral pneumonitis with tachypnoea may occur before the appearance of the rash

7 **Long-term immunity follows naturally acquired infection with:**
A measles
B rubella
C tetanus
D pertussis
E mumps

8 **The duration of the incubation period of:**
  A rubella is 7–10 days
  B measles is 8–11 days
  C chickenpox is 3–5 days
  D mumps is 7–10 days
  E malaria is 9–30 days

9 **Viruses involved in respiratory tract infection of infants include:**
  A adenovirus
  B parainfluenza
  C *Herpesvirus hominis*
  D respiratory syncytial virus
  E cytomegalovirus

10 **Pubertal development is abnormal when:**
  A testicular enlargement occurs in a boy of 8 years
  B there are no signs of testicular enlargement in a boy of 12 years
  C menarche does not occur until 16 years
  D there are no signs of breast enlargement in a 14-year-old girl
  E pubic hair appears in a 9-year-old girl

11 **The following conditions are more common in patients of immigrant origin compared with those of indigenous origin:**
  A unsatisfactory housing
  B unemployment
  C threadworms
  D non-pulmonary tuberculosis
  E iron deficiency anaemia

12 **Which of the following could cause an infant not to bend the right elbow and shoulder?**
  A lumbar meningomyelocele
  B hydrocephalus
  C right Erb's palsy
  D fracture of right humerus
  E right cephalhaematoma

13 **Frank blood in the stools of a 6-month-old child may be due to:**
  A anal fissure
  B intussusception
  C Meckel's diverticulum
  D appendicitis
  E shigella gastroenteritis

14 **Abdominal pain in childhood may be associated with:**
  A lobar pneumonia
  B Henoch-Schönlein purpura
  C school phobia
  D diabetes insipidus
  E lead poisoning

15 **Congenital dislocation of the hip:**
  A is commoner in girls than boys
  B is commoner in infants with spina bifida
  C cannot be detected at birth
  D may run in families
  E always requires an operation

16 **Deafness occurs following:**
  A meningococcal meningitis
  B measles
  C mumps
  D 'glue' ear
  E congenital syphilis

17 **In the following 3 questions indicate whether each statement is true or false.**
  A conductive nerve deafness is a sign of kernicterus
  B hypothyroidism may cause prolonged neonatal jaundice
  C plasma unconjugated bilirubin levels below 340 μmol/l are not associated with kernicterus in preterm infants
  D bruising may cause hyperbilirubinaemia
  E hypoglycaemic convulsions have a better prognosis than hypocalcaemic convulsions

18 A cyanosis of hands and feet occurs in many healthy babies
  B subconjunctival haemorrhage is associated with intracranial haemorrhage
  C infants of poorly-controlled diabetics are prone to respiratory distress syndrome
  D anaemia may cause respiratory distress
  E meconium aspiration indicates intrapartum asphyxia

19
A small-for-gestational-age term infants are liable to intraventricular haemorrhage
B cow's milk has a higher protein content than human milk
C cow's milk has a higher vitamin D content than human milk
D *Staphylococcus aureus* is the commonest cause of neonatal septicaemia
E modern artificial baby milks are not allergenic

20 Which of the following could cause bile-stained vomiting?
A overfeeding
B malrotation of the gut
C oesophageal atresia
D pyloric stenosis
E Hirschsprung's disease

21 Hydrocolpos:
A usually presents during the neonatal period
B is best managed by abdominal exploration
C may be due to excessive oestrogen secretion in the child .
D regresses spontaneously in many instances
E causes retention of urine

22 Evaluation of every child who has enuresis should include the following:
A family history
B urine culture
C intravenous urography
D a test of renal function
E physical examination

23 Immunisation against whooping cough is contra-indicated in:
A a child with acute otitis media
B a child whose birth weight was less than 2500 g
C the child who is allergic to eggs
D a child with a history of neonatal convulsions
E a child with eczema

24 In rubella:
A the rash usually appears on the third day
B the rash spares the face
C arthropathy may occur
D the rash is never vesicular
E the occipital adenopathy is an important diagnostic feature

25 In chickenpox:
A the lesions should heal without scarring
B the rash is centrifugal in distribution
C routine immunisation is offered to all children at one year
D hyperimmune gammaglobulin may be a common adjunct to therapy if the patient is taking steroids
E acquired in the first 5 days of life has approximately a 20% mortality

26 Strawberry naevi:
A are usually present at birth
B are hamartomas
C commonly undergo malignant change
D may be associated with an intracranial haemangioma on the same side
E should be excised

27 In iron poisoning:
A no symptoms occur until 8 hours after ingestion
B may cause an encephalopathy
C penicillamine is the treatment of choice
D if symptom free after 24 hours the patient may be discharged
E scarring of the pylorus may occur as a late complication

28 The risk of developing malignant disease in childhood is:
A 1:100
B 1:200
C 1:600
D 1:2000
E 1:10 000

29 The health visitor:
A can be a state enrolled nurse (SEN)
B is an employee of the general practitioners with whom she works
C must have some experience in obstetric nursing

D works solely with antenatal mothers and children up to the age of 15

E can prescribe treatment for simple medical conditions

30 An infant's size at birth:
A relates equally to maternal and parental size
B may be greater than expected if mother is diabetic
C correlates well with his adult height
D is not affected by sex
E is likely to be reduced if there is a congenital malformation

31 Vaginal bleeding in childhood is:
A commonest between 4 and 6 years of age
B often due to a blood dyscrasia
C caused by a foreign body in the vagina
D often associated with precocious puberty
E sometimes due to a malignant tumour of the vagina

32 Would you be worried about a child's development if:
A there was head lag on pull to sit at 5 months
B he was not sitting alone by 7 months
C he was not speaking in sentences by 18 months
D he was not walking alone by 18 months
E there was no tuneful babble with consonants by 10 months

33 The commonest malignant solid tumour of childhood is:
A nephroblastoma
B brain tumour
C Hodgkin's disease
D rhabdomyosarcoma
E osteogenic sarcoma

34 Vulvovaginitis in a child is:
A common in the neonatal period
B usually due to vaginal foreign bodies
C the result of poor vaginal acidity
D responsive to local oestrogen cream
E an allergic phenomenon

35 A 3-year-old cannot sleep at night and goes into his parents' bed. You should:
A admit him to hospital
B use a night sedative as first line of treatment
C discuss with the parents what has been happening in the family
D help the parents to be firm in putting the child back to bed
E explain that this is normal

36 Cystic fibrosis:
A occurs in one in 4000 Caucasian infants
B is commoner in African than Chinese peoples
C is commoner in males than females
D is inherited as an autosomal recessive
E has a gene carrier rate of one in 100

37 The common sites of presentation of soft tissue sarcomas in childhood are:
A head and neck
B retroperitoneum
C genito-urinary tract
D central nervous system
E lung

38 In the neonatal period:
A breast swelling in little girls is a serious problem calling for early treatment
B a vaginal discharge is often evident
C vaginal bleeding is never encountered
D cystic vulval swellings call for early excision
E vulval congestion and oedema are common

39 Most children of 3 years should:
A speak using short sentences
B give name and address
C play appropriately with miniature toys
D build a bridge of three cubes from memory
E remain clean and dry, day and night

40 Acute leukaemia in childhood may mimic:
A rheumatoid arthritis
B streptococcal tonsillitis
C irritable hip syndrome
D iron deficiency anaemia
E infectious mononucleosis

41 The following features suggest handicap:
A Moro reflex present at 6 months
B easily elicited asymmetrical tonic neck reflex
C hand preference present by 2 years
D mouthing toys at 18 months
E hand regard at 3 months

42 Significant bacteruria:
A is indicated by $>10^3$ bacteria/ml urine
B is always accompanied by pyuria
C may be asymptomatic
D in most cases involves the upper urinary tract as well as the bladder
E is an indication for a micturating cysto-urethrogram

43 In normal pubertal development:
A the pubertal growth spurt occurs earlier in boys than in girls
B testicular enlargement is the first sign of puberty in the male
C at the time of onset of menstruation in girls the height spurt is almost complete
D gynaecomastia may occur in boys
E aprocrine sweat activity, oiliness of the hair and acne are androgenic changes

44 In immunological reactions:
A T lymphocytes manufacture antibodies
B IgG may mediate type 1 hypersensitivity
C histamine is released from eosinophils
D IgA reduces antigen absorption through epithelial surfaces
E activation of the complement system produces cell lysis

45 The prescriber should:
A generally use liquid preparations for children under 8 years
B limit tetracyclines to topical use only in children under 12 years
C only use inhalational drug forms if oral forms are unavailable
D always check the weight and age of the child before prescribing
E use parenteral preparations in only those occasions when the child is vomiting

46 Rickets is more common in the following immigrant groups than in the indigenous population:
A Asian children over the age of two
B Chinese children
C African children
D Asian mothers
E Asian babies around the age of 6 months

47 The following vaccines are normally given by subcutaneous or intramuscular injection:
A measles
B poliomyelitis
C tuberculosis
D smallpox
E tetanus

48 Infantile eczema:
A may improve on a cow's-milk-free diet
B is less common in breast-fed babies
C is made worse by frequent baths
D on the face should never be treated with topical fluorinated steroids
E is made worse by heat

49 Children on cytotoxic chemotherapy are at particular risk from:
A nutritional deficiency
B skin infections
C chickenpox and measles
D sleep disturbance
E fungal infections

50 A five-year-old-boy has never spoken. You should:
A refer him for hearing tests
B see if there is any abnormal behaviour such as stereotypies
C take a detailed developmental history
D take a detailed family history
E check maternal rubella antibody titres

51 The following are associated with hypertension:
A coarctation of the aorta
B end-stage renal disease
C acute renal failure

D acute post-streptococcal glomerulonephritis

E acute gastroenteritis

52 **A 6-year-old girl has been dry at night but is now wetting again. You should:**

A restrict her night time fluid intake

B discuss possible family upsets with her parents

C keep her home from school

D set up an award system for dry nights

E culture her urine

53 **The following are common precipitants of wheeze in asthmatic children:**

A *Dermatophagoides pteronyssinus*

B exercise

C *Aspergillus fumigatus*

D adenovirus

E egg ingestion

54 **Three months after entering the UK a 3-year-old girl from a rural community in Pakistan develops a fever 39°C, vomiting and loose stools. She passed five round-worms in her stool:**

A her symptoms are due to heavy infestation with *Ascaris lumbricoides*

B she should be suspected of suffering from *P. vivax* malaria and this must be confirmed by examining a blood film

C she should be given a course of chloroquine immediately as cerebral malaria is a likely complication

D stool examination for *Giardia lamblia* and *Entamoeba histolytica* are unlikely to be positive

E she should be investigated for salmonellosis and shigellosis.

55 **In acute haemolysis:**

A the urine is brown due to methaemoglobin

B loin pain and myalgia occur

C reticulocytes and nucleated red cells are seen in the blood in the acute phase

D ascorbic acid as an antioxidant can limit the haemolysis in G6PD deficient patients

E testing for G6PD deficiency is best done during the acute haemolytic episode

56 **Vesico-ureteric reflux:**

A is an abnormal finding

B may disappear spontaneously

C is attributed to an abnormally long intramural course of the ureter

D should always be corrected surgically

E implies bladder neck obstruction

57 **In a retarded child with bilateral cataracts you might expect to find the following:**

A aminoaciduria and glycosuria

B a continuous heart murmur

C polydactyly

D warts

E deafness

58 **The children of social class IV parents:**

A include the sons of hotel porters

B make more use of immunisation services than do children of social class I parents

C make more use of the diagnostic and therapeutic services that the general practitioner offers, than do children of social class I parents

D have a greater chance of dying in the first year of life than do children of social class I parents

E are more likely to suffer from dental caries than the children of social class I parents

59 **The following conditions fulfill the criteria necessary for screening:**

A undescended testes

B hypothyroidism in the newborn

C plantar warts

D hypertension

E conductive deafness

60 **A 14-year-old is missing school, because of abdominal pain. You should:**

A see his parents and discuss ways of getting him to school

B admit him to hospital for investigations

C see if his mother is depressed or anxious

D test his urine

E contact educational welfare officer

61 **In an infant with a ventricular septal defect:**

A the shunt of blood through the VSD is from left to right

B there may be a diastolic murmur in the left mid-parasternal area

C the murmur is soft in quality and occupies only the first half of diastole

D the pulmonary circulation is congested on chest X-ray

E failure to thrive is common

62 In rheumatic fever:

A there may be a rash consisting of rings of normal skin surrounded by a raised erythematous margin

B an apical diastolic murmur might be heard

C there may be a prolonged PR interval on ECG

D the knees are often swollen for some weeks

E steroids are the treatment of choice

63 In infancy, heart failure:

A never occurs in the first day of life

B commonly presents with peripheral oedema

C causes enlargement of the liver

D may be caused by paroxysmal tachycardia

E should never be treated with digoxin

64 The following may occur in childhood lead poisoning:

A purpura

B reticulocytosis

C anaemia

D abdominal colic

E blue lines on the gums

65 The following diseases are correctly placed against their causes:

A neonatal tetanus: hypocalcaemia

B acute infantile bronchiolitis: respiratory syncytial virus

C *Haemophilus influenzae* meningitis: influenza virus

D oral thrush: *Oxyuris vermicularis*

E infective hepatitis: Epstein-Barr virus

66 Which of the following may be features of hypothyroidism in an 8-week-old infant?

A umbilical hernia

B dry skin

C prolonged physiological jaundice

D poor peripheral circulation

E hypotonia

67 Atopy:

A may be reduced by breast feeding

B may be influenced by month of birth

C is common in cystic fibrosis

D is associated with high IgD levels

E is always symptomatic

68 In haemolytic disease of the newborn which of the following are true?

A blood film showing 4 per cent nucleated red cells is diagnostic

B death *in utero* may be due to cardiac failure associated with haemolytic anemia

C Rhesus haemolytic disease is completely preventable by antenatal screening

D ABO disease occurs when maternal IgM antibodies are involved causing complete red cell lysis

E exchange transfusion may have to be repeated several times in severe cases of Rhesus disease

69 Defects of immune systems:

A frequently lead to development of atopy

B may be associated with absent tonsils and adenoids

C commonly occur in cystic fibrosis

D may occur following measles infection

E can be detected by a positive tuberculin test

70 Feeding:

A breast-fed infants are seldom grossly obese

B cereals should be introduced in the second month of life

C gastroenteritis is less common in bottle-fed babies

D infants with phenylketonuria should not be fed with goat's milk

E phenindione anticoagulant therapy in the mother is a contra-indication to breast feeding

71 The steroid-responsive nephrotic syndrome is associated with:

A microscopic haematuria

B reduced albumin synthesis

C highly selective proteinuria

D hypovolaemia if the PCV falls

E girls more commonly than boys

72 The following statements are true of imported childhood disease in the UK:

A visceral leishmaniasis can mimic acute leukaemia

B folate deficiency anaemia is associated with heavy hookworm infestation

C iron deficiency anaemis, tenesmus and rectal prolapse are features of heavy infestation with *Trichuris trichiuria*

D the majority of cases of childhood malaria are due to *P. falciparum*

E anaemia and splenomegaly are features of haematological inherited disease

73 In β-thalassaemia:

A dietary iron deficiency frequently exacerbates the anaemia of β-thalassaemia trait

B when both parents have β-thalassaemia trait no normal offspring will be produced

C blood transfusions should be avoided in β-thalassaemia major to prevent iron overload

D in β-thalassaemia, major death commonly occurs in the second or third decade from heart failure

E a serum ferritin of 13 μg/l is diagnostic of β-thalassaemia major

74 After a cot death, parents:

A usually receive much support from a variety of social and medical agencies

B will blame themselves for their child's death

C will continue to hear their child crying, especially at night

D soon recover from their grief, especially if another pregnancy quickly follows

E usually talk openly about their loss

75 Which of the following are associated with constipation:

A sugar intolerance

B anal fissure

C pyloric stenosis

D hypothyroidism

E Crohn's disease

76 Antihistamines are useful treatment for:

A contact dermatitis

B angio-oedema

C asthma

D coeliac disease

E chronic granulomatous disease

77 An 8-month-old male Chinese infant born in Vietnam is failing to thrive because he is not taking his feeds. He is listless, pale and underweight and his spleen is palpable 1 cm below the costal margin:

A he should be investigated for primary disseminated tuberculosis

B a blood film should be examined and a specimen sent for haemoglobin electrophoresis

C thalassaemia is not likely, if both parents are not anaemic

D his parents should be asked about exposure of their baby to naphthalene because of the danger of haemolysis in G6PD deficient infants

E if this baby was not jaundiced during the neonatal period, he is unlikely to be G6PD deficient

78 In an 8-year-old child complaining of recurrent episodes of mid-abdominal pain without obvious cause, it would generally be accepted as wise to:

A examine the urine for infection

B review the child's emotional and psychological status

C remove the appendix

D reassure the parents

E X-ray the spine

79 In unilateral talipes equinovarus:

A the forefoot is adducted

B the heel is everted

C there is overactivity of tibialis anterior muscle

D there may be an associated myelodysplasia

E a posteromedial release operation may be required

80 A 16-year-old girl has secondary amenorrhoea: You should:

A weigh her

B put her on the 'pill'

C arrange an immediate psychiatric opinion
D reassure her and her parents
E do a pregnancy test

81 Undiluted fresh cow's milk when compared with human breast milk contains more of the following:
A protein
B lactose
C fat
D phosphorus
E sodium

82 A 5-year-old English boy develops headache, vomiting cough and fever 40°C, 5 weeks after a holiday in Kenya. He had taken chloroquine 150 mg weekly whilst on holiday and for 3 weeks on return to the UK:
A he is unlikely to be suffering from malaria because he has been taking chloroquine
B malaria should be suspected as the most likely diagnosis
C Lassa fever is a likely diagnosis
D the presence of anaemia and splenomegaly on examination support the diagnosis of *P. falciparum* malaria
E if he has continuous fever and jaundice he probably has hepatitis

83 Rickets:
A always responds to oral vitamin D
B is less common in Asian immigrant children
C is excluded if the serum calcium level is normal
D may be associated with retarded motor development
E causes an angular stomatitis

84 Congenital adrenal hyperplasia of the 21-hydroxylase type:
A is inherited as an autosomal dominant
B can be diagnosed pre-natally
C may present as primary amenorrhoea
D if inadequately treated the excess androgens cause rapid linear growth and tall stature as adults

E may cause neonatal death due to severe hyponatraemic dehydration

85 Headache:
A the longer the history of headache the more serious is the cause likely to be
B erogotamine derivatives do not make a major contribution to the treatment of headache in childhood
C headaches due to raised intracranial pressure are acute but often brief
D the pain associated with tension headache in childhood has no organic basis
E the treatment of choice for headache in children under the age of 10 is soluble aspirin

86 Clumsy children:
A do not usually have an abnormal birth history
B are usually of normal birth weight
C are best identified by the performance scale of the WISC
D are difficult to identify reliably at the age of school entry
E respond well to stimulant drugs

87 The 3-week-old baby should:
A gain 20–30 g daily
B require 50 ml of milk/kg daily
C require 10 μg (400 iu) vitamin D daily
D take 5 minutes for a feed
E be given iron supplements routinely

88 Nasal polyps:
A occur commonly in cystic fibrosis
B are always bilateral
C are associated in some cases with an increased sensitivity to aspirin
D are associated with intestinal polyps
E may be mistaken for a meningocele

89 In juvenile rheumatoid arthritis (IgM Rh factor positive):
A boys are more affected than girls
B chronic arthritis is common
C the commonest age of onset is less than 2 years
D erosions may occur on X-ray

E HLA B27 tissue type antigen is present in 75%

90 **Iron deficiency in children:**
A is less common than megaloblastic anaemia
B is sometimes a presenting feature of coeliac disease
C is common in preterm infants
D causes a macrocytic hypochromic anaemia
E may be associated with hookworm infestation

91 **Feeding difficulties in the neonatal period may be due to:**
A prematurity
B hiatus hernia
C cerebral birth trauma
D intrauterine growth retardation
E congenital heart disease

92 **Stridor in the first 2 weeks may be caused by:**
A subglottic stenosis
B haemangioma of trachea
C laryngomalacia
D milk allergy
E cystic hygroma

93 **Reduced height velocity in the pre-pubertal child may be a feature of:**
A hypothyroidism
B congenital adrenal hyperplasia
C long-term steroid therapy
D simple obesity
E coeliac disease

94 **Nephroblastoma occurs with increased frequency in association with the following anomalies:**
A imperforate anus
B hemihypertrophy
C aniridia
D hypoplastic lung
E phocomelia

95 **Which of the following agents are β_2 stimulants and useful in asthma:**
A disodium cromoglycate
B beclomethasone propionate
C terbutaline
D aminophylline
E salbutamol

96 **In bleeding disorders:**
A prolonged prothrombin time, kaolin cephalin coagulation time and low platelet count suggest disseminated intravascular coagulation
B fresh frozen plasma is the treatment of choice in an acute joint bleed in a patient with haemophilia
C in a child with spontaneous bruising a platelet count of $202 \times 10^9/l$ suggests that non-accidental injury is a more likely cause than thrombocytopenia
D heparin treatment has dramatically reduced the mortality of the haemolytic-uraemic syndrome
E a history of recent viral infections should be sought in children presenting with thrombocytopenia

97 **Childhood asthma:**
A is always associated with atopy
B may be confused with an inhaled foreign body
C invariably remits in adolescence
D may respond to atropine
E is associated with eczema in less than 20% of cases

98 **Immediate priorities in the management of severe gastroenteritis are:**
A give a broad spectrum antibiotic
B stop oral feeding
C use an anti-emetic drug
D begin to restore fluid and electrolyte balance
E administer intravenous potassium

99 **The following activities represent secondary prevention:**
A immunisation against poliomyelitis
B amniocentesis for spina bifida
C the Guthrie test for phenylketonuria
D screening for hypertension
E the administration of anti D gamma-globulin postnatally in the Rhesus-negative

mother who has given birth to a Rhesus-positive baby

100 Which of the following statements are true:
A most drugs are metabolised at faster rates in children than adults
B for most drugs, mothers on therapy should be discouraged from breast feeding
C oxytetracycline is one of the drugs of choice for children with *Haemophilus influenzae* infections
D tricyclic antidepressant drugs are the first line in the general management of nocturnal enuresis
E Using an appropriate fluid and electrolyte mixture is a better approach to viral gastroenteritis management in the infant than using a kaolin paediatric mixture

101 The majority of tumours of the central nervous system in childhood:
A occur in structures above the tentorium
B are glioblastomas
C present with severe headaches
D cause a block in the CSF pathway
E respond well to cytotoxic chemotherapy

102 Under the National Health Service in the UK, a general practitioner:
A is employed by the local health authority
B is responsible for the care his patients receive from his deputy, even when he himself is not on call
C is more likely to be working single-handed than in partnership
D is responsible for providing the premises from which he works
E can obtain from the local district hospital the simple diagnostic equipment that he needs to do his work

103 The following statements are true:
A antibacterial prophylaxis should be limited to children with recurrent urinary tract infections or previous rheumatic fever
B most commonly used drugs are best given after meals
C intramuscular therapy will always prove

more effective than that given by the oral route
D children generally require less frequent drug dosing than adults
E compliance should be better with single rather than multiple therapy

104 Which of the following are associated with Turner's syndrome:
A dysplastic nails
B short stature
C pulmonary stenosis
D cubitus valgus
E primary amenorrhoea

105 In the treatment of imported diseases:
A chloroquine is the drug of choice for all types of acute malaria
B piperazine citrate is the drug of choice for ascaris infestation
C piperazine citrate is a safe drug and can be given in multiple doses
D thiabendazole is effective against hookworm and trichuris
E metronidazole is effective against *Entamoeba histolytica* and *Giardia lamblia* but a higher dose is required for the former

106 The following may cause malabsorption:
A threadworm infestation
B tuberculosis of the gut
C *Giardia lamblia* infection
D gluten sensitivity
E Hirschsprung's disease

107 The following convey a greater than 10% risk of epileptic seizures in later childhood and adolescence:
A reflex anoxic seizures in the first year
B two febrile convulsions in the first 3 years
C one parent affected by idiopathic epilepsy
D idiopathic infantile spasms
E head injury aged 5 with post-traumatic amnesia of 6 hours

108 The following are recognised adverse effects of sodium valproate:
A permanent alopecia
B thrombocytopenia

C induction of barbiturate metabolism
D liver failure
E depression and irritability

109 Febrile convulsions:
A can be prevented by intermittent treatment with phenobarbitone
B are the commonest seizure type under the age of 6 months
C are commoner in children with history of perinatal problems
D affect the sexes equally
E a positive family history favours a better outcome

110 A 25-year-old woman develops rubella during the third month of her pregnancy:
A the chances of a major fetal abnormality are greater than 50 per cent
B cardiac abnormalities in the fetus are unlikely
C the affected baby may excrete the virus for more than one year
D deafness is the commonest congenital abnormality at this stage
E giving immunoglobulin prevents any complication

111 In primary tuberculosis in children:
A the infection may be silent
B miliary TB cannot result
C erythema nodosum is never a feature
D the treatment of choice is isoniazid on its own for at least one year
E Mantoux conversion takes 3 weeks

112 The following are classical features of congenital rubella infection:
A jaundice
B hypoglycaemia
C purpura
D microphthalmia
E patent ductus arteriosus

113 Infantile gastroenteritis:
A is due to bacterial infection in over 70% of cases
B may be caused by coliform organisms

C is rare in wholly breast-fed infants
D is usually associated with metabolic alkalosis
E may present with meningism

114 Croup:
A is never a serious condition
B is characterised by expiratory stridor
C is often associated with an upper respiratory tract infection
D principally affects children over the age of 3 years
E may be caused by an acute epiglottitis

115 Cerebral palsy:
A in school age the incidence is about 2.5 per 1000
B spasticity is present from birth
C sensory loss is always present
D in bilateral hemiplegia the upper limbs are more severely affected than the lower
E hearing impairment occurs more frequently in dyskinesia than other forms of cerebral palsy

116 Transposition of the great vessels:
A is a form of non-cyanotic heart disease
B produces pulmonary oligaemia
C is incompatible with life unless there is also a VSD or a patent ductus arteriosus
D is associated with an increased heart size
E requires urgent treatment in the first few days of life

117 The following are associated with non-accidental injury to children:
A the degree of injury is out of keeping with the history
B bruises that appear to have a similar time aetiology
C retinal haemorrhages
D no delay between the injury and the seeking of medical advice
E spiral fractures of the long bones

118 Cerebral palsy:
A is a progressive condition
B is always associated with mental handicap

C is often associated with squint

D may be genetically determined

E can usually be diagnosed soon after birth

119 Severe visual handicap:

A may result from congenital cataracts

B can usually be detected at six weeks of age

C may cause delays in other areas of development

D in prenatal rubella is usually caused by retinopathy

E is not associated with premature birth

120 Delayed speech development:

A should be considered when a child uses only two words with meaning at one year of age

B may be due to hearing impairment

C is a common presenting symptom of mental handicap

D may be due to deprivation

E may be due to tongue-tie

121 Severe mental handicap:

A affects 3% of children

B is usually associated with late walking

C is usually associated with delayed language

D may cause early plateauing of development

E is usually the result of biological factors rather than normal variation

122 Clumsiness:

A is not a significant handicap to a child

B may be associated with specific learning difficulties

C may be associated with poor school progress

D is commoner following perinatal problems

E is readily apparent on brief neurological examination

123 Most children of 12 months should be able to:

A walk alone at least 10 steps

B sit alone

C move independently, e.g. by crawling

D find a toy that has rolled out of sight

E select familiar life-size objects on naming

124 A 3-year-old should be able to:

A pedal a tricycle

B build a 3-brick bridge

C select 3 objects on naming

D speak in short 3-word sentences

E ask questions

125 The risk of the same disorder recurring in siblings is greater than 1 in 10 if:

A the index child is a mutant for an autosomal dominant condition

B the index child has microcephaly for which no cause can be found

C the sibling shares one haplotype with the index child, who has congenital adrenal hyperplasia

D the index child has a de novo chromosomal translocation

E the index child has the fragile-X syndrome

126 It is useful to have the following when assessing the carrier status of the sister of a boy with Duchenne muscular dystrophy:

A blood from the affected boy for DNA studies

B blood from his unaffected brother for DNA studies

C blood from the affected boy's father for DNA studies

D blood from the sister for creatine kinase estimation

E a family history

127 Acute leukaemia in childhood:

A is usually myeloid in type

B often presents with bone pain

C can cause raised intracranial pressure

D will be associated with mediastinal widening in 10–15% of cases

E is always accompanied by a constitutional chromosomal anomaly

128 Brain tumours in childhood:

A occur most frequently in the cerebral hemispheres

B never produce metastases

C occasionally present with grand mal epilepsy

D may be associated with growth failure
E can cause unilateral blindness

129 Neuroblastoma:

A is commoner in the older child
B has a variable prognosis dependant on age
C can present with subcutaneous nodules
D may be associated with Horner's syndrome
E never spreads to bone marrow

130 Histiocytosis X (Langerhans cell histiocytosis):

A has a characteristic skin rash
B may present with polyuria and polydipsia
C has a relapsing course in most cases
D is a true malignancy
E often involves the bowel wall

131 Germ cell tumours:

A are associated with raised alfafetoprotein levels
B are unresponsive to cytotoxic drugs
C are found only in the gonads
D may be one element of a teratoma
E may be treated by surgery alone

132 Cot death:

A is more likely to occur in the child of an elderly primapara
B is associated with maternal smoking
C has a 50% risk of recurrence in subsequent siblings
D is more frequent in girls than boys
E there is good evidence that apnoea monitors can prevent cot deaths if used properly

133 The following are contraindications to pertussis vaccination:

A a serious general reaction in an older sibling
B a local reaction to a previous injection
C a strong family history of atopy
D a history of anaphylaxis after eating an egg
E a history of cystic fibrosis

134 The following are notifiable diseases:

A acquired immuno-deficiency syndrome (AIDS)
B rubella
C scarlet fever
D mumps
E viral meningitis

135 The following can be detected in pregnancy:

A cerebral palsy
B cretinism
C transposition of the great arteries
D congenital toxoplasmosis
E Down's syndrome

136 In a suspected case of child abuse:

A the GP's duty of confidentiality makes it difficult for him to disclose anything that parents have told him
B no undue importance should be placed on the word of a young child
C frequently there is a discrepancy between the parents' story and the apparent nature of the injury
D if parents bring their child to seek medical help straight away, it means that there is little risk of non-accidental injury
E the first doctor to see a child should immediately take forensic samples so as not to lose valuable evidence

137 The following statements regarding a child's behaviour are true:

A bed-wetting at the age of 4 is an indication for concern
B soiling at the age of 5 is a sign which needs thorough examination and investigation, including barium studies
C soiling at the age of 4 is harmless and the parents can be reassured accordingly
D of those 3-year-olds with moderate or severe behaviour problems, two-thirds will still have problems at the age of 8
E persistent crying in a 3-month-old baby is usually a sign of maternal depression

MCQ ANSWER KEY

Q	1	2	3	4	5	6	7	8	9	10	11	12	13	14	15
A	T	T	T	F	F	F	T	F	T	T	T	T	F	T	T
B	T	F	F	F	T	T	T	T	T	F	T	F	T	T	T
C	F	T	T	T	F	F	F	F	F	F	T	T	T	T	F
D	F	T	F	F	T	T	F	F	T	F	T	T	F	F	T
E	F	F	T	T	F	T	T	T	T	F	T	F	T	T	F

Q	16	17	18	19	20	21	22	23	24	25	26	27	28	29	30
A	T	F	T	F	F	T	T	T	T	T	F	F	F	F	F
B	T	T	F	T	T	F	T	F	F	F	T	T	F	F	F
C	T	F	T	T	F	F	F	F	T	F	F	F	T	T	F
D	T	T	T	F	F	F	F	T	T	T	F	F	F	F	F
E	T	F	T	F	T	T	T	F	T	T	F	T	F	F	T

Q	31	32	33	34	35	36	37	38	39	40	41	42	43	44	45
A	F	T	F	F	F	F	T	F	T	T	T	T	F	F	F
B	F	F	T	F	F	T	F	T	F	F	T	F	T	T	T
C	T	F	F	T	T	F	T	F	T	F	T	T	T	F	F
D	T	T	F	T	T	T	F	F	F	F	T	F	T	T	T
E	T	T	F	F	T	F	F	T	F	T	F	F	T	T	F

Q	46	47	48	49	50	51	52	53	54	55	56	57	58	59	60
A	T	T	T	T	T	T	T	T	F	T	T	T	T	T	T
B	F	F	T	F	T	T	T	T	F	T	T	T	F	T	F
C	F	F	F	T	T	T	F	F	F	T	F	F	T	F	T
D	F	F	T	F	T	T	T	F	F	F	F	F	T	T	T
E	T	T	T	T	F	F	T	F	T	F	F	T	T	T	T

Q	61	62	63	64	65	66	67	68	69	70	71	72	73	74	75
A	T	T	F	F	F	T	T	F	T	T	F	T	F	T	F
B	T	T	F	F	T	T	T	T	T	F	F	F	T	T	T
C	F	T	T	T	F	T	T	F	F	F	T	F	F	T	T
D	T	F	T	T	F	T	F	F	T	T	F	F	T	T	T
E	T	F	F	F	F	F	F	T	F	T	F	T	F	F	F

Q	76	77	78	79	80	81	82	83	84	85	86	87	88	89	90
A	F	T	T	T	T	T	T	F	F	F	T	T	T	F	F
B	T	T	T	F	F	F	T	F	T	T	T	F	F	T	T
C	F	F	F	F	F	F	F	F	T	T	F	T	T	F	T
D	F	T	T	T	F	T	T	T	F	F	T	F	F	T	F
E	F	F	F	T	T	T	F	F	T	F	F	F	T	F	T

Q	91	92	93	94	95	96	97	98	99	100	101	102	103	104	105
A	T	T	T	F	F	T	F	F	F	T	F	F	F	T	F
B	T	F	F	T	F	F	T	T	T	F	F	T	F	T	T
C	T	T	T	T	F	F	F	F	T	F	F	F	T	F	T
D	F	F	F	F	F	T	T	T	F	F	T	T	T	T	T
E	T	T	T	F	T	T	F	F	F	T	F	F	T	T	T

Q	106	107	108	109	110	111	112	113	114	115	116	117	118	119	120
A	F	F	F	F	T	T	T	F	F	T	F	T	F	T	F
B	T	F	T	F	F	F	T	T	F	F	T	F	F	T	T
C	T	F	F	T	T	T	T	T	T	F	F	T	T	T	T
D	T	T	T	F	T	T	T	F	F	T	T	F	T	F	T
E	F	F	T	T	F	T	T	T	T	T	T	T	F	F	F

Q	121	122	123	124	125	126	127	128	129	130	131	132	133	134	135
A	F	F	F	T	F	T	F	F	F	T	T	F	F	F	F
B	F	T	T	T	T	T	T	F	T	T	F	F	F	T	F
C	T	T	T	T	F	T	T	T	T	T	F	F	F	T	T
D	T	T	T	T	F	T	T	T	T	F	T	F	F	T	T
E	T	F	F	T	T	T	F	T	F	F	T	F	F	T	T

Q	136	137
A	F	F
B	F	F
C	T	F
D	F	T
E	F	F

Appendix

Normal paediatric values

BIOCHEMICAL AND PHYSIOLOGICAL DATA

The Système International d'Unités (or SI unit system) is now commonly used in the UK. Reference values are given in SI units followed by traditional units. A multiplication factor is included; traditional units are multiplied by this factor to convert to SI units (thus, if the values in SI units are divided by this factor, the result will be given in traditional units). The unit of volume commonly used is the litre.

The SI unit of quantity is the mole.

Normal blood, serum and plasma values

	Traditional units normal ranges	Multiplication factor	SI units normal ranges
Bicarbonate or total CO_2 (plasma)			
Newborns	18–23 mEq/l	1.0	18–23 mmol/l
Thereafter	18–25 mEq/l		18–25/mmol/l
Bilirubin (serum)			
Cord blood	up to 2.9 mg/100 ml	17.1	up to 50 μmol/l
Cord blood (preterm infants)	up to 3.4 mg/100 ml		up to 58 μmol/l
First 24 hours (higher in preterm infants)	up to 6.0 mg/100 ml		up to 103 μmol/l
2–5 days	up to 12 mg/100 ml		up to 205 μmol/l
(In the newborn period virtually all the bilirubin is present as free (unconjugated) bilirubin)			
After 1 month (mainly conjugated)	0.1–0.8 mg/100 ml		1.7–14 μmol/l
Calcium (serum)			
Cord blood	9.3–12.2 mg/100 ml	0.25	2.33–3.05 mmol/l
1st week — breast fed	8.2–12.2 mg/100 ml		2.05–3.05 mmol/l
— bottle fed	7.4–11.0 mg/100 ml		1.85–2.75 mmol/l
Thereafter	8.8–11.0 mg/100 ml		2.20–2.75 mmol/l
Carbon dioxide P_{CO_2} (arterial)	35–45 mmHg	0.133	4.7–6.0 kPa
Chloride (serum)	98–106 mEq/l	1.0	98–106 mmol/l
Cholesterol (serum)			
Cord blood	23–135 mg/100 ml	0.0259	0.6–3.5 mmol/l
1–6 weeks	93–217 mg/100 ml		2.4–5.6 mmil/l
Increasing gradually until 1 year and older	119–263 mg/100 ml		3.1–6.8 mmol/l
Cortisol (plasma)			
Children 0800 h	8–26 μg/100 ml	27.6	200–720 mmol/l
2200 h (usually less than 50% of 0800 h value)	below 10 μg/100ml		below 275 mmol/l

Normal blood, serum and plasma values (continued)

	Traditional units normal ranges	Multiplication factor	SI units normal ranges
Creatinine (serum)	0.4–1.3 mg/100 ml	88.4	35–106 μmol/l
Glucose (blood)			
Fasting	60–100 mg/100 ml	0.0556	3.3–5.5 mmol/l
Newborn	40–80 mg/100 ml		2.2–4.4 mmol/l
Transiently low values below 2.2 mmol/l are commonly seen on the first day of life. Persistently low values should be investigated			
Iron (serum)			
3 years of age	60–175 μg/100 ml	0.179	10.7–31.3 μmol/l
Iron binding capacity (serum) — (TIBC)			
after 6 months	250–500 μg/100 ml	0.179	44.8–89.5 μmol/l
Lead (blood)	up to 40 μg/100 ml	0.0483	up to 1.9 μmol/l
Magnesium (serum)			
Newborns	1.40–2.45 mg/100 ml	0.41	0.58–1.00 μmol/l
Older children	1.45–2.32 mg/100 ml		0.60–0.95 mmol/l
Osmolality (serum)	275–295 mosmol/kg	1.0	275–295 mmol/kg
pH (arterial blood)	7.35–7.42		
Po$_2$ — oxygen tension (arterial blood)			
Umbilical vein	12.8–32.0 mmHg	0.133	1.7–4.3 kPa
Newborns after first 24 hours	77–100 mmHg		9.3–13.3 kPa
Older children	85–100 mmHg		11.3–13.3 kPa
Phenylalanine (plasma)			
Newborns	0.7–2.8 mg/100 ml	60.5	42–170 μmol/l
Transient values above 2.8 mg/100 ml may be found in the newborn period. Plasma concentrations are usually maintained at between 84 and 300 μmol/l in the treatment of phenylkentonuria			
Phosphorus, inorganic (serum)			
Newborns, 1st week	5.8–9.0 mg/100 ml		1.87–2.91 mmol/l
Newborns, 2nd week	4.9–8.9 mg/100		1.58–2.87 mmol/l
Up to 1 year	4.8–6.2 mg/100 ml		1.55–2.00 mmol/l
Thereafter	3.6–5.9 mg/100 ml		1.16–1.91 mmol/l
Phosphorus values in the newborn period vary greatly depending very much on the type of milk feed; lower values are found in breast-fed infants			
Potassium (plasma)			
Newborns	4.3–7.6 mEq/l		4.3–7.6 mmol/l
Older children	3.5–5.6 mEq/l		3.5–5.6 mmol/l

Proteins (serum) (values in g/100 ml)	Total	Albumin	Globulins α^1	α^2	β	γ
1 year	5.6–7.3	3.5–5.0	0.2–0.4	0.4–1.0	0.5–1.0	0.5–13
4 years and over	6.4–7.5	3.7–5.0	0.2–0.4	0.4–1.0	0.6–1.1	0.5–1.8
1 year (values in g/l (using muliplication factor of 10))	56–73	35–50	2–4	4–10	5–9	4–12
4 years and over	64–75	37–50	2–4	4–10	6–10	5–12

Immunoglobins (serum)	IgG mg/100 ml	g/l	IgA mg/100 ml	g/l	IgM mg/100 ml	g/l
Newborns	650–1450	6.5–14.5	0–10	0–0.1	0–20	0–0.2
1–3 months	200–650	2.0–6.5	5–40	0.05–0.4	10–50	0.1–0.5
4–6 months	150–800	1.5–8.0	10–60	0.1–0.6	10–80	0.1–0.8
1 year	300–1200	3.0–12.0	20–80	0.2–0.8	20–100	0.2–1.0
3 years and older	500–1500	5.0–15.0	30–300	0.3–3.0	40–200	0.4–2.0

Normal blood, serum and plasma values (continued)

	Traditional units normal ranges	Multiplication factor	SI units normal ranges
Immunogloblin values vary widely in children particularly in the first 6 months of life. Care should be taken in interpreting marginal differences from the normal			
Sodium (plasma)	136–145 mEq/l	1.0	136–145 mmol/l
Standard bicarbonate (blood)			
Newborns	18–25	1.0	18–25
Thereafter	21–25		21–25
Thyrotrophin or thyroid stimulating hormone (TSH) (serum)	<1–5.8 μU/l	1.0	<1–5.8 μU/l
(1 represents the lower level of sensitivity of most present assay methods. Many euthyroid children may have TSH values which are less than 1 μU/1)			
Thyroxine — T4 (serum)			
Cord blood and newborns	5.5–18.2 μg/100	12.9	71–235 nmol/l
Thereafter	5.8–11.6 μg/100 ml		75–150 nmol/l
Urea (blood)	14–40 mg/100 ml	0.166	2.5–6.6 mmol/l
Higher values are commonly seen during the first 6 months of life in infants on unmodified milks, i.e. those whose protein concentration is substantially above that of breast milk			

Normal haematological values (all values shown are means with the ranges in parentheses)

Age	Red blood cells per litre	per mm³	Haemo-globin (%)	Haema-tocrit (%)	White blood cells per litre	per mm³	Neutro-phils (%)	Lympho-cytes (%)	Eosino-phils (%)	Mono-cytes (%)	Reticulo-cytes (%)	Platelets per litre	per mm³	MCV (fl)	MCH (pg)	MCHC (g/dl)
Birth	$5.0\text{-}6.0 \times 10^{12}$	$5.0\text{-}6.0 \times 10^{6}$	17 (14-20)	55 (45-65)	18×10^{9} ($9\text{-}30 \times 10^{9}$)	18 000 (9-30 000)	60 (40-80)	32	2	7-14	5 (3-7)	100×10^{9} to 300×10^{9}	100 000 300 000	94-118	32-40	34-36
1 week	Values fall within 3 months to		17 (13-21)	54 (43-66)	12×10^{9} ($6\text{-}22 \times 10^{9}$)	12 000 (6-22 000)	39 (30-50)	46	3	7-14	2 (0-4)			88-108	32-40	34-36
2 weeks	months to		16.5 (13-20)	50 (42-66)	12×10^{9} ($5\text{-}21 \times 10^{3}$)	12 000 (5-21 000)	40 (30-50)	48	3	6-12	1 (0-2)	150×10^{9} to	150 000 to	86-106	32-40	34-36
6 months	$3.5\text{-}5.6 \times 10^{12}$	$3.5\text{-}5.6 \times 10^{6}$	12 (10.5-14)	38 (33-42)	10×10^{9} ($6\text{-}15 \times 10^{9}$)	10 000 (6-15 000)	42 (35-52)	51	2-3	4-8	1 (0-2)	450×10^{9}	450 000	76-88	24-30	30-36
6 years–Adult F	$3.9\text{-}5.6 \times 10^{12}$	$3.9\text{-}5.6 \times 10^{6}$	14 (12-16)	42 (37-47)	7.5×10^{9} ($5\text{-}10 \times 10^{9}$)	7500 (5-10 000)	60 (40-75)	30 (20-45)	1-6	2-10	0-2			76-98	27-32	30-35
M	$4.5\text{-}6.5 \times 10^{12}$	$4.5\text{-}6.5 \times 10^{6}$	16 (14-18)	46 (42-52)										76-96	27-32	30-35

Up to 34-36 weeks of fetal life 90–95% of haemoglobin is fetal haemoglobin. Thereafter the proportion of fetal haemoglobin decreases at rate of 3–4% per week, until 40 weeks when mean is 75% and range 50% to 85%.

Thereafter slow fall to <60% at 2 months after birth (range 40–60%)

Then more rapid fall to: <30% at 3 months after birth
<15% at 4 months after birth
<5% at 6 months after birth
<2% at 3 years after birth

(See also Matoth Y, Zaizov R, Versano I 1971 Postnatal changes in some red cell parameters. Acta Paediatrica Scandinavica 60: 317–323)

Index